THE TEMPOROMANDIBULAR JOINT: A Biological Basis For Clinical Practice

THE TEMPOROMANDIBULAR JOINT: A Biological Basis For Clinical Practice

FOURTH EDITION

BERNARD G. SARNAT, M.D., M.S., D.D.S, F.A.C.S.

Adjunct Professor of Oral Biology and Plastic Surgery
Schools of Dentistry and Medicine, UCLA
Senior Research Scientist and Formerly
Chief of Plastic Surgery
Cedars-Sinai Medical Center, Los Angeles, California

DANIEL M. LASKIN, D.D.S., M.S.

Professor and Chairman
Department of Oral and Maxillofacial Surgery
Director, Temporomandibular Joint and Facial Pain Research Center
Medical College of Virginia, Richmond, Virginia

W.B. SAUNDERS COMPANY

Harcourt Brace Jovanovich, Inc.

Philadelphia • London • Toronto • Montreal • Sydney • Tokyo

W. B. SAUNDERS COMPANY
Harcourt Brace Jovanovich, Inc.

The Curtis Center
Independence Square West
Philadelphia, PA 19106

Library of Congress Cataloging-in-Publication Data

The Temporomandibular joint: a biological basis for clinical
practice / edited by Bernard G. Sarnat and Daniel M. Laskin.—
4th ed.

   p. cm.

ISBN 0–7216–7928–5

1. Temporomandibular joint—Diseases. 2. Temporomandibular
joint. I. Sarnat, Bernard G. (Bernard George). II. Laskin,
Daniel M. [DNLM:
1. Temporomandibular Joint.
2. Temporomandibular Joint Syndrome. WU 140 T287]

RK470.S27 1992

617′.522–dc20

DNLM/DLC   91-13859

Editor: John Dyson
Designer: Joan Sinclair
Production Manager: Frank Polizzano
Indexer: Diana Witt

THE TEMPOROMANDIBULAR JOINT: A Biological Basis   ISBN   0–7216–7928–5
For Clinical Practice

Printed in the United States of America.

Last digit is the print number: 9   8   7   6   5   4   3   2   1

Contributors

SANFORD L. BLOCK, D.D.S. LL.B

Associate Professor, Oral and Maxillofacial Surgery, University of Illinois College of Dentistry; Director of Dentistry and Oral Surgery, Swedish Covenant Hospital, Chicago, Illinois

Differential Diagnosis of Craniofacial-Cervical Pain; Differential Diagnosis of Masticatory Dysfunction

ALPHONSE R. BURDI, Ph.D.

Professor, Department of Anatomy and Cell Biology, and Research Scientist, Center for Human Growth and Development, and Director, Integrated Premedical-Medical Program, The University of Michigan, Ann Arbor, Michigan

Morphogenesis

HENRY M. CHERRICK, D.D.S., M.S.D.

Dean and Professor, University of California at Los Angeles School of Dentistry, Los Angeles, California

Pathological Aspects of Developmental, Inflammatory, and Neoplastic Disease

GLENN T. CLARK, D.D.S., M.S.

Professor and Associate Dean of Research, and Acting Director of Dental Research Institute; Co-Director, Pain Management Clinic, University of California at Los Angeles School of Dentistry, Los Angeles, California

Diagnosis and Nonsurgical Treatment of Masticatory Muscle Pain and Dysfunction; Diagnosis and Nonsurgical Treatment of Internal Derangements

STEPHEN L. CREANOR, B.D.S., Ph.D.

Clinical Lecturer, Oral Biology Group, University of Glasgow Dental School; Honorary Registrar, Greater Glasgow Health Board, Glasgow, Scotland

Comparative Functional Anatomy

SUZANNE E. DAVIS, M.M.S.

Research Associate, Department of Oral and Maxillofacial Surgery, University of Texas Health Science Center, San Antonio, Texas

Temporomandibular Disorders: Psychological and Behavioral Aspects

E. LLOYD DuBRUL, D.D.S., Ph.D.

Professor Emeritus, Department of Oral Anatomy, University of Illinois College of Dentistry, Chicago, Illinois

Origin and Adaptations of the Hominid Jaw Joint

DONALD H. ENLOW, Ph.D.

Thomas Hill Distinguished Professor Emeritus, Department of Orthodontics, Case Western Reserve University School of Dentistry, Cleveland, Ohio

The Condyle and Facial Growth

JEFFREY T. FUJIMOTO, D.D.S., M.A.

Assistant Clinical Professor, University of California at San Francisco School of Dentistry; Attending Staff, Davies Medical Center, San Francisco, California

Experimental Studies

ELLIOT N. GALE, Ph.D.

Professor, Department of Behavioral Sciences, State University of New York at Buffalo School of Dental Medicine, Buffalo, New York

Epidemiology

CHARLES S. GREENE, D.D.S.

Clinical Professor, Department of Orthodontics, Northwestern University Dental School, Chicago, Illinois

Temporomandibular Disorders: The Evolution of Concepts

TORE L. HANSSON, D.D.S., Odont. Dr.

Adjunct Assistant Clinical Professor, Department of Restorative Dentistry, University of California at San Francisco School of Dentistry; Director, Clinic for Craniomandibular Disorders and Facial Pain, St. Joseph's Hospital and Medical Center, Phoenix, Arizona

Pathological Aspects of Arthritides and Derangements

GUSTAF HELLSING

Associate Professor, Department of Clinical Oral Physiology, Department of Oral Surgery, Karolinska Institute, Huddinge, Sweden

Arthroscopy

ANDERS B. HOLMLUND, D.D.S., Ph.D.

Associate Professor, Department of Oral Surgery, Karolinska Institute; Department of Oral Surgery, Huddinge University Hospital, Huddinge, Sweden

Arthroscopy

WILLIAM L. HYLANDER, D.D.S., Ph.D.

Professor of Biological Anthropology and Anatomy, Duke University Medical Center, Durham, North Carolina

Functional Anatomy

SIGVARD KOPP, D.D.S., Odont. Dr.

Professor, School of Dentistry, Karolinska Institute; Chairman, Department of Clinical Oral Physiology, Huddinge Hospital, Huddinge, Sweden

Diagnosis and Nonsurgical Treatment of the Arthritides

DANIEL M. LASKIN, D.D.S., M.S.

Professor and Chairman, Department of Oral and Maxillofacial Surgery, Medical College of Virginia, Richmond, Virginia

History and Physical Examination; Temporomandibular Disorders: Diagnosis and Etiology; Surgical Considerations

MURRAY C. MEIKLE, B.D.S., M.S.D., Ph.D., F.D.S.R.C.S.

Senior Lecturer and Consultant, Department of Orthodontics, and Director, Connective Tissue Research Unit, University of London Institute of Dental Surgery; Research Scientist, Cell and Molecular Biology Department, Strangeways Research Laboratory, Cambridge, England

Remodeling

ROBERT L. MERRILL, D.D.S.

Lecturer and Research Associate, Section of Orofacial Pain, University of California at Los Angeles School of Dentistry, Los Angeles, California

Diagnosis and Nonsurgical Treatment of Masticatory Muscle Pain and Dysfunction; Diagnosis and Nonsurgical Treatment of Internal Derangements

HENRY W. NOBLE, Ph.D., F.D.S.

Senior Research Fellow, University of Glasgow Dental School, Glasgow, Scotland

Comparative Functional Anatomy

DAVID E. POSWILLO, C.B.E., D.D.S., D.Sc., M.DHC, F.D.S., F.R.C. Path.

Professor and Chairman, Oral and Maxillofacial Surgery, United Medical and Dental Schools of Guy's and St. Thomas's Hospitals, University of London; Honorary Consultant, Oral and Maxillofacial Surgery, Guy's and Lewisham Hospitals, London, England

Congenital and Developmental Anomalies

PAUL ROBINSON, B.D.S., M.B., B.S., F.D.S.R.C.S.

Lecturer, Department of Oral and Maxillofacial Surgery, United Medical and Dental Schools of Guy's and St. Thomas's University of London; Senior Registrar, Department of Oral and Maxillofacial Surgery, Guy's and Lewisham Hospitals, London, England

Congenital and Developmental Anomalies

JOHN D. RUGH, Ph.D.

Professor, and Director, Division of Research, Department of Oral and Maxillofacial Surgery, University of Texas Health Science Center, San Antonio, Texas

Temporomandibular Disorders: Psychological and Behavioral Aspects

J. PHILIP SAPP, D.D.S., M.S.

Professor, Section of Oral Diagnosis and Oral Medicine and Oral Pathology, University of California at Los Angeles School of Dentistry; Consultant, Veterans Hospital, Sepulveda, California

Pathological Aspects of Developmental, Inflammatory, and Neoplastic Disease

BERNARD G. SARNAT, M.D., M.S., D.D.S., F.A.C.S.

Adjunct Professor of Oral Biology and Plastic Surgery, University of California Los Angeles

Schools of Dentistry and Medicine; Senior Research Scientist and formerly Chief of Plastic Surgery, Cedars-Sinai Medical Center, Los Angeles, California

History and Physical Examination; Surgical Considerations

BARRY J. SESSLE, B.D.S., M.D.S., B.Sc., Ph.D

Dean, Faculty of Dentistry, and Professor, Faculty of Medicine, Department of Physiology, University of Toronto, Toronto, Canada

Neurobiology of Facial and Dental Pain

ARTHUR T. STOREY, D.D.S., M.S., Ph.D.

Professor and Chairman, Department of Orthodontics, University of Texas at San Antonio Health Science Center, San Antonio, Texas

Neurophysiology

WILLIAM H. WARE, D.D.S., M.S.

Professor and Chairman Emeritus, Division of Oral and Maxillofacial Surgery, University of California at San Francisco School of Dentistry; Attending Staff, Davies Medical Center, San Francisco, California

Experimental Studies

PER-LENNART WESTESSON, D.D.S., Ph.D.

Associate Professor of Radiology and Clinical Dentistry, University of Rochester; Senior Research Associate of Orthodontics, Eastman Dental Center, Rochester, New York

Imaging

ROBERT YEMM, B.D.S., B.Sc., Ph.D., F.D.S.R.C.S.(Ed.)

Professor of Dental Prosthetics Science, and Head, Department of Dental Prosthetics and Gerontology, and Dean of Dentistry, University of Dundee Dental School; Honorary Consultant, Dundee Dental Hospital; Tayside Health Board, Dundee, Scotland

Pathophysiology of the Masticatory Muscles

Foreword

As one with primarily a basic science background, it has been a great pleasure to read the scholarly contributions which this exceptionally well illustrated book contains. Forty years have passed since the appearance of the first edition of the *Temporomandibular Joint*, in 1951, and this presentation of the biomedical information with the clinical aspects concerning the temporomandibular joint continues to be unique in the world literature.

The contents of this multiauthored book provide the fundamental information necessary to both diagnose and treat the various conditions that affect the masticatory apparatus. Some of the chapters presenting the biological basis for rational therapy of disorders of the temporomandibular joint include descriptions of comparative functional anatomy, condylar and craniofacial growth, neurophysiology, and pathologic aspects of various diseases and anomalies. The reader also learns that the temporomandibular joint is an extraordinary example illustrating some of the principles of phylogeny, the primary temporomandibular joint of amphibians and reptiles having evolved to a combined gliding and hinge joint in humans. Understanding this enables one to appreciate better the biomechanics of this complex structure.

Considerable attention is also given to the masticatory musculature. Because of their involvement both as primary and secondary causes of mandibular dysfunction and temporomandibular joint disorders, great emphasis is placed on the physiology and pathology of these structures. This serves as an excellent prelude in determining correct etiology, forming an accurate differential diagnosis, and establishing appropriate methods of treatment.

The particular presentation used in this book has an obvious advantage in that it correlates current information from biology with the various clinical aspects, including new perspectives. Without any question, the reader will find that this integration will make it less difficult to understand some of the perplexing problems of the temporomandibular joint.

The editors are to be commended on the choice of material, organization, and format. The text is written in a lucid style and extremely well edited. Each of the chapters is contributed by a world authority in the particular field. Although each chapter is an entity in itself, it is intimately integrated with the rest of the book. Fourteen chapters are updated and, with the additional 12 new chapters, reflect a great sum of current information on the various subjects. There is something for everyone in this comprehensive book: student, teacher, scientist and clinician. The editors as well as the authors and publishers are to be congratulated on having prepared a volume of this magnitude, with so many excellent qualities.

GERT-HORST SCHUMMACHER, DR. SC. MED., D. MED. DENT.

Foreword

A benchmark of a publication's success is the credibility of its contents. The fourth edition of this very popular and substantive text on the temporomandibular joint and related structures continues to meet this high standard. In this edition the skills, knowledge and expertise of major internationally recognized authorities on the subject are again brilliantly combined. The format is logically divided into two parts: Part I, entitled "Biological Basis" and Part II, entitled "Clinical Practice: Diagnosis and Treatment." This structuring, with related correlations, provides an accurate summation of the most current scientifically accepted theory and concept, and forms the basis for a rational approach to therapy. As a clinician with a basic science background, I find this method of presentation extremely beneficial.

The two editors have a long and enviable record related to the temporomandibular joint. Over the years their dedicated efforts, knowledge, and research have opened vistas for the thoughtful and credible management of this complex apparatus. Forty years ago, at midcentury, when this book was first published as a monograph, our basic and clinical understanding of this single facet of the stomatognathic system was woefully meager. The dental and medical professions were groping in their diagnostic and treatment protocols. In that early era of discovery, Drs. Sarnat and Laskin were among the very first to develop and present both a scientific and clinically sound basis for our comprehension of this complex subject. Certainly, as in other scientific endeavors, there were some errors of interpretation, presentation, or omission. These were recognized early and conscientiously altered, corrected, or eliminated by the incorporation, in subsequent editions, of the most current, accurate information from authoritative authors. Thus, we have continued to witness, in these sequential editions, a unique correlation of basic science and clinical information addressed to the important needs of practitioners and their patients not found in other textbooks on the subject.

The proper practice of either dentistry or medicine is based on the factual foundations of basic and clinical science. This text offers this valuable data to those desirous of enhancing their knowledge and skills related to the temporomandibular joint and associated structures. The exceptionally broad coverage of the subject, presented by a wide spectrum of recognized and reputable contributors in a rational progression throughout the text, provides the serious student, interested scientist, and dedicated practitioner a wealth of integrated, valuable current information. Any individual attempting to gain this material independently from research reports, journals, continuing education courses, or specialty meetings, would have to expend months and years of personal time. The accumulated information so beautifully presented in this fourth edition accomplishes the task for the reader in an organized and authoritative manner. The editors are to be congratulated on providing us with another landmark edition of this classic text.

HAROLD T. PERRY, D.D.S., PH.D.

Preface

In the preface to the first edition of this book (1951), the need was recognized for valid information about the temporomandibular joint and its associated structures. Since then many excellent, well-documented scientific studies have appeared in the literature, and these have strengthened our knowledge base significantly. The dimensions and complexity of problems involving the temporomandibular joint, coupled with the veritable explosion of new knowledge in the past decade, warrant a fourth edition.

The chosen title indicates our philosophy. As in earlier editions, we have developed and emphasized a basic biological approach to the difficult and, in many instances, unanswered clinical problems involving the temporomandibular joint and, in the broader context, the masticatory apparatus. There are two parts to the book. Part I emphasizes the biology of the temporomandibular joint region, and incorporates clinical correlations. This serves as a foundation for Part II, which is devoted almost entirely to clinical evaluation, accurate diagnosis, and proper treatment, reinforced by reference to the basic science aspects. We are not aware of another book on the temporomandibular joint that takes this approach.

Since publication of the last edition, much has changed. Thus, in this fourth edition, many former concepts have been modified in the light of recent knowledge. Outdated information has been eliminated and the most recent findings in this rapidly expanding area have been added, making the breadth and scope of the book much greater. Although it is indeed a thoroughly revised work, with new contributors and new contents, we have made a concerted effort to maintain our previous standards of excellence. Our hope is that this will be *the authoritative and definitive* work in this field.

Because no one person can be expert in all aspects of such a broad subject, we have invited contributions from those whom we consider highly knowledgeable in specific areas. Thus, basic scientists and clinicians have pooled their knowledge and experience to provide a unique view of temporomandibular joint disorders. We welcome and thank the following new contributors and co-contributors: Stephen Creanor (Comparative Functional Anatomy), Alphonse Burdi (Morphogenesis), Arthur Storey (Neurophysiology), Barry Sessle (Neurobiology of Facial and Dental Pain), Robert Yemm (Pathophysiology of the Masticatory Muscles), Philip Sapp (Pathologic Aspects), Tore Hansson (Pathologic Aspects of Arthritides and Derangements) Paul Robinson (Congenital and Developmental Anomalies), Jeffrey Fujimoto (Experimental Studies), Eliot Gale (Epidemiology), Per-Lennart Westesson (Imaging), Anders Holmlund and Gustav Hellsing (Arthroscopy), John Rugh and Suzanne Davis (Temporomandibular Disorders: Psychological and Behavioral Aspects), Glenn Clark and Robert Merrill (Diagnosis and Nonsurgical Treatment of Masticatory

Muscle Pain and Dysfunction Syndrome; Diagnosis and Nonsurgical Treatment of Internal Derangements), and Sigvard Kopp (Diagnosis and Nonsurgical Treatment of Arthritides). And, of course, we continue to appreciate those who contributed to the previous edition and now join us once again—Sanford Block, Henry Cherrick, E. Lloyd DuBrul, Donald Enlow, Charles Greene, William Hylander, Murray Meikle, Henry Noble, David Poswillo, and William Ware.

The main purpose of this book is to distill the enormous accumulation of biological and clinical data into a unified text that will provide an accurate basis for clinical practice. In any multiauthored book, however, particularly one dealing with such a complex subject, there are bound to be some differences of opinion and interpretation. As editors, we have attempted to encourage such diversity, when controversy still exists. We see this as an advantage because, by presenting more than one expert point of view, readers may reach their own conclusions on the basis of the information provided. Such interpretation is aided by the comprehensive basic biologic background that is included.

In closing, we wish to thank those students, practitioners, teachers, and researchers whose enthusiastic reception of previous editions has encouraged us to make this new effort. We acknowledge the staff at the W.B. Saunders Company for their dedicated support, which contributed so much to the value of this book.

BERNARD G. SARNAT

DANIEL M. LASKIN

Preface to the Third Edition

Time brings change. Since the publication of the second edition of this book much has changed. Thus, a new edition is justified to modify past concepts in the light of current knowledge, to eliminate information that is outdated or less useful, and to add recent or more useful information. This publication not only reflects such changes, but also provides a depth and scope far greater than in the past. The third edition is indeed a new book with many new contributors and contents but with the same high editorial and professional standards. As in previous editions the basic science approach to clinical practice has been emphasized. Our hope is that this will be the authoritative, definitive work related to the temporomandibular joint and masticatory system.

There are two parts to the book. Part I pertains primarily to the biology of the temporomandibular joint with some clinical correlations. Part II is devoted essentially to concepts of clinical practice, accurate diagnosis, and proper treatment, re-inforced by reference to the basic science aspects. In this edition further emphasis has been given to complex clinical problems and in particular to the myofascial pain-dysfunction syndrome. Because of the many new correlations between the basic and clinical sciences, the title has been modified to *The Temporomandibular Joint: A Biological Basis for Clinical Practice*.

Unfortunately, in the care of many complex problems of the temporomandibular joint and related structures, iatrogenic disease is not uncommon. A cardinal principle in effective treatment is first to do no harm—*primum non nocere*. In this book emphasis has been on this theme as well as on the use of therapy that does not produce irreversible changes.

In any multi-authored book there may be differences of opinion and interpretation of findings. No editorial privileges were exercised when such situations existed. This is as it should be. Thus, in some chapters varying and differing thoughts are expressed. For example, the role of the condyle as a primary site of growth has been challenged by some of the contributors. Is this position the correct one or is it possible that at different times the growth function of the condyle changes? At present there is neither unanimity of opinion nor sufficient valid evidence for a positive decision. Because of many important basic clinical relationships, this problem merits continued study. Hopefully, by the time of publication of the fourth edition there will be further clarification.

Although a multi-authored book, the selection of topics and their order of presentation provide a continuity enabling the reader to progress from one section to the next using the previous information as a basis of understanding. At the same time, individual chapters can be reviewed when specific questions arise. The various chapters are extensively referenced, thus offering a source of additional information for those interested in greater detail. Each contributor is an expert in the field so that the material presented is not only authoritative but also current.

Of the distinguished contributors to the first edition, most have died. Our sincere respects and thanks are given to them for their contributions to our fundamental knowledge of the masticatory apparatus. For this third edition we would like to thank all of the current contributors, as well as the many others involved directly or indirectly in its development, for their excellent cooperation, patience, and understanding. Finally, permit me (BGS) the opportunity to welcome with pleasure a colleague and former student, Daniel M. Laskin, as the co-editor of this volume.

BERNARD G. SARNAT
DANIEL M. LASKIN

Preface to the Second Edition

The Temporomandibular Joint, which is part of a higher unit of structure, the masticatory system, represents a unique functional adaptation to the evolutionary changes in the mammalian skull. It differs from other joints of the body in several ways. First, it is a complex joint with an articular disc and it is capable of an unusual combination of hinging and gliding movements. Second, it is exceptional because the spatial relations of the component parts are influenced not only by muscular balance and structural morphology but also by the occlusion and malocclusion of the teeth. Third, it is unique because the joints cannot operate independently; both act as a single functional unit. Any alteration in the activity of one side will therefore affect the other, an important factor frequently overlooked in the analysis of disturbances in this region. Last, the articular surfaces of this joint are not covered by hyaline cartilage but by avascular fibrous tissue with a few scattered cartilage cells. Just beneath this layer on the condyle is an epiphyseal-like growth center. This serves as both the pacemaker and organizer for growth of the mandible. All these morphological and functional variations contribute to the complex problems in both the diagnosis and the treatment of temporomandibular joint disease.

Along with the contributors, the editor is grateful for the opportunity to acknowledge the cordial reception given the First Edition of this book. It was a source of special pleasure to learn of its acceptance not only by the medical and dental professions, but also by those in the basic sciences.

The same general purpose has been kept in mind in the preparation of this edition as in the previous one, namely to present and correlate the latest authoritative information, both basic and clinical, pertaining to the temporomandibular joint and related structures. The original contributors have had the privilege of revising and adding new material. In addition, several new chapters have been included. They are Evolution of the Temporomandibular Joint, by Dr. E. Lloyd Du Brul; Embryological Development of the Temporomandibular Joint, by Dr. Barnet M. Levy; Roentgenography of the Temporomandibular Joint, by Dr. Robert M. Ricketts; and Surgery of the Temporomandibular Joint, by Drs. Bernard G. Sarnat and Daniel M. Laskin.

It is with deep regret that a contributor to the First Edition has been claimed untimely by death. This opportunity is taken to pay final respects to our personal friend and longtime colleague, Dr. Joseph P. Weinmann.

BERNARD G. SARNAT

Preface to the First Edition

There is an increasing need for a critical examination and evaluation of our knowledge pertaining to the temporomandibular articulation and related structures. Although there is considerable literature on the clinical aspects of the temporomandibular joint, some of it is based upon interpretations which are not entirely valid. Unfortunately, this misinformation has been prepetuated by being "handed down" from one report to another. The need for correct information is evidenced by the number of difficult clinical problems in terms of diagnosis and treatment directly or indirectly associated with this region.

The purpose of this monograph is to bring some of our knowledge up to date and to correct some of the misconceptions by a review and analysis of the temporomandibular articulation from the point of view of both the basic and clinical sciences. Most disturbances of the temporomandibular joint are either congenital, inflammatory, traumatic, or neoplastic in nature. Congenital absence or deficiency of the condyle, containing the most important growth site of the mandible, is associated with marked deformity of the face. In the past, middle ear infection has been the most common inflammatory lesion which spread to the temporomandibular joint and not only affected the condylar growth site but also caused an ankylosis. Arthritis of the temporomandibular joint may be on either an inflammatory or traumatic basis. The latter is usually a result of faulty occlusion. Benign tumors of the condyle are not common and malignant tumors are rare.

The following will be considered in relation to the temporomandibular joint: 1) the masticatory apparatus from a gross anatomical and functional point of view; 2) the growth and development of the jaws and face; 3) histologic, pathologic and experimental aspects; and 4) treatment by means of corrective dentistry. This monograph, however, is not intended to serve as a complete review and summary of the subject, but rather as a basis for critical evaluation of the literature and for further study.

Articulations are part of a higher functional unit. The temporomandibular joint is part of the masticatory apparatus, comprised not only of this joint, but also of the teeth and their supporting structures, the jaws and their musculature. Alteration in the functions of any one of these structures will be reflected in all other parts of the masticatory apparatus.

The temporomandibular joint is a delicately balanced structure, and its functional and anatomic integrity is dependent upon the normal relations and functions of the rest of the masticatory apparatus. It is well known, for example, that traumatic arthritis can be caused by an occlusal disharmony. The correct diagnosis and proper treatment of such conditions, however, are dependent upon an understanding of the normal structure and function as well as of the pathologic physiology of the masticatory apparatus.

In order to clarify some of the problems related to the temporomandibular joint, a series of symposia and lectures were organized by the editor. In selecting the faculty and subject matter the following objectives were set up: 1) to present the latest authoritative basic science information including correlative material pertaining to the entire masticatory apparatus; and 2) on the basis of this knowledge to interpret the clinical findings, diagnosis, and treatment of these disorders.

This program was offered through the Postgraduate Division of the University of Illinois College of Dentistry during April and May of 1949 and much of it will be included in the Postgraduate Long Distance Telephone Extension broadcasts of December 10, 1951 and January 14, 1952. The 1949 course was received most enthusiastically by all who attended, namely, general dental and medical practitioners, otologists, prosthodontists, orthodontists and oral, plastic and orthopedic surgeons. Many students who took the course, and others who had heard about it, indicated a desire to have this information made available in permanent form. Because of these requests, the material has been published.

This monograph represents the combined efforts of many individuals. With their willing and splendid cooperation, the organization, development, and realization of this publication has been a source of especial pleasure. I also wish to express my thanks to Miss Claire Stanton for her assistance.

BERNARD G. SARNAT

Contents

PART II *Clinical Practice: Diagnosis and Treatment*

PART I

Biological Basis

ORIGIN AND ADAPTATIONS OF THE HOMINID JAW JOINT*

E. LLOYD DuBRUL, D.D.S., M.S., Ph.D.

INTRODUCTION

Jaws and jaw joints hold particular importance in the history of vertebrates. A complete vertebrate is a beast not only with a backbone but also with biting jaws. Furthermore, complete mammals have long been distinguished from all other vertebrates—and from animals very nearly mammalian—largely on the basis of their jaw-ear structure. However, there is an even greater significance to jaw joints in vertebrate evolution. Fishes swim with swift, undulating, lateral waves of the body axis. These movements may be powerful at top speed, but the length of movement at each vertebral joint is slight. When jaws were devised, they were the first, speedy, wide-swinging, vigorous appendages protruding from the body. The true diarthrodial joint was first formed in fishes, and its basic structure remained essentially unchanged when it was appropriated by the limbs of land animals.

"Eudiarthrodial joints probably were devel-

oped first in the common ancestors of the bony fishes in Silurian times, and may have been an essential part of the mechanism that differentiated the Gnathostomata from the Agnatha" (Haines, 1942). Thus, jaw joints apparently originated in all joint evolution.

This chapter attempts to sketch a clear, simplified, but consistent picture of what is currently known about the origin, evolution, and functions of this extraordinary articular complex. The account traces how those crucial diagnostic structures—the jaws, their joints, and associated ear and cranial parts—arose in primitive fish-like forms, gradually emerging as a basic mammalian arrangement. It highlights the underlying mechanisms through which this basic blueprint was modified to produce certain subsequent divergent mammalian feeding adaptations. Stemming from this solid basis, it tracks the trail of the hominid line to the present form. In following this course, recent studies of fossil remains have revealed surprising biomechanical contrivances in the oral systems of the earliest known hominids. The significance of these findings in refining concepts of craniomandibular function emerges with a clarification

---

*See Chapters 2, 3, 5, 9, 10, 12, 18, and 24.

of certain puzzling gyrations of the jaw joint of modern man.

The origin and homologies of the jaws in all vertebrates were clearly outlined in the last century by Gegenbauer (1872). These general notions were based upon still earlier work, as far back as that of Carus in 1818 and Meckel in 1820, until a definitive statement of the thesis was made by Reichert in 1837. This general concept, called *Reichert's Theory*, has been solidly substantiated by investigations continuing into the beginning of the present century (Broom, 1912; Gaupp, 1911; Goodrich, 1930; van der Klaauw, 1924) and the known facts are usually reviewed, at least cursorily, in the literature (Romer, 1970).

The latter part of the account is new. Paleoanthropology, comparative anatomy, muscle physiology, and biomechanics afford an eclectic attack on the subtleties of jaw joint function in modern man. The story tracks the cranial adaptations of the earliest hominids known from exceptionally well-preserved fossil crania. It examines extant crania with detailed dissections of a wide variety of mammals and probes muscle action to derive the biomechanics of modern human jaws. From this extended vista the logic of pathological anatomy looms and the essence of the clinical problems in joint function becomes clear. The wide latitude in current literature on the working of the human jaw joint encompasses much unverified speculation. The present analysis emphasizes the tangible features of anatomic function.

ORIGIN OF THE VERTEBRATE HEAD

The skeleton of the higher vertebrates is composed mostly of bone, which can arise in two ways. *Dermal bone*, as the name implies, arises directly in the dermis. Such bone is near the surface, under the skin. *Cartilaginous bone* is preformed in cartilage, the early cartilage model being replaced by mature bone. Bones of this origin are deeper in the body, most of them being related to the axial skeleton or its extensions. The *visceral arches*, another source of cartilaginous bone, are not contributed by the axial skeleton but by the structures that support the viscera, i.e. the gut. The skeleton of the head of higher vertebrates is a complex of all three of these elements—dermal bone, axial skeleton, and visceral arches. The visceral arches are now, for the most part, transitory in embryologic development.

The structural ground plan of vertebrates is distinctive. Every vertebrate begins life with a *notochord*, a long, flexible, central body axis. The adults of most vertebrates then develop a *vertebral column*, whereby the bony bodies of a series of vertebrae surround and replace the notochord. The spinal cord of a central nervous system lies closely dorsal to the chain of vertebral bodies, which send up bony arms called *neural arches* to embrace and protect this delicate neural cable along the back. The gut lies ventral to the vertebral axis. Each side of the body is essentially a mirror image of the other, making it bilaterally symmetrical. There is a fore, or head region, and an aft, or tail region. This arrangement is quite different from the radial symmetry of some invertebrates. It results in an active, swift locomotive life.

Vertebrate bodies are essentially segmented, as can be seen in their metameric vertebrae, but this has become exceedingly complex in the head region. After exhaustive study for nearly two centuries, it has finally been concluded that the vertebrate head is the result of persistent differentiation of the anterior segments of an originally uniform series. This process of cephalization has all but obscured the traces of the primitive segmentation, but when the present product is explained in these terms, much of the complexity becomes simple and is clearly a remarkable reminder of the past. The first vertebrates had no biting apparatus, but the process of cephalization also produced the singular structures called jaws.

Once jaws were operant and available to the evolutionary process, further complexities of the head region continued through fish, amphibian, and reptilian stages. Life on land offered strange metabolic possibilities. This was expressed in the wide divergence of vertebrates into birds and mammals, as well as in the intricate divergences within each of these major divisions. At this time, special feeding behaviors were prerequisites for the rise in metabolic activity, and so jaw mechanics blossomed in a variety of basic patterns.

From the comparative microscopic study of the soft as well as hard tissues of extant animals, joints are classically arranged in a morphological series that runs from the simplest to the most complex. It has been conceded that this series coincides more or less with a true evolutionary sequence (Haines, 1942; Lubosch, 1910).

The simplest joints are *synarthroses*, in which the parts are made slightly movable by a binding of cartilage, fibrocartilage, or tendinous connective tissues between them. Next, *schiz-*

arthroses are joints made more mobile by several small, separated splits or joint spaces interrupting these bonding tissues. *Diarthroses* are the most complex joints, with the wide single articular cavity surrounded by a specialized sleeve lined with a synovial layer.

These major types have been further subdivided according to histologic details. The last category, particularly, is separated into two types, the *hemidiarthroses* (Halbegelenke) and the *eudiarthroses* (the definitive diarthrodial joint), based on the degree of specialization of coverings and capsules (Lubosch, 1910; 1938).

Some of the fossil reptiles show characteristics of structure that led to the term *mammal-like reptiles*. The biologic migration across this chasm to the true mammal, strange and complex as it has been, is often seen clearly in the cranial morphology of these forms. The crucial morphological features marking the mammalian skull are as follows:

1. The lower jaw is composed of one bone on each side, homologous with the old dentary bone of reptiles, to which all the lower teeth are attached. It is now known as the *mandible*.

2. The lower jaw is joined to the skull by a dentary-squamosal articulation. The squamous is that part of the temporal bone complex that forms the upper part of the joint, which is now known as the *temporomandibular joint* (TMJ).

3. The old jaw joint of reptiles, the articular-quadrate joint, which came from a front gill arch, now has no part in jaw support. These two bones, in addition to a third bone, are now the ossicles of the middle ear and subserve the sense of hearing. Hence, the articular bone is the *malleus*; the quadrate is the *incus*; and the hyomandibular is the *stapes*.

Clinicians have long suspected that certain ear disturbances are related to a particular type of jaw dysfunction. Some of the asserted functional relationships, however, are not credible to the biologist (see Chapter 18). However, the jaw and ear evolved together, and the history of the process is quite revealing. Amazing motor relationships still remain between the jaw and ear, and have great clinical significance. Only by a careful unraveling of the evolutionary past can comprehension be made of such matters.

Agnatha: Vertebrates Without Jaws

The front end of this earliest and most simple of vertebrates had its nervous system elaborated in a longitudinal series of swellings, which were collectively called the brain. Special transducers

were connected by cables to these swellings. They were the sense organs—nose, eyes, and ears—that scanned the environment for vital information to signal to the brain. The skull, a skeletal strengthening around the brain and sense organs, was a forward continuation and projection of the vertebral axis. The front of the gut opened at the mouth just below the fore part of the brain. This led through an oropharyngeal channel to the gut proper, which continued caudally, ventral to the vertebral axis. Slits in the pharyngeal wall opened to the outside. They were stiffened by skeletal braces called gill arches, but these were not connected with the body axis or skull. This series of louvered slits was used both for respiration and food filtering (Fig. 1–1A).

The epiceratobranchial joint at the bend of a gill arch in a modern shark probably most closely represents the form of the earliest jaw joint. Microscopic studies show a thin plate of

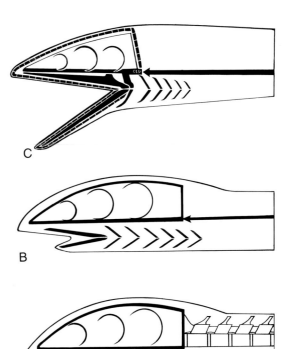

FIGURE 1–1. Origin of the Jaws. *A,* Agnatha: sedentary animal; skull in heavy outline. Oral opening at left (dark arrow) sucks food in from mud; food is filtered and debris squirted out through gill slits (small arrows). *B,* Gnathostome: more active animal; anterior gill arch enlarged as first set of jaws. Forward thrust of swimming body indicated by horizontal arrow. *C,* Osteichthyes: speed swimmer; increased thrust from body axis indicated by heavy horizontal arrow; great development of jaws braced by second gill arch (interrupted dark outline covering skull under skin represents dermal bone plates).

flexible fibrocartilage connecting the two carti-laginous joint elements. At the periphery, this layer gradually merges with the perichondrium of each cartilage (Haines, 1942). This is a simple synarthrosis.

Fossil Agnatha of the type previously de-scribed are found from the Silurian Period. Lampreys are the living, primitive representa-tives, which have a basic arrangement similar to the known fossils. Although their skeletons are only cartilaginous, they represent good ex-amples of how the original ancestors must have behaved. The extinct forms sucked mud from which food was filtered. The living forms feed somewhat similarly as larvae, but as adults they are specialized parasites that suck blood and meat rasped from their hosts by a horny tongue (Denison, 1961).

Gnathostomes: The First Jawed Vertebrates

The gill arch cage began as a respiratory filter-feeder pump (Fig. 1–1A). Muscles pulling on the arch bars caused expansion and contrac-tion of the buccopharyngeal space. Food clumps sucked into the mouth were caught by appro-priately named *gill rakers*, as water was pumped out through the respiratory gill slits of the pharynx. Gill arches bent most vigorously at the epiceratobranchial joint in this activity. Clamping of the arch bars could help in holding mobile bits of food. Thus, through selection, the ventilation system became a specialized feeding apparatus near the front of the buccal cavity.

It has been suggested recently that the fore-most arches were incorporated into the brain-case above, but the third and fourth arch bars were caught up more and more in the service of prehension and less in that of respiration (Thomson, 1971). Hence, the grabbing jaws of gnathostomes gradually appeared as these arch bars became renovated for tighter biting (Fig. 1–1B). As these jaw arches increased in size and changed in shape, the stretched skin rolling over their edges became modified and enlarged in localized pockets to produce hard barbs, the teeth. During embryologic development in modern man, the process is repeated precisely in the form of small enamel organs arising from pouches poked into the jaws from the oral mucosa.

The modern shark most closely represents a simplified blueprint of the first vertebrate with jaws. There are three major parts to this con-struct: the housing of the brain, the housing of

the sense organs, and the scaffolding of the jaws. A cartilaginous trough jointed directly in series with the vertebral axis runs forward to a terminal projection called the *rostrum*. This cradles the brain in which bulbous swellings nestle into the closely adapted floor. Three open cartilaginous baskets are hung out like carriage lamps from each side of the trough. They house the sense organs, and, from front to back, they are the olfactory, optic, and otic capsules. The enlarged and modified third gill arch is slung immediately below the cranial overhang from the vertebral column. As the mouth enlarged for biting larger prey, this jaw gill arch crowded back against the arch behind. This process is well-demonstrated in the modern shark. Though less enlarged and less modified, the fourth arch makes for somewhat of a gradual transition to the following monotonous repeti-tion of the gill arch series diminishing in size behind (Fig. 1–1C).

The microscopic picture of this jaw joint is that of the classical schizarthrosis. A rather thickened mass of connective tissue binds the cartilage bars. Peripherally, this tissue is con-tinuous with the perichondrium, which is more dense around the joint. Centrally, numerous small fluid-filled cavities are found distributed more or less randomly between the articulating surfaces.

The oldest and most informative fossils, hav-ing most of the above components in their skull construction, are the spiny sharks of the extinct order *Acanthodii* from the late Silurian and Devonian Periods. "The skull is partly ossi-fied—important evidence that the boneless condition of elasmobranchs was not typical of all early gnathostomes" (Young, 1955). How-ever, as they were only partly ossified, this also suggests that earlier ancestors, still to be found, may well have had only an inner skull scaffold-ing of cartilage, perhaps calcified, but not true bone.

Knowledge about the whole vertebrate body is suggested by the architecture of the skull, which is the most prominently preserved in fossils. One principle of biological construction becomes clear because, as the skull evolved, its form varied directly with change in total body structure, and of course, as body form changed so did general behavior. The brain developed in an ever-increasing complexity of neural cir-cuits to drive the animal to greater activity and speedy movement. From a bottom-living, sed-entary mudsucker, the beast became a speedy, nomadic predator, and biting jaws were a ra-pacious part of this whole locomotor adaptation.

The skull has been shown to arise from two sources, but both are cartilaginous. The first is a forward extension of the vertebral body axis, which forms the skull base with its projecting sockets for the sense organs. The second is the forward extensions of the gill arch series; these are the jaws and their hyoid accessories. Both of these cartilaginous contributions are replaced, at least in part, by bone in the higher vertebrates.

There is a third source of bone in the definitive vertebrate. It is the dermal bone derived from the membrane or connective tissue of the skin. Concomitant with the increase in vigor of the swimming behavior or the need for protection from the predator, a helmet of outer bony plates arose. It encased the entire head and pectoral girdle. Thus, in modern bony fish, there is an inner bony skeleton that arises in cartilage for the base of the brain and the jaws and an outer complete covering that develops from dermal bone for the head and pectoral area. The remnants of this early armor plate are retained in all mammals. In man, dermal bones cover the cranium, house the facial organs, and form the adult jaws. Remnants of the cartilaginous upper jaw have been described in the human embryo (Fawcett, 1924), and Meckel's cartilage is the well-known embryonic vestige of the lower jaw. Even the human pectoral girdle recalls the past, for the clavicle, a dermal bone once incorporated in the early skull, is one of the earliest bones to appear in the fetus.

The primary jaws made from modified, ossified gill arches were connected at their caudal ends by a simple hinge joint. There was an obvious mechanical deficiency in this sort of arrangement, because the joint was left hanging free, protruding slightly on each side like the bowlegged elbows of a primitive reptile, though still within the body wall. This was corrected when the fourth or hyoid arch was commandeered as an accessory strut, properly bracing the jaw joint to the skull. The jaws were further strengthened, stiffened, and protected by the armor of numerous dermal, bony plates plastered to their outer surface. Some of these bones at the edge of the mouth also developed teeth. These outer tooth-bearing plates, braced by adjacent dermal bones, are known as secondary jaws. However, the primary jaws still formed the single joint on each side for the entire jaw complex (Fig. 1–1C).

Microscopically, the suggestion of several slight steps leading to the eudiarthrodial joint is found within the group of true bony fish. *Lepisosteus*, or the garpike, has a well-ossified quadrate bone that is the upper element of the jaw joint. The convex articular end of the bone is covered by a layer of calcified cartilage, which is, in turn, covered by a thick layer of hyaline cartilage. The actual articular surface is composed of a thin acidophilic layer of fibrocartilage. The ossified end of Meckel's cartilage forming the lower joint element, the *articular bone*, is similarly constructed. Between the two surfaces is a broad, well-defined joint cavity. It is lined on the sides by a complete synovial membrane composed of two parts. The stratum intimale lies on the inner surface and is supported in this position by a surrounding stratum subsynoviale. This closely associated outer layer carries the nerve and vascular supply. The whole is wrapped peripherally in a strong fibrous tissue cuff, which is continuous with the periosteum of the bones (Becht, 1953). Other joints in the fishes' bodies (fins, gill arches, and similar structures) are never as highly developed as the jaw joint. Thus, the definitive, true eudiarthrodial construction, later seen in all mammalian joints, was established phylogenetically in the jaw joint initially.

All further complicating features of the jaws and their joints leading to those of mammals have been derived by selective playing with adaptive modifications of these several original elements. In doing so, however, many complex problems had to be solved by amphibians and reptiles, then resolved by mammals. It took the evolutionary process approximately 130 million years to stabilize this composite, basic vertebrate head skeleton with its built-in pincers called jaws.

Amphibia: The Single Joint for Double Jaws

One of the boldest vertebrate ventures was the invasion of the land. Major mechanistic changes obviously were involved; in particular, a shift from gill- to lung-breathing and a shift from sinuous swimming to four-footed walking. Fish already possessed the prerequisites for this in their primitive lungs or swim bladders. Thus, the first amphibians: long, slim, possibly still slimy, were, except for the absence of median fins, air-breathing, four-legged fish.

But early air-breathing mechanisms required the concerted action of buccal and lung chambers. A pulse-pumping device took a given volume of air or water into the buccal cavity. The mouth was closed and the cavity compressed, squirting the buccal contents either into the lung, in the case of air, or through the gill slits, in the case of water. The volume of intake depended on the size of the buccal space, which also ". . . figures prominently in feeding and prey capture" (Gans, 1970). Further adaptation to land life produced a separation of the two activities; a suction pump aspirated air into the lungs, and the oral apparatus was freed entirely for specialization in feeding.

An essential functional feature of the jaw apparatus in amphibians and reptiles must be mentioned at this point, because it involves the problem of feeding in the new air medium. The jaws of these creatures were used only for prehension. There was as yet no agile tongue, and as the prey was swallowed whole, it had to be maneuvered into the gullet without permitting it to escape. Thus, the skull became *kinetic;* that is, new movable joints appeared within the cranium. This ingenious device was a shuttling pterygopalatine component coordinated with joints between the frontal and nasal bones. It then ensured that some link in the jaw complex remained clamped on the struggling prey, while other parts shifted forward to hook and drag the prey back along this conveyor system into the gut. As a consequence, in some extant reptiles, the musculature of the kinetic system often exceeds that of the jaw-closing muscles (Frazzetta, 1966).

Proliferation of loose, movable parts impairs the architectural stability of the skull. Thus, kinesis has disappeared in the crania of reptiles such as turtles and crocodiles, which feed in water. The density of the medium is used to hold the food, as the captor simply swims forward onto his prey or rotates rapidly to twist a chunk of meat out of the victim. With the development of true mastication, structural stability was again essential, and cranial kinesis is absent in mammalian forms.

The skull of a primitive amphibian tends to be long, wide, and remarkably flat. The changes of importance were mainly in the covering of dermal bone. Because it is quite complex, only bones intimately involved with the jaws and joints are considered here; a part of the roof shield and the lower jaw.

The roof shield, composed of numerous bone plates that were seamed at sutures, was functionally a flat protective top, rolling down steeply on all sides. It was breached only by the small openings for nostrils, eyes, and a tiny median "eye." A notch cutting in from the posterior rim of the skull on each side was the only other defect in an otherwise complete carapace. The margins of the notch anchored the tympanic membrane of a primitive auditory apparatus. Being bilaterally symmetrical, the bones were generally paired. Those necessary in this discussion are at the edge of the front and sides. A small premaxilla bearing anterior teeth lay at the front; the maxilla, bearing the majority of the marginal teeth, was sutured to it on the side. Next, the jugal bone extended back to continue the margin of the upper jaw and to form the lower border of the orbit. The quadratojugal then extended the jaw backward to the last bone, the quadrate, which was the ossified end of the palatoquadrate cartilage protruding from under its dermal bone shield (Fig. 1–2A). The squamosal bone, which was not on the jaw margin, was later to become important. It lay above and in contact with the jugal, quadratojugal and quadrate bones.

The lower jaw was complex, similar to the cranium. The inner cartilaginous core of the old primary jaw was wrapped tightly in a blanket of numerous dermal bony plates. The primary jaw was also exposed only at its back end, where it poked out posteriorly from under its bony shield. In fossil amphibians, the structure can be likened to a scabbard of some eight polished plaques that sheathe the blade of a renovated lower jaw gill arch in which the protruding handle was the articular head (Fig. 1–2A). On the outer surface, the dentary bone held the marginal teeth. This worked against the maxilla and its teeth in the upper jaw. Below the dentary, and sutured to it, two splenials and an angular bone formed the lower jaw margin. Posterior to the dentary and above the angular, the surangular continued the upper jaw margin back to the exposed end of the mandibular (Meckel's) cartilage. On the medial side, three coronoid bones closed the gap between the splenials and the dentary. Farther back, a prearticular bone filled the gap between the angular below and the surangular above. Thus, the jaws of each side were doubled, one inside the other.

The important thing to observe at this point is that the major joint of the jaw, the one of primary interest, had not changed. Although the old palatoquadrate cartilage became ossified at certain growth sites, the posterior site (presently called the quadrate bone) still articulated with its old partner, the now-ossified hind end of Meckel's cartilage (appropriately called the articular bone). Together they functioned as before in a firm hinge joint for the double jaw (Fig. 1–2A). The microscopic anatomy of the joint was also that of the eudiarthrodial type, previously established in the bony fish. It remained unchanged up to the mammalian level.

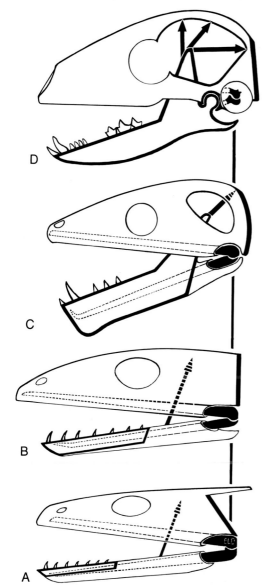

FIGURE 1–2. Evolution of Mammalian Jaw Joint. Posterior wall of skull and dentary bone with teeth in heavy outline; dotted line represents cartilage jaws under dermal bone; joints in black; arrows represent muscle vectors. A, Amphibian: note notch in rear margin of skull. B, Reptile: note increase in dentary bone, loss of notch in rear margin of skull. C, Mammal-like reptile: note further increase in dentary bone with addition of coronoid process and opening in skull roof (temporal fossa). D, Mammal: note that dentary bone connects with cranium to form dentary-squamosal joint (TMJ); primitive jaw joint now malleolar-incus joint of ear ossicles.

Reptilia: Loss of Bony Parts

The first notable change from the amphibian structure was the disappearance of the otic notch that supported the tympanum of the primitive ear. Thus, there is no skeletal clue to the eardrum (Allin, 1975). It may have been pushed down and back toward the second gill arch area. The old cartilaginous hyomandibular bone, whose proximal end stuck into the auditory capsule, was involved in sound transmission. It was called the *columella* and later became the stapes. Still articulating with the quadrate bone, it conducted vibrations from the tympanic membrane to the inner ear.

At this time, the side and straight rear margin of the skull made a rigid vertical support over the jaw joint because the tympanum no longer interfered (Fig. 1–2B). Many associated changes appeared with the better bracing. The teeth began to lose their continuity of repetition; that is, different segments along the dental line developed teeth of different sizes and incipient functions. Concomitantly, the muscles grew in size and mechanical advantage (Barghusen, 1973). The jaws may then have been used for more than mere prehension. All these features strongly suggest that, with the increase in metabolic activity that was needed to hold the body up out of water, more food, more efficiently utilized, was certainly needed. This turned the tide toward a mammalian way of life in which much food is burned and a high, constant body temperature is maintained.

Amphibian fossils have not shown any great advance in skull mechanics over the crossopterygian fish. Apparently, several more urgent defects had first to be settled to ensure survival of the system out of water. On the other hand, some of their reptilian descendants seem well-suited to live on land. They are appreciably advanced over modern amphibians in the normal dryness of the skin, in devices for preventing water loss, and in methods of reproduction out of water. The fossil record reveals that no terrestrial type lasts unchanged for more than a few million years. Then, as previously pointed out, these major changes in general body form and function had soon to be reflected in the architectonics of the skull.

The history of reptilian skull renovation leading to the general mammalian arrangement is largely one of a progressive reduction in number of bony components. As this continued, the skull became deeper and narrower so that it lost the extreme flatness of contour characteristic of the early amphibians. Then a curious thing began to happen to the originally intact cranial roof shield: holes formed in special spots, exposing the muscular fossae beneath (Fig. 1–2C). There has been some difficulty in defining an adaptive aspect to these fenestrations. Explanations seem to center on three proposals primarily based on muscle attachments.

The jaw-closing muscles in the early forms took origin from the under surface of the cranial roof on each side of the braincase. They ran in a strongly horizontal, slanting course to their mandibular insertions. This afforded the necessary fiber length for a reasonable gape in a flat skull. It was first suggested that the openings developed simply to allow bulging in the forceful contraction of progressively enlarging muscles (Gregory, 1915). It is doubtful, however, that the fossae were ever composed completely of muscle. The infratemporal fossae in man are amply filled with fatty clumps and venous plexuses, which accommodate free muscle bulging, slimming, and sliding. Bone recedes from regions of net tension to be replaced by suitable fascia (Oxnard, 1971). Tension might well be expected from orthogonal pull on the cranial roof, but a tug on a fascial roof would lower the roof rather than raise the jaw. Furthermore, tension from the same muscles seems to have advanced a coronoid process on the jaw, and the tension here would seem to have a higher net value.

What seems a more reasonable view looks not at the holes, which are boneless spaces, but at the bony rims arching around the openings. These are seen as essential buttresses resisting the complicated interplay of pressures and tensions imposed by shifting muscle action (Frazzetta, 1966). This suggests that, since tough connective tissue resists tension superbly, angular tendinous attachment to the edges of bony arches transmits the muscle tug on bone in line with its periosteal fibers, which then take up the tension. The bony flying buttresses thus resist bending, which imposes alternate tensions and pressures on the buttresses. Thus, as skull and musculature changed, forces on bones shifted; bone was built where functional and removed where unessential under the strict auspices of natural selection.

The story of jaw joints now divides into two parts. First, among the wide diversity of reptilian forms that radiated throughout the Mesozoic, the Age of Reptiles, those leading to mammals showed a continuous enlargement of the marginal tooth-bearing bones at the front of the jaws. This is clearly a corollary of the consistent loss of separate bony elements; the expanding bones grew back to fulfill jaw function. In the upper jaw, the premaxilla, and especially the maxilla, increased in length and vertical depth. In the lower jaw, the dentary bone on the outer side of the old Meckel's cartilage jaw expanded relentlessly backward, crowding out the diminishing bones behind it.

When the dentary reached the level of jaw muscles slanting down from the cranial roof, it gained anchorage on it. A single bone makes a stronger and more rigid lever than a series of many bones that must give, however slightly, at each connecting suture. Hence, the dentary finally came in contact with the cranium at the squamosal bone (Fig. 1–2D). In this way, the back end of the dentary bone came to lie in the same transverse plane as the old primary jaw joint and became closely attached to it. At this time then, two bones came to form the condyle of the mandible. Surprisingly, and most fortunately, many of the details of these extraordinary developments are remarkably well-recorded in numerous fossil remains (Crompton, 1963; Romer, 1969).

The second part of the story traces concomitant occurrences at the back of the jaw. It concerns the destiny of the unit of postdentary bones that composed the primitive jaw joint. Here, while the new dentary-squamosal (temporomandibular) joint was becoming increasingly stabilized in feeding function, the old joint was gradually being released from feeding commitments. In a long, adaptive crescendo, the primary jaw joint gained efficiency in a different performance, the transmission and tempering of the energy of airborne vibrations (Allin, 1975; Hotton, 1959; Thomson, 1966; Webster, 1966). This phenomenon may portray a complicated compromise between selection acting on jaws for both feeding and hearing adaptations. Contrary to the prevalent view, which deems dominance of the dentary as primarily a feeding adaptation, it has been proposed that it actually ". . . was to an important extent a reflection of auditory adaptation" (Allin, 1975). In either case, the jaw joints and ears have been intimately associated since the beginning of mammalian emergence.

It had long been predicted that somewhere in mammalian phylogeny animals must have existed with double-boned jaw condyles. The fossils were finally found; one was appropriately named Diarthrognathus, (Crompton, 1958; Kermack, 1958) and additional such fossils continue to be uncovered (Romer, 1969). Thus, at the time of transition from reptiles to mammals, a hinge movement of the jaws was swinging on combined quadrato-articulare and dentary-squamosal joints, since they lie in line in a manner similar to hinges on a barn door.

In the very late mammal-like reptiles, the small temporal opening in the cranial roof became greatly enlarged. It opened more and more toward the top of the skull so that the fenestrae of both sides almost met, leaving but a slim strip of parietal between them. Ventrally, only a bony bar was left. This was comprised of the jugal and squamosal bones, called the zygomatic arch in mammals. The opening increased so much in mammals that the bar separating the orbit from the temporal fenestra disappeared, and most mammals have a continuous orbitotemporal fossa. The maxilla also increased, especially in its vertical dimension, to accommodate an elongated canine. This pushed the lacrimal bone back to the eye socket. It also pushed the outer nasal openings forward to come together at the midline and open in one doubled outer aperture.

There is no living specie that truly represents the mammal-like reptile. Monotremes, the duck-billed platypus and echidna, are apparently deviants from the modern mammalian line.

MAMMALIAN ARCHITECTURAL THEME

The great diversity of animal forms has arisen only by the reworking of a surprisingly few fundamental architectural themes. The theme of mammalian body structure is a horizontal fore-and-aft layout featuring head-neck-torso-tail. This sequence is strung along a sturdy horizontal girder, the backbone, or vertebral column. The whole edifice is supported by four vertical pillars, the paired limbs.

Structuration of the head segment is still too often presented as if it, or its component parts, could really be understood without reference to the total animal. The head is but an integral part of the organism; it is a tightly fitted composite of organ complexes laid out in strict harmony with the total body plan. The skull is the consolidating framework that holds the organ complexes together. Its architectural theme can be sketched as a trusswork in three parts (Fig. 1–3), (DuBrul, 1974).

First, the *viscerocranium* in front is an elongated pyramid laid flat on its side. Its apex is the nasal vent and its base abuts the tapered projection of the neurocranium behind. The viscerocranium houses the upper airway, provides roofs and walls to the upper foodway, supports the special sense organs of smell, sight, and taste, and its base forms the front walls of the orbits. Thus, its upper surface is formed by the nasal bones, its sides by the premaxillae and maxillae, and its undersurface by premaxillae, maxillae, palatine, and pterygoid bones.

Second, the *neurocranium* in back is a truncated cone also laid horizontally on its side. Its narrow apex butts into the base of the viscerocranium between the orbital fossae. Its own base is the flat occipital plane facing squarely backward to connect with the neck. The neurocranium houses the brain, provides the opening for passage of the spinal cord, and forms the broad surface by which the skull is cantilevered from the vertebral column. Its upper curved surface is formed by the frontal and parietal bones, its curving sides by the parietal, sphenoid, and temporal bones, and its underside by the sphenoid, occipital, and temporal bones. Its base is the flat posterior part of the occipital bone. Because visceral and neural components join in an extremely constricted midline between the orbits, sturdy lateral bracing is required. This need is met by wide-flung flying buttresses, the zygomatic arches, spanning the constriction on each side.

Third, the *mandible* below is a long, straight, level bar with its fulcrum, the jaw joint, at the back end. The mandible also spans the cranial constriction contacting the visceral component at the front through the dentition and the neural component at the back through the jaw joint. A high coronoid flange rises from the basal bony bar where the biting muscles attach. It lies between the tooth row and the joint. The mandible walls the upper foodway, which is roofed above by the palate and floored below by a muscular hammock hung between the bony bodies of both sides.

This is the basic blueprint of the familiar long, low, flat, cranial contour characteristic of the mammalian skull (Fig. 1–3). From it, two adaptive feeding modifications have been repeatedly developed in mammalian phylogeny. These forms have been loosely labeled *carnivores* as opposed to *herbivores*. This elaboration has occurred in lines of unrelated species and it appears to be particularly pertinent in explaining early hominid fossils.

Of special interest is the architecture of the viscerocranium. It is dominated by the feeding

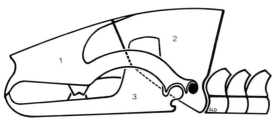

FIGURE 1–3. Mammalian Model. Viscerocranium (1), neurocranium (2), mandible (3).

mechanics of the oral apparatus that is based on the distinctive lever system of mammalian jaws.

Lever Systems

The lever is a mechanical contrivance found universally in living locomotor systems. Arms, legs, wings, and backbones are basically strung out sequences of levers. Lever action is based on the *principle of moments*. The principle defines the tendency of a rigid bar, balanced on a pivot or turning axis, to rotate when a load is hung on one arm of the balance. The turning force is the product of the load and its distance from the pivot (Load × Distance). The measure is called a *moment of force*. The bar is brought back to balance when an equal moment of force is hung on the opposite arm. In this way a load of one pound, 10 inches from the pivot, can balance a load of 10 pounds one inch from the pivot! A lever, living or inanimate, is a system used to overcome a resistance. Thus an effort force applied to one arm of the lever is thrust across a fulcrum (pivot) to move a resistance force at the end of the opposing lever arm. From this it follows that the force a lever can deliver can be increased in three ways: (1) by applying more effort force, (2) by lengthening the effort arm, and (3) by shortening the resistance arm.

Three classes of levers are recognized. Defining advantages and disadvantages of each class clarifies the functional potentials and limitations of the mammalian system.

Class I—The fulcrum lies between the effort force and the resistance force. Therefore, shortening or lengthening either arm is unrestricted, a mechanical advantage. But both forces act against the fulcrum. Excessive pressure in a joint is a biological disadvantage.

Class II—The fulcrum lies at one end, the effort force at the other, and the resistance force lies between. Lengthening the effort arm is unrestricted, but its shortening is restricted. Lengthening the resistance arm is also restricted, sometimes a disadvantage (see further on). But now the forces act in opposite directions; only the resistance force acts against the fulcrum. Lessened pressure in a joint is a biological advantage.

Class III—The fulcrum lies at one end, the resistance force at the other, and the effort force lies between. Lengthening the effort arm is now restricted and it is always shorter than the resistance arm, which is a distinct mechanical disadvantage. Again both forces act in opposite

directions, with only the effort force acting against the fulcrum. Lessened pressure in a joint is a biological advantage, but because lengthening the resistance arm is now unrestricted, an unexpected biological advantage emerges. A jaw with a short effort arm has muscles close to the joint. Muscles need to lengthen only slightly to open a long jaw in a wide gape. A widely swung resistance arm with stabbing canines at its end will move farther and faster than a short effort arm in the same period of time! The momentum thus developed with a minimum of muscle contraction is a decided biological advantage for a snapping predator such as a wolf.

The Carnivorous Adaptation

Feeding behavior in carnivores is characterized by speedy, violent prehension followed by leisurely tearing and cutting up of the relatively soft, unresistant meat diet (see Chapter 2). This adaptation requires a wide gape and therefore emphasizes the temporalis muscle, since the masseter must be shoved far back to expose the cutting cheek teeth. This is best illustrated in the dog skull, which has differentiated little from the basic mammalian plan (Fig. 1–4). The crucial characteristics are:

1. Projecting jaws, used for grabbing prey, house long canines in strong buttresses but relatively shorter, though sharp, cheek teeth.

2. Long lower jaw with no ramus provides a lever with long resistance arm for speed in snapping; greater momentum at the front, where resistance is concentrated on one pene-

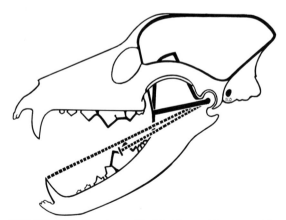

FIGURE 1–4. Carnivore Model. Note wide gape with emphasis on temporalis muscle. Temporal fossa and coronoid process in heavy outline. Dark black bar extending from jaw joint to anterior edge of temporalis is lever arm of effort force; resistance arms (dashed lines) extend from joint to canine and molar.

trating canine point, compensates for lessened power.

3. The joint is firmly fitted for stability of the fulcrum in violent predatory action.

4. A large coronoid process increases the effort arm and insertion area for a large temporalis muscle.

5. There is a horizontally expanded temporal fossa for the origin of an enlarged temporalis muscle and a short zygomatic area of attachment for the retruded masseter.

6. Long canines are at the front, where the snapping speed is fastest, and bladed carnassials are at the back, where the resistance arm for cutting is shortest.

The Herbivorous Adaptation

Feeding behavior in herbivores is characterized by leisurely prehension followed by forceful and prolonged milling of the relatively hard, resistant cellulose in the vegetable diet (see Chapter 2). This adaptation demands little gape and, therefore, a short oral opening. A long oral slit extending past the back teeth is distinctly disadvantageous for containing and controlling the cud or bolus. Thus emphasis is on the masseter complex, which can now expand forward. This is best illustrated in the much-modified horse skull (Fig. 1–5). The crucial characteristics are:

1. Long jaws for cropping are greatly deepened for housing long cheek teeth, but there are no canines (or merely vestigial ones), hence no canine buttresses.

2. A lower jaw with a high, bent, vertical ramus, widened below, provides a great area for masseter insertion and vertical depth of the jaw for long cheek teeth.

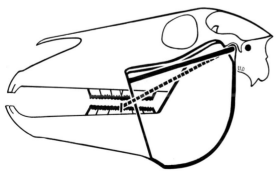

FIGURE 1–5. Herbivore Model. Note narrow gape with emphasis on masseter muscle. Masseter attachments on zygoma and ramus in heavy outline. Dark black bar extending from jaw joint to anterior edge of masseter is lever arm of effort force; resistance arm (dashed line) extends from joint to center of cheek tooth row.

3. The joint is fitted for wide, gliding, horizontal movements in lateral grinding.

4. There is a small coronoid process for the diminished temporalis muscle.

5. A greatly decreased temporal fossa again expresses deemphasis of the temporalis muscle; an enormously lengthened masseter origin that extends far forward of the zygomaticomaxillary suture to the midlevel of the tooth row results in tremendous lengthening of the effort arm.

6. There are broad cropping incisors but no canines; long, high, cheek teeth are set well back where the resistance arm in grinding is shortest.

EMERGENCE OF HOMINID HEAD FORM

Three overriding influences have reworked this phylogenetically plastic construct to change it from its original elongated flatness to the shortened roundness of the human skull. In their evolutionary sequence these are: (1) upright locomotion, (2) modified oral apparatus, and (3) burgeoning brain. The intricate interplay adjusting the different engineering requirements for each of these impingements has produced confused concepts concerning the basis of skull form in the past. But now, accumulating fossil finds make it possible to isolate the effects of each influence, and the logic of human skull form emerges.

Exceptionally well-preserved early hominid fossil skulls fall into two distinct groups. A small, relatively delicate form called the gracile type has been labeled *Australopithecus africanus*. A large, massive form labeled *Australopithecus boisei* is called the robust type.

Two of the influences reworking the skull are clearly evident in both australopithecine types. Therefore, they have produced the same cranial changes in each. These are the locomotion and brain effects. The modified oral effects are divergent in the two types. Thus the variables are isolated and the oral divergence parallels the carnivorous and herbivorous trends in other mammals.

Upright Locomotion

Fully upright locomotion was acquired early in hominid evolution. Consequently, it is present in both australopithecine types (Broom, 1946; Clark, 1964; Napier, 1967; Robinson, 1972). It had the heaviest impact on the renovation of the hominid skull. The most obvious

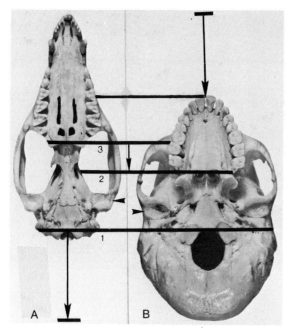

FIGURE 1–6. Postural Adaptations of the Skull (basal view). Note severe reduction and retraction of viscerocranium and downward and forward rotation of posterior cranial base. Mammalian skull model (*A*), human skull (*B*). Both skulls oriented at level of basion (1), level of hard palate of human skull (2), level of hard palate of mammalian skull (3).

effect is a severe bending between visceral and neural components that considerably shortens the skull. This satisfies two requirements imposed by the now-vertical body. It brings the sense organs and oral apparatus down in front, preserving their orientation to the surrounding environment. It brings the neural component down in back to maintain its orientation with the spinal cord and vertical vertebral column. This balanced the skull on the vertebral column and the head could then make a horizontal rotation to scan the surrounding environment.

Bending the skull produced an effect similar to bending a bar of taffy. The top curved and the bottom buckled. The cranial effects were therefore: (1) curving of the cranial roof, (2) buckling of the cranial floor (at sella turcica), (3) extreme retrusion of snout and jaws, (4) deepening of the mandible with outward flaring of its lower border, especially at the chin, and (5) downward and forward swing of the nuchal plane carrying the foramen magnum and occipital condyles forward toward the center of the skull.

The final effect is a severe crowding of the skull base (Fig. 1–6). Because this is clearly demonstrated in the skulls of both australopithecine types, whose postcranial skeletons are

clearly adapted to upright posture, it is isolated from the effects of a bulging brain. The brain was still no larger than a gorilla brain.

Modified Oral Apparatus

Although modification of the oral apparatus is partly an adjustment to upright locomotion, the two australopithecine types show a distinct divergence in feeding adaptations.

A. africanus is the least differentiated. The skull dorsum is vaulted in a long, uniformly rounded arc with no superstructures. Projecting supraorbital ridges are prominent but slender. The jaws protrude sharply below the infraorbital rims to extend the oral apparatus forward rather than downward. Thus the jaws are relatively shallow, housing short cheek teeth. The upper jaw has outstanding canine buttresses reaching from the frontal bone to the canine sockets. The zygomatic buttresses reach the level of the second molars. They are slender and less impressive. The lower jaw is fairly shallow, with a moderate ramus much like the human jaw, but with a sturdier coronoid process (Fig. 1–7).

Faint temporal lines that remain separated on the dorsum of the skull outline low, oval temporal fossae. The zygomatic arches are quite slender. The teeth are larger than those of modern man, especially the broad, spatulate, upper incisors. Upper canines are broad, bulky, and long-rooted as they project from their sturdy buttresses. The biting edges of the crowns extend well below the occlusal plane when not worn. The lower canines are more

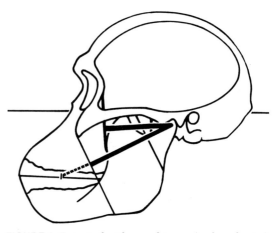

FIGURE 1–7. Australopithecus africanus (oral mechanics). Upper heavy line is moment arm of temporalis muscle, lower heavy line is moment arm of masseter muscle; dotted line is resistance arm from joint to center of cheek tooth row.

interesting. Their crowns are longer than the upper canine crowns. They are asymmetrical, with a short anterior occlusal slope and a long distal slicing slope ending at the cervix in a tiny distal cusp. Posterior teeth are small and narrow. These peculiarities all suggest cutting and tearing adaptive specializations (Robinson, 1954a; 1954b; 1956).

Consequently, A. *africanus* had a jaw-lever arrangement that seems much like the carnivorous form. Effort force (muscle mass) seems greater in the temporalis than in the masseter. The ratio of effort arms relative to resistance arms appears adequate but not unusual (Fig. 1–7). Considering the large anterior teeth, especially the specialized canines, the oral mechanics in this gracile form tend to favor the carnivorous construct (see previous). The animal was most probably omnivorous and therefore not excessively differentiated (Robinson, 1968).

A. *boisei* is considerably differentiated. The skull dorsum is deeply vaulted in a short asymmetrical arch flattened posteriorly. Superstructures rise in a thick sagittal crest, highest in the middle third of the dorsal outline. The supraorbital ridges are so bulky that they seem less projecting than the ridges on the gracile form. The enormous jaws are severely retruded, but extend far downward to house huge, long-rooted cheek teeth. Surprisingly, there are no distinct canine buttresses, but massive zygomatic buttresses have been thrust so far forward that they engulf the canine eminences and give the face a dished-in frontal plane (Fig. 1–8).

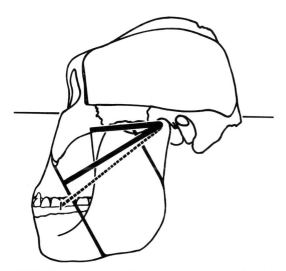

FIGURE 1–8. Australopithecus boisei (oral mechanics). Upper line is moment arm of temporalis muscle; lower heavy line is moment arm of masseter muscle, dotted line is resistance arm to center of cheek tooth row.

The entire cranium is short, but excessively broadened. The temporal lines forming the sagittal crest outline a high temporal fossa. The zygomatic arches are broad and bulky. They expand at the anterior root, which extends downward on the face at the dominating zygomatic buttresses. The arches bow widely to encompass the deep, temporal fossae.

The teeth are startling; there is a striking contrast between anteriors and posteriors. All front teeth, including canines, are diminutive in this context. They are not only smaller than the gracile teeth, but also fall within the size range of modern man! In contrast, the cheek teeth are enormous. Their occlusal surfaces are *more than three times greater* than these surfaces are in modern man. These peculiarities indicate heavy grinding herbivorous adaptations.

Manipulating this bulky complex, A. *boisei* had a jaw-lever arrangement that was highly differentiated. Thus the effort force was massive and greatest in the masseter area. Effort arms are lengthened, particularly that of the masseter muscle (Fig. 1–8). Along with the tremendously enlarged posterior teeth, the oral mechanics of this robust type reflects specialization in the direction of heavy herbivory. Even with its drastically shortened snout, this form resembles the horse in that the masseter was expanded forward as far as possible (see Fig. 1–5). Its origin was pushed forward beyond the level of the rest of the face, causing the dished-in facial surface.

Even from this curtailed survey it is evident that the structural contrasts between the two australopithecine types imply divergent jaw mechanics that partially parallel the carnivorous and herbivorous feeding adaptation previously discussed.

Burgeoning Brain

Although the brain has played a determining role in human evolution, and has impressed early investigators most, it has had the least impact on basic skull architecture. It merely ballooned the top of the head! At the australopithecine stage, it had not even begun the expansion that rapidly tripled in the later stages. Thus the brains of both types were ". . . essentially similar in size and form" (Tobias, 1967). The estimated cranial capacities of the specimens are about 500 milliliters, the same as that of the gorilla. Brain expansion, therefore, had minimal influence on skull architecture at this level. This variable, then, is obviously isolated from the other two.

NATURAL EXPERIMENT

A most striking and unexpected parallelism is to be found between the living bears and the extinct australopithecines. The bones, muscles, jaw joints, and teeth all reflect this parallelism. It thus emerges as a natural experiment (DuBrul, 1950; 1954; 1958; 1965), a test case substantiating the validity of the biomechanical analysis of hominid feeding adaptations presented here.

The Bones

Although classified in the order Carnivora, bears in general are now omnivorous. Their diet is primarily vegetable matter, but they will eat whatever is available (Murie, 1944). Thus, in respect to feeding behaviors, bears as a group are not considered highly specialized carnivores.

Ursus horribilis (Grizzly Bear): The skull is long and narrow, the jaws are relatively narrow and shallow, and the cheek teeth are narrow. In dorsal view, the snout projects strongly, so that the narrow skull tapers toward the front. The zygomatic arches slant slightly away from the cranium as they run posteriorly to outline a narrow, triangular, infratemporal space on each side (Fig. 1–9A).

Ailuropoda (Giant Panda): In a penetrating and definitive study, the giant panda has been shown to be actually a highly specialized herbivore (Davis, 1964). This animal is thus a contradiction; in nature it eats only bamboo shoots, some of which are up to 1½ inches thick (Sheldon, 1964), and this must be as extreme as herbivory can be. This requires tremendous force applied in long transverse grinding movements. In this case, the skull is short and broad, the jaws are deep, and the zygomatic arches are extremely deep from upper to lower borders. In dorsal view, the snout projects only moderately so that the cranium is short and round, almost completely spherical. The zygomatic arches are widely bowed to outline broad, circular temporal spaces (Fig. 1–9B).

When the skulls of the australopithecines are seen in dorsal view (Figs. 1–9 C and D), the remarkable similarities to the ursines are unmistakable.

A. africanus: The snout projects well beyond

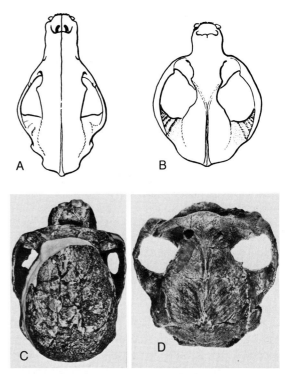

FIGURE 1–9. Parallelism in Cranial Adaptations. A, *Ursus:* note long narrow skull, protruding viscerocranium, and flattened zygomatic arches. B, *Ailuropoda:* note greatly broadened skull, shortened viscerocranium, wide bowing of zygomatic arches. C, *A. africanus:* note relatively narrow skull, protruding viscerocranium, flattened zygomatic arches. (Sts 5 Wenner-Gren cast). D, *A. boisei:* note extremely broadened skull, wholly retracted viscerocranium, extremely wide bowing of zygomatic arches (OH 5 Wenner-Gren cast).

the supraorbital rim of the narrow skull. Though the zygomatic arches stand out laterally at the front, they run straight posteriorly to outline a narrow, triangular, temporal space on each side.

A. boisei: The snout is barely visible at the front, so that the skull outline is practically a perfect sphere. The zygomatic arches jut out anterolaterally at the front, and are extremely widely bowed to outline the wide, circular temporal spaces.

The Muscles

Ursus horribilis: The jaw muscles of the grizzly bear exemplify the standard pattern of carnivores; the temporalis muscle is the dominant component representing ". . . at least half the total mass of the masticatory muscles" (Davis, 1964). It arises from a long, oval temporal fossa and inserts on a high, broad coronoid process. The masseter is considerably smaller. It arises from the lower border of the zygomatic arch and runs down behind the tooth row to insert at the angle of the jaw. It is displaced posteriorly so that its posterior fibers run behind the back of the jaw and must find attachment on a raphe, the meatoangular ligament (Scapino, 1974). The medial pterygoid is about half the size of the masseter, and the lateral pterygoid is diminutive. The zygomaticomandibular is an important muscle in carnivores. It arises from the entire inner surface of the zygomatic arch and inserts on the outer surface of the coronoid process. Thus, it takes over most of the function of the lateral pterygoid in shifting the jaw laterally.

Ailuropoda: All the jaw muscles of the giant panda are enormously enlarged. The temporalis muscle is exceptionally large. It arises from a greatly expanded temporal fossa, which encroaches forward on the facial area to make the snout seem shortened. The muscle is complex and highly pennated. Its fibers converge to insert on both surfaces of the coronoid process. In this case, the masseter is also extremely large. It arises from the anterior three quarters of the lower border of the zygomatic arch and inserts on the outer side of the lower jaw border below the coronoid process. It has been shifted anteriorly since the front of the zygomatic arch has been swung out and forward beyond the frontal plane. The posterior fibers do not insert as far back as the meatoangular or stylomandibular ligament, as they do in *Ursus* and all other carnivores (Davis, 1964). The medial pterygoid muscle is thin and smaller than in other carnivores, but the lateral pterygoid is short and thick and fitted with special alternate tendons of insertion. From this origin on the pterygoid plate, it runs straight laterally in the frontal plane to insert in a deep pit on the inner surface of the jaw condyle. The zygomaticomandibular muscle is also greatly expanded, relatively larger than in all other carnivores (Davis, 1964). It arises from the entire inner surface of the greatly expanded zygomatic arch. Its fibers converge medially to insert on the lower lateral surface of the large coronoid process by multiple tendons that raise numerous strong bony crests on the mandibular surface. Thus, both the lateral pterygoid and zygomaticomandibular muscles pull powerfully in a transverse plane.

Parallels in development, positioning, and orientation of the jaw muscles are also quite distinct in the australopithecines.

A. africanus: The jaw muscles in this form could only have been moderately developed since attachment surfaces are small and there are no outstanding scars of muscle attachments on the skull or jaw, as the term gracile implies. The temporal fossa afforded a modest origin for the temporalis muscle. The coronoid process of the jaw, however, seems more sturdy than that of the modern European mandible. The slender zygomatic arch suggests a less massive masseter. This also indicates a diminished development of the zygomaticomandibular muscle. The position of the lateral pterygoid plate anterior to the foramen ovale, and the infratemporal articular surface (preglenoid plane) of the sphenoidal wing anterior to the jaw joint, indicate a strong anterior component to the anteromedial pull of the lateral pterygoid muscle (Fig. 1–10).

A. boisei: All of the jaw muscles are enormously enlarged. The temporal fossa, though shortened anteroposteriorly, is expanded superoinferiorly and further extended by a heavy, raised, sagittal crest along the middle third of the cranial vault. The coronoid process of the mandible is high and wide. The long, deep zygomatic arch indicates a heavy, anteriorly extended masseter muscle and an advanced development of the zygomaticomandibular muscle, which pulls the jaw in a transverse plane. An extraordinary posterior extension of the lateral pterygoid plate medially and posteriorly to the foramen ovale indicates an almost

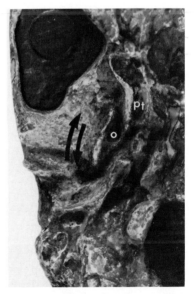

FIGURE 1–10. Parallelism Reflected in Jaw Joints of Hominids. *A. africanus:* temporal articular surface. Foramen ovale (o). Lateral pterygoid plate (pt). Note shallow glenoid fossa, low articular eminence extending forward as preglenoid plane. Foramen ovale posterior to pterygoid plate (as in man). Arrows indicate excursions of condyle during lateral movement to opposite side (Sts 5 Wenner-Gren cast).

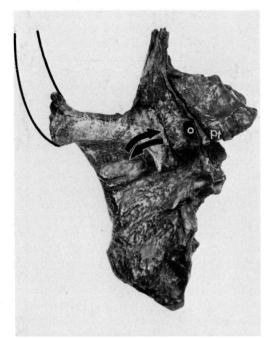

FIGURE 1–11. Parallelism Reflected in Jaw Joints of Hominids. *A. boisei:* temporal articular surface. Foramen ovale (o). Lateral pterygoid plate (pt). Note deep glenoid fossa, high articular eminence, no preglenoid plane, extensive medial glenoid plane. Foramen ovale anterior to extended rear edge of pterygoid plate. Arrows indicate excursions of condyle during lateral movements to opposite side. Extended lines at left represent outline of missing zygomatic arch. (OH5 Wenner-Gren cast).

completely transverse pull of the lateral pterygoid muscle (Fig. 1–11).

The Joints

In carnivores the craniomandibular joint works like a hinge that slides sideways in its slot. The condyle is a cylinder tapering gently medially. It supports a spiral articular surface that curls from anterolaterally across the top and then down and back posteromedially and inferiorly. The condyle fits fairly snug in the mandibular (glenoid) fossa, which is a reciprocally transverse trough on the undersurface of the temporal squama. The fossa is walled and subtly narrowed posteromedially by a bulky, forwardly curved, postglenoid process that hooks under the taper of the condyle. A smaller preglenoid process on the anterolateral side continues medially as a slim lip to complete the deep transverse slot anteriorly. In simple opening and closing, the jaw rotates around a common transverse axis almost continuously with the longitudinal axes of the mandibular condyles (see Fig. 1–4).

Ursus horribilis: The jaw joint of the grizzly bear matches this standard quite closely. At rest, the lower cheek tooth row lies partially inside the upper row. Therefore, to cut meat or crush vegetation, the lower jaw must be shifted bodily laterally to line up the lower carnassial blades with the uppers on the chewing side. Thus, the chewing movement at the joint has two major components: a simple hinge swinging of the condylar cylinder and a transverse slide in the groove of the fossa. The result is a spiral or screw movement (Sicher, 1944).

Ailuropoda: Given this structural inheritance, the change from scissor-like slicing to heavy transverse grinding was evolved simply by a gradual blunting and broadening of the buccal carnassial cusps into wide occlusal milling surfaces and a lengthening of the transverse joint trough. This was closely correlated with the broadened skull and zygomatic arches and the reordering of muscle vectors and power. Comparison of the transverse movement of the condyle between grizzly bear and giant panda reveals a lateral shift in *Ursus* of about 3 mm, whereas it is doubled in *Ailuropoda*, about 6 mm (Davis, 1964). This, of course, is in perfect coordination with the heavily developed and transversely oriented zygomaticomandibular and lateral pterygoid muscles.

In hominids, the craniomandibular joint acts as a roving fulcrum. The cylindrical condyles tend not to run directly in the transverse plane; they are twisted so that extension of their long axes to the midline forms a variable angle open anteriorly. At rest, the jaw condyles lean against the posterior slopes of the articular eminences on the temporal bone. In simple opening and closing movements, the condyles rotate around a transverse axis passing through the centers of the eccentric condyles as they slide forward on the variably steep articular eminences. Thus, in the hominids, even simple opening usually has two major components: a hinge swinging of the condyle and a downward and forward slide on a convex articular slope. The key to predicting possible joint movements in the fossils lies in the structure of the temporal articular surface.

A. africanus: The articular contour of the temporal bone is low and undulating, the articular fossa is shallow, and the low articular eminence flattens anteriorly to a preglenoid plane. Laterally, the eminence is bounded by a raised articular tubercle and medially by a distinct, raised entoglenoid plate, making the eminence strongly saddle-shaped (DuBrul, 1974). The entoglenoid process separates the articular surface from the foramen ovale, which is situated posterolateral to the lateral pterygoid plate, as in modern man. At rest, the lower cheek tooth row lies partially inside the upper row, but the teeth come into occlusal contact on complete closure. To chew, the lower jaw must be swung to the chewing side. This was probably done by rotating the jaw in the horizontal plane around a vertical axis near the back of the condyle of the chewing side. To do this, the condyle on the opposite side would have to ride forward and inward on the preglenoid plane. Apparently, no directly transverse medial movement of this condyle was possible, since the articular fossa was walled medially by the entoglenoid process (see Fig. 1–10).

A. boisei: The articular contours of the temporal bone in this hominid are in sharp contrast to those of the gracile type. The articular fossa is deep, and the eminence descends in an extremely steep, long slope. It terminates abruptly at its summit in a sharp anterior rim. This bounds the posterior margin of the wide temporal fossa opening above. There is no preglenoid plane since the narrow braincase does not extend laterally over the area.

Laterally, the articular eminence curves back to terminate in a strong crest-like articular tubercle. Medially, the eminence is quite different from that of the gracile type. The medial wall rolls over a thick edge onto a wide medial glenoid plane. This is clearly a medial expansion of the articular surface reaching the rim of the foramen ovale. Only a low, roughened ridge separates this surface from the opening of the foramen ovale. Furthermore, the foramen is not only entirely walled medially by the lateral pterygoid plate, but also the plate extends well posterior to the foramen (Fig. 1–11) (DuBrul, 1974). The chewing movement is accomplished by an almost completely transverse lateral slide to the chewing side. The jaw cannot rotate around a vertical axis at the working condyle, as in *A. africanus*, because there is no preglenoid plane on which the contralateral condyle can ride forward; the condyle would dislocate into the temporal fossa. The opposite condyle therefore slides medially on the extensive medial glenoid plane. The flat, vertical articular eminence in front acts as a wall to prevent forward displacement. Curiously, as in the carnivore, this hominid mandible also performs a screw-like movement; it rotates around a horizontal axis as it slides medially. The only difference is that the condyle slides downward and inward on a convex medial eminence, giving a lateral rocking movement to the jaw in the frontal plane (Fig. 1–12).

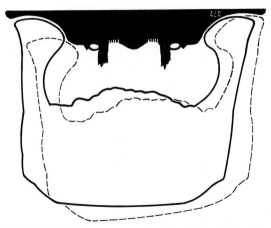

FIGURE 1–12. Transverse section through jaw joints of *A. boisei* to show extraordinary rocking of jaw in lateral movements.

Thus, once again, even though given the different structural inheritance of the primate type of jaw joint, the adaptive adjustment was essentially the same as in bears. An anteromedial swing of the contralateral condyle rotating around a vertical axis at the condyle of the chewing side, as in *A. africanus*, was changed to a long, transverse rocking roll on the medial glenoid plane. As has been seen, the muscles were developed and reoriented to pull the joint in the transverse plane, paralleling the movement in the giant panda.

The Teeth

The teeth of purely carnivorous feeders are adapted for piercing, tearing, and cutting. In cats, the number of cheek teeth is severely reduced, as is the transverse diameter of each tooth in the row. These cheek teeth are developed into cutting bladed carnassials by the formation of a high, jagged, sharp ridge running along the outer side of the remaining premolars and molars. When the lower jaw is raised, the upper blades slice past the lowers on the outside.

In *Ursus horribilis,* the anterior premolars are degenerate and peg-like, while the remaining teeth in the row are moderately broadened. An outer raised sharp ridge still prevails in the upper row (Fig. 1–13A). *Ailuropoda,* on the other hand, has a tremendously broadened cheek tooth row that extends to the anterior premolars. The cusps of these teeth are all of a relatively more rounded uniform height (Fig. 1–13B).

In *A. africanus*, the cheek tooth row is moderately broad. There is nothing particularly

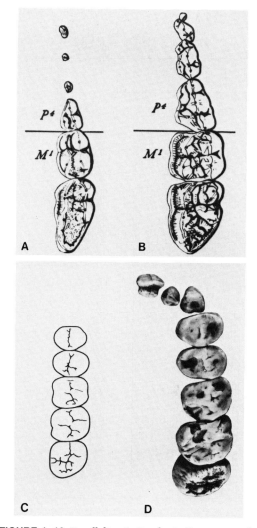

FIGURE 1–13. Parallelism in Teeth. *A. Ursus:* note relatively narrow cheek tooth row. *B, Ailuropoda:* note extreme broadening of entire cheek tooth row. (From Davis, D., 1964. Courtesy of Field Museum of Natural History, Chicago, IL). *C, A. africanus:* note relatively narrow cheek tooth row (tracing made from published photographs). *D, A. boisei:* note extreme broadening of entire cheek tooth row (OH5 Wenner-Gren cast).

distinctive in this dentition (Fig. 1–13*C*). In *A. boisei*, the whole cheek tooth row is enormously broadened. This also includes the premolars, where it is especially striking (Fig. 1–13*D*).

Once again, parallelism between ursines and australopithecines is extraordinary and correlates closely with all of the other features involved in the evolution of specialized, transverse grinding movements (DuBrul, 1977).

SUMMARY

Just as the clinician needs the medical history of a patient to make a logical diagnosis, so too the evolutionary history of a biological construct is essential for a logical explanation of its function and dysfunction. The preceding account traces the evolution of the jaws and their joints.

Jaws, hyoid bone, larynx, thyroid cartilage, and similar structures all arose from the gill arch sequence in primitive jawless vertebrates. This process is still imitated by the visceral arches in the human embryo. The primitive jaw, now represented by the embryonic Meckel's cartilage, is covered and resorbed by the dermal bone of the mandible. The only remnants of the cartilage are the miniature bones in the middle ear. The joints and muscles of these ossicles and the mandible are still innervated by branches of the same fifth cranial nerve. It is possible, therefore, that specific ear symptoms, such as tinnitus, that are associated with some jaw joint dysfunctions, can result from spasm of the musculature that moves the ossicles.

The evolution of man's erect bipedal posture is associated with specific clinical manifestations such as flat feet, distortion of the spinal column, hemorrhoids, hernias, prolapsed uteri, and the like. This account demonstrates how the rigorous reduction and retrusion of the jaws in adjusting the skull to an erect vertebral column has also made the jaw joint vulnerable to a disarray of structures.

REFERENCES

Barghusen, H. R.: The adductor jaw musculature Dimetrodon (Reptilia, Pelycosauria). J. Paleontol. *47*:823–834, 1973.

Becht, G.: Comparative biologic-anatomical researches on mastication in some mammals, pts. I and II. Proc. K. Ned. Akad. Wet. (Biol Med) *56*:508–527, 1953.

Broom, R.: On the structure of the internal ear and the relations of the basicranial nerves in Dicynodon, and on the homology of the mammalian auditory ossicles. Proc. Zool. Soc. Lond. 419–425, 1912.

Broom, R. and Schepers, G. W. H.: The South African Fossil Ape-Men: The Australopithecinae. Pretoria, South Africa, Transvaal Museum, 1946.

Carus, C. G.: Lehrbuch der Zootomie. Leipzig. Gerhard Fleischer dem Jungern, 1818.

Clark, W. E. L.: The Fossil Evidence for Human Evolution, 2nd Ed. Chicago, University of Chicago Press, 1964.

Crompton, A. W.: The cranial morphology of a new genus and species of Ictidosauran. Proc. Zool. Soc. Lond. *130*:183–216, 1958.

Crompton, A. W.: On the lower jaw of Diathrognathus and the origin of the mammalian lower jaw. Proc. Zool. Soc. Lond. *140*:697–750, 1963.

Davis, D. D.: The giant panda: A morphological study of evolutionary mechanisms. Fieldiana Zool. Mem. *3*:1–339, 1964.

Denison, R. H.: Feeding mechanisms of Agnatha and early Gnathostomes. Am. Zool. *1*:177–181, 1961.

DuBrul, E. L.: Posture, locomotion and the skull in La-gomorpha. Am. J. Anat. 87:277–314, 1950.

DuBrul, E. L. and Sicher, H.: The Adaptive Chin. Spring-field, IL, Charles C Thomas, 1954.

DuBrul, E. L.: Evolution of the Speech Apparatus. Spring-field, IL, Charles C Thomas, 1958.

DuBrul, E.L.: The skull of the lion Marmoset Leontideus rosalia Linnaeus: A study in biomechanical adaptation. Am. J. Phys. Anthropol. 23:261–271, 1965.

DuBrul, E. L.: Development of the hominid oral apparatus. In Schumacher, G. (Ed.): Morphology of the Maxillo-mandibular Apparatus. Leipzig, VEB George Thieme 1967.

DuBrul, E. L.: Origin and evolution of the oral apparatus. In Kawamura, Y. (Ed.): Physiology of Mastication. Fron-tiers of Oral Physiology Series, vol. 1. New York, S. Karger, 1974, pp. 1–29.

DuBrul, E. L.: Early hominid-feeding mechanisms. Am. J. Phys. Anthropol. 47:305–320, 1977.

Fawcett, E.: The Development of the Bones Around the Mouth. London, Dental Board of the United Kingdom, Ballantyne Press, pp. 1–21, 1924.

Frazzetta, T. H.: Studies on the morphology and function of the skull in the Boidae (Serpentes). Part II. Morphol-ogy and function of the jaw apparatus in Python sebae and Python molurus. J. Morphol. 118:217–296, 1966.

Furstman, L.: Embryology. In Sarnat, B. G., and Laskin, D. M. (Eds.): The Temporomandibular Joint, 3rd Ed. Springfield, IL, Charles C Thomas, 1980.

Gans, C.: Respiration in early tetrapods—The frog is a red herring. Evolution 24:740–751, 1970.

Gaupp, E. Von: Beiträge zur Kenntnis des Unterkiefers der Wirbeltiere. III. Das Problems der Entstehung eines "sekundaren" Kiefergelenkes bei den Säugern. Anat. Anz. 39(23–24):609–666, 1911.

Gegenbauer, C.: Untersuchungen zur vergleichenden An-atomie der Wirbeltiere. III. Das Kopfskelet der Sela-chier. Leipzig, 1872.

Goodrich, E. S.: Studies on the Structure and Development of Vertebrates, vol. 1. New York, Dover, 1930, p. 404.

Gregory, W. K., and Adams, L. A.: The temporal fossae of vertebrates in relation to jaw muscles. Science 41:763–765, 1915.

Haines, R. W.: Eudiarthrodal joints in fishes. J. Anat. 77:12–19, 1942.

Hotton, N.: The pelycosaur tympanum and early evolution of the middle ear. Evolution 13:99–121, 1959.

Kermack, K. A., and Mussett, F.: The jaw articulation of the Docodonta and the classification of Mesozoic mam-mals. Proc. R. Soc. Lond. (Biol.) 149:204–215, 1958.

Lubosch, W. Von: Bau and Ensteung der Wirbeltiergel-enke. Jena, East Germany, Gustav Fischer, 1910.

Lubosch, W. Von: C. Vergleichende anatomie der skelet-verbingungen. Handbuch der Vergleichenden Anatomie der Wirbeltiere. 5:305–332, 1938.

Meckel, J. F.: Handbuch der Menschlichen Anatomie.

Wierter Band: Besondere Anatomie; Eingeweidlehre und Geschichte des Fötus. Halle und Berlin, in der Buch-andlung des hallischen Waisennauses, 1820, p. 47.

Murie, A.: The wolves of Mount McKinley. Fauna of the National Parks of the United States, Grizzly Bear. Fauna Series, No. 5, 1944, p. 189.

Napier, J. R.: The antiquity of human walking. Sci. Am. 216:56–66, 1967.

Oxnard, C. E.: Tensile forces in skeletal structures. J. Morphol. 134:424–436, 1971.

Reichert, C.: Ueber die Visceralbogen der Wirbelthiere im Allgemeinen und deren Metamorphosen bei den Vögeln und Sägethieren. Archiv für Anatomie, Physiologie und Wissenschaftliche Medicin, 120–222, 1837.

Robinson, J. T.: The genera and species of the Australo-pithecinae. J. Phys. Anthropol. 12:181–200, 1954a.

Robinson, J. T.: Prehominid dentition and hominid evolu-tion. Evolution 8:324–334, 1954b.

Robinson, J. T.: The Dentition of the Australopithecinae. Transvaal Museum Memoir, no. 9. Pretoria, South Africa, Transvaal Museum, 1956.

Robinson, J. T.: The origin and adaptive radiation of the Autralopithecines. In Kurth, G. (Ed.): Evolution und Hominisation. Stuttgart, Gustav Fisher Verlag, 1968, pp 150–175.

Robinson, J. T.: Early Hominid Posture and Locomotion. Chicago, University of Chicago Press, 1972.

Romer, A. S.: Cynodont reptile with incipient mammalian jaw articulation. Science 166:881–882, 1969.

Romer, A.: The Vertebrate Body, 4th ed. Philadelphia, W. B. Saunders, 1970.

Scapino, R. P.: Function of the masseterpterygoid raphe in carnivores. Anat. Anz. 136:430–446, 1974.

Sheldon, W. G.: Notes on the giant panda. J. Mammal. 18:13–19, 1937. In Davis, D. D.: The giant panda. Fieldiana Zool. Mem. 3:1–339, 1964.

Sicher, H.: Masticatory apparatus in the giant panda and the bears. Zoology Series of the Field Museum of Natural History 29:61–73, 1944.

Thomson, K. S.: The evolution of the tetrapod middle ear in the Rhipidistian-Amphibian transition. Am. Zool. 6:379–397, 1966.

Thomson, K. S.: The adaptation and evolution of early fishes. Biol. Rev. 46:139–166, 1971.

Tobias, P. V.: The cranium and maxillary dentition of Australopithecus (Zinjanthropus) Boisei. In Leakey, L. S. B. (Ed.): Olduvai Gorge, vol. 2, Cambridge, MA, Cambridge University Press, 1967.

van der Klaauw, C. J.: Bau und Entwickelung der Gekörk-nöchelchen. Ergeb Anat Entwicklungsgesch 25:565–622, 1924.

Webster, D. B.: Ear structure and function in modern mammals. Am. Zool. 6:451–466, 1966.

Young, J. Z.: The Life of Vertebrates. Oxford, Oxford University Press, 1955, p. 182.

2

COMPARATIVE FUNCTIONAL ANATOMY*

*HENRY W. NOBLE, PH.D., F.D.S.,
and STEPHEN L. CREANOR, B.D.S., PH.D.*

INTRODUCTION

Functional anatomy is the study of the manner in which anatomical structures perform physiological functions. The physiological activities in which the temporomandibular joint (TMJ) plays a part may be voluntary or reflex and may range from mastication, deglutition, and phonation to such momentary actions such as gasping and yawning. The TMJ is a form of articulation found only in mammals, so the various jaw joints found in other vertebrates are not considered in this chapter (see Chapter 1).

In some animals, certain teeth may serve powerful functions not directly concerned with mastication. The beaver's use of the gnawing ability of its incisors in the construction of a habitat and the carnivore's use of its canines as weapons are but two examples of specialized activities in which both the teeth and TMJ are involved. The most important action, however, is mastication.

There can be no doubt about the need for a close correspondence between a diet and the physiological actions that prepare it for digestion. These specialized actions are, in turn, the result of variations in the direction and magnitude of the muscle forces that produce them.

*See Chapters 1, 3, 4, 5, 6, and 11.

These variations of the musculature produce modifications of the bones that transmit the forces and the TMJ that forms part of this masticatory apparatus. Any TMJ is therefore a result of the continuing development of a close relationship between a diet and the masticatory apparatus of which the joint forms a part. It may thus be beneficial to look first at the treatment required by different diets to prepare them for ingestion and digestion, and then the principal modifications of the masticatory apparatus that attempt to cater efficiently to these special requirements. A consideration of the ways in which the different parts of the masticatory apparatus have reached this intimate functional relationship with a particular diet would then lead to a clearer appreciation of the role of the TMJ in this process.

VARIATIONS IN DIET ACCOMMODATED BY THE MAMMALIAN MASTICATORY APPARATUS

General Remarks

The nature of the diet has always had the greatest effect upon the evolving structure and pattern of functional activity of the masticatory apparatus (see Chapter 1). Ever since the primitive vertebrate abandoned the role of a relatively stationary, passive feeder, the masticatory apparatus has been progressively modified to deal effectively with the increasingly wider range of sources of nourishment that became available. A number of functional power strokes were developed by varying combinations of the activity of muscles that move the mandible in directions predominantly vertical to the occlusal plane with those that tend to move the mandible horizontally in directions essentially parallel to the occlusal plane (Fig. 2–1). It is possible to classify the sources of nourishment and discern corresponding types of masticatory apparatus that function in distinctly different ways to prepare the food for ingestion.

Diet of Flesh

The diet of flesh is probably the most complete diet in the sense that animals are most likely to find in animal cells the correct range and proportions of nutritive factors. It is also probably the diet that makes least demands upon the masticatory and digestive systems. In

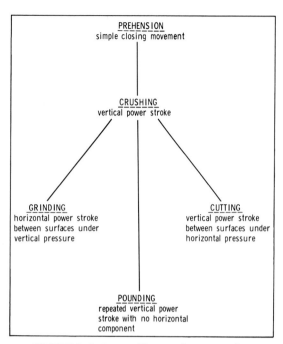

FIGURE 2–1. Range of functional power strokes.

a carnivore, the swift slicing action between the sharp edges on upper and lower cheek teeth severs a portion that is immediately swallowed without further masticatory preparation.

Diet of Fish

In the case of aquatic carnivores such as the seal, sea lion, and sea leopard, an enlarged canine is associated with a simple tritubercular type of cheek tooth that interlocks, securely catching a slippery prey. The mandible shows some slight evidence of processes for muscle attachment, but the TMJ shows little evidence of specialization.

The masticatory apparatus may be considered to have regressed to a most primitive state of function and development in the case of the order Cetacea. In the dolphin, for instance, the tooth is reduced to the simplest form of cone, with no variation in morphology throughout the series. The mandible is lacking in processes for muscle attachment and can be regarded only as an alveolar element supported by a basal element that terminates in a condylar-articulating surface posteriorly (Fig. 2–2). The functional activity is at its simplest level in that only prehension is attempted. The aquatic environment of this animal counteracts the normal effect of gravity on the mandible and greatly reduces whatever demands this force usually makes upon the jaw musculature.

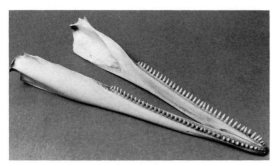

FIGURE 2–2. Extreme simplification of tooth form and jaw structure in the dolphin.

Diet of Vegetation

Large quantities of vegetation must be ingested to obtain an adequate level of nutrition. Such a diet also requires greater preparation by the masticatory apparatus and a more elaborate digestive system. The masticatory apparatus of the herbivore, which deals with soft vegetation and foliage, differs from that of the rodent, which is designed to gnaw and grind the tougher forms of vegetation and fruit in the form of nuts. In each case, muscles capable of continuously producing great force and teeth capable of withstanding it throughout a lifetime are required. The different rates of wear of the three calcified dental tissues forming alternating layers of the tooth provide a constant unevenness to the occluding surface. When two such surfaces are slowly but powerfully moved horizontally while in contact, they grind efficiently any food particles between them.

Mastication in the order Sirenia, including manatees and dugongs, might be described most like that of the aquatic herbivores, as their diet consists entirely of marine vegetation. The dentition is adapted for continual wear by means of successive eruption of teeth at the back of the jaw and their movement anteriorly until the worn remains are shed at the front. This is described as a form of exaggerated physiologic mesial drift, in which the entire process of eruption is horizontally oriented. The distribution of the muscle processes and the height of the condyle relative to the occlusal plane are similar to the arrangement in terrestrial herbivores.

Diet of Insects

Mammals subsisting on insects tend to be small and have difficulty eating with sufficient frequency to produce energy and maintain body temperature. A crushing action is adequate to make the nourishment available to the digestive juices. A precise arrangement of alternating cusps, pits, ridges, and grooves on the teeth of one jaw is opposed by a similarly precise arrangement in the opposite jaw. Every elevation in one fits accurately into a corresponding depression in the other. Repetition of a simple vertical power stroke thus operates a battery of mortars and pestles in a most efficient manner.

Omnivorous Diet

In many of the larger mammalian orders, there are members who have resisted the tendency to specialize or have reverted to a less-specialized form of masticatory apparatus. Carnivores such as the bear, ungulates such as the pig family, and primates such as man, have this ability to adapt to a wider range of environments. Although unaccompanied by any obvious lack of specialization in the masticatory apparatus, the diet of many rodents, such as rats or mice, may also be mixed (see Chapter 1).

MANNER IN WHICH SPECIAL RELATIONSHIPS BETWEEN THE DIET AND THE MASTICATORY APPARATUS DEVELOP

Priorities and Order in the Sequence of Changes

The close relationship between each food supply and the modified masticatory apparatus that deals with it is probably still developing slowly over the ages. These relationships are the culmination of many small changes that involve the dental tissues, the teeth, the jaws, and the musculature. Before the period when mammals evolved, there is evidence that fossil reptiles possessed dentitions that were adapted to a particular diet. It is believed that further adaptation of a functional nature was restricted by limitations imposed by the primitive vertebrate jaw joint. The replacement of this joint by the more flexible temporomandibular articulation was the first crucial step in the development of many later modifications. The adaptive nature of the TMJ enables it to conform to the movements required by the teeth, jaws, and musculature. The teeth specialize when the potential is available in the jaws and musculature to utilize a particular modification. Change in the musculature, with its demands for bone attachment to ensure effective action, is probably the fundamental variation that must occur before any of the others can effectively proceed. It is therefore likely that, in many cases, the order in which changes were initiated is as follows:

1. Availability of a particular diet
2. Simple variations of tooth form to suit the diet
3. Replacement of mechanical rigidity of primitive jaw joint by an articulation with greater adaptive flexibility
4. Adaptation of the musculature to the dietary requirements
5. Response of bone to demands of musculature
6. Occurrence of further dental variations that improve efficiency of jaw actions
7. Coordination of activity of jaws and dentition by patterns of movement controlled by the TMJ and designed to ensure effective mastication.

Replacement of the Primitive Jaw Joint by the Temporomandibular Joint

An appreciation of the evolutionary history of the TMJ clearly shows that this was not a transformation into bone of an ancient cartilaginous skeletal interface (see Chapter 1). This joint represents an area of frictional contact between two hitherto unrelated membrane bones. It has been created by migrating muscles and ligaments as they attempted to introduce a greater range of functional movements into the masticatory activity of the tooth-bearing portion of the lower jaw and escape from the simple Class III lever operation. The subdivision of the primitive adductor musculature, which was believed to be present in early vertebrates, into the masseter, medial pterygoid, and temporalis muscles; and the development of an angle, sometimes in excess of 90 degrees, between the direction of action of the more oblique part of the masseter and the more posterior part of the temporalis, brought with it the possibility of increased range of movement. They also brought the possibility of the application of a rotary movement to the mandible. In Figure 2–3, an estimate is made of the effects this change had in partially relieving the joint surfaces from the heavy pressures they would otherwise have to sustain if a simple Class III lever arrangement were still present. Such a static analysis of the distribution of the muscle pull suggests that, although greater forces may be required, the subdivision of their point of

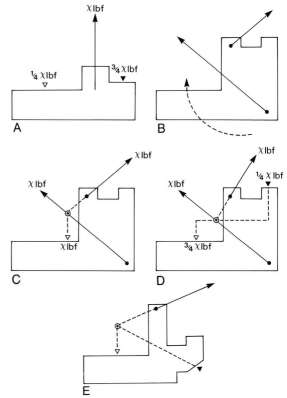

FIGURE 2–3. *A*, Class III lever with undivided muscle pull unfavorably distributed between joint force at fulcrum and biting force in tooth-bearing region. *B*, Rotary movement imparted by divided muscle pull at different points. *C*, In certain circumstances, rotary movement is balanced by a biting force in which the line of action passes through the center of activity of the other two forces. *D*, More favorable distribution of muscle pull between joint and biting forces. *E*, Replacement of the pulling force of masseter muscle by resistance in same direction offered by the enlarged postglenoid process in the case of the shrew (*S. minutus*).

application to the mandible and the direction of muscle pull might, in some cases, result in a more favorable distribution of load between the joint and the biting surface.

Subdivision and Diversification of the Action of the Jaw Musculature

Any attempt by the jaw musculature to deal with a particular item in a diet more efficiently has usually required a new force in a new direction. This modification of the magnitude and direction of the muscle forces that can be applied to the jaws may either increase the range, restrict it, or by a combination of these processes, replace one force with another. Thus, a characteristic pattern of activity is associated with each of the main forms of diet.

Most muscles contain a large reserve that can be called upon by muscle-building activities or the demands of some particular element in the diet. Therefore, the increase (or decrease) in the force that can be developed as a result of the existing directions of muscle fiber bundles is not difficult to envisage. The manner in which a muscle may develop a force in a different direction is more difficult to understand. In its earliest stage of development, the muscle is related to the fibrous tissue within which the bone is developing, rather than to the bone itself. It is possible that reorientation may be accomplished by an adjustment at this stage. Enlargement of the developing bone in a particular direction may carry the investing fibrous tissue with the developing muscle attached to it to a new position and thus effectively alter the direction of the muscle fibers.

When any group of muscle fibers operating in a slightly different direction to the main body of the muscle contracts as a unit with sufficient frequency, it is probable that in time a fibrous septum will intervene and give this part of the muscle an anatomical as well as a functional identity. In the human masseter muscle, there is a certain degree of separation posteriorly between the superficial oblique and the deep vertical portions. In some rodents, the deep portion is completely separate from the rest of the muscle and runs along the floor of the orbit within a greatly enlarged infraorbital foramen to be attached to the lateral surface of the bones forming the nasal passage.

Growth of Bone to Provide New Areas of Attachment and the Development of Muscle Processes

The growth of those parts of the bone regarded as muscle processes has long been regarded as a response to functional demands. Indeed, the concept of a functional matrix regards the development of all bone as a response to demands for support by the investing connective tissues. It is thus to be expected that the bones of the jaw and the skull should respond to demands for support from new directions of pull by the musculature. This is generally achieved by permitting the area of attachment to extend further over an existing surface or by increasing the area of surface available for attachment by the formation of crests, spines, and processes.

The morphology of the jaws and skull is, however, also dependent upon other factors, such as the number, size, and positions of the teeth that demand support; the size of the tongue and its actions; the dimensions of the nasal passages; the existence of other functions apart from mastication; and the variation in the size and position of other organs, such as the eyes and the brain. These factors influence the length and direction of action of the muscles of mastication and the location of the ligaments and the joint which, in turn, guide the path of occlusion.

The osseous structure of the masticatory apparatus in any animal reflects the degree to which an ancient, genetically controlled structure has gradually responded to the influence of the functional demands imposed upon it. The variations that thus adapt one masticatory apparatus to a particular diet include the response of the bone to the attempt by the muscles to function more effectively.

Modification of the Dentition

There are few ways in which the tooth crowns, formed long before eruption, can be adaptively modified during use to suit a particular diet. The degree and pattern of attrition may substantially improve the biting edge or grinding surface in certain teeth, but the hard tissues no longer possess the ability to respond, and so only minor protective changes in the dentin and pulp and adjustments to the rate of eruption result.

A different process of modification is responsible for the close degree of adaptation that often exists between a dentition and the particular diet for which it is best suited. The most suitable variation is constantly selected from among a large number of random, chance mutations, and thus, a progressively closer adaptation is achieved. In considering the normal stages in tooth development, one can perceive where successive mutations might arise. At the earliest stage of initiation, when the tooth germs arise from the dental lamina, variations in the number and spacing of teeth in an arch may occur. During the succeeding stages of proliferation, histodifferentiation, and morphodifferentiation, variations in size, shape, arrangement of cusps and fissures, and in the distribution of the various dental tissues over the crown and root might arise. Only minor variations in the histology of the dental tissues occur; these take place during the stages of apposition and mineralization. The process of eruption is described as being continuous, semicontinuous, or limited, in accordance with the rate of formation of the tissues and the rate of wear as a result of attrition.

Although each of the preceding small variations is the product of a chance mutation, it either confers an advantage or a disadvantage in a most important aspect of the struggle for survival and so tends to be speedily adapted or eliminated. The ability of the musculature and bony tissues to adapt to functional stimuli should not overshadow the fact that similar variations may also occur in these tissues.

Factors that Limit the Range of Mandibular Movements

The muscles controlling the range of movement of the mandible relative to the base of the cranium, and relating to other structures such as the tongue and hyoid bone, determine the greater part of the space envelope within which the mandible moves in function (see Chapter 5). In certain directions, movement is restricted by the application of isometric tension by ligaments. In other directions, static pressure is provided by the bony surface of the glenoid fossa and articular eminence, which similarly limits mobility. In this context, the bolus also constitutes a temporary limit to mobility that is overcome as it yields to the muscular force that carries the mandible in the direction of interocclusal contact. The occlusal surfaces of the teeth and any prominent intercuspal relations determine the final limitation to movement in this direction.

Variations in Height of Joint Relative to the Occlusal Plane

There are considerable variations in the height of the TMJ relative to the occlusal plane of the dentition among mammals. Reference is frequently made to the fact that, in carnivores, the hinge-like joint is in line with the occlusal plane. Similarly, in the human mandible at birth, the condyle is situated at a low level, in line with the upper border of the body, and here a simple hinge-like action is present initially. In many ungulates, however, the joint is situated high above the plane of occlusion (Fig. 2–4).

The main consideration seems to be to ensure that the joint is neither too near the area of insertion of the major elevating muscle nor in line with the direction in which it is acting. The joint, therefore, tends to be located as far from the principal area of muscle attachment on the

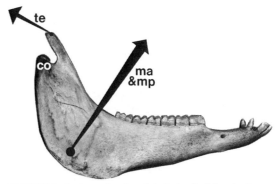

FIGURE 2–4. Example of condyle (co) at high level relative to plane of occlusion in the horse. Note the distance between line of action of masseter (ma) and medial pterygoid (mp) and condyle in comparison with smaller distance in the case of the temporalis muscle (te).

mandible and as much to one side of the line of action of this muscle as possible.

The lateral pterygoid muscle does have an area of attachment to the neck of the condyloid process, which is close to the articulating surface. Those fibers inserted into the anterior edge of the articular disc act in a direction that is in line with the joint cavities. This muscle, of course, does not produce any levering advantage with the joint as fulcrum; instead, it is more concerned with altering the position of the condyle in the anteroposterior direction by unilateral or bilateral action.

The Possibility of a Symphyseal Joint

In many mammals, the tissue in the midline between the two halves of the mandible remains unossified for a considerable time, if not the entire lifetime of the animal. This arrangement is believed to be advantageous in the human in that molding of the mandible is possible at birth. Thereafter, some midline growth may occur until ossification unites the two halves at the end of the first year.

The question of whether lack of bony union confers any advantages in other animals remains unanswered. It is possible that in carnivores the force couple consisting of the zygomaticomandibular and the medial pterygoid muscles, which ensures edge-to-edge contact when the sectorial teeth slice together, operates by virtue of the movement permitted in the midline. If this occurs, a movable articulation, i.e. a joint, develops between two separate centers of intramembranous ossification in accordance with the demands of the musculature, jaws, and dentition, similar to that in which the TMJ evolved.

Much more information is required concerning the functional significance of movements occurring at this site before any final interpretation of their importance can be made.

CLASSIFICATION OF MAMMALIAN MASTICATORY FUNCTION

The pattern of muscular activity is the connecting link among the variations in size, shape, and position, which are found in the teeth, jaws, muscles, and TMJs of mammals. Attempts to observe, record, and describe a particular pattern of muscle activity in detail are probably as difficult in the process of mastication as in the swinging of a golf club. It is possible, however, to attempt a broad classification of mammals into one generalized and four spe-

cialized groups. Each specialized group is differentiated because, in its extreme form, its members have ceased to be able to deal efficiently, if at all, with the diet of any of the other specialized groups. In the case of the generalized group, the masticatory apparatus has retained the ability to prepare for ingestion of a wider range of food sources than is possible in the case of any of the specialized groups. Studies of masticatory action in primitive man give some indication of the most recent changes in the human.

The Flesh-Shearing Action of the Carnivore

In addition to a generalized mesiodistal elongation of the crowns of the sectorial cheek teeth, the carnassial tooth (last upper premolar) pos-

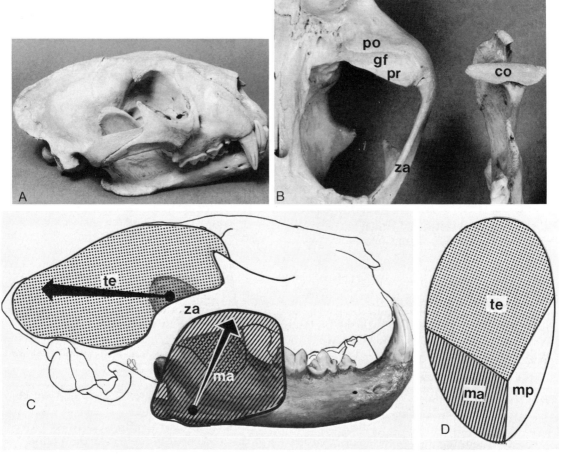

FIGURE 2–5. *A,* Lateral view of skull and jaws of member of the cat family. *B,* Glenoid fossa (gf) with prominent preglenoid process (pr) laterally, and postglenoid process (po) medially. Condyle (co) shows convex surface anteroposteriorly. Note wide zygomatic arch (za) for prominent temporalis muscle. *C,* Representation of area of attachment and direction of pull of masseter (ma), and temporalis (te) muscles upon mandible zygomatic arch (za). *D,* Proportion of mass of each of the main muscles contributing to the closing effort. Masseter (ma), temporalis (te), and medial pterygoid (mp) muscles.

sesses a blade-like ridge that meets a similarly sharp ridge on the first lower molar. These slice together as the jaws close in a hinge-like manner.

The features of the TMJ are most clearly seen in the cat family. A laterally elongated condyle with a rolled, convex, articular surface fits closely into a deeply concave, laterally elongated glenoid fossa with accentuated preglenoid and postglenoid processes (Fig. 2–5). These processes are not in the same parasagittal plane, and when viewed from the side, they appear to form the circumference of a circle in some species. The action of the joint is that of a hinge, except for the slight tilting that brings the sharp dental edges together as they shear. For the shearing action to be progressive from the back to the front of the cheek teeth, the condyle must be situated posteriorly in line with the occlusal plane (Fig. 2–5A). An articular disc is present, but the lateral pterygoid muscle has neither the same mandibular insertion nor function that it has in other mammals, since no unilateral or bilateral protrusive movements are permitted. Speed in snapping the jaws together is of greatest importance in this dentition, and the temporalis muscle, with its greater fiber length, is more efficient in this action than are the shorter fibers of the masseter.

The temporalis muscle extends upward and posteriorly from its insertion into a large area of the prominent coronoid process to an area over the greater part of the cranium. It meets its counterpart at a sagittal crest and extends back to meet the neck muscles at an occipital crest. The wide zygomatic arch is at once a measure of the bulk of the temporalis muscle, which passes beneath it, and also of the strength of the force transmitted to it by the masseter. The medial pterygoid meets the masseter at the lower border of the mandible; between them, the angle of the mandible lies in a muscular sling.

The Grinding Action of the Herbivore

The complex infoldings of enamel in the crowns of the cheek teeth of horses and cattle ensure a continually rough grinding surface as the crown is gradually worn throughout the lifespan. A steady rate of eruption compensates for the loss of tooth substance. The grinding action occurs unilaterally as the mouth opens and the mandible shifts to the same side to which the bolus is displaced, and then powerfully closes in an upward and medial direction, crushing and grinding the vegetable fibers between the rough opposing surfaces. After several strokes on one side, the bolus is displaced to the other side and the action shifts smoothly across to the teeth on the opposite side.

The high position of the condyle of the mandible relative to the occlusal plane favors the action of the masseter and medial pterygoid muscles rather than that of the temporalis muscle. The masseter tends to be the most powerful closing muscle, assisted in its action by a prominent medial pterygoid muscle. They provide the slow, powerful, grinding action required by these animals. The lateral pterygoid muscle is also particularly well developed, displacing the opening jaw laterally at the beginning of every masticatory stroke according to the side on which the bolus is located. The temporalis muscle is attached to a relatively slender coronoid process, which curves posteriorly in line with most of the fibers that insert on the upper and posterior surfaces of the cranium.

The condyle has a relatively large, flattened articular surface, faintly convex anteroposteriorly and slightly concave laterally. The glenoid fossa is shallow, with a slight postglenoid process to resist backward displacement (Fig. 2–6). Anteriorly, the articular surface of the fossa blends imperceptibly with the articular eminence, which is little more than a slight convexity of the articular surface. There is a well-developed articular disc in this joint where sliding forms an important part of the movement.

In the majority of herbivores, the ridges of enamel exposed by attrition are arranged mesiodistally; therefore, the most effective direction for a grinding stroke is lateral. In the elephant, however, the ridges of enamel are arranged laterally and the direction of the grinding stroke is posteroanterior.

The Gnawing-Grinding Action of the Rodent

The cheek teeth of the rodent have much in common with those of an herbivore. Provision of a continuously rough grinding surface is associated with powerful horizontal movements. A unique addition, however, is the presence of opposing pairs of exceedingly sharp central incisors. The dentition is completely divided anatomically and functionally into the incisors and cheek teeth. Each has a distinctive method of growth, rate of eruption, histological structure, and function to perform. Each part of the den-

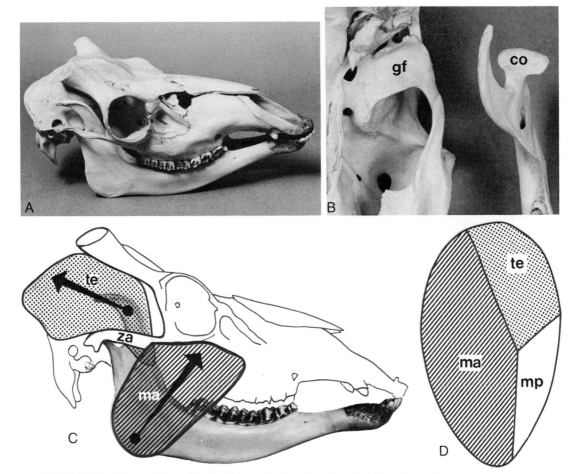

FIGURE 2–6. *A,* Lateral view of skull and jaws of a deer. *B,* Relatively shallow glenoid fossa (gf), and condyle (co), typical of articulation in cattle. *C,* Representation of area of attachment and direction of pull of masseter (ma), and temporalis (te) muscles upon mandible; zygomatic arch (za). *D,* Proportion of mass of each of the main muscles contributing to the closing effort. Masseter (ma), temporalis (te), and medial pterygoid (mp) muscles.

tition has its own pattern of muscular activity and must operate separately from the other. Two functionally distinct dentitions exist in the mouth, and yet the TMJ harmonizes successfully with the anatomical and functional requirements of each. The condyle is a rounded knob with a convex articular surface facing upward. It is located in an open-ended, anteroposteriorly directed groove with prominent medial and lateral flanges that represent the glenoid fossa (Fig. 2–7).

When the animal uses the incisors, the lower incisors move in a down-forward-up-and-backward power stroke. In changing to the use of the cheek teeth, the condyle moves to a more posterior position in the glenoid groove. The cheek teeth now follow a down-backward-up-and-forward power stroke.

An articular disc is present, but the capsular ligament surrounding the joint must be more lax than usual to permit the large shift between the different positions at which the condyles operate in the grooves. The condyle is situated well above the level of the occlusal plane, as in the herbivore. The dominant muscle is the masseter, which plays an important part in the powerful approximation of the chisel-edged incisors. The medial pterygoid again assists the masseter in a powerful manner, while the lateral pterygoid is responsible not only for lateral grinding excursions but also for the forward shifting or protrusion of the mandible when the incisors come into use. The temporalis muscle is overshadowed by the other muscles in this group of animals and contributes the smallest force to the closing effort of the jaws.

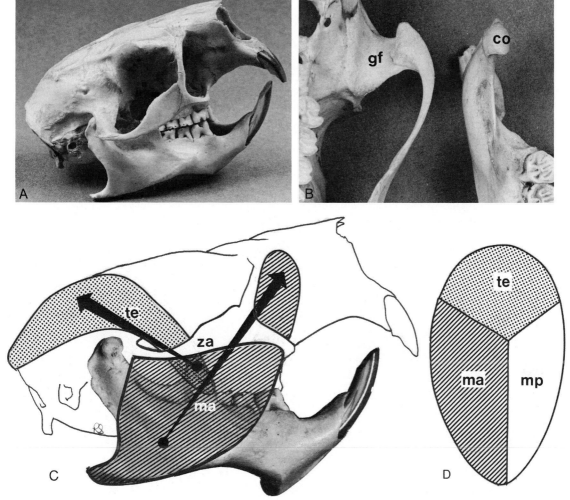

FIGURE 2–7. *A*, Lateral view of skull and jaws of a porcupine. *B*, Glenoid fossa (gf) and condyle (co) typical of articulation. *C*, Representation of area of attachment and direction of pull of masseter (ma), and temporalis (te) muscles upon mandible; zygomatic arch (za). *D*, Proportion of mass of each of the main muscles contributing to the closing effort. Masseter (ma), temporalis (te), medial pterygoid (mp) muscles.

The Piercing-Crushing Action of the Insectivore

Sharp, pointed cusps and deep pits on the occlusal surfaces of the cheek teeth interdigitate in an interlocking manner in this group of animals. The sharp, pointed cusps are buttressed by shearing edges that slice against each other as the predominantly vertical power stroke brings the jaws together. The crowns of these teeth are short and do not permit compensation for wear. The coronoid process is large and gives attachment to a powerful temporalis muscle in which fibers are directed in a backward direction. The zygomatic arch and the angle of the mandible are poorly developed in keeping with the underdevelopment of the masseter and medial pterygoid muscles.

Although the movement is predominantly vertical, the joint is not as specialized as in the carnivore. The absence of the violent resistance of a struggling prey may render a tight hinge-like joint unnecessary. Because of the interlocking nature of the occlusion and the anatomy of the insectivore TMJ, no large horizontal movement can occur.

Certain features that are of particular interest when the functional anatomy of the joint is being considered are clearly illustrated when an animal is examined in which the TMJ is not typical of the entire class. The complex nature of the TMJ of the pygmy shrew *(Sorex minutus)* was first described by Fearnhead, Shute, and Bellairs (Fearnhead, 1955). The predominantly posterior direction of the fibers of the large temporalis muscle (Fig. 2–8A) and the almost total absence of masseter and medial pterygoid fibers have created a great need for a supporting force acting from a posterior and inferior direction. The enlarged postglenoid tubercle that supplies this support articulates with a downward and backward extension from the neck of the condyloid process to form a second, separate, inferior joint cavity (Fig. 2–8B).

This most interesting variation of the mammalian TMJ demonstrates three fundamental principles. First, it shows how easily a joint-like arrangement of the tissues can arise between two membrane bone surfaces that are brought intermittently against each other throughout their period of growth. There is a separate joint cavity for each cartilage-covered articular facet on the condyle, but there is no articular disc in the lower joint (Fig. 2–9). Second, the arrangement shows the probable manner in which the missing oblique fibers of the masseter and the fibers of the medial pterygoid muscle normally would act in conjunction with the posterior fibers of the temporalis. Also shown is the way in which this role can be taken by bone processes forming an articulation when necessary (Fig. 2–9). Third, the articular cartilage in a stress-bearing joint is not normally covered by a fibrous perichondrium. The lack of a layer of fibrous tissue covering the cartilage in this articulation is an indication of the degree to which it has assumed a stress-bearing role in the absence of the masseter and medial pterygoid muscles. In other mammals, including man, the muscle forces combine to reduce the load on the joint, and a layer of fibrous tissue

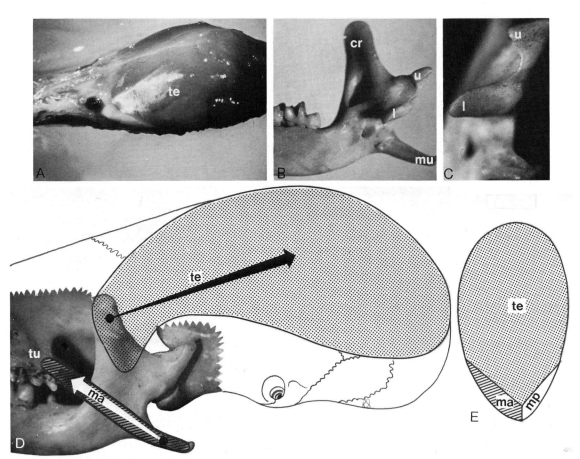

FIGURE 2–8. *A*, Lateral view of skinned head of a shrew (*S. minutus*) showing relatively large temporalis muscle (te). *B*, Medial view of right mandible showing upper (u) and lower (l) condylar facets, relatively large coronoid process (cr), and small muscle process (mu) at angle of mandible. *C*, Posterior view of two condylar facets, upper (u) and lower (l), with nonarticular isthmus intervening. *D*, Representation of area of attachment and direction of pull of masseter (ma), and temporalis (te) muscles upon the mandible. Note absence of a zygomatic arch and attachment of a few fibers of the masseter to tuberosity on maxilla (tu). *E*, Proportion of mass of each of the main muscles contributing to the closing effort. Masseter (ma), temporalis (te), and medial pterygoid (mp) muscles.

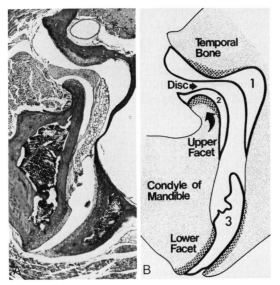

FIGURE 2–9. *A*, Parasagittal section through temporomandibular joint of the shrew *(S. minutus)*. *B*, The rarely found areas of cartilage on articular surfaces are darkly shaded and the cavities of the upper joint are numbered 1 and 2, while the single cavity in the lower joint is numbered 3. (Note: *B* is a diagram of *A*.)

covering the condylar cartilage is normally present.

In the pygmy shrew, in which mastication does not require a lateral component of force and a simple vertical pounding action suffices, the simpler but less efficient lever system with the normal upper articulation as a fulcrum is not used. It appears that a more economic use of force is the main advantage obtained.

Masticatory Action in Primitive Man

Changes in the masticatory apparatus of primitive man were not only the result of his omnivorous diet, but also of the adoption of the upright posture that necessitated a change in the position of the head relative to the spine. The inclusion of a protrusive mandibular movement and modification of the associated musculature are characteristic of the hominoid masticatory apparatus (see Chapter 1).

It is readily accepted that loss of tooth specialization, and modification of the musculature in primitive man resulted from the increased range of diet that he was now able to collect and consume. With improved manual dexterity, there was no longer a need, for example, to catch and hold prey with the aid of large canines, and no need to grind vast amounts of vegetation with highly differentiated cheek teeth.

Modifications of the muscular elements of the apparatus were evident in the specialization of the lateral pterygoid muscle and a decrease in bulk of the temporalis muscle. Bilateral contraction of the lateral pterygoid muscles permitted a modification of condylar movement within the glenoid fossa to include a protrusive excursion. It has been suggested that primitive man's protrusive movements have merely been a bilateral sequel to the individual forward movement of each balancing condyle during lateral excursions of the mandible. Nevertheless, this was fundamental to his success since mastication had to incorporate both incisive and grinding functions. The potential to perform both functions became possible only with an ability to alter the anteroposterior position of the mandible within a shallower and larger glenoid fossa. A detailed examination of early fossils has indicated that the wear pattern of early hominoid species had resulted from a lateral rotary movement, previously not possible in the great apes because the large canines prevented lateral excursions and did not permit protrusive mandibular movements. The decrease in the mass of the temporalis muscle is not pronounced. In monkeys and apes the temporalis muscle comprises two distinct heads—a superficial and a deep head. The deep head alone would appear to correspond with the classical description of the human temporalis muscle. The muscular component of the superficial head is lost, leaving the temporal fascia as the only evidence of its previous existence. These changes are the result of a diminished requirement for a powerful snapping and gripping action.

There is little doubt that a combination of these modifications to the masticatory apparatus, together with increased manual dexterity and higher intelligence, played an important part in ensuring the successful survival of primitive man.

The Unspecialized Action of the Omnivore

Animals such as the pig, bear, and humans can masticate a variety of foods to a satisfactory degree. In each case, however, the efficiency with which the masticatory process is carried out falls far short of the result achieved by the appropriately specialized masticatory apparatus. The crowns of the cheek teeth possess rounded cusps capable of crushing and grinding. If wear of the cusps occurs, the occlusal surfaces present an irregular pattern of enamel ridges until the wear exhausts the enamel at the depths of the fissures. The forceful power stroke incorporates a horizontal element as the jaw is returned to a more centric position after each lateral excursion. Each joint performs a combination of hinge and sliding movements under the influence of a balanced effort from the temporalis, masseter, and medial pterygoid muscles. The lateral pterygoid muscles are well developed and contribute protrusive movements if both act together or contralateral excursions if each acts separately. The TMJ of an omnivore is characterized by an obvious glenoid fossa with an articular eminence as its anterior border. The condyle is laterally elongated and the articular surface is more convex anteroposteriorly than in the lateral direction. The articular disc is a well-developed component of the joint.

The TMJ is seen to be an arrangement of joint surfaces in harmony with the nature of the demands for support transmitted to it by the muscles as they attempt to use the jaws to operate the dentition in an efficient and effective manner.

CLINICAL CONSIDERATIONS

The manner in which nature has modified the TMJ in response to the different requirements of each type of specialized diet shows how sensitive the tissues have been to functional stress during evolution. It can also be seen that the morphology of the skeleton and the degree of development of the different muscles of mastication have also varied in accordance with the functional demands of the type of diet adopted by each of the specialized groups.

It is readily accepted that muscle attachments in the human depend upon the functional activity of the individual for their development and that muscle development can, within limits, reflect the exercise and activity that each muscle experiences. It must also be accepted that the TMJ in each individual responds to the presence or absence of functional stresses and strains transmitted to it.

Orthodontic intervention often modifies functional activity, and by altering the occlusal movements and articulation of the teeth must also affect the TMJ to some degree (see Chapter 6). The changes that occur in the human facial skeleton and in the muscles of mastication with advanced age reflect declining function and must also be accompanied by less readily rec-

ognizable variations in the structure and morphology of the TMJ surfaces (see Chapters 6 and 11). The gradual or sudden loss of the dentition must also impose especially severe strains upon the TMJ. These strains may be diminished or considerably exacerbated by prosthodontic replacement of the missing dentition.

An appreciation of the rich variation in the range of actions and degrees of development of this joint in the animal kingdom must make clinicians aware of the adaptability of the tissues concerned. An analysis of the actions involved in attempts by the masticatory apparatus to deal with items in a diet should always form part of a clinical examination of any patient.

It must, of course, be remembered that nature has evolved satisfactory modifications over countless periods of time and that adequate adaptation may not be possible in a single lifetime. Indeed, with observation of the wide range of functional activities that have been satisfactorily accommodated by modification of this joint in the animal kingdom, one is drawn to the belief that it is the lack of time to respond that is in most cases responsible for masticatory dysfunction.

SUMMARY

The masticatory apparatus is concerned with the procurement and the earliest stages of mechanical and chemical preparation of food for digestion. The differing requirements for each type of food have resulted in several well-defined, adaptively specialized, and highly successful types of masticatory apparatus in different groups of mammals. The close interrelationship among diet, tooth form, musculature, bone structure, and functional activity in the development of each modified masticatory apparatus is noted.

SUGGESTED REFERENCES

Becht, G.: Comparative biologic anatomical researches on mastication in some mammals. Proc. K. Ned. Akad. Wet. [Biol. Med.] 56:508–527, 1953.
Biegert, J.: Das Kiefergelenk der Primaten, seine Altersveranderungen und Specialisationen in Gestaltung und Lage. Morphol. Jb. 97:249–404, 1956.
Davis, D. D.: The giant panda. A morphological study of evolutionary mechanism. Fieldiana Zool. Mem. 3:1–339, 1964.
Fearnhead, R. W., Shute, C. C. D., and Bellairs, A.: The temporomandibular joint of shrews. Proc. Zool. Soc. Lond. 125:795–807, 1955.

Fox, S. S.: Lateral jaw movement in mammalian dentitions. J. Prosthet. Dent. *15*:810–825, 1965.

Gillbe, G. V.: A comparison of the disc in the craniomandibular joint of three mammals. Acta Anat. (Basel) *86*:394–409, 1973.

Hiiemae, K. M.: Masticatory function in the mammals. J. Dent. Res. [Suppl.] *46*:883–893, 1967.

Hiiemae, K. M., and Houston, W. J. B.: The structure and function of the jaw muscles in the rat. I. Their anatomy and internal architecture. Zool. J. Linn. Soc. *50*:75–99, 1971.

Maynard-Smith, J., and Savage, R. J. G.: The mechanics of mammalian jaws. School Sci. Rev. *40*:289–301, 1959.

Mills, J. R. E.: The functional occlusion of the teeth of the Insectivora. Zool. J. Linn. Soc. *47*:1–25, 1966.

Scapino, R. P.: Adaptive radiation of mammalian jaws. *In* Schumacher, G. H. (Ed.): Morphology of the Maxillo-Mandibular Apparatus. Proceedings of the Ninth International Congress of Anatomists. Leipzig, VEB Georg Thieme Verlag, 1972, pp. 33–39.

Starck, D.: Kaumuskulatur und Kiefergelenk der Ursiden, Untersuchungen an verschiedenen Altersstadien. Morphol. Jb. *76*:104–146, 1935.

Stocker, L.: Trigeminus muskulatur und Kiefergelenk von *Elephas maximus*. L. Morphol. Jb. *98*:35–76, 1957.

Storch, G.: Functional types of the temporomandibular articulation of mammals. Nature Museum, Frankfurt *98*:41–46, 1968.

Turnbull, W. D.: Mammalian masticatory apparatus. Fieldiana Geol. *18*:147–356, 1970.

van Vendeloo, N. H.: On the correlation between the masticatory muscles and the skull structure in the muskrat *Ondatra zibethica*. L. Proc. K. Ned. Akad. Wet. [Biol. Med.] *56*:116–127, 265–277, 1953.

Zuckerman, S.: Myths and methods in anatomy. J. R. Coll. Surg. Edinb. *11*:87–114, 1966.

3

MORPHOGENESIS*, **

ALPHONSE R. BURDI, PH.D.

INTRODUCTION

With increasing interest in the natural history, clinical delineation, and management of temporomandibular joint (TMJ) dysfunctions, as well as in the more severely anomalous joint conditions in such craniofacial disorders as mandibulofacial dysostosis and hemifacial microsomia, there has also developed a renewed interest in a better understanding of TMJ morphogenesis. A brief review of human TMJ morphology at birth and throughout the lifespan should help set the stage for an even greater appreciation of the types of coordinated morphogenetic phenomena that must take place before birth to produce the recognizably human TMJ (Fig. 3–1) (see Chapter 5). It is interesting to consider how the many discrete structures comprising the TMJ take on their characteristic appearance over time. This is especially so when clear signs of TMJ morphology progressively emerge from within a seemingly homogeneous field of mesenchymal cells and related tissues located at the junction between the maxillary and mandibular processes in the embryo's face 42 days after implantation into the uterine wall.

MORPHOGENESIS OF THE PRIMARY TEMPOROMANDIBULAR JOINT

In the prenatal and postnatal continua of human development there are two distinct sets of articulations between the lower jaw and the cranium, or the primary and secondary TMJ.

The terms primary and secondary describe the chronological appearance of these two types of joints that share important roles in the understanding of TMJ morphogenesis.

The sequential existence of both the primary and secondary TMJ in human development may be more fully appreciated from a brief phylogenetic or evolutionary perspective (see Chapter 1) (Crompton, 1985; Moffett, 1966). While vertebrate animals with jaws include the fishes, amphibia, reptiles, birds, and mammals, the adult human TMJ is found only in mammals and represents a distinguishing characteristic. Before the phylogenetic emergence of mammals, the vertebrate mandible consisted of several dermal-like bones that articulated with the cranium at a joint formed by two bones derived from the cartilage bars within the first branchial arch. With the phylogenetic emergence of mammals, only one dermal bone, the dentary bone, was retained as the mandible. The two bones derived from cartilage in nonmammalian animals did not persist as parts of the mandible. They instead became incorporated in the middle ear cavity as the malleus and incus ear ossicles (Crompton, 1985; Gaupp, 1911; Moffett, 1966).

Development and Fate of Meckel's Cartilage

The early process of human primary TMJ development is one in which the embryonic

---

*See Chapters 1, 2, 4, 5, 12, and 24.

**Supported in part by NIDR grant DE-03610-22. Assistance by Dan Cohan is gratefully acknowledged.

36

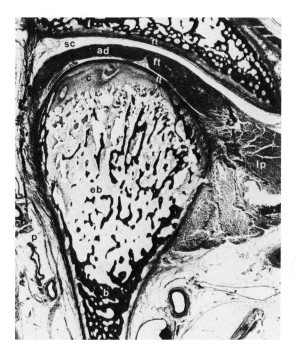

FIGURE 3–1. A frontal section through the TMJ at birth showing the temporal bone (t), the superior compartment (sc), the articular disc (ad), the condyle (c) in stages of endochondral bone formation (eb), membrane bone (b), the parotid gland (p) lateral to the joint, and fibers of the lateral pterygoid muscle (lp) attached to the disc. The inferior joint compartment (unlabeled) is the white cleft below the disc. The outer surface of the condyle and fossa are covered by a thin, fibrous, connective tissue layer (ft). (From Furstman, L.: Embryology. *In* Sarnat, B.G., and Laskin, D.: The Temporomandibular Joint, 3rd ed. Springfield, IL, Charles C Thomas, 1980.)

Meckel's cartilage and the first branchial arch ear ossicles play most significant roles. It is this early embryonic joint that is superseded over time by the secondary or definitive joint that gradually emerges into the characteristic human TMJ of postnatal life.

Up through the eighth prenatal week, the mandibular arch portion of the embryo's first branchial arch is supported by right and left cylindrical rods known as Meckel's cartilages. At six weeks, the cartilages extend upward and posteriorly from the facial midline to the otic capsule of the developing middle ear region in a horseshoe-shaped arrangement. The Meckel's cartilages are not continuous at the facial midline but are separated by a thin zone of mesenchyme. The upper ends of the cartilages are continuous with two islands of cartilage within the middle ear cavity. A relatively large island of cartilage differentiates into the first of the three ear ossicles, known as the malleus (Fig. 3–2A). The malleus in turn connects with the second cartilaginous island, called the incus

(Fig. 3–2B). These progressively undergo endochondral ossification at about 16 weeks and become the definitive malleus and incus ear ossicles within the petrous portion of the temporal bone that evolves from the embryonic otic capsule. The third ear ossicle in the series is the stapes. Unlike the malleus and incus, which develop within the first branchial arch, the stapes develops from within the morphogenetic field of the embryonic second branchial arch.

The joint between the incus and the malleus comprises and serves as the primary TMJ up through about 16 weeks of prenatal life. Unlike the multiple actions allowed by the secondary, or definitive, TMJ, this primary TMJ is a uniaxial hinge joint capable of little or no lateral action. Beyond 16 weeks, there is a progressive development of the secondary TMJ, which is the articulation between the mandibular condyle and mandibular fossa of the temporal bone. It is this secondary joint that functions throughout life as a synovial joint.

Early Development of the Mandible

The mandible is a composite bone having its early beginnings in several source tissues and structures. One of the first indications of mandibular development, seen at about six and one-half weeks, is a sheet of densely staining mesenchyme lateral to each Meckel's cartilage in the future canine region. This is where the incisive and mental nerves branch from the inferior alveolar nerve, which is recognizable at that time. This mesenchymal sheet progressively expands anteroposteriorly and, at about seven weeks, undergoes intramembranous bone formation eventually to form the body of the mandible. From this initial ossification site, new bone is laid down anteriorly toward the mandibular midline and posteriorly toward that point where the inferior alveolar nerve, which lies between Meckel's cartilage and the newly ossifying mandibular body, joins with the lingual nerve (Fig. 3–3A). This ossification of the mandibular body eventually forms a canal for the inferior alveolar nerve and bony alveoli for the developing tooth germs.

As intramembranous ossification of the mandibular body occurs lateral to Meckel's cartilage, beginning at about six and one-half weeks, the distalmost regions become progressively smaller in circumference, with a concomitant atrophy of cartilage cells. At about 16 weeks, when the malleus and incus ear ossicles are ossifying, that segment of Meckel's cartilage between the point of the developing mandibular

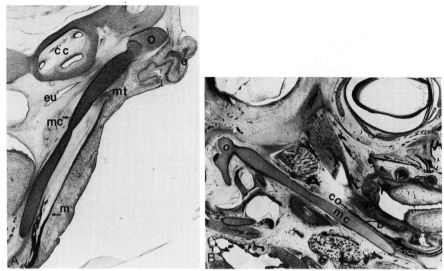

FIGURE 3–2. *A,* A frontal section through the TMJ at 10 weeks prenatal showing the external ear (e), the medial location of Meckel's cartilage (mc), the upper end of Meckel's cartilage next to the malleus ear ossicle (o), the cochlea (cc), the mandible (m), and the eustachian tube (eu). Note the mesenchymal tissue field (mt) for the mandibular body lateral to Meckel's cartilage (magnification, × 12.5). *B,* A parasagittal section through lower jaw of 13-week (72-mm CRL) fetus showing Meckel's cartilage (mc) running diagonally upward and posteriorly toward the malleus (o), ear ossicle. Note that Meckel's cartilage is separated from the mandibular membrane bone (b) and condyle (co) (magnification, × 9). (From Furstman, L.: Embryology. *In* Sarnat, B.G., and Laskin, D.: The Temporomandibular Joint, 3rd ed. Springfield, IL, Charles C Thomas, 1980.)

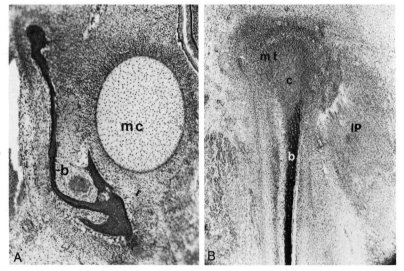

FIGURE 3–3. *A,* A frontal section through the lower jaw at 10 weeks (45-mm CRL) showing the position of the relatively large Meckel's cartilage (mc) medial to intramembranous bone of the mandibular body (b) (magnification, × 55). *B,* A frontal section through 10-week fetus (45-mm CRL) showing a deeply staining mesenchymal field (mt) above the superior region of the mandible. Also shown is the first evidence of the condylar cartilage (c) and its contiguity with the mandibular body (b). Fibers of the lateral pterygoid muscle (lp) are seen streaming upward to the dense field of condylar mesenchyme (mt) (magnification, × 75). (From Furstman, L.: Embryology. *In* Sarnat, B.G., and Laskin, D.: The Temporomandibular Joint, 3rd ed. Springfield, IL, Charles C Thomas, 1980.)

foramen (i.e., at the bifurcation of the lingual and inferior alveolar nerves) and the region of the future mandibular fossa of the temporal bone transforms into the sphenomandibular ligament. This ligament continues within the middle ear cavity as the sphenomalleolar ligament. The anteriormost region of each Meckel's cartilage undergoes endochondral ossification and is incorporated within the menton or chin region of the mandible. It is at this specific site where Meckel's cartilage actually contributes cellular substance to the development of the bony mandible. Finally, at about 18 to 20 prenatal weeks, the only other remaining sign of Meckel's cartilage ever being in place is the mylohyoid line to which the mylohyoid muscle attaches along the medial surface of the mandibular body (Avery, 1987; Perry, 1985; Richany, 1956; Ten Cate, 1980).

At about eight weeks, the ramus of the future mandible appears as a relatively large mesenchymal field showing the progressive differentiation of muscle fibers within it. While bone occurs relatively late in this ramal morphogenetic field (Spyropoulos, 1977; 1988), the mesenchymal field takes on the definitive shape of the ramus. Muscle fibers of the lateral and medial pterygoid muscles appear to differentiate first within this field, followed by the first signs of intramembranous ossification of the ramus. This early appearance of muscle fibers plays a primary role in shaping the mesenchymal field in which the expected components of the TMJ will subsequently develop. Ossification of the ramus spreads posteriorly into the dense mesenchyme of the first branchial arch following a course that diverges from Meckel's cartilage and toward the developing external ear and its auricular hillocks surrounding the cleft between the embryo's first and second branchial arches.

Beginning with the 10th gestational week (30–40 mm crown-rump length [CRL]), the membrane bone of the mandibular body and ramus shows considerable enlargement while still following the contour of Meckel's cartilage that, in a sense, serves as the shape-size morphological template for the embryonic mandible. While most intramembranous ossification occurs within the mandibular body at this particular time, the mesenchymal field surrounding the ossifying ramus continues to differentiate and enlarge. Although both the mandibular body and ramus are evident, except for the appearance of dense mesenchyme, there are few morphological signs of a bony condyle (Fig. 3–3B).

The basic shape of the embryonic mandibular body and ramus seen at 10 weeks is modified over time by the appearance and enlargement of several secondary growth cartilages, including the coronoid, symphyseal, and condylar. Development of the condylar cartilage is a most important and integral step in the morphogenesis of the definitive TMJ.

PRENATAL DEVELOPMENT OF THE SECONDARY TEMPOROMANDIBULAR JOINT

With the developmental obsolescence of the primary joint between Meckel's cartilage and the incus and malleus ear ossicles, there is a progressive shift to a secondary human TMJ during fetal development. This secondary joint eventually becomes the recognizable postnatal TMJ. The major morphogenetic events in human TMJ morphogenesis occur during the critical period of about seven to 11 weeks of gestation. At about the ninth prenatal week, a condensation of mesenchyme appears surrounding the upper posterior surface of the rudimentary ramus. At this stage, the mesenchymal cells rapidly proliferate and take on a more regular orientation. While initially seen as an indefinitely shaped mesenchymal field, it soon becomes more definitive. The concept of developmental fields in mammalian morphogenesis, as described by Spemann and Mangold (1924), has taken on new emphasis in recent years as related to the anomalous development of related body structures (Opitz, 1986). As pointed out by Spyropoulos (1977) in studies on the developing mandible, an embryonic block of mesenchymal tissue can be considered as a morphogenetic or developmental field whose normal morphogenesis into discrete anatomical structures can be interfered with in some significant and timely manner. Thus the structures that are expected to emerge from the field can show a range of abnormalities.

The shape of this mesenchymal field, in a sense, acts as an early developmental template for the subsequent development of the condylar cartilage and related joint components. The apex of this cone-shaped field is directed toward, and is contiguous with, the developing ramus. This mass progressively chondrifies at about 10 to 11 weeks to form the cartilaginous mandibular condyle (Fig. 3–4). At its earliest appearance, the mandibular condyle consists of a convex cluster of cartilage cells surrounded by a perichondrium. With the continuing interstitial proliferation of cartilage cells, however,

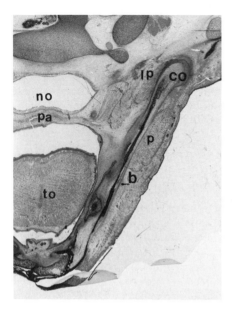

FIGURE 3–4. A frontal section through jaw of 11-week fetus (48-mm CRL) showing the spatial relations of the tongue (to), palate (pa), nasal cavity (no), lateral pterygoid fibers (lp), parotid gland (p), condyle (co), and bone of the mandibular body (b). The condensed field of mesenchyme seen above the superior region of the mandible in Figure 3–3A is clearly along the superior edge of the mandible in this plane of section (magnification, × 12.5). (From Furstman, L.: Embryology. *In* Sarnat, B.G., and Laskin, D.: The Temporomandibular Joint, 3rd ed. Springfield, IL, Charles C Thomas, 1980.)

the condyle significantly increases in size. Although Meckel's cartilage lies medial to this cone-shaped cartilage, it does not contribute structurally to the morphogenesis of the mandibular condyle. The upper, or distalmost re- gion, of the cone-shaped cartilage enlarges to take on the shape of the condyle, which maintains its connective tissue covering. With progressive endochondral ossification, the apical portion of the cone-shaped cartilage fuses with

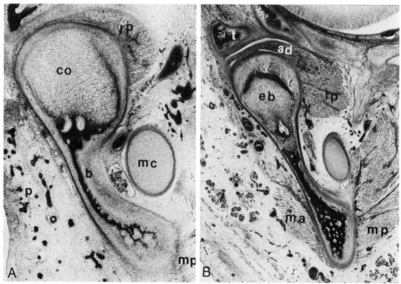

FIGURE 3–5. *A*, A frontal section through 12-week fetus (65-mm CRL) showing the relations of Meckel's cartilage (mc) and joint components. Lateral pterygoid muscle fibers (lp) are seen coursing toward the relatively large mandibular condyle. Medial pterygoid muscle fibers (mp) are seen along inferior edge of body near mandibular angle. The parenchyma of the parotid gland (p) is lateral to the condyle (co) and mandibular body (b) (magnification, × 35). *B*, A frontal section through 14-week fetus (90-mm CRL) showing further ossification of the mandibular fossa of the temporal bone (t) above the articular disc (ad). Endochondral bone of the condyle (eb) is much more pronounced. Muscle fibers of the lateral pterygoid (lp), medial pterygoid (mp), and masseter (ma) are seen attaching to the ramus (magnification, × 15). (From Furstman, L.: Embryology. *In* Sarnat, B.G., and Laskin, D.: The Temporomandibular Joint, 3rd ed. Springfield, IL, Charles C Thomas, 1980.)

the posterior part of the bony mandibular body. From the 12th week on, the entire condylar cartilage enlarges even further to become the most conspicuous part of the ramus. This mass of cartilage is rapidly transformed into bone by endochondral ossification so that at 20 weeks only the head region of the condyloid process remains as cartilage, which persists throughout most of postnatal life. In terms of spatial arrangements, Meckel's cartilage lies medial to the developing mandible, the secondary TMJ, and related soft tissues (Fig. 3–5A, B).

At about nine to 10 weeks, the muscle fibers noted earlier in the ramal morphogenetic field become even more differentiated and can be

recognized as the lateral pterygoid muscle, including its upper sphenomeniscus portion that attaches to the developing articular disc and its lower portion that blends into the condylar neck region. As described by Furstman (1963), branches of the trigeminal nerve and fibers of the auriculotemporal nerve become increasingly distinguishable among the soft tissues as early as the 12th gestational week (Fig. 3–6A, B, and C). Blood vessels are clearly present and organized, surrounding the joint region in the embryo at 10 weeks.

The appearance of the mandibular fossa of the temporal bone is somewhat earlier than that of the condyle. At seven to eight weeks, the

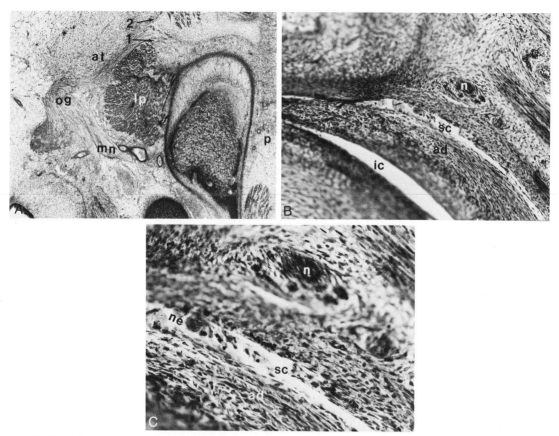

FIGURE 3–6. A, A frontal section through condylar region at 12 weeks (65-mm CRL). A branch of the auriculotemporal nerve (at) is seen coming from the otic ganglion (og) as it returns from the TMJ among fibers of the lateral pterygoid muscle (lp). One branch (1) goes into the future region of the articular disc; the other (2) passes into the temporal region. Also seen is the mandibular nerve (mn) as it passes laterally and inferiorly toward the mandibular ramus (magnification, × 35). B, This section through a 22-week fetus (180-mm CRL) shows a large nerve fiber (n) immediately above the superior joint cavity (sc). Note the relatively large inferior joint cavity (ic) below the articular disc (ad) (magnification, × 125). C, A higher magnification of the same fetus as in B shows a small nerve end organ (ne) in the superior compartment (sc) relative to its parent nerve trunk (n) articular disc (ad) (magnification, × 150). (From Furstman, L.: Embryology. In Sarnat, B.G., and Laskin, D.: The Temporomandibular Joint, 3rd ed. Springfield, IL, Charles C Thomas, 1980.)

42 / I Biological Basis

fossa is first seen as a mass of deeply staining mesenchymal cells along the upper edge of the tissue block that give rise to the TMJ synovial elements. Beginning ossification of the fossa above the future disc region is most prominent at 10 to 11 weeks. From this time on, ossification of the fossa is more advanced than that of the condyle in terms of increasing cortical bone thickness and density of bone trabeculae. Ossification continues in this temporal bone region so that at 22 weeks the mandibular fossa shows both medial and lateral bony walls. It is at this time that the articular eminence becomes evident. The shape of the developing fossa is convex through the ninth week, after which it takes on its definitive concave shape that will provide a reciprocal match for the convex condyle.

The remaining portion of the joint developmental field is a mass of differentiating mesenchymal cells interposed between the developing condyle and the mandibular fossa. These cells eventually give rise to the capsular and intracapsular structures of the secondary TMJ, including the articular disc, the articular capsule, the superior and inferior joint cavities, and synovial linings.

The articular disc is first seen at about seven

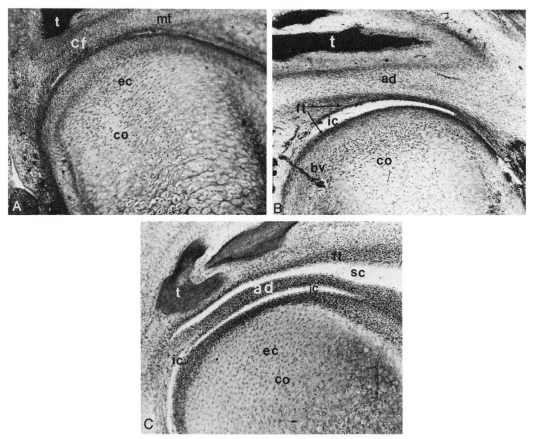

FIGURE 3–7. *A,* A frontal section through 12-week fetus (65-mm CRL) showing the beginning of the inferior joint compartment above the mandibular condyle (co). The first signs of bone spicules in the temporal bone (t) are seen above the block of mesenchyme tissue (mt) that will give rise to the articular disc, beginning of cleft formation (cf). The mandibular condyle shows advanced stages of endochondral bone formation (ec) (magnification, × 75). *B,* This photomicrograph at 13 weeks (72-mm CRL) shows the further enlargement of the inferior compartment (ic), the passing of a small blood vessel (bv) into the condyle (co), disc (ad), and a heavy layer of temporal bone tissue (t) (magnification, × 75). *C,* At 14 weeks (82-mm CRL) both superior (sc) and inferior (ic) joint compartments are well formed, and the articular disc (ad) is prominent. Both the temporal bone (t) and the condyle (co) are covered with dense fibrous tissue. Note the mass of embryonic cartilage (ec) remaining in the condyle (magnification, × 75). (From Furstman, L.: Embryology. *In* Sarnat, B.G., and Laskin, D.: The Temporomandibular Joint, 3rd ed. Springfield, IL, Charles C Thomas, 1980.)

and one-half weeks as a deeply staining, horizontal band of mesenchyme oriented transversely within the block of mesenchymal tissue separating the cranial and condylar portions of the joint. Although there is some variation, a more definite band of presumptive disc cells can be identified at eight and one-half weeks. Interestingly, this disc primordium appears before there are any definite signs of cavitation for the superior and inferior joint cavities. The first signs of collagenous fibers within the disc appear at about 10 weeks and become progressively more pronounced by 12 weeks. From about 19 to 20 weeks, the disc increasingly takes on its definitive fibrocartilage tissue composition. Even at this early time, and before the first signs of upper and lower joint cavities, the developing disc already shows a pattern of differential cell proliferation in which the central region becomes thinner than the periphery. The newly formed disc also shows signs of being more vascular in its peripheral regions than in its central portion. Only after the central portion of the disc is compressed between the condyle and temporal bone does it become avascular (Moffett, 1957).

As with the articular disc, there is some variation with regard to timing and early initiation of the development of the articular cap-

sule. The capsule first appears at about nine to 11 weeks as a very thin and deeply stained zone surrounding the presumptive joint region. This zone becomes more fully differentiated at about 17 weeks so that the capsule is then seen as a fully formed tissue boundary between the intracapsular and extracapsular components of the joint. The expected cellular morphology of the articular capsule and its synovial lining are well differentiated at 26 weeks. At this time, lateral pterygoid muscle fibers are conspicuous and show definite insertions into the thickened medial portion of the capsule.

The superior and inferior joint cavities progressively appear as groups of small spaces or clefts within the mesenchymal tissue block that, at an earlier time, had given rise to the condylar cartilage, the articular disc, and the mandibular fossa. Initiation of both joint cavities is not synchronous. Small, coalescing interstitial spaces for the inferior joint cavity can be seen at about 10 weeks (50- to 58-mm CRL), whereas beginning cavitation for the superior joint cavity is seen at about 12 weeks (60- to 70-mm CRL). The small spaces between the mesenchymal cells below the disc region gradually enlarge and coalesce into larger spaces that will eventually form a pronounced inferior joint cavity (Fig. 3–7A). From 13 weeks on (72-mm CRL),

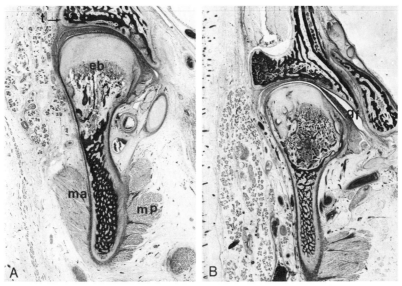

FIGURE 3–8. *A*, This frontal section at 16 weeks (110-mm CRL) shows the typical formation of the articular disc along with both increased intramembranous ossification of the temporal bone (t), mandibular fossa, and endochondral ossification (eb) of the condyle. Masseter (ma) and medial pterygoid (mp) muscle fibers are seen attaching to the angle region of the mandibular ramus (magnification, × 12). *B*, A frontal section at 22 weeks (185-mm CRL) showing further enlargement of the mandibular or glenoid fossa (gf). Note the relatively large size of the condyle region relative to the size of the mandibular ramus (magnification, × 9). (From Furstman, L.: Embryology. *In* Sarnat, B.G., and Laskin, D.: The Temporomandibular Joint, 3rd ed. Springfield, IL, Charles C Thomas, 1980.)

the lower cavity has significantly enlarged while the superior joint cavity begins to become more evident (Fig. 3–7B). Both cavities are fully evident at about 14 weeks (Fig. 3–7C). From that time on, and especially at 16 to 22 weeks, the joint cavities merely increase in size to conform to the size and shape of the bony articular elements, the condyle and the mandibular fossa (Fig. 3–8A and B). The shapes of the joint cavities are generally reciprocal at this early time. When the upper joint cavity is concave, the lower cavity is convex.

By referring to Figures 3–9 and 3–10 the gross development of the human TMJ can be observed through its various fetal stages from nine to 20 weeks of prenatal age.

CLINICAL CONSIDERATIONS

With the recognition that timing is one of the most important variables in the understanding of normal and abnormal morphogenesis (Wilson, 1977; Persaud, 1977), it is important to

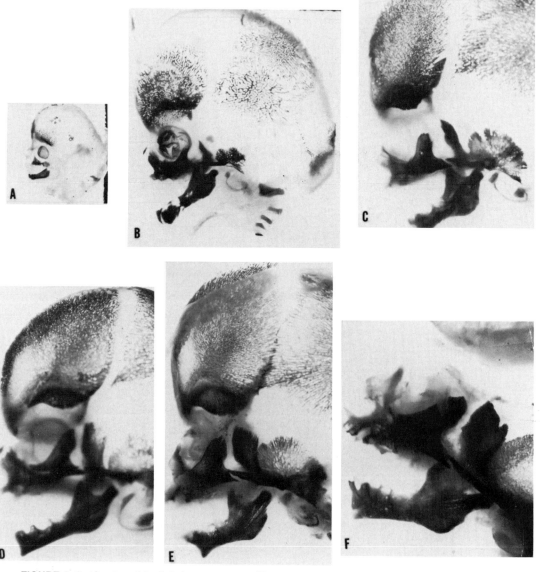

FIGURE 3–9. Alizarin red Spalteholz preparations of hemisections of human fetal heads. A, Nine weeks. B, 11 weeks. C, 14 weeks. D, 15 weeks. E, 18 weeks. F, 20 weeks. The shape of the condyle is not clearly defined in the nine-week specimen, but by the 11th week, all bones of the TMJ are well demarcated. (From Levy, B.: Embryological development. In Sarnat, B.G.: The Temporomandibular Joint, 2nd ed. Springfield, IL, Charles C Thomas, 1964.)

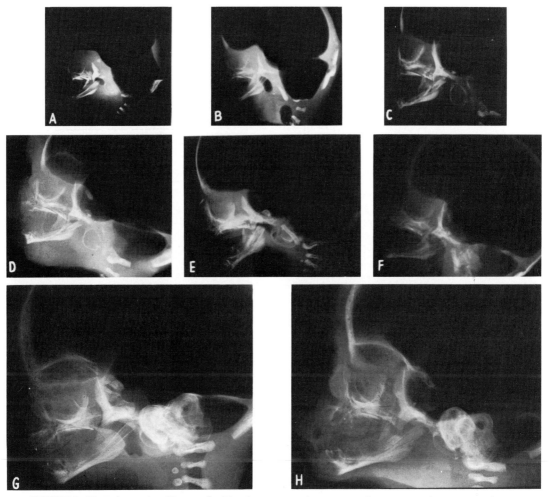

FIGURE 3–10. Radiographs of human fetal heads. *A*, 11 weeks. *B*, 12 weeks. *C*, 13 weeks. *D*, 14 weeks. *E*, 15 weeks. *F*, 16 weeks. *G*, 18 weeks. *H*, 20 weeks. The growth of the condyle in relation to the mandible and other skeletal landmarks is readily seen. (From Levy, B.: Embryological development. *In* Sarnat, B.G.: The Temporomandibular Joint, 2nd ed. Springfield, IL, Charles C Thomas, 1964.)

recognize that the crucial time period in initiating each of the anatomical components of the human TMJ is between seven to 11 gestational weeks (Van der Linden, 1987) (Fig. 3–11). Following this critical four-week period, when TMJ morphogenesis is extremely vulnerable to teratogens, the major changes in each of the joint components that do occur before birth deal with increasing size, changes in shape, continuing ossification, and the beginning of recognizable joint functions.

Given these perspectives on developmental timing and critical periods as related to TMJ development, it is interesting to cite just one or two examples on how a better appreciation of the chronology of TMJ development can be used to understand better the early structure and function of the joint. The classical works of Hooker (1954) and Humphrey (1968) show that active mouth-opening actions in live human fetuses are observable as early as seven to eight weeks of gestation. The timing in TMJ development (Baume, 1962; Furstman, 1963; Moffett, 1957; Perry, 1985; Symons, 1952; Van der Linden, 1987), however, generally shows that only scattered muscle fibers of the jaw-opening lateral pterygoid muscle are clearly discernible in the TMJ field at seven to eight weeks. The mandibular fossa, condyle, and articular disc are only in their earliest developmental stages. Therefore, the prenatal jaw-opening activity that both Hooker (1954) and Humphrey (1968) observed, chiefly as elicited reflexes, appears to have involved articulations of the primary TMJ, which is Meckel's cartilage and the malleus and incus ear ossicles, rather than compo-

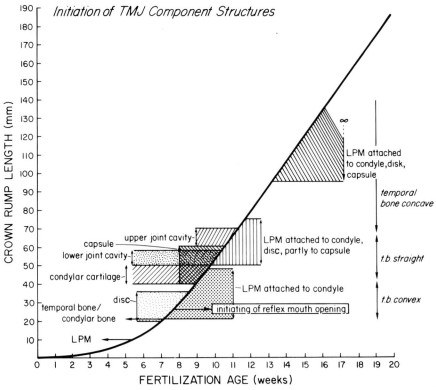

FIGURE 3–11. Summary of the sequential appearance of the TMJ components and regions, demonstrating that the known crucial period for early TMJ morphogenesis is between seven and 11 gestational weeks. This graph also shows the time discrepancy between the appearance of mouth-opening reflexes as reported by Hooker (1954) and Humphrey (1968). (From Van der Linden, E.J., Burdi, A.R., and de Jongh, H.J.: Critical periods in the prenatal morphogenesis of the human lateral pterygoid muscle, the mandibular condyle, the articular capsule, and medial articular capsule. Am. J. Orthod. *91*:22–28, 1987.)

nent structures of the relatively late-forming secondary TMJ.

As an example of how an understanding of developmental timing and critical periods can relate to structural development, one can draw upon many clinical examples in the vast literature of human birth defects (Goodman, 1983; Gorlin, 1976; Smith, 1976; Warkany, 1971). They address just when in human embryonic and fetal morphogenesis a given group of cells, tissues, and structures within a developmental field was affected by environmental or genetic disturbances of significant magnitude to produce the birth defects. A more specific and especially relevant example to emphasize further the importance of developmental timing comes from a report that shows that the typical facies of mandibulofacial dysostosis, with deformed Meckel's cartilage and mandible, abnormal TMJ, and aberrant malleus and incus ear ossicles seen postnatally, is already quite evident by the 15th week of gestation (Behrents, 1977).

SUMMARY

The human TMJ seen after birth reflects the summation of a series of morphogenetic or developmental processes occurring early in prenatal life. From a biological point of view, it is fascinating to know that such a complex mammalian joint as the TMJ involves many cell and tissue types that show chronological stages and morphogenetic patterns in their progressive differentiation leading to final joint morphology and function. Knowing that there is this prenatal and postnatal timeline in the development of the TMJ may make it somewhat easier for clinicians, dysmorphologists, and developmental biologists to understand at what crucial point or points along this timeline birth defects involving the joint are initially expressed.

The picture of TMJ development presented in this chapter is based on a blend of information coming chiefly from direct observations of over 50 human prenates and corroborated by information derived from pertinent literature, and emphasizes that from seven to 11 prenatal weeks is the crucial developmental period for laying down each of the discrete morphological components of the postnatal TMJ. This does not imply, by any means, that the myriad of morphological changes occurring in joint tissues before or after this time are of any less importance.

This picture of human TMJ morphogenesis necessarily includes both phylogenetic and ontogenetic perspectives. Following an earlier embryonic time when Meckel's cartilage and related malleus and incus ear ossicles were prominent structures serving as the primary or first-appearing TMJ, there is a gradual unfolding of the secondary TMJ, beginning with the late embryonic period (seven weeks) and extending into the fetal period, which will result in the TMJ as it is structured postnatally (see Figs. 3–9 and 3–10). With the establishment of the complete picture of TMJ morphology by about 11 weeks, subsequent changes in joint structure deal chiefly with growth and development of the joint in preparation for the functional demands placed upon it after birth, throughout the lifespan.

REFERENCES

Avery, J. A.: Oral Development and Histology. Baltimore, Williams & Wilkins, 1987.

Baume, L. J.: Ontogenesis of the human temporomandibular joint. I. Development of the condyles. J. Dent. Res. 41:1327–1339, 1962.

Behrents, R. G., McNamara, J. A., and Avery, J. K.: Prenatal mandibulofacial dysostosis (Treacher Collins syndrome). Cleft Palate J. 14:13–34, 1977.

Crompton, A. W.: Origin of the mammalian temporomandibular joint. In Carlson, D. S., McNamara, J. A., and Ribbens, K. A. (Eds.): Developmental Aspects of Temporomandibular Joint Disorders. Monograph 16: Craniofacial Growth Series. Center for Human Growth and Development, Ann Arbor, MI, University of Michigan, 1985.

Furstman, L.: The early development of the human temporomandibular joint. Am. J. Orthod. 49:672–682, 1963.

Gaupp, B.: Beitrage zur kenntnis des unterkiefers der wirbeltiere. Anat. Anz. 39:609–666, 1911.

Goodman, R. M., and Gorlin, R. J.: The Malformed Infant and Child. New York, Oxford University Press, 1983.

Gorlin, R. J., Pindborg, J. J., and Cohen, M. M., Jr.: Syndromes of the Head and Neck, 2nd ed. New York, McGraw-Hill, 1976.

Hooker, D.: Early human fetal activity, with a preliminary note on double simultaneous fetal stimulation. Res. Publ. Assoc. Res. Nerv. Ment. Dis. 33:98–113, 1954.

Humphrey, T.: The development of mouth opening and related reflexes involving the oral area of human fetuses. Ala. J. Med. Sci. 5:126–157, 1968.

Moffett, B.: The prenatal development of the human temporomandibular joint. Carnegie Contributions to Embryology 36:19–28, 1957.

Moffett, B.: The morphogenesis of the temporomandibular joint. Am. J. Orthod. 52:401–415, 1966.

Opitz, J. M.: The developmental field concept. In Opitz, J. M., Reynolds, J. F., and Spano, L. (Eds.): The Developmental Field Concept. New York, Alan R. Liss, Inc., 1986.

Perry, H. T., Xu, Y., and Forbes, D.P.: The embryology of the temporomandibular joint. J. Craniomandib. Pract. 3:126–132, 1985.

Persaud, T. V. N.: Problems of Birth Defects. Baltimore, University Park Press, 1977.

Richany, S. F., Bast, T. H., and Anson, B. J.: The development of the first branchial arch in man and the fate of Meckel's cartilage. Q. Bull. Northwestern U. Med. School 30:331–356, 1956.

Smith, D.: Recognizable Patterns of Human Malformation, 2nd ed. Philadelphia, W. B. Saunders, 1976.

Spemann, H., and Mangold, H.: Uber induktion von embryonanlagen durch implantion artfremder organisatoren. Arch. Mikrosk. Anat. 100:599–638, 1924.

Spyropoulos, M.: The morphogenetic relationship of the temporal muscle to the coronoid process in human embryos and fetuses. Am. J. Anat. 150:395–410, 1977.

Spyropoulos, M., and Burdi, A.R.: Morphogenetic fields in craniofacial biology. In Vig, K. W. L., and Burdi, A. R. (Eds.): Craniofacial Morphogenesis and Dysmorphogenesis. Monograph 21: Craniofacial Growth Series. Center for Human Growth and Development, University of Michigan, Ann Arbor, MI, 1988.

Symons, N. R.: The development of the human mandibular joint. J. Anat. 86:326–333, 1952.

Ten Cate, A. R.: Oral Histology: Development, Structure and Function. St. Louis, C. V. Mosby, 1980.

Van der Linden, E. J., Burdi, A. R., and de Jongh, H. J.: Critical periods in the prenatal morphogenesis of the human lateral pterygoid muscle, the mandibular condyle, the articular capsule, and medial articular capsule. Am. J. Orthod. 91:22–28, 1987.

Warkany, J.: Congenital Malformations. Chicago, Year Book Medical, 1971.

Wilson, J. G., and Fraser, F. C.: Handbook of Teratology, Pt. 1. General Principles and Etiology. New York, Plenum Press, 1977.

4

THE CONDYLE AND FACIAL GROWTH*

DONALD H. ENLOW, Ph.D.

INTRODUCTION

Growth of the Face and Cranium

Two basic types of growth change are involved for each of the many separate bones comprising the craniofacial skeleton. One of these is a process termed *displacement* (or translation) and is a physical movement of each whole bone in conjunction with the progressive growth of the soft tissues enclosing it. As the muscles, connective tissues, epithelia, and cartilages expand, the bones associated with these soft tissue masses move along with them, thus tending to separate the various bones at their articulations (sutures, condyles, and synchondroses). As this process of displacement occurs, each bone is triggered to undergo simultaneously its own process of proportionate enlargement, thereby keeping the bones in constant articulation and providing size increases to match the extent of the increases for the soft tissues (Fig. 4–1). How these changes are regulated and carried out is presently a subject of great controversy among researchers.

The second change, *remodeling growth,* is the enlargement process for the various bones of the face and cranium. It is carried out not only at the articulations previously mentioned, but also throughout all other parts of the individual bones by activity of the periosteum and

the endosteum. Remodeling is involved as a part of the growth process, because widespread changes are required in all regions of each bone for the bone to enlarge, as explained further on. The displacement process and the remodeling process together constitute the growth mechanisms of the craniofacial skeleton.

One of the basic and most important considerations in craniofacial biology today is the source of the actual force and the nature of the control process that carry out, respectively, these displacement and remodeling activities. One of biologists' great goals is to be able to control clinically the growth process. It was once widely believed that the different bones push themselves apart at sutures by the act of depositing new bone at the sutural edges and that this is the force that causes displacement. It is now realized, however, that the compression-sensitive membranes of the sutures cannot accommodate a pushing force of one bone against another. The suture, rather, is a traction-adapted growth site. That is, as the bones all become displaced away from one another, presumably by the force of expansion of the muscles, brain, or other soft tissues, tension is set up in the sutural membranes. This is currently believed to be the trigger that stimulates deposition of new bone by the sutural membrane on the sutural edges. The amount of new formation appears to be determined by the corresponding extent of the displacement movement.

---

*See Chapters 3, 6, 10, 12, 13, and 24.

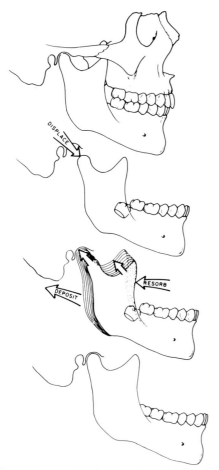

FIGURE 4-1. Two basic types of growth *movement* are illustrated. The entire mandible is progressively *displaced* anteroinferiorly away from its condylar articulation in the glenoid fossa. Simultaneously, the condyle and ramus *remodel* in an opposite posterosuperior direction. The magnitude and direction of the displacement movement interrelate with the corresponding extent but opposite direction of the remodeling movement. While only ramus remodeling, as visualized two-dimensionally, is represented here, the entire mandible participates in the three-dimensional remodeling process as shown in Figure 4-4. Examples of adjustments in the remodeling process to accommodate changing morphogenetic conditions are illustrated in Figures 4-9 through 4-13.

Similarly, it was long held that the endochondral growth mechanism exerts a pushing effect that thrusts the bones apart at the various cartilaginous growth sites (the condyles and synchondroses). This was a reasonable idea, because it has long been known that cartilage represents a special pressure-tolerant tissue well adapted to the functional and morphogenetic environment involved in certain compressive types of tissue relationships. Many experimental studies have been carried out in attempts to identify any regulatory role of car-

tilage in the displacement process, but this has been found to be an especially difficult and complex conceptual and procedural problem. A similar situation also exists with regard to the displacement of the nasomaxillary complex and the role of the septal cartilage. As a result of these studies over a period of years, some investigators now maintain, as a generalization, that both bone and cartilage growth are secondary in nature. That is, the rate and extent of bone and cartilage growth are in response to other intrinsic and extrinsic control factors, rather than their acting as primary pacemakers. There is still uncertainty, however, as to just how much genetic programming actually is present within cartilage, especially among the different types of cartilage, and this remains a controversial topic among researchers. It is generally accepted that formation of bone tissue itself is indeed secondary in nature, and that its growth activity is not programmed within the hard part of the bone. However, the bone provides essential feedback information to the other tissues responsible for regulating its progressive growth and remodeling. It is generally realized, also, that the mode of operation of all the factors involved in the growth control process is not currently understood.

One of the most familiar phrases in facial biology is that the face grows downward and forward. When serial headfilm tracings are superposed on the cranial base, i.e., registered at the sella and superposed on a line drawn from sella to nasion, the apparent anterior and inferior mode of facial growth can be clearly visualized. This is a morphologically realistic way to demonstrate facial growth, however, only if certain misrepresentations and limitations are understood. The face does not simply grow downward and forward, and the cranial base is not fixed, as implied by this overlay procedure. The superposition demonstrates, rather, the successive locations held by each enlarging facial part relative to the points of registration used and at the respective ages observed. These locations are produced by the aggregate of all the growth changes that have occurred in all parts of the face and cranium. The growth process itself is multifactorial, and many regional changes and localized morphogenetic processes contribute to the cumulative composite that can be seen as the downward-and-forward result. Each separate bone enlarges by bone deposition and resorption in a complex three-dimensional variety of anterior, posterior, superior, inferior, and lateral directions. Some of the growth vectors involved relate to major changes and others to only relatively slight alterations. All, however, are required for normal growth. As each of these regional, multidirectional remodeling changes takes place, the bones simultaneously become displaced, and it is the composite of all these regional processes that produces growth.

Another important concept is that the growth changes in the different parts of the face and cranium do not proceed in an isolated and regionally independent manner. Close morphogenetic interrelationships exist, and growth changes in any one part accommodate the nature of growth changes in other parts. For example, the vertical enlargement of the nasal chambers is carried out, in part, by a downward direction of remodeling growth of the palate and the bony maxillary arch. The expansion of one part thus directly involves growth changes in other parts. The vertical growth of both the nasal chambers and the maxillary arch, in turn, is accommodated by the vertical enlargement of the mandibular ramus, which thereby lowers the mandibular arch to keep pace with the downward growth of the nasomaxillary complex. Similarly, as the horizontal dimension of the pharynx increases, the breadth of the mandibular ramus enlarges to keep pace with it.

MANDIBULAR GROWTH AND DEVELOPMENT

As the entire mandible is displaced in an anterior and inferior direction, its predominant size increases are in the opposite superior and posterior direction. That is, as it moves forward and downward, it grows upward and backward at the same time by an equal amount. The process of mandibular growth is complex, however, and of course does not merely involve condylar growth to accomplish these changes. Each regional part of the whole mandible actively participates, and a widespread distribution of remodeling fields blanket the entire bone, inside and out. About half of the periosteal surfaces of the mandible (and most other bones in the face and cranial floor as well) have fields that are characteristically resorptive in character, and about half are depository. The bone undergoes remodeling to relocate its component parts. The mandibular ramus, for example, grows posteriorly, with about half of the outside surfaces undergoing resorption and about half deposition (Fig. 4–2). This relocates the whole ramus in a posterior direction, and the area that was once part of the ramus be-

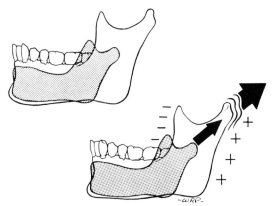

FIGURE 4–2. In this overlay at two random age levels, the mandibular outlines were superposed so that the surface fields of resorption and deposition are expressed. The mandible enlarges predominantly posteriorly and superiorly. The actual growth vector may vary somewhat in different individuals, and it also undergoes variable regional changes during the growth of any given person. In three dimensions, the growth process is seen to be more complex than can be represented in a simple two-dimensional outline drawing (compare with Fig. 4–4).

comes remodeled into a new addition for the corpus. The corpus grows longer as a result. The ramus, at the same time, also becomes proportionately more broad, because the amount of posterior deposition exceeds the extent of anterior resorption on the various surfaces.

As the ramus grows posteriorly, the mandibular condyle simultaneously grows upward and backward by an endochondral mode of bone formation, in contrast to the intramembranous manner of growth in the other parts of the ramus. The condyle thus becomes relocated into progressively new positions in conjunction with the growth of the whole ramus. The bone located where the condyle used to be during past growth stages is remodeled, successively, into the mandibular neck and a part of the ramus.

Because the mandibular neck is narrower than the condyle itself, the periosteal surfaces on the lateral and medial sides of the neck are resorptive, and the endosteal surfaces are depository. The endosteal surface of the mandibular neck, rather than the outer surface, is oriented so that it faces the upward and backward direction of condylar growth. It is thus the endosteal surface that actually receives the bone deposits (Fig. 4–3). In Figure 4–4, the coronoid processes are seen to grow upward and backward by progressive bone deposition on the medial (lingual) surfaces, with resorption from the lateral (buccal) sides, because it is the

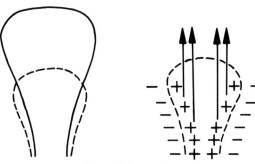

FIGURE 4–3. As the condylar cartilage grows posterosuperiorly, the condylar neck keeps pace by intramembranous bone deposition and resorption. Note that the lateral cortices of the neck have resorptive surfaces; the endosteal sides are depository because it is the inside surfaces that face the direction of progressive growth.

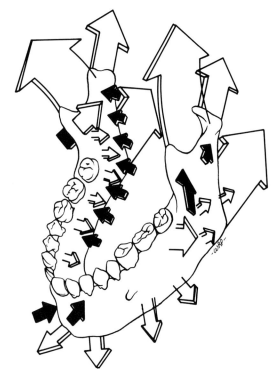

FIGURE 4–4. The three-dimensional directions of mandibular growth are summarized. Surfaces that are depository in nature are represented by light arrows; resorptive periosteal surfaces are shown by black arrows (compare with Fig. 4–6).

medial surface that faces the direction of growth. Note that this arrangement of remodeling surfaces also provides another basic remodeling change. As mentioned above, the ramus is remodeled into new additions for the elongating corpus as it grows posteriorly. The ramus, however, is positioned well lateral to the corpus, and the conversion process must thus relocate this part in a medial (lingual) direction (Fig. 4–5). New bone deposition on the medial side of the ramus accomplishes this.

THE CONDYLE AS A MAJOR GROWTH SITE

Throughout all parts of the mandible there are many regional sites of localized growth and remodeling, and all actively participate to develop the regional shapes and dimensions needed to carry out the multiple functions of the mandible as a whole (Fig. 4–6). A key point in the rationale underlying the distribution and the nature of these growth sites is that the morphology and the morphogenetic processes in each regional area represent direct adaptations to the localized functional, developmental,

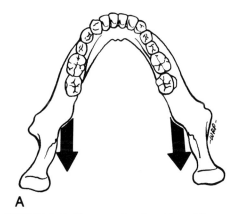

A

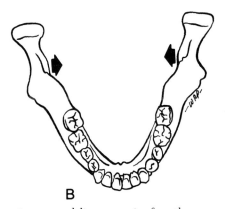

B

FIGURE 4–5. The posterior elongation of the corpus (A) requires a remodeling conversion from the ramus, which is growing and relocating posteriorly at the same time. Because the ramus is lateral to the principal axis of the corpus, it must relocate medially by bone deposition on the medial side (B).

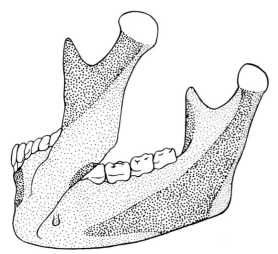

FIGURE 4–6. The principal fields of periosteal resorption *(dark)* and deposition *(light).*

biomechanical, and physiological circumstances that are present. The condyle is such a growth site, as are the coronoid process, the alveolar bone housing the teeth, the posterior border of the ramus, the gonial region, the mental protuberance, and so on. No growth field is any less involved than any other, since all are required to produce the functional bone. However, historically, the condyle has been singled out as a special site (or center) because it has a distinctive growth cartilage, and this cartilage has been believed to provide certain special functions during growth. Because of clinical relevance, the matter has received a great deal of research attention and is currently a subject of major interest in several clinical fields.

Cartilage is a tissue that is adapted to a number of different functional circumstances; one of these involves its capacity to tolerate great levels of pressure and, at the same time, provide for continued growth in such an environment. This is the basis for the role of the endochondral mode of ossification, in contrast to intramembranous bone formation in areas involving surface membrane tension. The posterior and superior manner of growth of the mandibular ramus requires an endochondral type of bone formation at its condylar junction with the cranial floor because of the surface compression involved. Intramembranous bone growth takes place in the other areas of the ramus because of the tensile relationships of the periosteum with the muscles of mastication. The membranes covering the mandibular neck, for example, are not subject to direct surface pressure, and bone growth thereby proceeds

by periosteal and endosteal activity. The special function of the condylar cartilage, essentially, is to provide a regional growth mechanism that can accommodate a particular local need, just as all other regional growth sites utilize processes of growth adapted to their own localized situations.

Phylogenetically, the original articular part of the mandible (derived from Meckel's cartilage) was utilized for conversion into an auditory ossicle (see Chapters 1 and 3). In humans and other mammals, a new cartilage was secondarily added to carry out this articular function. It is believed that the original periosteum in this altered part of the mandible, under the influence of pressure at its new articular contact with the basicranium, was transformed into a cartilage-forming membrane (Hall, 1970). Thus, the cartilage of the condyle has been introduced as a *secondary* or *adventitious* cartilage; that is, it was developed secondarily after the original primary cartilage was modified for a different function elsewhere in the skull. A key conceptual question has arisen with regard to the secondary nature of the condylar cartilage. Some investigators now hold that it is secondary not only in phylogenetic origin, but in its growth behavior as well. The growth cartilages of long bones (epiphyseal plates) have long been presumed, correctly or incorrectly, to function as pacemakers for the growth of the limbs, and this concept quite reasonably was extended to include the mandibular condyle. It has been believed that the genetic capacity of the chondrocyte provides a primary determinant of overall mandibular growth rate and amount. Further, because of the pressure-adapted nature of cartilage construction, it was logically assumed that the upward and backward growth of the condyle has a resultant push effect against the basicranium, with a subsequent displacement of the entire mandible forward and downward. This was the classic *condylar-thrust* concept that was adopted everywhere and used as a working principle for many years. Recently, however, these explanations have been questioned, and the state of the matter is presently one of uncertainty with alternative theories under active study. These considerations are evaluated in later pages.

MICROSCOPIC STRUCTURE OF THE CONDYLE

The cells within the fibrous covering of the condyle, under the influence of surface pressure

and a resultant increase in the extent of ischemia, undergo differentiation into chondroblasts
rather than osteoblasts, as demonstrated by Hall
(1970). The covering fibrous layer is highly
cellular early in development but becomes
much more dense with increasing age. It is
sparsely vascularized. Just deep to the fibrous
articular layer is a chondrogenic zone of *prechondroblasts* (Fig. 4–7). This is the major site
for proliferative activity within the condyle (Duterloo, 1967; Meikle, 1973). It is here that
repeated cell divisions that result in the posterosuperior growth of the condylar cartilage
proceed. That is, it grows by appositional proliferation just deep to the capsular covering as,
simultaneously, removal of cartilage with bone
replacement takes place on the internal side of
the cartilage mass. The entire cartilage plate
thereby moves upward and backward, while
providing for the bone formation that lengthens
the ramus behind the moving cartilage. Only
an endochondral growth process could be op-
erational here.

The cells within the proliferative zone are
densely arranged with very little intercellular
matrix because of the rapid nature of the proliferative activity. Significantly, the continued
formation of daughter cells does not result in
linear columns of cell groups, as is characteristic
of the isogenous lines of chondrocytes in the
epiphyseal plate cartilages of long bones. In the

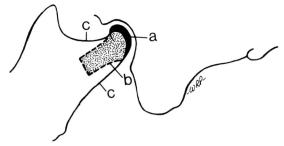

FIGURE 4–8. As the condylar cartilage (*a*) proliferates in
an upward and backward direction, it is progressively
replaced by a medullary core of endochondral bone (*b*).
The cortical bone of the mandibular neck and other parts
of the ramus (*c*) undergo remodeling growth by periosteal
and endosteal activity.

latter, cell proliferation is adapted to, essentially, a unidirectional course of growth. The
condylar cartilage, in contrast, is not committed
to such a restricted capacity for its growth
direction. The cartilage of the mandibular condyle, importantly, is able to respond to growth
changes in other parts of the craniofacial composite. A range of growth directions can be
produced to adapt mandibular growth to the
growth changes taking place elsewhere. This is
necessary because of the architectural and morphogenetic complexity of the craniofacial composite in comparison with a long bone. A built-
in latitude also exists in the capacity of the
condyle to adapt its rate and amount of growth,
although, as pointed out previously, the extent
is controversial.

Deep to the proliferative zone is a region of
maturing chondroblasts. While there is some
increase in the amount of intercellular matrix,
the cells remain closely packed. The chondroblasts undergo progressive hypertrophy within
this zone. In the deepest part, the scant intercellular matrix becomes calcified. The erosive
zone follows the region of hypertrophied cells,
and chondroclastic resorption of the calcified
matrix takes place. Appositional bone formation
then proceeds within the resorbed areas, and
the mandibular neck thereby extends into a
region previously occupied by the condylar
cartilage. The process of endochondral bone
growth produces a core of fine cancellous bone
located specifically in the medullary part of the
condyle and its neck (Fig. 4–8). As previously
mentioned, the membranes of the cortical bone
in the nonarticular parts of the condyle and
mandibular neck are not exposed to the compressive forces of joint contact, and the cortices
here are thus formed by intramembranous ossification.

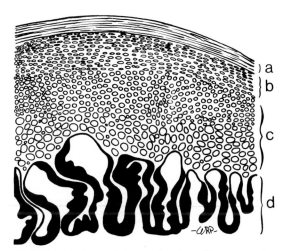

FIGURE 4–7. The condylar cartilage has a fibrous covering
(*a*) that overlays a region of rapidly proliferating prechondroblasts (*b*). In area *c*, the cells have become chondroblasts
that mature in the deeper part of the zone. Each cell
undergoes hypertrophy, and a limited deposition of intercellular matrix occurs. Near zone *d*, the matrix calcifies,
and cartilage resorption with subsequent bone deposition
begins along the posterosuperior moving interface between
c and *d*.

INTERRELATIONSHIPS BETWEEN CONDYLAR GROWTH AND GROWTH OF THE REMAINDER OF THE FACE AND CRANIUM

The structural function of the mandibular ramus, in addition to providing attachments for masticatory muscles, is to bridge the span of the floor of the middle cranial fossa, placing the lower arch in proper occlusal position relative to the upper arch. The horizontal dimension of the ramus must adapt to the anteroposterior size of this part of the basicranium.

The ramus is often involved as a growth and remodeling site that provides compensatory adjustments in the placement of the mandibular arch into a functional occlusal position (Enlow, 1982). The breadth of the ramus can become wider or remain narrow during growth in order to place the mandibular corpus in a more protrusive or retrusive position. Remodeling rotations of the ramus can also accommodate rotations in other areas or otherwise compensate for individualized growth circumstances. In all cases, the condyle is a major participant in these growth events. Two examples are given.

The angle between the ramus and the corpus normally progresses to close as a child's face continues to grow. The reason is schematized in Figure 4–9. Note that the ramus increases in height much more than in breadth. This is to accommodate the considerable extent of vertical expansion of the nasal region and the eruption of the teeth. As seen in the diagram, the ramus must become more upright to do

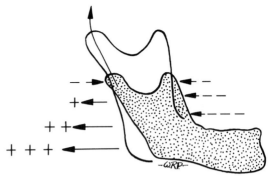

FIGURE 4–10. A more upright ramus is achieved by a change in the direction of condylar growth, as shown by the arrow. Corresponding changes in the distribution and the amount of resorption (−) and deposition (+) accompany the altered growth of the condyle.

this. It is the ramus, rather than the corpus, that must carry out most of the remodeling changes involved. As long as the ramus is actively undergoing a posterior growth movement and also increasing in breadth (to match the growth of the middle cranial fossa), this alteration in ramus angle is achieved simply by following a more upright direction of condylar growth (Fig. 4–10). However, significant vertical midfacial growth, with corresponding vertical lengthening of the ramus, continues after the horizontal growth movements of the ramus have slowed or ceased. When this begins to happen, a more complex remodeling process can be required on the part of the ramus, as schematized in Figure 4–11.

The direction of condylar growth becomes even more vertical and can even proceed some-

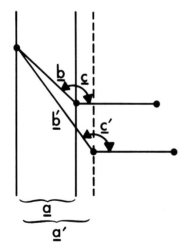

FIGURE 4–9. Schematic basis for a progressive closing of the ramus-corpus angle during mandibular growth. Because the vertical lengthening of the ramus from b to b' greatly exceeds its horizontal enlargement from a to a', angle c must necessarily become reduced to that at c'.

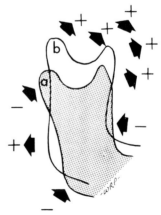

FIGURE 4–11. The ramus in some individuals can apparently undergo the illustrated remodeling changes, particularly at older age levels. Note that the condyle has a slight anterior growth direction and that the superior part of the anterior edge of the ramus is depository.

what anteriorly, with corresponding changes in the combinations of resorption and deposition in the other parts of the ramus. When the ramus and condyle are placed in their actual anatomical positions, it can be seen that this elaborate remodeling process has achieved several results. These include a more vertical alignment of the ramus without any actual increase in its breadth, a vertically longer ramus, and an increase in the horizontal dimension of the mandibular corpus to allow room for the eruption of the last molar (Fig. 4–12).

In the preceding example of ramus accommodation to changing growth circumstances involved in craniofacial enlargement, note especially that the multidirectional capacity of the condylar cartilage is a basic feature that makes these changes possible (Fig. 4–13). As previously stated, the lack of an orientation of the proliferating cells into unidirectional linear columns is a feature that reflects a latitude for growth directions by the condyle.

The ramus and condyle play a major role in providing intrinsic compensations that tend to offset partially the tendencies for malocclusions present in most individuals. Persons with a dolichocephalic head form, for example, have a built-in predisposition for a retrusively positioned mandible. The ramus can become broadened during growth, however, placing the mandibular arch in a more favorable occlusal position and preventing a severe Class II type of malocclusion (Enlow, 1982). To do this, the condyle appears to respond by an increased amount of posterior growth to achieve a better functional relationship between the upper and lower arches. Conversely, the mandible can, intrinsically, respond to a predisposition for a

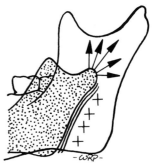

FIGURE 4–13. The condylar cartilage is believed by many researchers to have the capacity for multidirectional growth movements, thus providing for the ramus an intrinsic adaptability that allows for the progressive, functional positioning of the lower arch to accommodate the childhood changes in maxillary and basicranial growth.

Class III malocclusion by a retardation of its horizontal ramus growth and cartilage proliferative activity to produce a more narrow ramus. This converts a possible severe facial imbalance into a Class I or at least a much less severe Class III malocclusion. Should these intrinsic mechanisms fail to function, a full expression of the malocclusion then necessarily follows. Thus, not only can the direction of condylar growth become altered as a normal process during the course of progressive facial development, but apparently some degree of latitude exists in its amount of growth as well.

ROLE OF THE CONDYLAR GROWTH SITE

Because of the great clinical importance of the mandibular condyle and the real need to understand the biological basis for its mode of growth and the regulatory factors involved, much research attention has been, and is being, given to it (see Chapters 12, 13, and 24). One of the great historical controversies in the field of facial growth has developed as a result of the efforts of many investigators attempting to account for the functional nature of the condylar growth mechanism. The arguments have centered on two essential points: (1) whether the condyle is a primary pacemaker for mandibular growth with a self-contained genetic capacity to regulate the rates, amounts, and directions of its own growth or, conversely, whether it behaves in an entirely secondary, responsive, and adaptive way; and (2) whether the growth of the condylar cartilage pushes the whole mandible anteriorly and inferiorly or, conversely,

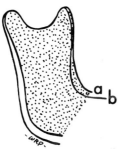

FIGURE 4–12. The growth and remodeling of the ramus by the process illustrated in Figure 4–11 produce an anatomical placement of the mandible, as shown here. The ramus is vertically longer but not horizontally wider. Resorption at the anterior border in the inferior part of the ramus in mandible a provides continuing corpus lengthening in b to allow for completion of molar eruption. The ramus-corpus area has been closed.

whether the condyle itself is incidental, with the mandible becoming displaced by a pull caused either by the expansion of the soft tissues enclosing it or by some other currently unrecognized force. In all cases, the issues at hand are far more than merely theoretical in importance. Recent work has shown that control mechanisms for the condyle are multifactorial in nature, and this is one reason the pioneer experiments necessarily encountered procedural and interpretive difficulties. The studies of McNamara (1972), for example, have demonstrated that sensory nerve input from the periodontal membrane and other parts of the face influences the musculature, which in turn, appears to influence the direction and rate of condylar proliferation. Experimental work by a number of investigators suggests that the condyle, while pressure-tolerant, is sensitive and responsive to changes in the amount of compression exerted on it. An increase in pressure is believed to retard the growth of the condylar cartilage, but a relief in the amount appears to stimulate condylar growth. The investigations of Koski (1971) provide experimental evidence that the condylar cartilage is intrinsically programmed to undergo continued cellular divisions but that their rate, duration, and direction are subject to extrinsic regulatory influences. It is the possible adaptive capacity of the condyle, in contrast to a primary type of role, that has been emphasized by many researchers (Durkin, 1973; Petrovic, 1972), although this interpretation remains controversial.

A number of experimental procedural problems have been encountered that make it difficult, and perhaps even impossible, to resolve thoroughly the problems involved as they are now defined. Sarnat (1971), for example, has been able to show that experimental condylar resections can have effects in adult animals that are similar to those in growing animals, thus making it clear that the results of all such experiments must be interpreted with caution. Changes in the functional relationships among the various bones, muscles, cartilages, and other anatomical parts, caused by the experiment itself, can mask any normal or experimentally altered growth control processes that might or might not also be occurring at the same time and that, therefore, makes any conclusions uncertain.

The functional matrix concept of Moss (1969) has often been used to account for the biological basis for answers to these difficult growth control questions. The usefulness of this concept, which has had great impact in the field, should not be overextended, however. The functional matrix is a special application of the classic structure-function principle of biology. It explains what happens during growth, but is not intended to account for how the histogenetic mechanisms at the cellular level actually carry it out. In just what way the control processes function for the condyle, and for mandibular growth in general, at best remains incompletely understood. When this becomes better known, the old arguments previously mentioned will likely cease to exist. The experimental work by many investigators during the 1960s, in the 1970s and 1980s, and to date has given some of the key information needed to begin to redefine questions and to pose new hypotheses.

SUMMARY

There exist two principal categories of craniofacial skeletal *growth movement*. One is a displacement type of movement in which an entire bone becomes moved progressively away from its articular contacts. The other, which occurs simultaneously, is remodeling. The latter growth movement provides several basic functions, including size increases, shaping, and continuous adjustments to allow fitting among all separate soft and hard tissue parts. Both movement processes are involved in any TMJ dysplasia in which growth and anatomical structuring are underlying factors. They are also involved as a part of any treatment procedure involving TMJ and craniofacial adaptations. Establishment of morphological interrelationships that affect the TMJ extends throughout the craniofacial complex. The development and growth of all the various regional parts are involved in the nature of the composite functional and structural balance that is achieved progressively throughout childhood and beyond.

The mandibular condyle is a structure of particular importance because its pressure-tolerant cartilage provides a means for endochondral enlargement of the mandible in a functional location where intramembranous growth is not possible. It also provides a latitude of morphogenetic adaptability allowing for directional variations in mandibular growth in response to the ongoing, changing conditions that prevail throughout the growth period. Together with the condyle, the progressive development and the remodeling of the whole ramus provide for the vertical and anteroposterior positioning of the corpus and lower dental arch, all the while functioning with its attached musculature. A corresponding latitude of developmental adjustment also characterizes the entire ramus that, with its condyle, can undergo individualized remodeling adaptations to give functional mandibular fitting with the midface on one side and the basicranium on another. That most of us are not afflicted with TMJ problems underscores the versatile adaptability of such morphogenetic adjustment potential. There exists, however, some as yet undefined limit to this potential. This is because, in part, human anatomical conditions have imposed certain developmental constraints on mandibular, midfacial, and basicranial adaptive structuring and positioning. These appear to exceed, in some individuals, the adjustive capacity of all of the various craniofacial parts that allow interrelated accommodation, either during growth or in response to pathological conditions or trauma.

ACKNOWLEDGMENT: The illustrations in this chapter have been adapted from Enlow, D. H.: *Handbook of Facial Growth*, 2nd ed. Philadelphia, W.B. Saunders, 1982.

REFERENCES

Durkin, J. F., Heeley, J. D., and Irving, J. T.: The cartilage of the mandibular condyle. Oral Sci. Rev. 2:29–99, 1973.
Duterloo, H. S.: In Vivo Implantation of the Mandibular Condyle of the Rat. Unpublished dissertation. Nijmegen, the Netherlands, University of Nijmegen, 1967.
Enlow, D. H.: Handbook of Facial Growth, 2nd ed. Philadelphia, W.B. Saunders, 1982.
Hall, B. K.: Differentiation of cartilage and bone from common germinal cells. J. Exp. Zool. 173:383–393, 1970.
Koski, K.: Some characteristics of craniofacial growth cartilages. In Moyers, R. E., and Krogman, W. M. (Eds.): Cranio-facial Growth in Man. Oxford, Pergamon, 1971, pp. 125–128.
McNamara, J. A., Jr.: Neuromuscular and Skeletal Adaptations to Altered Orofacial Function. Craniofacial Growth Series. Monograph no. 1. Center for Human Growth and Development, University of Michigan Press, Ann Arbor, MI, 1972.
Meikle, M. C.: In vivo transplantation of the mandibular joint of the rat: An autoradiographic investigation into cellular changes at the condyle. Arch. Oral. Biol. 18:1011–1020, 1973.
Moss, M. L.: The primary role of functional matrices in facial growth. Am. J. Orthod. 55:566–577, 1969.
Petrovic, A.: Mechanisms and regulation of condylar growth. Acta. Morphol. Neerl. Scand. 10:25–34, 1972.
Sarnat, B. G., and Muchnic, H.: Facial skeletal changes after mandibular condylectomy in growing and adult monkeys. Am. J. Orthod. 60:35–45, 1971.

SUGGESTED REFERENCES

Bassett, C. A. L.: A biological approach to craniofacial morphogenesis. Acta Morphol. Neerl. Scand. 10:71–86, 1972.
Baume, L. J.: Cephalofacial growth patterns and the functional adaptation of the temporomandibular joint structures. Eur. Orthod. Soc. Trans. 1969:79–98, 1970.
Baume, L. J.: Differential response of condylar, epiphyseal, synchondrotic, and articular cartilages of the rat to varying levels of vitamin A. Am. J. Orthod. 58:537–551, 1970.
Bell, W. H., and Levy, B. M.: Revascularization and bone healing after anterior mandibular osteotomy. J. Oral. Surg. 28:196–203, 1970.
Beresford, W. A.: Schemes of zonation in the mandibular condyle. Am. J. Orthod. 68:185–195, 1975.
Björk, A.: The face in profile. Sven. Tandlak. Tidskr. No. 5B [Suppl.]. 40:1947.
Björk, A.: Variations in the growth pattern of the human mandible: Longitudinal radiographic studies by the implant method. J. Dent. Res. 42:400–411, 1963.
Björk, A.: Prediction of mandibular growth rotation. Am. J. Orthod. 55:585–599, 1969.
Björk, A.: The role of genetic and local environmental factors in normal and abnormal morphogenesis. Acta Morphol. Neerl. Scand. 10:49–58, 1972.
Björk, A., and Kudora, T.: Congenital bilateral hypoplasia of the mandibular condyles. Am. J. Orthod. 54:584–600, 1968.
Blackwood, H. J.: Vascularization of the condylar cartilage of the human mandible. J. Anat. 99:551–563, 1965.
Blackwood, H. J.: Growth of the mandibular condyle of the rat studied with tritiated thymidine. Arch. Oral. Biol. 11:493–502, 1966.
Bowden, C. M., and Kohn, M. W.: Mandibular deformity associated with unilateral absence of the condyle. J. Oral. Surg. 31:469–472, 1973.
Bremers, L. M. H.: De Condylus Mandibulae In Vitro. Unpublished dissertation. Nijmegen, the Netherlands, Katholieke Universiteit te Nijmegen, 1973.
Brodie, A. G.: On the growth pattern of the human head. Am. J. Anat. 68:209–262, 1941.
Brodie, A. G.: Facial patterns: A theme on variation. Angle. Orthod. 16:75–87, 1946.
Brodie, A. G.: The growth of the jaws and the eruption of the teeth. Oral Surg. 1:334–341, 1948.
Brodie, A. G.: Late growth changes in the human face. Angle Orthod. 23:146–157, 1963.
Bruce, R. A., and Hayward, J. R.: Condylar hyperplasia and mandibular asymmetry. J. Oral Surg. 26:281–290, 1968.
Burdi, A. R.: Morphogenesis of mandibular dental arch shape in human embryos. J. Dent. Res. 47:50–58, 1968.
Charlier, J. P.: Les facteurs Mácaniques dans la croissance de l'arc basal mandibulaire a la lumière de l'analyse des caractères structuraux et des propriétés biologiques du cartilage condylien. Orthod. Fr. 38:177–186, 1967.
Charlier, J. P., and Petrovic, A.: Recherches sur la mandibule de rat en culture d'organs: Le cartilage condylien a-t-il un potentiel de croissance indépendant? Orthod. Fr. 38:165–175, 1967.
Charlier, J. P., Petrovic, A., and Hermann-Stutzmann, J.: Déterminisme de la croissance mandibulaire: Effets de l'hyperpulsion et ce l'hormone somatotrope sur la croissance condylienne de jeunes rats. Orthod. Fr. 39:567–579, 1968.
Charlier, J. P., Petrovic, A., and Hermann-Stutzmann, J.: Effects of mandibular hyperpulsion on the prechondroblastic zone of young rat condyle. Am. J. Orthod. 55:71–74, 1969.
Charlier, J. P., Petrovic, A., and Linck, G.: La fronde mentonniere et son action sur la croissance mandibulaire. Recherches expérimentales chez la rat. Orthod. Fr. 40:99–113, 1969.
Collins, D. A., Becks, H., Simpson, M. E., and Evans, H.

M.: Growth and transformation of the mandibular joint in the rat. I. Normal female rats. Am. J. Orthod. *32*:431–442, 1946.

Crelin, E. S., and Koch, W. E.: An autoradiographic study of chondrocyte transformation into chondroclasts and osteocytes during bone formation in vitro. Anat. Rec. *158*:473–483, 1967.

Cunat, J. J., Bhaskar, S. N., and Weinmann, J. P.: Development of the squamoso-mandibular articulation in the rat. J. Dent. Res. *35*:533–546, 1916.

Dibbets, J.: Juvenile Temporomandibular Joint Dysfunction and Craniofacial Growth. Unpublished dissertation. Groningen, Sweden, University of Groningen, 1977.

Droel, R., and Isaacson, R. J.: Some relationships between the glenoid fossa position and various skeletal discrepancies. Am. J. Orthod. *61*:64–78, 1973.

Durkin, J. F.: Secondary cartilage: A misnomer? Am. J. Orthod. *62*:15–41, 1972.

Durkin, J. F., Irving, J. T., and Heeley, J. D.: A comparison of the circulatory and calcification patterns in the mandibular condyle in the guinea pig with those found in the tibial epiphyseal and articular cartilages. Arch. Oral. Biol. *14*:1365–1371, 1969.

Duterloo, H. S., and Jansen, H. W. B.: Chondrogenesis and osteogenesis in the mandibular condylar blastema. Eur. Orthod. Soc. Trans. *1969*:109–118, 1969.

Duterloo, H. S., and Wolters, J. M.: Experiments of the significance of articular function as a stimulating chondrogenic factor for the growth of secondary cartilages of the rat mandible. Eur. Orthod. Soc. Trans. *1971*:103–115, 1972.

Engel, M. B., and Brodie, A. G.: Condylar growth and mandibular deformities. Surgery *22*:976–992, 1947.

Engel, M. B., Richmond, J. B., and Brodie, A. G.: Mandibular growth disturbance in rheumatoid arthritis of childhood. Am. J. Dis. Child. *78*:728–743, 1949.

Enlow, D. H.: Role of the temporomandibular joint in facial growth and development. In Laskin, D., Greenfield, W., and Gale, F. (Eds.): The President's Conference on the Examination, Diagnosis, and Management of Temporomandibular Disorders. Am. Dent. Assoc. Publ., pp 13–16, 1983.

Frommer, J.: Prenatal development of the mandibular joint in mice. Anat. Rec. *150*:449–461, 1964.

Furstman, L.: The early development of the human temporomandibular joint. Am. J. Orthod. *49*:672–682, 1963.

Gans, B. J., and Sarnat, B. G.: Sutural facial growth of the *Macaca rhesus* monkey: A gross and serial roentgenographic study by means of metallic implants. Am. J. Orthod. *37*:827–841, 1951.

Gianelly, A. A., and Moorrees, C. F. A.: Condylectomy in the rat. Arch. Oral. Biol. *10*:101–106, 1965.

Glasstone, S.: Differentiation of the mouse embryonic mandible and squamo-mandibular joint in organ culture. Arch. Oral. Biol. *16*:723–727, 1971.

Greenspan, J. S., and Blackwood, H. J.: Histochemical studies of chondrocyte function in the cartilage of the mandibular condyle of the rat. J. Anat. *100*:615–626, 1966.

Hall, B. K.: In vitro studies on the mechanical evocation of adventitious cartilage in the chick. J. Exp. Zool. *168*:283–306, 1968.

Jarabak, J. R., and Thompson, J. R.: Cephalometric appraisal of the cranium and mandible of the rat following condylar resection. J. Dent. Res. *28*:655–656, 1949.

Kanouse, M. C., Ramfjord, S. P., and Nasjleti, C. E.: Condylar growth in rhesus monkeys. J. Dent. Res. *48*:1171–1176, 1969.

Koski, K.: Cranial growth centers: Facts or fallacies? Am. J. Orthod. *54*:566–583, 1968.

Koski, K.: The mandibular complex. Eur. Orthod. Soc. Trans. 53–67, 1974.

Koski, K., and Makinen, L.: Growth potential of transplanted components of the mandibular ramus of the rat. I. Suom. Hammaslaak. Toim. *59*:296–308, 1963.

Koski, K., and Mason, K. E.: Growth potential of transplanted components of the mandibular ramus of the rat. II. Suom. Hammaslaak. Toim. *60*:209–218, 1964.

Koski, K., and Rönning, O.: Growth potential of transplanted components of the mandibular ramus of the rat. III. Suom. Hammaslaak. Toim. *61*:292–297, 1965.

Latham, R. A.: Maxillary development and growth: The septo-premaxillary ligament. J. Anat. *107*:471–478, 1970.

Levy, B. M.: Growth of mandibular joint in normal mice. JADA *36*:177–182, 1948.

Long, R., Greulich, R. C., and Sarnat, B. G.: Regional variations in chondrocyte proliferation in the cartilaginous nasal septum of the growing rabbit. J. Dent. Res. *47*:505, 1968.

Meikle, M. C.: The role of the condyle in the postnatal growth of the mandible. Am. J. Orthod. *64*:50–62, 1973.

Melcher, A. M.: Behaviour of cells and condylar cartilage of foetal mouse mandible maintained in vitro. Arch. Oral. Biol. *16*:1379–1391, 1971.

Moffett, B. C., Johnson, L. C., McCabe, J. B., and Askew, H. C.: Articular remodeling in the adult human temporomandibular joint. Am. J. Anat. *115*:119–142, 1964.

Moss, M. L.: Embryology, growth and malformations of the temporomandibular joint. In Schwartz, L. (Ed.): Disorders of the Temporomandibular Joint. Philadelphia, W.B. Saunders, 1959.

Moss, M. L.: Functional analysis of human mandibular growth. J. Prosthet. Dent. *10*:1149–1159, 1960.

Moss, M. L.: The functional matrix. In Kraus, B. S., and Riedel, R. A. (Eds.): Vistas of Orthodontics. Philadelphia, Lea & Febiger, 1962.

Moss, M. L.: Neurotrophic processes in orofacial growth. J. Dent. Res. *50*:1492–1494, 1971.

Moss, M. L., and Salentijn, L.: The primary role of functional matrices in facial growth. Am. J. Orthod. *55*:566–577, 1969.

Perry, H. T.: The temporomandibular joint. Am. J. Orthod. *52*:399–400, 1966.

Perry, H. T.: Relation of occlusion to temporomandibular joint dysfunction: The orthodontic viewpoint. JADA *79*:137–141, 1969.

Petrovic, A., and Hermann-Stutzmann, J.: Le muscle pterygoidien externe et la croissance du condyle mandibulaire. Recherches experimentales chez je jeune rat. Orthod. Fr. *43*:271–281, 1972.

Petrovic, A., Hermann-Stutzmann, J., and Oudet, C.: Control processes in the postnatal growth of the mandibular condylar cartilage. In McNamara, J. A., Jr. (Ed.): Determinants of Mandibular Form and Growth. Craniofacial Growth Series. Monograph no. 4. Center for Human Growth and Development, University of Michigan Press, Ann Arbor, MI, 1975.

Petrovic, A., Oudet, C., and Gasson, N.: Effects des appareils de propulsion et de retropulsion mandibulaire sur le nombre des sarcomeres en serie du muscle pterygoidien extrene et sur la croissance du cartilage condylien de jeune rat. Orthod. Fr. *44*:191–212, 1973.

Pimenidis, M. A., and Gianelly, A. A.: The effects of early postnatal condylectomy on the growth of the mandible. Am. J. Orthod. *62*:42–46, 1972.

Poswillo, D. E.: The late effects of mandibular condylectomy. Oral Surg. *33*:500–512, 1972.

Rees, L. A.: The structure and function of the temporomandibular joint. Br. Dent. J. *96*:125–133, 1954.

Robinson, I. B., and Sarnat, B. G.: Growth pattern of the

pig mandible. A serial roentgenographic study using metallic implants. Am. J. Anat. 96:37–64, 1955.

Rönning, O.: Observations on the intracerebral transplantation of the mandibular condyle. Acta Odontol. Scand. 24:443–457, 1966.

Rönning, O., and Koski, K.: The effect of the articular disc on the growth of condylar cartilage transplants. Eur. Orthod. Soc. Trans. 1969:99–108, 1970.

Rönning, O., and Koski, K.: The effect of periostomy on the growth of the condylar process in the rat. Proc. Finn. Dent. Soc. 70:28–29, 1974.

Rönning, O., Paunio, K., and Koski, K.: Observations on the histology, histochemistry and biochemistry of growth cartilages in young rats. Suom. Hammaslaak. Toim. 63:187–195, 1967.

Salzmann, J. A.: Practice of Orthodontics. Philadelphia, J. B. Lippincott, 1966.

Sarnat, B. G.: Facial and neurocranial growth after removal of the mandibular condyle in the Macaca rhesus monkey. Am. J. Surg. 94:19–30, 1957.

Sarnat, B. G.: Postnatal growth of the upper face: Some experimental considerations. Angle. Orthod. 33:139–161, 1963.

Sarnat, B. G.: The Temporomandibular Joint, 2nd ed. Springfield, IL, Charles C Thomas, 1964.

Sarnat, B. G.: The face and jaws after surgical experimentation with the septovomeral region in growing and adult rabbits. Acta Otolaryngol. [Suppl.] 268:1–30, 1970.

Sarnat, B. G.: Clinical and experimental considerations in facial bone biology: Growth, remodeling, and repair. JADA 82:876–889, 1971.

Sarnat, B. G.: Surgical experimentation and gross postnatal growth of the face and jaws. J. Dent. Res. 50:1462–1476, 1971.

Sarnat, B. G.: Growth pattern of the mandible: Some reflections. Am. J. Orthod. Dentofacial Orthop. 90:221–233, 1986.

Sarnat, B. G., and Engel, M. B.: A serial study of mandibular growth after the removal of the condyle of the rhesus monkey. Plast. Reconstr. Surg. 7:364–380, 1951.

Sarnat, B. G., and Greeley, P. W.: Effect of injury upon growth and some comments on surgical treatment. Plast. Reconstr. Surg. 11:39–48, 1953.

Sarnat, B. G., and Muchnic, H.: Facial skeletal changes after mandibular condylectomy in the adult monkey. J. Anat. 108:323–338, 1971.

Sarnat, B. G., and Shanedling, P. D.: Postnatal growth of the orbit and upper face in rabbits. Arch. Ophthalmol. 73:829–837, 1965.

Sarnat, B. G., and Wexler, M. R.: Growth of the face and jaws after resection of the septal cartilage in the rabbit. Am. J. Anat. 118:755–767, 1966.

Silbermann, M., and Frommer, J.: Further evidence for the vitality of chondrocytes in the mandibular condyle as revealed by ^{35}S-sulfate autoradiography. Anat. Rec. 174:503–511, 1972.

Silbermann, M., and Frommer, J.: Vitality of chondrocytes in the mandibular condyle as revealed by collagen formation. An autoradiographic study with ^{3}H-proline. Am. J. Anat. 135:359–370, 1972.

Silbermann, M., and Frommer, J.: The nature of endochondral ossification in the mandibular condyle of the mouse. Anat. Rec. 172:659–667, 1972.

Thilander, B.: The structure of the collagen of the temporomandibular joint disc in man. Acta Odontol. Scand. 22:135–149, 1969.

Washburn, S. L.: The relation of the temporal muscle to the form of the skull. Anat. Rec. 99:239–248, 1947.

Wright, D. M., and Moffett, B. C.: The postnatal development of the human temporomandibular joint. Am. J. Anat. 141:231–250, 1974.

Yuodelis, R. A.: The morphogenesis of the human temporomandibular joint and its associated structures. J. Dent. Res. 45:182–191, 1966.

5

FUNCTIONAL ANATOMY*,**

WILLIAM L. HYLANDER, D.D.S., PH.D.

TEMPOROMANDIBULAR JOINT PROPER

Articulating Bodies

The temporomandibular, or craniomandibular, articulation is the articulation between the lower jaw and the cranium. The bony elements of this articulation are the mandibular condyles below and the squamous temporal bones above. This articulation consists of two synovial joints: a left and right *temporomandibular joint (TMJ)*.

The TMJ is a complex joint both morphologically and functionally. An articular disc composed of dense fibrous tissue is interposed between the temporal bone and the mandible, dividing the articular space into an upper and lower compartment. Gliding movements occur primarily in the upper compartment, while the lower compartment primarily functions as a

---

*Based in part on Harry Sicher's Chapter, Functional Anatomy of the Temporomandibular Joint. *In* Sarnat B.G. (Ed.): The Temporomandibular Joint, 2nd ed. Springfield, IL, Charles C Thomas, 1964.
**See Chapters 1 through 7, 9, 11, 19, 21, 23, 24, 26.

hinge joint. Therefore, the TMJ is often classified as a hinge joint with a movable socket.

Most synovial joints have hyaline cartilage
lining their articulating surfaces. In contrast,
the articulating surfaces of the TMJ are lined
by dense, avascular, fibrous connective tissue.
The presence of this type of tissue has often
been interpreted as indicating that the TMJ
must not bear any stress because known stress-
bearing synovial joints are lined by hyaline
cartilage. Over the last 15 to 20 years, however,
a considerable amount of evidence has accumulated indicating that the TMJ is a stress-
bearing joint (Hylander, 1985b). If so, then why
does this joint have such peculiar articular tissues? The answer to this question is directly
related to the evolutionary history of this joint
(see Chapter 1), which in turn is reflected in
its early ontogeny.

The bones of a typical synovial joint are
cartilage-replacement bones that are initially
preformed in hyaline cartilage. Most of this
cartilage is eventually lost and replaced by bone
during ontogeny, but the cartilage lining the
articular surfaces persists, although in a modified form. In contrast, the bones of the TMJ
are dermal bones. Rather than being preformed
in cartilage, they are formed directly from intramembranous centers of ossification. These
developing bones become completely surrounded by periosteum, including the areas that
eventually form the articular surfaces of the
TMJ. The periosteum lining these articular surfaces is gradually transformed during its early
development into the dense fibrous articular
tissues of the TMJ, and articular forces acting
through the TMJ play an important role in this
gradual transformation. Articular forces also
continue to play a major role in the development of these tissues well into adult life (Bouvier, 1982).

Thus, the lack of hyaline cartilage on the
articular surfaces of the TMJ simply reflects its
unique ontogenetic (and phylogenetic) development, rather than indicating that this joint is
incapable of bearing articular reaction force.
Parenthetically, although there is a secondary
cartilage in the condyle of the growing mandible, this cartilage does not form part of the
articular surface because it is also covered by
the periosteum-derived fibrous articular tissues
(Duterloo, 1970).

Mandibular Condyle

The articular surface of the mandible is the
upper and anterior surface of the condyle (Fig.

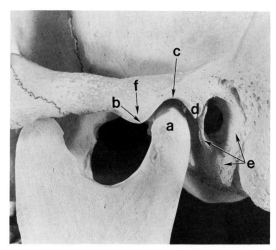

FIGURE 5–1. Lateral view of the skull with the mandibular
condyle pulled out of the glenoid fossa: mandibular condyle
(a), crest of the articular eminence (b), roof of the glenoid
fossa (c), postglenoid process (d), tympanic portion of the
temporal bone (e), and location of the articular tubercle (f).

5–1). The adult condyle is about 15 to 20 mm
from side to side and 8 to 10 mm from front to
back. Its long axis is at right angles to the plane
of the mandibular ramus. Because of the flare
of the ramus, however, the long axes of the left
and right condyles cross approximately at the
anterior margin of the foramen magnum, forming an obtuse angle varying from 145 to 160
degrees.

The articular surface of the condyle is strongly
convex when viewed from the side and less so
when viewed from the front. The articular surface faces upward and forward so that in side
view the neck of the condyloid process seems
to be bent forward. The articular convexity, seen
from in front, often resembles a tent-like configuration that is divided into a medial and lateral
slope by a variably prominent crest. The lateral
pole of the condyle extends slightly beyond the
outer surface of the ramus and is roughened for
the attachment of the articular disc and the
temporomandibular ligament (TML). The medial
pole of the condyle juts considerably beyond
the inner surface of the ramus and is also slightly
roughened for the attachment of the articular
disc. Variations in the shape of the condyle are
frequent. Some of the irregularities of the articular surface apparently are obscured and
smoothed by the thick covering of fibrous tissue
that is derived from and directly continuous
with the mandibular periosteum.

Glenoid or Mandibular Fossa, Articular
Fossa, and Articular Eminence

Frequently the names *glenoid fossa*, *mandibular fossa*, and *articular fossa* are used inter-

changeably. The glenoid, or mandibular, fossa is the concavity within the temporal bone that houses the mandibular condyle. Its anterior wall is formed by the articular eminence of the squamous temporal and its posterior wall by the tympanic plate, which also forms the anterior wall of the external acoustic meatus. The bony roof of the glenoid fossa is quite thin and often appears translucent when held against the light. This is but one indication that the roof of this fossa is not a major stress-bearing portion of the TMJ.

The articular fossa is that portion of the glenoid fossa that is lined by articular tissues. It is formed entirely by the squamous temporal (Figs. 5–1 and 5–2). The posterior part of the articular fossa is elevated to a ridge called the *posterior articular lip*. In most individuals the posterior articular lip is higher and thicker at its lateral end and thus is seen from the side as a cone-shaped process between the articular fossa and tympanic plate (Figs. 5–1 and 5–3). This structure is the *postglenoid process*. The lateral border of the articular fossa is sometimes marked by a narrow, low ridge. Medially, the articular fossa is bounded by a bony plate that leans against the spine of the sphenoid bone (Fig. 5–2). This medial plate is sometimes drawn out into a triangular process, the *temporal spine*.

In the back and lateral part of the glenoid fossa, a fissure separates the tympanic portion from the squamous portion of the temporal bone. This fissure, which is called the *tympa-*

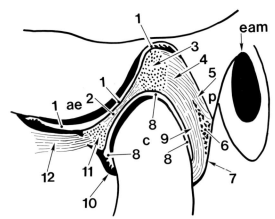

FIGURE 5–3. Parasagittal section of the TMJ: mandibular condyle (c), postglenoid process (p), external auditory meatus (eam), articular eminence (ae), upper joint compartment (1), the intermediate zone (2), the posterior band (3), the bilaminar zone (4), upper portion of bilaminar zone (5), spongy tissue with a profuse nerve and blood supply (6), posterior portion of joint capsule (7), lower joint compartment (8), lower portion of bilaminar zone (9), anterior portion of joint capsule (10), anterior band (11), and small portion of the superior head of the lateral pterygoid muscle (12). Note the thick dense fibrous avascular tissues covering the articular eminence and the mandibular condyle.

nosquamosal fissure, separates the articular from the nonarticular portion of the glenoid fossa (Fig. 5–2). Medial to this fissure a bony plate of the petrous temporal, the tegmen tympani, protrudes between the tympanic and squamous portions. Therefore, instead of a tympanosquamosal fissure along the medial aspect of the glenoid fossa, there is an anterior *petrosquamosal fissure* and a posterior *petrotympanic fissure*. The petrotympanic fissure is slightly widened laterally to permit the passage of the chorda tympani nerve and the anterior tympanic blood vessels.

It is important to make a distinction between the *articular eminence* and the *articular tubercle*. The articular eminence is the transverse bar of dense bone that forms the posterior root of the zygomatic arch and the anterior wall of the articular fossa. It has a large articular surface. The articular tubercle is the small bony projection situated laterally to the articular eminence. The articular tubercle is not an articular surface. Instead, it serves as the attachment area for portions of the TML.

The articular eminence is somewhat saddle-shaped. It is strongly convex in a side view and moderately concave when viewed from the front or back. The degree of this convexity and concavity is highly variable. The medial and lateral borders of the articular eminence are often accentuated by fine bony ridges. The anterior

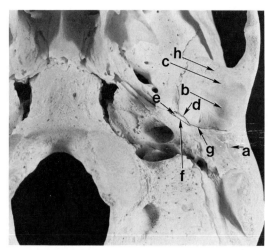

FIGURE 5–2. Basal view of left side of human cranium: external auditory meatus (a), glenoid fossa (b), articular eminence (c), petrosquamous fissure (d), tegmen tympani (e), petrotympanic fissure (f), tympanosquamous fissure (g), and preglenoid plane (h); (d), (f), and (g) have been darkened with an ink pen.

slope of the eminence, the *preglenoid plane*, rises gently from the infratemporal surface of the cranial base; its precise anterior boundary is often indistinct. The condyle and disc move anterior to the summit of the eminence and onto the preglenoid plane during wide opening. The gentle anterior slope facilitates movements of the mandibular condyle and disc posteriorly from this anterior position.

Although the roof of the glenoid fossa is covered by a thin layer of fibrous tissue, the fibrous tissue covering the articular eminence is thicker and quite firm (Fig. 5–3). Moreover, unlike the roof, the articular eminence is composed of a fairly thick layer of dense bone. These morphological characteristics reinforce the hypothesis that the articular eminence transmits most of the routine joint reaction force developed between the mandible and the squamous temporal.

Articular Disc

The articular disc is derived ontogenetically from a mesenchymal block of tissue that also gives rise to the capsule of the TMJ and the lateral pterygoid muscle (Van der Linden, 1987). This tissue mass is positioned between the developing squamous temporal and mandibular condyle. In adults the uppermost portion of the lateral pterygoid muscle usually, but not always, still retains its original connection to the capsule and articular disc of the TMJ (Harpman, 1938).

The articular disc is a firm, oval, fibrous plate positioned between the mandibular condyle and the articular fossa and eminence (Fig. 5–3). Its central part, the intermediate zone, is considerably thinner than its periphery, the anterior and posterior bands. Anteriorly the disc is fused to the capsule of the TMJ. Posteriorly the disc continues as the bilaminar zone, a thick double layer of vascularized connective tissue. The bilaminar zone splits into two parts: (1) an upper fibroelastic layer that attaches to the postglenoid process, posterior articular lip, and tympanosquamosal fissure; and (2) a lower fibrous layer that attaches to the posterior portion of the condylar neck immediately below the articular tissues. Posteriorly these two layers are separated by loose connective tissues that attach to the posterior wall of the joint capsule (Fig. 5–3). Both the bilaminar zone and the loose connective tissues have a profuse supply of nerves and blood vessels (Griffin, 1960; Rees, 1954).

The disc is not attached to the capsule later-ally or medially. Instead, it is tightly bound directly to the medial and lateral poles of the mandibular condyle. It is these attachments of the disc that cause it to move with the mandibular condyle. It is often stated that the position of the disc relative to the condyle may be influenced by the pull of the superior head of the lateral pterygoid muscle because a small portion of this muscle often attaches to the disc. Thus, contraction of the superior head of the lateral pterygoid is thought to protract the disc anteromedially or limit posterolateral retraction movements of the disc. The influence of this muscle on the articular disc, however, is not a settled issue. Since the superior head of the lateral pterygoid also attaches to the mandibular condyle, it has been suggested that this muscle has no special influence on movements of the articular disc relative to the condyle (Meyenberg, 1986; Wilkinson, 1988).

Blood vessels and nerves are absent in the intermediate zone, i.e., the firm central region of the articular disc, as well as in the avascular fibrous layers covering both the mandibular and temporal articular surfaces of the joints. The lack of these neurovascular structures is compatible with the hypothesis that there is considerable reaction force along this portion of the joint.

Articular Capsule and Ligaments

The fibrous capsule of the TMJ is attached to the squamous temporal along the limits of the articular surface of the articular eminence and fossa. Posteriorly, the capsule arises from the postglenoid process, posterior articular lip, and tympanosquamosal fissure. Whereas the articular capsule is quite thin anteromedially, medially, and posteriorly, it is thicker anterolaterally and laterally where it attaches to the articular tubercle (DuBrul, 1988). This reinforced lateral portion of the capsule is called the temporomandibular ligament (TML) (Fig. 5–4).

The anatomy of the capsular and TMLs of the TMJ is somewhat controversial. The TML has been described by DuBrul as being divided into two layers: a wide, fan-shaped superficial portion and a narrow deep portion. The broad origin of the superficial portion and its narrow attachment to the mandibular neck account for its fan-shaped morphology. Its anterior fibers run obliquely down and back, while the posterior fibers have a more vertical orientation. Fibers of the deep portion are said to run horizontally, and this portion is described as a

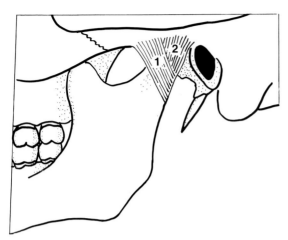

FIGURE 5–4. Lateral view of the temporomandibular (1) and capsular (2) ligaments. Most of the fibers of these ligaments are either aligned vertically or downward and backward, although some are also aligned horizontally.

ligamentous band that attaches along the lateral pole of the mandibular condyle and extends to a crest situated along the articular tubercle (DuBrul, 1988).

In contrast to DuBrul's descriptions, Savelle (1988) suggests that the morphology of the lateral portion of the temporomandibular capsule is highly variable, and that in most instances (13 of 16 dissected joints) the lateral aspect of the capsule is not reinforced by a well-developed TML. The author's (WLH) recent dissections indicated a well-developed TML in

all five specimens examined. In addition, the TML in these dissections extended along the anterolateral portion of the TMJ and therefore, unlike most descriptions, it is not limited to only the lateral aspect of this joint. The anterolateral portion passes in close proximity to the anterior part of the lateral pole of the condyle. The deep horizontal band described by DuBrul (1988) is apparently part of the lateral aspect of the joint capsule (Wilkinson, 1988).

The joint capsule and its TML function to limit movements of the mandible (Fig. 5–5). These structures help prevent the mandibular condyle from being pulled away from the articular eminence, and the horizontally aligned fibers prevent excessive retrusive movements of the condyle. Finally, the anterior part of the capsule and the anterolateral part of the TML may help limit the amount of condylar rotation during mouth opening.

The synovial membrane, a highly vascularized layer of connective tissue, lines all structures of the articulation that do not experience compressive reaction force. The largest area of synovial lining covers the upper and lower surfaces of the bilaminar zone and the loose connective tissue binding the posterior border of the disc to the capsule. Synovial tissue also lines the inner aspect of the fibrous capsule. When the condyle is positioned in the glenoid fossa, the synovial membrane forms rather heavy folds posteriorly. As the condyle is pro-

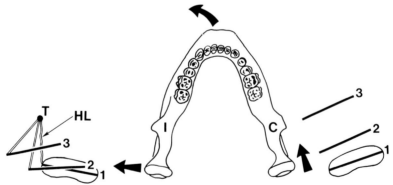

FIGURE 5–5. Mandible during left lateral movement. I and C indicate position of ipsilateral and contralateral sides, respectively. HL indicates the horizontal components of the temporomandibular capsular ligament that attach to the lateral pole of the mandibular condyle and the articular tubercle (T). Position 1: The ipsilateral and contralateral condyles just before movement. Position 2: The left lateral movement is initiated. The ipsilateral condyle first rotates about a vertical axis that passes through its center. Then, the horizontal component of the temporomandibular ligament becomes taut and prevents the lateral pole of the ipsilateral condyle from moving any further posteriorly. This condyle now shifts slightly laterally. The contralateral condyle translates medially, anteriorly, and downward. Position 3: With continued movement, the ipsilateral condyle now has shifted further laterally, slightly anteriorly, and downward along the articular eminence. The horizontal components of the temporomandibular ligament guide this movement. The contralateral condyle continues to translate medially, anteriorly, and downward. The relative amount of rotation of the ipsilateral condyle has been exaggerated. The arrows indicate the direction of movement of the chin and the ipsilateral and contralateral mandibular condyles. (Redrawn from DuBrul, 1988.)

truded toward the summit of the articular eminence, the folds disappear as these tissues are stretched.

The blood supply to the capsule and disc of the TMJ is supplied mainly by branches from the superficial temporal artery. The sensory nerves for proprioception and pain are branches of the auriculotemporal, deep temporal, and masseteric nerves (see Chapter 7). Blood vessels and nerves are numerous in the posterior portions of the articular disc and fibrous capsule (see Chapter 3).

Accessory Ligaments

Two structures have been described as accessory ligaments of the temporomandibular articulation: the sphenomandibular and the stylomandibular ligaments.

Sphenomandibular Ligament

The *sphenomandibular ligament* is derived from Meckel's cartilage. It arises from the spine of the sphenoid bone and is directed downward and outward (Fig. 5–6). It inserts on the mandible at the mandibular lingula, which is located along the upper border of the mandibular foramen. It also inserts along the lower border of the groove of the condylar neck. In most individuals the sphenomandibular ligament is a thin

layer of connective tissue with indistinct anterior and posterior borders. It has been suggested that this ligament protects the blood vessels and nerves passing through the mandibular foramen from tensile stress during mouth opening and closing (Moss, 1959).

Stylomandibular Ligament

The *stylomandibular ligament* is a reinforced sheet of cervical fascia that extends from the styloid process and stylohyoid ligament to the region of the mandibular angle (Fig. 5–6). Some of its fibers are attached to the lower part of the mandibular ramus, but the majority continue onto the fascia along the medial surface of the medial pterygoid muscle. The upper border of the stylomandibular ligament is often thickened considerably. This ligament is loose when the mouth is both closed and wide open; it is tense only when the mandible is maximally protruded. Thus, this ligament appears to limit excessive protrusive movements.

MUSCLES OF THE MANDIBLE

Four powerful muscles, the masseter, the temporalis, the medial pterygoid, and the lateral pterygoid, are often referred to as the muscles of mastication. These muscles, in conjunction with groups of muscles of the face, tongue, palate, and hyoid bone, function in a coordinated manner during mastication. This chapter will not attempt to deal with all these muscle groups, although it will consider the morphology and function of the most important muscles that play a role in mandibular movements.

Masseter

The *masseter* muscle (Figs. 5–7 and 5–8) stretches as a rectangular plate from the zygomatic arch to the outer surface of the mandibular ramus. The muscle is divided into a superficial portion and a smaller deep portion. The superficial portion arises from the lower border of the zygomatic bone as strong tendinous fibers. The most anterior fibers may arise from the outer corner of the zygomatic process of the maxilla. Posteriorly the origin of the superficial portion ends along the zygomaticotemporal suture. In side view the muscle fibers of the superficial masseter are directed downward and backward to insert along the angle of the mandible. In a frontal view it can be seen that the

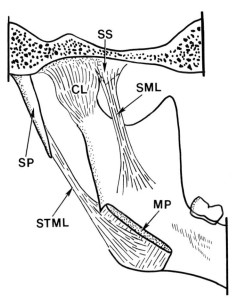

FIGURE 5–6. A medial view of the mandible and the sphenomandibular and stylomandibular ligaments: sphenoidal spine (SS), sphenomandibular ligament (SML), styloid process (SP), stylomandibular ligament (STML), capsular ligament (CL), and medial pterygoid muscle (MP).

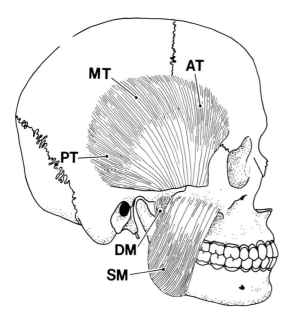

FIGURE 5–7. The masseter and temporalis muscles: deep masseter (DM), superficial masseter (SM), anterior temporalis (AT), middle temporalis (MT), and posterior temporalis (PT).

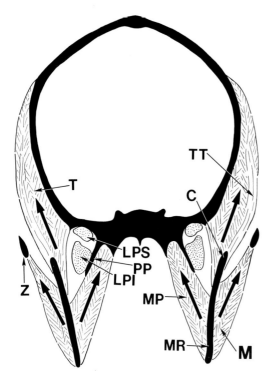

FIGURE 5–8. Coronal section of the muscles of mastication: temporalis (T), tendon of temporalis (TT), zygomatic arch (Z), coronoid process (C), mandibular ramus (MR), masseter (M), medial pterygoid (MP), pterygoid process (lateral) (PP), lateral pterygoid-superior head (LPS), and lateral pterygoid-inferior head (LPI). The large arrows indicate the general direction of pull of the anterior temporalis, superficial masseter, and medial pterygoid muscles.

masseter is directed downward and medially (Fig. 5–8). The mandibular attachment of the superficial masseter extends along the lower third of the posterior border of the ramus and along the lower border of the mandible anterior to the level of the third molar, and it covers, more or less, the lower half of the outer surface of the ramus. The field of insertion has ridges into which the tendons insert and grooves between the ridges into which the fleshy fibers insert.

The superficial masseter is covered on its outer surface by a strong tendinous layer that extends down from the zygomatic bone over the upper third or half of the muscle. The tendon ends with a downwardly convex border or in a zigzag line. If the overlying tissues are not too thick, the border of this tendon can be seen during mastication as the flat tendon contrasts with the muscle bundles bulging below the tendon. Alternating tendinous and fleshy bundles are present within the superficial portion. Thus, the structure of this muscle is rather intricate, and it is often referred to as a multipinnate muscle.

If the superficial masseter muscle is strongly developed, the area of its insertion is slightly widened, giving the anterior border of the muscle a concave appearance when viewed from the side. Posteriorly the fibers of the superficial masseter may wrap around the angle of the mandible, joining fibers of the medial pterygoid muscle in a tendinous raphe. This muscular arrangement is called the pterygomasseteric sling.

The deep and superficial portions of the masseter fuse anteriorly, but posteriorly the two can be separated. The fibers of the deep portion arise from the entire length of the zygomatic arch up to the anterior slope of the articular eminence. Some of its fibers may also arise from the lateral wall of the TMJ capsule (Meyenberg, 1986; Widmalm, 1987). The deep masseter inserts above the superficial masseter along the mandibular ramus as a triangular-shaped insertion field. The base of this triangle faces posteriorly while the apex faces anteriorly. In side view the fibers of the deep masseter, which have a near vertical alignment, pass downward at an angle of about 30 to 40 degrees to the fibers of the more obliquely aligned superficial masseter.

The masseter muscle is a powerful elevator of the mandible. When viewed from the side it is evident that the deep masseter exerts primarily a vertical force on the mandible. In contrast, the superficial masseter exerts a vertical and slightly anteriorly directed force on the mandible that is approximately perpendicular to the occlusal plane of the molars (Fig. 5–7). The entire masseter, particularly the deep portion, also exerts a lateral component of force on the mandible.

The masseter muscle is derived from the first branchial arch, and therefore it is innervated by the fifth cranial nerve, the trigeminal (V). More specifically, it is innervated by the masseteric nerve, which is a small branch from the mandibular or third division of the trigeminal (V_3). The masseteric nerve passes above the lateral pterygoid muscle, and then, after passing through the mandibular notch behind the tendon of the temporalis muscle, it enters the medial surface of the deep masseter muscle. The masseteric nerve supplies the deep masseter, perforates it, and then enters the superficial masseter.

Temporalis

The fan-shaped *temporalis* muscle (Figs. 5–7, 5–8, and 5–9) has its origin along the lateral surface of the skull and the dense fascia overlying this muscle. The bony attachment field, the temporal fossa, is encircled above by the inferior temporal line. This attachment field includes a narrow strip of the parietal bone, the greater part of the temporal squama, the temporal surface of the frontal bone, and the temporal surface of the greater wing of the sphenoid bone. Muscle fibers and tendons also arise from the postorbital septum, which is the bony par-

tition separating the temporal fossa from the orbit. Both the zygomatic and frontal bones and the greater wing of the sphenoid contribute to the formation of the postorbital septum. The bony field of origin of the temporalis reaches downward to include the infratemporal crest of the sphenoid.

Many of the temporalis muscle fibers originate from the inner surface of the temporalis fascia. The temporalis fascia is set in a frame formed by the superior temporal line and the upper border of the zygomatic arch. Passing downward from the superior temporal line, the temporalis fascia thickens considerably and then splits into two layers; the superficial layer continues into the periosteum of the zygomatic arch along its outer surface, and the deep layer extends into the periosteum of the zygomatic arch along its inner surface. Superficial and deep layers are joined by irregular bands of connective tissue. The outer layer is stronger and, when palpated, gives the impression of bone. The inner layer is thin and, in some areas, is strengthened by aponeurotic fibers from which bundles of the temporalis muscle originate.

The bundles of the temporalis muscle converge toward the opening between the zygomatic arch and the lateral surface of the skull, in the center of which the tip of the coronoid process is situated. The anterior fibers of the temporalis, which form the major bulk of this muscle, are vertical; the fibers in the center of the muscle are increasingly oblique (Fig. 5–7). The most posterior fibers run forward almost horizontally, bend around the posterior root of the zygomatic arch in front of the articular eminence, and pass downward vertically to the mandible. The flesh of the temporalis muscle is divided unequally by a tendinous plate that is partially visible along the lateral aspect of this muscle (Figs. 5–8 and 5–9). Most of the fibers of the temporalis are situated medially to this plate. Muscle fibers arise from the temporalis fascia laterally and the skull medially and insert into this plate. Therefore, this muscle is often characterized as being bipinnate. The fibers of the temporalis muscle are actually much shorter than most illustrations indicate, although they are longer than those of the masseter muscle.

The middle and posterior portions of the temporalis muscle are attached, respectively along the apex of the coronoid process and along its posterior slope to the deepest point of the mandibular notch. The more superficial fibers of the anterior temporalis muscle insert along the apex of the coronoid process and

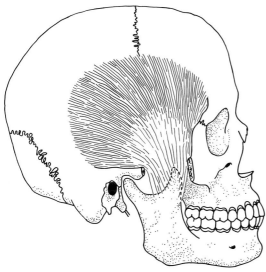

FIGURE 5–9. The temporalis muscle. The masseter muscle and the zygomatic arch have been removed.

along the anterior surface of the coronoid process and mandibular ramus. The deeper fibers of the anterior temporalis attach along the medial surface of the mandibular ramus. These two groups of fibers send two tendons far down toward the posterior end of the alveolar process and are separated from each other by a downwardly widening cleft. The inner or deep tendon, which juts medially from the mandibular ramus and reaches downward into the region of the lower third molar, is stronger and longer than the superficial tendon, which is attached to the anterior border of the coronoid process and mandibular ramus. The area of the mandible between the superficial and deep tendons is the retromolar fossa.

Similar to the masseter muscle, the temporalis muscle mainly elevates the mandible. Its fan-shaped morphology indicates that its direction of pull can vary considerably, depending on which muscle fibers are active. It appears that its most posterior fibers should be able to retract the mandible because of their horizontal orientation along the side of the skull; however, these fibers are bent around the posterior root of the zygomatic arch and thus are oriented essentially in a vertical manner. Therefore, this portion of the temporalis muscle exerts primarily an upward or vertical force on the mandible. Because its fibers pass close to the articular eminence, it probably also functions as a stabilizer of the TMJ. The middle oblique portion of the temporalis muscle is capable of exerting a vertical and retracting force on the mandible. Most of the anterior portion is capable of a vertical pull on the mandible. That portion of the anterior temporalis originating from the postorbital septum pulls the mandible upward and slightly forward. Finally, the deep fibers of the anterior temporalis that originate along and just above the infratemporal crest pull the mandible upward and somewhat medially. Thus, the morphology of the entire temporalis muscle indicates that its fibers are capable of considerable variability in their direction of pull.

The temporalis muscle is innervated by the deep temporal branches of the anterior trunk of V_3. Of the three deep temporal nerves ordinarily present, the posterior and middle branches arise as separate filaments from the anterior trunk immediately after the trigeminal nerve emerges through the foramen ovale. The anterior branch is initially united with the buccal nerve; this common trunk, which lies in a sulcus adjacent to the foramen ovale, runs close to the base of the skull anteriorly and laterally. It is held in place by a ligament that bridges the sulcus. If this ligament ossifies, it contributes to the formation of the temporobuccal foramen. The anterior temporal nerve usually separates from the buccal nerve after the buccal nerve has passed between the two heads of the lateral pterygoid muscle.

Medial Pterygoid

The *medial pterygoid* muscle (Figs. 5–8 and 5–10), which is situated on the medial side of the mandibular ramus, appears to be the anatomical counterpart of the masseter muscle when viewed from the side. It is a powerful rectangular muscle, although it is smaller than the masseter. Its main origin is in the pterygoid fossa, which is the depression that is located between the back edges of the medial and lateral pterygoid plates of the sphenoid bone. The innermost fibers arise by strong tendons, while others arise directly from the medial surface of the lateral pterygoid plate. A flat tendon covers the medial surface of the muscle at its origin, and it is as wide as the tensor veli palatini muscle, with which it is in contact. The most anterior fibers of the medial pterygoid arise from the outer and inferior surface of the pyramidal process of the palatine bone and from the adjacent parts of the maxillary tuberosity.

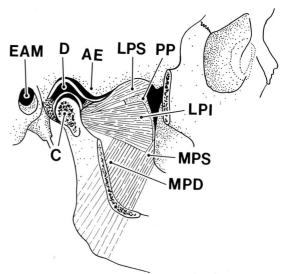

FIGURE 5–10. The medial and lateral pterygoid muscles: mandibular condyle (C), external auditory meatus (EAM), articular disc (D), articular eminence (AE), lateral pterygoid-superior head (LPS), pterygoid plate (lateral) (PP), lateral pterygoid-inferior head (LPI), medial pterygoid-superficial portion (MPS), and medial pterygoid-deep portion (MPD). The zygomatic arch and coronoid process have been removed and the TMJ has been sectioned parasagittally.

These fibers, which are referred to as the superficial head of the medial pterygoid, are positioned laterally to the lateral pterygoid muscle. The remaining and largest portion of this muscle, the deep head, is positioned medially to the lateral pterygoid muscle (Fig. 5–10).

The medial pterygoid muscle runs downward, backward, and laterally and is inserted along the medial surface of the angle of the mandible. The field of insertion is approximately triangular and is located between the mandibular angle and the mylohyoid groove. As noted earlier, the fibers of the medial pterygoid muscle often meet fibers of the masseter in a tendinous raphe behind and below the mandibular angle (the pterygomasseteric sling).

The internal structure of the medial pterygoid muscle is a complicated alternation of fleshy and tendinous parts similar to the temporalis and masseter. The muscle fibers, arising from one tendon and ending on another, are arranged at an angle to the general orientation of the muscle. This bipinnate or multipinnate arrangement gives the muscle fibers of the medial pterygoid (and also the masseter and temporalis) a braided appearance and tends to increase their capability for generating powerful forces.

The overall fiber orientation of the medial pterygoid muscle in side view is similar to the superficial portion of the masseter muscle, and therefore it is primarily an elevator of the mandible. However, unlike the masseter, which exerts a lateral component of force on the mandible, the medial pterygoid exerts a medial component of force on the mandible.

The nerve to the medial pterygoid arises from V_3 immediately before it divides into its anterior and posterior trunks. The medial pterygoid nerve, which also innervates the tensor tympani and tensor veli palatini muscles, reaches the medial pterygoid muscle at its upper posterior border.

Lateral Pterygoid

The *lateral pterygoid* muscle (Figs. 5–8 and 5–10) arises from two heads. The inferior head is about three times larger than the superior head (Honée, 1972; Schumacher, 1961). The superior head originates from the infratemporal surface of the greater wing of the sphenoid medial to the infratemporal crest. From its origin, the fibers of the superior head run almost horizontally backward and lateral in close relation to the external surface of the cranial base. The inferior head originates from the outer surface of the lateral pterygoid plate.

Although the fibers of the inferior head also run backward and laterally, they run upward at an angle of about 45 degrees relative to the superior head.

The two heads of the lateral pterygoid are separated at their origins by a wide gap but fuse in front of the TMJ. The fibers of the superior head are primarily attached to a roughened fossa on the anteromedial surface of the neck of the condylar process. This fossa is called the pterygoid fovea. In addition, a small portion of the superior head is frequently attached directly to the anteromedial portion of the TMJ capsule and to the anteromedial portion of the articular disc. All the fibers of the inferior head insert into or along the periphery of the pterygoid fovea. This description of the lateral pterygoid is based on the work of numerous authors (DuBrul, 1988; Meyenberg, 1986; Moritz, 1987; Sicher, 1964; Widmalm, 1987; Wilkinson, 1983; Wilkinson, 1988).

In contrast to this description of the lateral pterygoid, Griffin (1960) and Honée (1972) state that the two heads do not fuse in front of the TMJ, and that all of the superior head is attached to the capsule and disc. The latter two studies prompted the author to dissect five human TMJs. In all instances the two heads of the lateral pterygoid were fused in front of the joint, and a small flat portion of the superior head was attached to the capsule and disc.

Recent work, however, has indicated that the morphology of the human lateral pterygoid is somewhat more variable than the author's findings. Meyenberg (1986) recently dissected 25 TMJs and found that although the two heads of the lateral pterygoid were always fused in front of the joint, in 40 per cent of the joints the superior head of the lateral pterygoid did not attach to the articular disc. In these instances all of the lateral pterygoid attached to the pterygoid fovea. In the remaining 60 per cent of these joints a small portion of the superior head of the lateral pterygoid was attached to the anteromedial aspect of the articular capsule and disc. The remainder of the muscle was attached to the pterygoid fovea. Similarly, the work of Wilkinson (1988) confirms the results of Meyenberg (1986).

There is some EMG evidence indicating that the lateral pterygoid muscle is composed of two functionally distinct parts. The superior head is said to contract during jaw closing while the inferior head contracts during protraction, opening, and shifting the jaw to one side (Gibbs, 1983; Lipke, 1977; Wood, 1986b). Therefore, the probable functions of each head need to be discussed separately.

The resultant force of the superior head of the lateral pterygoid on the condyle is directed forward and medially. In side view it passes slightly below, but near perpendicular (70° to 90°) to the posterior slope of the articular eminence and to the articular surface of the condyle that faces this slope. Therefore, this part of the lateral pterygoid can function in stabilizing the mandibular condyle against the articular eminence during mastication and biting.

The resultant force of the inferior head on the condyle is directed forward, medially, and downward. Compared with the superior head, its direction of pull is more tangential to the articular surface of the TMJ. Bilateral contraction of the lower head of the lateral pterygoid muscle pulls the mandibular condyles and the attached articular discs down and over the articular eminences. This movement causes mandibular protrusion. Unilateral action of this part of the muscle shifts the mandible to the opposite side by pulling the condyle forward, inward, and downward along the articular eminence.

If the superior or inferior head is actively recruited during mandibular closure the muscle must experience an eccentric or lengthening contraction, i.e., it is stretched as it is generating tension because the condyles are translated backward at this time (Hylander, 1987; Wilkinson, 1988). Under these conditions the lateral pterygoid muscle would exhibit considerable stiffness and this would facilitate joint stability by controlling condylar movements (Rack, 1974).

The nerve to the lateral pterygoid muscle is usually a branch of the buccal nerve, which is a branch of the anterior trunk of V_3.

Digastric

As the name implies, the *digastric* muscle (Fig. 5–11) consists of two parts: an anterior and a posterior belly. These two straight, parallel-fibered muscle bellies are connected by a strong, round, intermediate tendon. The posterior belly arises from the mastoid notch medial to the mastoid process; the intermediate tendon is held to the body of the hyoid bone by a fascial loop. The anterior belly attaches to the digastric fossa of the mandible. This fossa is located along the lower border of the mandible slightly lateral to the midline on the lingual or inner surface of the symphysis. In side view the two bellies of the muscle form an obtuse angle. The posterior belly is much longer than the anterior belly and is slightly flattened in the mediolateral direction. Gradually tapering an-

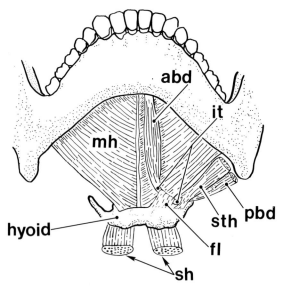

FIGURE 5–11. Hyoid muscles: Sternohyoid (sh), mylohyoid (mh), stylohyoid (sth), and anterior (abd) and posterior (pbd) bellies of the digastric. Note the fascial loop (fl) surrounding the intermediate tendon (it) of the digastric.

teriorly, the posterior belly continues into the round intermediate tendon. The shorter anterior belly, which arises from the intermediate tendon, generally is comprised of a thick lateral and thin medial portion. It is flattened dorsoventrally. Its insertion into the digastric fossa is partly fleshy and partly tendinous.

The intermediate tendon is attached to the hyoid bone by a condensation of fibers of the deep cervical fascia that forms a loop around the tendon and is sometimes separated from it by a synovial bursa. The fibers of this fascial loop are attached to the greater horn and the lateral part of the body of the hyoid. The length of the fascial loop varies, as does the distance of the tendon from the hyoid and the angle between the posterior and anterior bellies of the digastric muscle. The longer the loop and the greater the distance between the hyoid bone and the intermediate tendon, the more obtuse the angle between the two bellies of the muscle.

Frequent variations of the digastric muscle are almost entirely confined to the anterior belly. The most common deviation from its typical shape consists of connections between the two anterior bellies. Accessory muscle bundles may occupy some or all of the space between them.

It is usually stated that if the hyoid is fixed by the action of the infrahyoid muscles, activity of the digastric muscles pulls the front of the mandible back and down, and thus they function during retrusive and opening movements of the mandible. Although a study of hyoid movements during opening and closing of the mouth suggests that the hyoid bone is never completely fixed during mastication (Crompton, 1975; Hiiemae, 1985), the digastric muscles generally appear to function as stated. If the mandible and teeth are held in centric occlusion by the jaw-closing muscles, then contraction of the digastrics is associated with a vertical force on the hyoid.

The digastric muscle is derived from the first and second branchial arches, and therefore it is innervated by V_3 and the facial nerve (cranial nerve VII), respectively. The anterior belly, a first-arch derivative, is innervated by a branch of the mylohyoid nerve, which is a branch of the inferior alveolar nerve. The posterior belly, a second-arch derivative, is supplied by a branch of the facial nerve that enters the muscle close to its posterior end.

Mylohyoid

The *mylohyoid* muscle (Figs. 5–11 and 5–12) forms a muscular diaphragm or floor for most of the oral cavity. It is a flat, continuous, triangular sheet of muscle that is located deep to the anterior belly of the digastric. The base of this triangle attaches to the body of the hyoid bone, and the two sides attach to the lingual aspect of each mandibular corpus along the mylohyoid line. The apex of this triangle attaches to the midline symphysis. Its most posterior fibers, which originate at the level of the third molar, pass medially, downward and posteriorly to insert along the ventral aspect of the body of the hyoid (Fig. 5–11). The middle and anterior fibers have a similar orientation, although these fibers do not attach directly to the

hyoid. Instead, they attach to a midline mylohyoid raphe that connects the body of the hyoid with the lingual surface of the mandibular symphysis.

Occasionally the anterior belly of the digastric is fused to the ventral surface of the mylohyoid. This fusion reflects the embryologic origin of these two muscles from a common muscle mass derived from the first branchial arch. As expected, this muscle is innervated by V_3, via the mylohyoid nerve, which is a branch of the inferior alveolar nerve.

The anatomy of the mylohyoid suggests that it can slightly raise the hyoid (and tongue) and floor of the mouth. Moreover, if the mandible is stabilized, it can also pull the hyoid forward. In the event that the hyoid is stabilized or being pulled down and/or backward, this muscle can also depress the mandible.

Geniohyoid

The *geniohyoid* muscle (Fig. 5–12) is a strap-shaped muscle that runs from the ventral surface of the body of the hyoid to the lingual aspect of the mandibular symphysis immediately lateral to the midline. It is located deep to the mylohyoid. The muscle is composed of parallel fibers that run straight from origin to insertion. The anatomy of the geniohyoid indicates that if the mandible is fixed or stabilized (e.g., in centric occlusion) it can slightly raise the hyoid (and tongue), and it can pull these structures forward. Conversely, in the event that the hyoid is fixed or pulled downward and/or backward, the geniohyoids can help depress the mandible.

The geniohyoid muscles are not branchial arch derivatives. These muscles are the serial homologs of the rectus abdominis muscles, and this is why they are often described as belonging to the "rectus cervicis" group, the straight muscles of the neck. The geniohyoids are innervated by ventral rami of the first and second cervical nerves. These nerve fibers hook up with the left and right hypoglossal nerves to reach the floor of the mouth.

Stylohyoid and Infrahyoid

The *stylohyoid* muscle (Fig. 5–11) is a thin, round muscle with fibers that run between the styloid process of the temporal bone and the greater horn and body of the hyoid. Before its insertion on the hyoid it is split by, and therefore surrounds, the intermediate tendon of the digastric muscle. The stylohyoid is a derivative

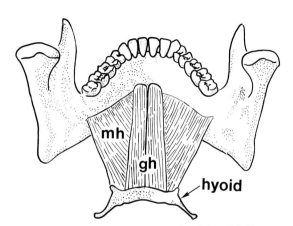

FIGURE 5–12. Geniohyoid (gh) and mylohyoid (mh) muscles.

of the second branchial arch and therefore is innervated by the facial nerve. It presumably functions as a stabilizer, retractor, and elevator of the hyoid bone. Very little is known about the actual function of this muscle, and it is unlikely to have much influence on mandibular movements.

There are four longitudinally arranged strap-shaped muscles in the so-called *infrahyoid* muscle group. These straight, parallel-fibered muscles, which contribute to the ventral body wall of the neck, are the remaining members of the rectus cervicis group. Two of these muscles form a deep layer and two form a superficial layer. The two muscles in the deep layer attach to the outer surface of the thyroid cartilage. The fibers of the thyrohyoid pass upward from the thyroid cartilage to attach to the ventral surface of the body of the hyoid; the fibers of the sternothyroid pass downward from the thyroid cartilage to attach to the deep surface of the manubrium of the sternum. The two muscles of the superficial layer both attach to the ventral surface of the body of the hyoid. The sternohyoid (Fig. 5–11) attaches to the manubrium of the sternum, and the omohyoid to the upper border of the scapula.

The infrahyoid muscles presumably have an important influence on both stabilizing and lowering of the hyoid. Moreover, they also may function to control or limit upward movement of the hyoid. Therefore, these muscles, working in conjunction with the so-called *suprahyoid* muscle group (i.e., the stylohyoid, mylohyoid, geniohyoid, and digastric muscles), function to control hyoid, tongue, and mandibular positions. Although the omohyoid attaches to the scapula, its small size precludes the possibility that it has an important influence on shoulder movements. The infrahyoid muscles are innervated by cervical ventral rami (first, second, and third cervical nerves) via a delicate loop of motor fibers known as the ansa cervicalis.

FUNCTIONAL ANALYSIS OF THE TEMPOROMANDIBULAR JOINT

The masticatory movements of the mandible can often be understood more easily if the free (or empty) movements are analyzed first. Free or empty movements are defined as those occurring without food in the oral cavity. These movements are contrasted with the masticatory movements of the jaw, which are those associated with the incision and chewing of food.

Free Movements of the Mandible

Two basic movements of the mandible can be distinguished: (1) the *rotary or hinge movement*, which is a rotation of the mandible around a transverse axis passing through the centers of the mandibular condyles, and (2) *the translatory or sliding movement*, which is a bodily movement of the mandible in the anteroposterior and/or mediolateral directions, respectively (Figs. 5–13 and 5–26). The rotating movement occurs between the disc and condyle in the lower joint compartment while anteroposterior and mediolateral translatory movements occur between the articular eminence and disc (and mandible) in the upper compartment of the temporomandibular articulation. The translation movements need not be symmetrical between left and right joints.

The free movements of the mandible, combining rotation and translation, include: (1) opening and closing, (2) protrusion and retrusion (symmetrical forward and backward movements), and (3) lateral shifts of the mandible. The extreme or outer limits of the various combinations of these movements define what have been called the border movements of the mandible (Fig. 5–14) (Posselt, 1968; Ramfjord, 1971).

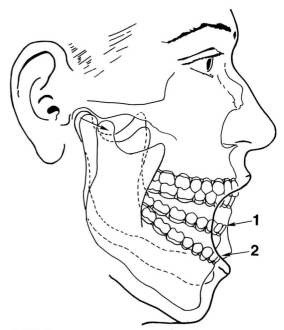

FIGURE 5–13. Rotation and translation of the mandibular condyle during opening. The arrow indicates the direction of condylar translation during opening. The initial stage of mouth opening (position 1) involves much less condylar translation than later stages of mouth opening (position 2).

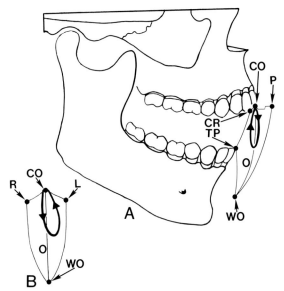

FIGURE 5–14. Border movements of the mandible in the sagittal (A) and frontal (B) planes. The thin dark lines indicate the movement of the tip of the mandibular central incisors relative to the maxillary teeth. A, centric relation (CR), centric occlusion (CO), maximum protrusion (P), and the border-movement lines drawn between these points are tooth-determined positions. WO is the wide-open position. TP is the transitional point where continued opening involves anterior translation of the condyle. The arc CR–TP involves pure rotation of the condyle with the condyle in the retruded position. The arc TP–WO combines condylar rotation and translation. The arc P–WO describes opening in the maximum protruded position. The arc O describes habitual opening and closing empty movements. The heavy lines with the arrows indicate mandibular incisor movements during chewing on the left side. B, CO, WO, and O as in A. L and R indicate maximum lateral positions along the left and right sides, respectively. R, CO, L, and arcs R–CO and CO–L are tooth-determined positions.

Opening and Closing

A combination of both translation and rotation is observable in the *opening* and *closing* movements of the mandible. Translation brings the disc and condyle forward and downward along the posterior slope of the articular eminence. The condyle and disc may even move anteriorly to the greatest height of the articular eminence onto the preglenoid plane (Fig. 5–13). The rotary movement is extensive and can normally go so far that the opening between the upper and lower incisors easily accommodates three fingers (40 to 60 mm).

If a finger is placed just in front of the tragus of the ear, the forward and downward sliding of the mandibular condyle can be felt. The soft tissues behind the moving condyle sink in slightly and a shallow groove often becomes visible during mouth opening. The movement of the mandibular condyle also influences the width of the cartilaginous part of the external acoustic meatus to a slight degree. If a finger is introduced into the external acoustic meatus, one can easily feel the prominence of the lateral pole of the mandibular condyle on the cartilaginous anterior wall of the meatus and the widening of this passage when the mouth is opened.

The translatory and rotatory components are not evenly combined during opening and closing (although see Merlini, 1988). The opening movement starts primarily with a rotatory movement. Then rotatory and translatory components combine in a smooth movement to complete opening (Fig. 5–13).

After maximal opening of the mouth, the closing movement commences with a phase in which the translatory backward movement predominates. In this way the mouth is closed to about two-thirds of its maximal opening, and, at the same time, the condyles and discs are brought either to the height or to the posterior slope of the articular eminences. Then, closing occurs in a smooth combination of translatory and rotatory movements until the rest position is reached. The occlusal position is then attained primarily, although not entirely, by a rotatory movement (Nevakari, 1956).

Protrusion and Retrusion

The forward and backward movements of the mandible are mainly translatory. From the rest position, the mandible can be pulled forward quite extensively, with the lower teeth remaining at a distance from the upper teeth. This movement is called *protrusion*. The mandibular condyles are pulled forward together with the articular discs at this time. Therefore, the movement occurs primarily in the upper compartment of the TMJ, and is symmetrical. The reversal of the forward movement, called *retrusion*, is also mainly translatory. These condylar movements can be confirmed easily by palpation.

Most people with a relatively normal masticatory apparatus can retrude the mandible 1 to 2 mm from the full occlusal position or *centric occlusion* (Fig. 5–14). The retrusion from this position is limited by the horizontally aligned component of the capsular ligament of the TMJ. This retruded position beyond centric occlusion is referred to as *centric relation*. It is not reached during normal masticatory movements in humans, although by definition this position falls along the border movements of the mandible.

Lateral Shift

A *lateral shift* of the mandible results if the condyle and disc of the opposite (*contralateral*) side are pulled forward, downward, and medially along the articular eminence (Fig. 5–5). The *ipsilateral condyle*, often called the *resting condyle*, executes limited movement. This movement primarily consists of a rotation of the mandible around a nearly vertical axis located immediately behind the ipsilateral condyle. This movement also results in a slight translation of the two condyles toward the ipsilateral side.

As previously noted, during the lateral shift of the mandible the ipsilateral condyle rotates about a vertical axis and moves slightly laterally. This rotational movement is influenced by the same limitations that are placed on the retrusive movement of the mandible from centric occlusion. That is, the lateral pole of the condyle can only move backward about 1 to 2 mm until it is checked by the capsular ligament of the TMJ. Thus, under guidance of this ligament, the center of the ipsilateral condyle is forced to move slightly forward, and laterally (Fig. 5–5). The lateral component of this movement is called the *Bennett movement*. The different movements of the ipsilateral and contralateral condyles can be palpated easily.

Action of Muscles in Free Mandibular Movements

Descriptions of muscle function in this and later sections primarily are based on electromyographic (EMG) data and on a muscle's presumed mechanical capabilities as determined from its overall morphology. As the EMG literature is quite extensive, the interested reader is referred to the works of Ahlgren (1966), Carlsöö (1952), Gibbs, (1983), Hannam (1981), Hiiemae (1978), Hylander (1985), Møller (1966; 1974), Stohler (1985a; 1985b), Vitti (1977), and Wood (1986a; 1986b).

The mandibular muscles combine in various patterns to execute the different movements of the mandible. It is especially important to realize that one muscle may act synergistically with different muscles at different times. Moreover, antagonistic muscles may act simultaneously so as to control jaw movements. In no instance does a muscle act independently; instead, muscles act in groups and almost always in surprisingly large groups. In addition, a single muscle may have portions that can function differentially.

The most important muscles that affect movements of the mandible can be divided into three groups: (1) *elevators*—the temporalis, masseter, and medial pterygoid muscles; (2) *depressors*—the digastric, mylohyoid, and geniohyoid muscles; and (3) *protractors*—the lateral pterygoid muscles. The retractors of the mandible do not constitute an independent group; they are represented by the middle temporalis and digastric muscles. If the hyoid is fixed by the stylohyoid and infrahyoid muscles, the mylohyoid and geniohyoid may also help retract the protruded mandible. The fibers of the posterior temporalis and the deep portion of the masseter also help retract the protruded mandible. Thus, both elevators and depressors may function as retractors of the mandible. The infrahyoid muscles function to control hyoid movements and therefore they function during both mouth opening and mouth closing.

Protrusion: Forward Movement

Protrusion of the mandible is primarily the result of contraction of the inferior heads of the lateral pterygoid muscles, although there is slight activity of the masseter and medial pterygoid muscles. The temporalis muscle is not usually active during this movement, and the depressors are only slightly active. The lateral pterygoid muscles pull the mandibular condyles (and discs) forward and downward along the articular eminences, while the elevators and depressors apparently stabilize the position of the mandible relative to the maxilla. The contraction of the elevators and the depressors in an unresisted forward thrust is often not noticeable when palpated. However, if the lower jaw is moved to the extreme forward position, contraction of the masseters can be demonstrated.

Retrusion: Backward Movement

In the retrusive movement the obliquely-aligned fibers of the middle temporalis muscle combine forces with the depressors, while the remaining elevators exhibit varying amounts of activity. The depressing component of the suprahyoid muscles on the mandible is apparently neutralized by the activity of the elevator muscles.

Opening Movement

The opening movement is caused by gravity, relaxation of the elevator muscles, and a combined action of the lateral pterygoid, geniohyoid, mylohyoid, and digastric muscles. The role of the infrahyoid muscles during opening is not known. Presumably they are slightly active so as to stabilize or lower the position of the hyoid during rapid wide opening.

If the opening movement occurs without resistance, the depressors act without any great force. If opening is only slight, this can be accomplished simply by relaxation of the elevators and the force of gravity. When wide opening occurs, the protracting force of the inferior heads of the lateral pterygoid muscles acting upon the condyles and discs combines with the depressing and retracting force of the geniohyoid and digastric muscles acting upon the chin and the action of the mylohyoid muscle upon the body of the mandible. These combined forces produce extensive rotatory and translatory jaw movements.

Closing Movement

The closing movement is executed by the elevators of the mandible. If the mouth is opened to its maximal extent, the timing of the activation and relaxation of the different parts of these muscles may be important for proper closure (DuBrul, 1988). Each disc and condyle glides anteriorly to the summit of the articular eminence onto the preglenoid plane during maximal mouth opening. At the beginning of closure the discs and condyles must be moved back from this anterior position. After this phase of the closing movement has been executed (in which the condyle glides sharply backward while only rotating to a small extent), the closing movement is completed by the elevators. This action returns the jaw to the rest or occlusal position.

Lateral Shift

Lateral shift of the mandible results from an asymmetrical variation of protrusion; that is, the contralateral lateral pterygoid muscle combines forces with the slightly active elevators. The middle portion of the ipsilateral temporalis muscle must assist in this movement by holding the resting condyle and preventing it from deviating anteriorly to any great extent.

Masticatory Movements of the Mandible

The masticatory movements of the lower jaw frequently involve the application of considerable muscle, tooth, and joint reaction force. Although there is a general overall pattern of movement of the mandible during mastication, the actual movements vary in detail both within and between individuals. In a given individual these movements are in part dependent on the shape and proportions of the jaws and teeth, the type of food masticated, and the stage of particle-size reduction of the bolus.

All masticatory movements of the mandible must occur within or along its so-called border movements. These movements are combinations of rotation and translation, the two basic mandibular movements previously described. The masticatory jaw movements are of two general kinds: a cutting movement, as in biting off a piece of food, and a crushing and grinding movement that comminutes a piece of food. The cutting of food into bite-sized pieces, referred to as *incision*, is carried out mainly by the action of the incisors and canines. Occasionally, premolars and molars are used for this purpose. Crushing and grinding of food, termed *mastication*, is carried out almost exclusively by the premolars and molars.

Incision: The Cutting Movement

Unlike movements during mastication, jaw movements during incision have received little attention and therefore are not well understood. The following account is primarily based on the work of Jankelson (1953) and Sheppard (1964).

Starting from the rest or occlusal position, incision is often divisible into three parts. First, the mouth is opened by depressing the mandible. The extent of the opening is primarily dependent on the dimensions of the food item. Second, the mandible is elevated. There is an upward and forward movement of the mandibular incisors and an upward and backward movement of the mandibular condyles during jaw closure, and this part of incision continues until the upper and lower incisors contact the food object. Third, the teeth continue to move upward with the simultaneous application of force to the food object. These three phases of incision can be referred to as the *opening*, *closing*, and *power strokes*, respectively. In many instances the closing stroke may not exist simply because the food object is so large (e.g., a whole apple) that the amount of mouth open-

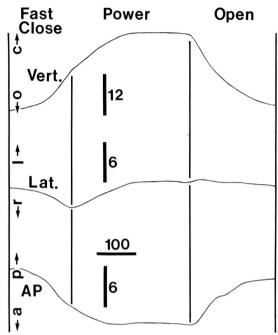

Fast
Close   Power   Open

Vert.

12

6

Lat.

100

AP

6

FIGURE 5–15. Movements of the tip of the mandibular central incisor during unilateral mastication of apple skin along the right side. Vert: vertical jaw movements; arrows labeled (c) and (o) indicate direction of closing and opening movements, respectively; Lat: lateral movements; arrows labeled (l) and (r) indicate direction of left and right movements, respectively; and AP: anteroposterior movements; arrows labeled (p) and (a) indicate direction of posterior and anterior movements. The tracing of vertical jaw movements indicates the fast close, power, and opening (O) strokes of mastication. The horizontal bar indicates 100 milliseconds. The vertical bars labeled 12 and 6 indicate either 12 or 6 mm of incisor movement, respectively. These jaw movements were recorded with a magnet-sensing jaw-tracking system.

ing is just enough to accommodate this object between the upper and lower incisors.

Mandibular movements during the opening and closing strokes of incision are presumably very similar to the free mandibular opening and closing movements. Jaw movements during the power stroke of incision, however, differ from simple jaw-closing movements, particularly in the presence of an incisor overbite. That is, as the anterior teeth approach the edge-to-edge position during incision, the entire mandible moves backward and upward as the edges of the lower incisors and canines glide along the lingual surfaces of the upper incisors and canines until centric occlusion is reached. The food item is cut and sheared with the upper and lower incisors acting as two blades that move past one another at this time. Once initial tooth contact has been attained during incision, the morphology of the anterior teeth influences mandibular movements to a considerable extent.

Patterns of incision are also influenced by use of the hands. In some instances food is vigorously pulled away from the mouth, while in other instances the hands play a less active role by simply positioning the food object between the upper and lower front teeth during incision.

Mastication: The Crushing and Grinding Movement

Mastication also can be described as consisting of three basic strokes: *opening, closing,* and *power* (Fig. 5–15) (Hiiemae, 1978). These three strokes combine to make up a single *chewing cycle,* and all chewing cycles associated with the mastication of a single piece of food are referred to as a *chewing sequence.*

A chewing cycle begins with opening of the mouth; as the lower jaw is depressed, the midline incisal point is ordinarily swung slightly to the nonchewing side and then back to the chewing side (Fig. 5–16). This movement is the

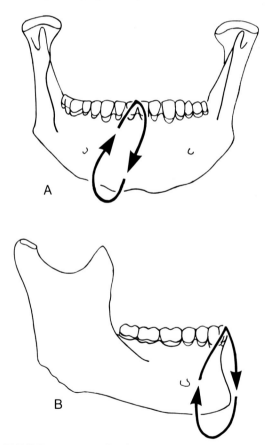

FIGURE 5–16. Frontal and lateral views of the mandible. Arrows in *A* and *B* describe the movement of the incisal contact point of the mandibular central incisors during unilateral mastication on the right side. The relative amount of movement has been exaggerated.

opening stroke. The amount of opening varies from one chewing cycle to the next, and it depends partly on the size and consistency of the food object. From the position of maximum opening, the mandibular incisors are moved upward, forward, and away from the midline. This portion of the upward jaw movement is called the *closing* or *fast stroke.* Completion of the closing stroke leads to the *power stroke,* which is the forceful contact of food between the occlusal surfaces of the molar and premolar teeth. The incisal point during the power stroke is moved back toward the midline. Note in Figure 5–14 that with the exception of those movements associated with contact between the upper and lower teeth, mandibular incisor movements during mastication do not occur along the border movements of the mandible. Instead, they are well within these border movements.

The power stroke of mastication often ends before the upper and lower teeth make contact. This type of power stroke is called *puncture-crushing.* In contrast to puncture-crushing, a power stroke can also involve direct contact between the upper and lower teeth. This type of power stroke is called *tooth-tooth contact.* Generally there is more transverse movement of the mandible and teeth during a tooth-tooth contact power stroke than during a puncture-crushing power stroke.

In a power stroke involving tooth-tooth contact there is an upward, slightly anterior, and medial movement of the lower molars (relative to the uppers) on the chewing side (Fig. 5–17)

and an upward, lateral, and slightly backward movement of the lower molars on the nonchewing side (Gibbs, 1969; 1971). The teeth either continue to be moved into centric occlusion, or these occlusal movements are abruptly terminated and the opening stroke begun. When viewed in the transverse or occlusal plane, the mandible is rotating around a vertical axis positioned somewhat behind the ipsilateral mandibular condyle during these occlusal movements.

The tooth contact movements described above are often called Phase I (or buccal phase) movements (Kay, 1974; Mills, 1955; 1978). Following a Phase I movement, one of two things can happen. Either the power stroke ends and tooth contact is lost as the mouth opens, or the power stroke continues into a Phase II (or lingual phase) movement (Kay, 1974; Mills, 1955; 1978). Prior to the Phase II movement, however, the teeth and jaws are held stationary in centric occlusion during what has been referred to as the motionless period of mastication (Gibbs, 1975). This period is said to last about 200 milliseconds (Gibbs, 1975), although data in Fig. 5–15 indicate that it is only about 50 to 75 milliseconds in this particular subject. Phase II movements occur when the chewing-side teeth, which are positioned in centric occlusion, are moved slightly downward, forward, and toward the nonchewing side of the jaw while maintaining occlusal contact. The Phase II movement then grades directly into the opening stroke of mastication as tooth contact is eventually lost (Kay, 1974; Yeager, 1978).

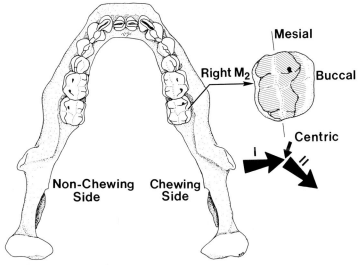

FIGURE 5–17. Occlusal view of the mandible demonstrating the direction of tooth movement during Phases I and II. The right mandibular second molar has been enlarged, and the hatched lines along its occlusal surface are aligned parallel to the orientation of movement relative to its antagonist. The arrows demonstrate the direction of movement of the right maxillary second molar relative to the right mandibular second molar. Note that movement of the mandibular second molar, relative to the maxillary molar, is opposite to the direction indicated by the arrows. Phase I starts at the initiation of tooth-tooth contact and terminates when the chewing-side mandibular molars have moved upward and medially into centric occlusion. The mandible is rotating about a variably-located vertical axis in the region of the ipsilateral mandibular condyle during Phase I. Phase II starts when the chewing-side mandibular molars are moved slightly downward, medially, and anteriorly out of centric occlusion, and this phase terminates when molar tooth contact is broken. (This figure was prepared with the assistance of Richard F. Kay.)

Action of Muscles During Masticatory Movements

Incision

The EMG activity of the jaw muscles has not been systematically analyzed throughout the entire incision cycle. It is assumed that muscle activity patterns during the opening and closing strokes of incision are very similar to those during the free opening and closing movements. If so, the opening stroke is initiated by activity of the depressor group of muscles followed by contraction of the inferior heads of the lateral pterygoid muscles. The mandible is depressed, and the condyles are translated forward at this time. The closing stroke is initiated by the medial pterygoids and then assisted by the remaining elevator muscles.

The elevator muscles contract more or less synchronously during the power stroke of incision, which is unlike the situation during mastication. Until recently it was thought that most of the force during incision was due to bilateral contraction of the medial pterygoid and masseter muscles, with the temporalis muscle contributing little or nothing (Hylander, 1975; 1979b). Recent experiments demonstrate, however, that all of the jaw-closing muscles are important for generating force during incision, including the temporalis muscles (Hylander, 1985). In contrast, only the medial pterygoid and masseter muscles exert much force during isometric incisor clenching (Greenfield, 1956; Latif, 1957; Møller, 1966; Pruzansky, 1952; Vitti, 1977).

The lateral pterygoid muscle is also thought to be active during the power stroke of incision. This suggestion is based on (1) the observation that both heads of the lateral pterygoid muscle are active during incisor clenching (Gibbs, 1983), (2) the assumption that the TMJ must be stabilized during incision, and (3) that this muscle is ideally positioned to perform the stabilizing function. The TMJ must be stabilized because the power stroke of incision often occurs when reaction and muscle forces are large and rapidly changing both in direction and amount. For example, when a large food object suddenly breaks in response to an incisal bite force, the holding force and stiffness of each lateral pterygoid muscle prevents an uncontrolled posterior and upward displacement of the mandibular condyles as the condyles and discs are balanced precariously near the summit of the articular eminence.

Mastication

In the description of muscle activity patterns, the side on which the food bolus is located is referred to as the *ipsilateral* or chewing side. Many authors also refer to this side as the working or active side. The side opposite to the location of the bolus is referred to as the *contralateral* or nonchewing side. This side is also referred to as the balancing, nonworking, or supporting side.

Muscle activity patterns of the jaw elevators during mastication are fairly well known, although many details have yet to be worked out. Much less is known about the activity patterns of the lateral pterygoid and depressor muscles, and virtually nothing is known about the stylohyoid and infrahyoid muscles. Much of the following description is based on the work of Ahlgren (1966), Hannam (1981), Møller (1966; 1974), Stohler (1985a; 1988), and Wood (1986a; 1986b).

The opening stroke is preceded by activity of the depressor group, with the mylohyoid contracting somewhat earlier than the digastric muscles (Fig. 5–18). This initial activity of the depressor group slightly overlaps the EMG activity of the elevator muscles (Møller, 1966; 1974; Stohler, 1985b; 1988; Winnberg, 1983). Shortly after the initial activity of the depressor group (about 80 milliseconds), the inferior heads of the lateral pterygoid muscles begin to contract, with activity on the ipsilateral side ordinarily preceding activity on the contralateral side. The mandible is slightly depressed when the opening moments of the depressor group exceed the closing moments of the relaxing elevator group. The mandible continues to rotate open, and the chewing side of the mandible shifts slightly toward the contralateral side as the condyles and discs are translated forward. The chewing side of the mandible then moves back toward the ipsilateral side during opening when the level of activity in the lateral pterygoid muscle (inferior head) on the contralateral side exceeds that of the ipsilateral muscle.

In many instances the beginning of mouth closing appears to precede electrical activity of the elevator muscles (Hiiemae, 1978). This observation, however, is probably due to inadequate amplification of the EMGs of the elevator muscles during low levels of activation (Stohler, 1985a). The depressor group muscles often exhibit low levels of EMG activity during the initial phase of closing. Presumably the simultaneous activation of elevators and depressors facilitates well-controlled and precise jaw movements during mastication.

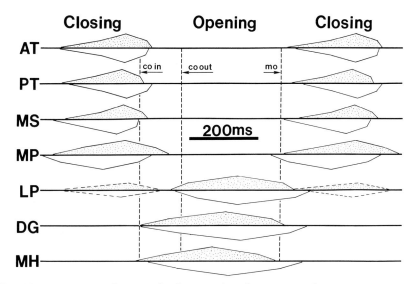

FIGURE 5–18. EMG activity of jaw muscles during unilateral mastication of gum: anterior temporalis (AT), posterior temporalis (PT), masseter (superficial portion) (MS), medial pterygoid (MP), lateral pterygoid (LP), digastric (DG), and mylohyoid (MH). The ipsilateral muscle (stippled) is above the solid black line and the contralateral muscle (not stippled) is below this line. This figure presents mean normalized EMG values and therefore does not indicate the considerable amount of EMG variability within and between subjects during mastication. Both the primary (solid lines) (lower head?) and secondary (dashed lines) (upper head?) activity patterns of the lateral pterygoid muscle have been included. The vertical dashed lines indicate when the teeth move into centric occlusion (co in), out of centric occlusion (co out), and when the mouth is maximally open (mo). Note the coactivation of elevator and depressor muscles during occlusion and at maximum opening. (Adapted from Møller, EL: The chewing apparatus: An electromyographic study of the action of the muscles of mastication and its correlation to facial morphology. Acta Physiol. Scand. [Suppl. 280] 69:1, 1966.)

The closing stroke is often initiated by contraction of the contralateral medial pterygoid muscle. The chewing side of the mandible continues to be moved laterally at this time, partly because of the activity of this muscle. Studies in both humans and nonhuman primates indicate that this lateral movement may also be assisted by the transversely aligned fibers of the ipsilateral deep masseter (Belser, 1986; Hylander, 1987). The ipsilateral medial pterygoid muscle is then activated, followed by the contralateral superficial masseter. This causes the chewing side of the mandible to be moved back toward the midline. Then the ipsilateral temporalis (anterior and posterior), the contralateral anterior temporalis, and the ipsilateral superficial masseter muscles are activated, in that order. Finally, the contralateral posterior temporalis muscle is activated. The combined effect of the elevators is closing of the mouth, with the chewing side of the mandible eventually moving back toward the midline. The inferior heads of the lateral pterygoid muscles continue to be active during the closing stroke (Fig. 5–18) (Gibbs, 1983; Wood, 1986b).

The closing stroke grades into the power stroke. When the upper and lower teeth are in forcible contact with food or with one another,

the EMG activity of the elevators reaches a maximum (Ahlgren, 1966; Møller, 1966; 1974). The period of maximum occlusal force is about 40 to 80 milliseconds after peak EMG activity and this period of maximum force occurs before or in the initial period of centric occlusion, i.e., during Phase I movements (Graf, 1975; Hylander, 1987). If loading and EMG patterns in humans are similar to those in macaques and opossums, then peak masticatory force correlates with the initiation of activity of the digastric and geniohyoid muscles (Hylander, 1987). Following peak occlusal force the jaws are rapidly unloaded as the jaw elevators relax and the jaw depressors develop tension. The entire cycle is now repeated with the activation of the depressor muscles being followed by the activation of the inferior head of the lateral pterygoid late in the terminal portion of the power stroke (Wood, 1986b).

Activity of the superior head of the lateral pterygoid muscle during the chewing cycle is said to occur during closing and/or the early part of the power stroke (Gibbs, 1983; Lipke, 1977; McNamara, 1973), although this is controversial. The behavior of this part of the lateral pterygoid is unclear because of problems that relate to verification of electrode position and the possibility of EMG cross-talk from adjacent muscles (Widmalm, 1987; Wood, 1986b).

There are some interesting and important details of muscle behavior during the power stroke that have not yet been discussed. Peak muscle activity in the contralateral superficial masseter and contralateral medial pterygoid muscles precedes peak activity in their ipsilateral counterparts during tooth-tooth contact. The temporalis muscles exhibit the reverse pattern, particularly the posterior portion, i.e. peak activity of the ipsilateral portions precedes the contralateral portions. In contrast, all these muscles reach peak activity simultaneously during puncture-crushing. These different timing patterns relate directly to different mandibular movements. Puncture-crushing is associated with relatively few mediolateral components of jaw movement as compared with jaw movements during tooth-tooth contacts. Puncture-crushing is primarily a series of up-and-down vertical strokes (Ahlgren, 1966). Hence, jaw muscle activity tends to be rather synchronous at this time. In contrast, tooth-tooth contact power strokes are often associated with extensive mediolateral movement of the mandible and this movement can be accomplished only by asynchronous muscle activity.

Compared with the temporalis and superficial masseter muscles, the medial pterygoids exhibit a relatively large degree of asynchronous activity (Hannam, 1981; Møller, 1966; 1974). Although both medial pterygoid muscles reach maximum EMG activity during the power stroke, the activity of the ipsilateral medial pterygoid peaks well after the contralateral medial pterygoid (Fig. 5–18). The behavior of these two muscles importantly is related to providing the necessary force to move the chewing-side teeth through the transverse movements of the power stroke. Moreover, the late persistent activity of the contralateral posterior temporalis is also thought to be important for effecting this movement.

If the behavior of the deep masseter of humans is similar to that of macaque monkeys (Hylander, 1987), then there is also a considerable amount of asynchronous behavior of this muscle in humans. In macaque monkeys, activity of the ipsilateral deep masseter peaks well before that of the contralateral deep masseter. Moreover, peak activity of the contralateral deep masseter correlates with peak activity of the ipsilateral medial pterygoid. This is of considerable significance because the direction of force of the ipsilateral medial pterygoid and the contralateral deep masseter are well aligned to

aid in driving the chewing-side lower molars across the upper molars during mastication. Moreover, this persistent activity of the contralateral deep masseter is correlated with the gradual relaxation of the contralateral superficial masseter, medial pterygoid, and anterior temporalis muscles, indicating that although vertical muscle force along the contralateral side is decreasing, there is a relative increase in laterally directed contralateral muscle force. Presumably this pattern of activity correlates with a relative increase in the transverse component of the bite force. The transverse component of masticatory force, particularly from the contralateral deep masseter, is thought to be responsible for the mandible being bent like a wishbone during the power stroke of mastication (Hylander, 1985a).

Another interesting aspect of jaw-muscle activity has to do with the relative amount of muscle force from the ipsilateral and contralateral sides during mastication. EMG data suggest that whereas the ipsilateral and contralateral temporalis and deep masseter muscles exhibit similar amounts of activity during unilateral mastication (Belser, 1986; Møller, 1966; 1974), the ipsilateral superficial masseter and medial pterygoid muscles are often much more active than their contralateral counterparts (Møller, 1966; 1974). The actual pattern of force recruitment for the superficial masseter and medial pterygoid muscles, however, is variable and probably related to the mechanical properties of the chewed food. EMG data on macaque monkeys indicate that chewing soft foods results in about three times more force from the ipsilateral masseter than from the contralateral masseter, whereas during the mastication of tough foods the contribution of force from the ipsilateral masseter is about 1.5 times greater than from the contralateral masseter (Hylander, 1983). This is important because the relative amount of muscle force from the two sides of the head has an important influence on TMJ reaction forces. This point will be developed in a later section.

Although it is not well known how patterns of muscle activity during Phase I movements differ from those of Phase II movements, presumably the lateral pterygoids play an important role in the protrusive movement associated with Phase II. It does appear, however, that the direction and magnitude of the bite force are quite different between Phase I and Phase II movements. It has been argued that powerful grinding of food occurs during Phase II movements (Kay, 1974), but recent experimental data on macaques suggest that the jaws are loaded very little during Phase II movements (Hylander, 1987). Whereas peak muscle and bite forces occur during Phase I, Phase II occurs during a period when occlusal forces are small and rapidly decreasing as the elevator muscles are relaxing and the depressor muscles are developing tension. Moreover, the sequence of jaw elevator relaxation patterns indicates that the bite force during Phase II may be more transversely aligned than during Phase I movements.

Functional Significance of Condylar Translation

TMJ instability during biting is influenced by the ability of the two condyles to translate freely. Presumably the direction and magnitude of the various muscular and reaction forces acting on the mandible are adjusted continuously so as to minimize this instability. If condylar translation contributes to jaw joint instability, and also possibly predisposes this joint to derangements of its disc (Smith, 1985), what is the functional significance of condylar translation, particularly anteroposterior translation?

The mandibular condyles of humans are capable of translation mediolaterally as well as anteroposteriorly. Mediolateral condylar translation apparently occurs in all mammals, even in those forms that experience little or no anteroposterior condylar translation. The main function of mediolateral condylar translation in mammals is probably to enhance occlusal function, i.e., to facilitate transverse movements of the lower teeth relative to the opposing upper teeth when they contact one another during mastication. Moreover, many mammals would be unable to bring their upper and lower teeth into occlusion without mediolateral translation simply because, unlike humans, their upper jaws are much wider than their lower jaws, i.e., they are anisognathic.

Unlike mediolateral condylar translation, anteroposterior translation of the condyle does not occur in all mammals. For example, it does not occur (or occurs only slightly) in carnivorans (members of the order Carnivora, such as dogs, cats, bears, raccoons). The apparent explanation for why carnivorans have little or no anteroposterior translation is that their TMJ must be designed to prevent dislocation of the mandible due to the erratic and unpredictable nature of the forces applied to their jaws when subduing struggling prey (Smith, 1959). One way to prevent jaw dislocation is by having a tightly fitted

TMJ that cannot translate anteroposteriorly because of its bony and ligamentous configuration. Although not all modern carnivorans subdue struggling prey, it is assumed that this behavior characterized the early members of that order, and that is why even the entirely herbivorous giant panda has a typical carnivoran TMJ, incapable of anteroposterior translation (Davis, 1964).

This brings us back to the question of why humans and many other mammals have a TMJ that is able to translate anteroposteriorly. An hypothesis that emphasizes the enhancement of occlusal function may explain the origin of anteroposterior translation but is inadequate to explain the full range of this type of translation. In humans and in many other mammals the amount of anteroposterior translation of the condyles during occlusal function, i.e., during the power stroke of mastication, is much less than what the condyles are actually capable of achieving. Most anteroposterior condylar translation occurs during wide mouth opening and during the initial phase of mouth closing from this wide-open position. Therefore, although anteroposterior translation may have initially evolved to enhance occlusal events, extensive translatory movements of the condyles must have evolved for a different reason.

There are a number of hypotheses to explain the functional significance of extensive anteroposterior condylar translation in humans and other noncarnivoran mammals (Smith, 1985). One of these can be referred to as the *airway-impingement hypothesis*. This hypothesis states that in mammals with a condyle positioned high above the occlusal plane (e.g., humans, gorillas, horses, and cattle), forward translation of the condyle during wide mouth opening prevents the tongue and angle of the mandible from rotating backward and pressing against the cervical airway, thereby disrupting its integrity (Smith, 1984; 1985). As noted in Figure 5–13, there is only a small amount of backward movement of the angle of the mandible (and tongue) during wide mouth opening in humans because the condyles translate forward at that time.

There are two major problems with the airway-impingement hypothesis. One is that it only attempts to explain condylar translation in mammals whose mandibular condyles lie well above the occlusal plane. It cannot account for why extensive anteroposterior condylar translation is also found in many mammals that have their mandibular condyles positioned low along the occlusal plane (e.g., insectivorans, and many strepsirrhine primates and marsupials), which presumably is the primitive condition for mammals. Since it is extremely doubtful that the tongue or mandible of the latter mammals would impinge on their airway even if they did not translate their condyles forward during mouth opening (Smith, 1985), it is more reasonable to believe that extensive anteroposterior condylar translation evolved for some other reason. The second problem with the airway-impingement hypothesis is that there is simply no convincing evidence indicating that the integrity of the human airway will be compromised by the mandible and tongue if condylar translation fails to occur during mouth opening.

DuBrul (1988) has implied a similar hypothesis to explain why there is anteroposterior condylar translation in humans, suggesting that extensive readjustments of the human skull to upright bipedal locomotion have resulted in a "... greatly narrowed space between jaw and mastoid process" and thus "A wide opening of the jaw in a pure, back-swinging hinge is therefore now impossible." The main problem with this explanation is that the capability for anteroposterior translation of the mandibular condyles is not confined to humans, and therefore the explanation for its presence cannot be plausibly linked to just upright posture in humans.

Another hypothesis, which will be referred to as the *sarcomere-length hypothesis*, states that anteroposterior condylar translation is a mechanism to minimize sarcomere length changes of the masseter and medial pterygoid muscles throughout a wide range of jaw gapes (Carlson, 1977; Hylander, 1978). In humans (and also in macaques and rabbits) the instantaneous axis of rotation (Fig. 5–19) during wide mouth opening (from the closed position) moves toward the masseter-medial pterygoid complex (Carlson, 1977; Grant, 1973; Weijs, 1989). This indicates that the origin and insertion of the masseter and medial pterygoid muscles are separated much less during wide mouth opening than they would be if the mandible was simply hinged open. In contrast, the origin and insertion areas of the posterior and middle portions of the temporalis are separated more when forward condylar translation is combined with mouth opening, whereas those of the anterior temporalis are more or less unaffected (Fig. 5–13). Thus, as the masseter-medial pterygoid complex is larger than the combined middle and posterior portions of the temporalis, this indicates that the overall elevator muscle mass in humans (as well as in monkeys and rabbits) is stretched less than it would be if the condyles did not translate forward during wide opening.

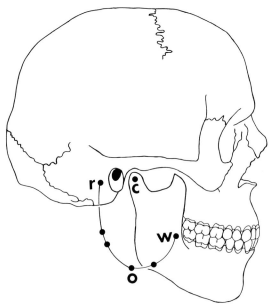

FIGURE 5–19. Path of the instantaneous center of rotation of the mandible during simple opening (Grant, 1973). c is the axis of rotation located in the center of the condyle; r, o, and w are the instantaneous centers of rotation in rest, moderately open, and wide open positions, respectively. See Gibbs (1969) for the various locations of the instantaneous center of rotation of the mandible during mastication.

Or conversely, most of the elevator muscle mass is compressed less than it would be if the condyles did not translate backward during mouth closing from the wide open position.

The reason it is important to minimize muscle stretch or compression during mouth opening and closing is that the amount of force a muscle fiber can generate is inversely proportional to how much it is stretched (or compressed) beyond its resting sarcomere length (Carlson, 1974). Minimizing the amount of sarcomere-length change beyond its resting length allows the masseter-medial pterygoid complex to function at a wide variety of gapes without causing a major reduction in the amount of force it can generate. Smith (1985), Carlson (1977), and Weijs (1989) have estimated that the amount of masseter stretch (in humans, macaques, and rabbits, respectively) during mouth opening would indeed greatly affect the ability of this muscle to generate force if the condyles did not translate forward.

It has been suggested by Smith (1984; 1985) that the sarcomere-length hypothesis must be false because it is based on the incorrect assumption that the mandibular elevators are capable of generating maximum force when the teeth are in or near occlusion (Carlson, 1977).

Actually, the sarcomere-length hypothesis need not be based on this admittedly erroneous assumption. The sarcomere-length hypothesis simply states that stretching and compressing of the masseter-medial pterygoid complex is minimized by extensive anteroposterior translatory movement of the condyles so that this powerful muscle mass is able to generate high levels of force at a wide variety of gapes. The exact point at which the jaw muscles are capable of generating maximum force is irrelevant to the argument.

The main problem with the sarcomere-length hypothesis is that it is incapable of providing a satisfactory explanation for the presence of extensive anteroposterior condylar translation in certain mammals. For example, unlike the situation in humans, the temporalis muscle of many bats and insectivorans (members of the order Insectivora, such as shrews, moles, and hedgehogs) is often larger than the masseter-medial pterygoid complex (Turnbull, 1970). Moreover, much of this relatively large temporalis is horizontally oriented. Therefore, if the above mammals experience extensive anterior translation of the condyles during mouth opening, this movement stretches most of their jaw muscle mass more than simple hinge opening of the mouth. Therefore, extensive anteroposterior condylar translation in these mammals, if it occurs, must result in most of the jaw elevator muscle mass being stretched or compressed more (not less) during mouth opening and closing.

It has been suggested that the published EMG data during incision supports the sarcomere-length hypothesis (Hylander, 1978) because it was once thought that only the masseter and medial pterygoid muscles exhibited significant levels of activity during incision. This was interpreted to indicate that the temporalis is stretched so much at large jaw gapes that it is not nearly as efficient for generating force as the masseter and medial pterygoid muscles; therefore, it is relatively inactive during incision. More recent work indicates, however, that all of the jaw elevators are active during incision (Hylander, 1985). Thus, jaw muscle EMG activity patterns do not provide any special support for this hypothesis.

Although mediolateral and anteroposterior condylar translation in mammals may have initially evolved so as to enhance occlusal function, i.e., to facilitate movements of the lower molars relative to the opposing upper molars during mastication, it can be concluded that this explanation does not account for why the mandibular condyles of many mammals are capable of such extensive anteroposterior movements. The two major hypotheses that attempt to explain the functional significance of these extensive movements, i.e., the airway-impingement and sarcomere-length hypotheses, are both inadequate to varying degrees. Nevertheless, it is clear that anterior condylar translation results in a reduction of sarcomere-length changes of the masseter and medial pterygoid muscles during wide mouth opening in humans. In contrast, it is not clear whether the failure to translate the condyles forward during mouth opening would have any effect whatsoever on respiratory function.

Mandibular Biomechanics

Lever Versus Nonlever Action of the Mandible

For well over 100 years, most researchers have assumed that the mandible functions as a lever both during biting and the power stroke of mastication, with the mandibular condyle acting as a fulcrum (Cuvier, 1805; Gysi, 1921; Picq, 1987; Ryder, 1878) (Fig. 5–20). This hypothesis, however, has been challenged by a number of researchers who have suggested, either directly or indirectly, that there is little or no reaction force at either mandibular condyle and, therefore, that the condyles do not act as fulcra during biting or mastication (Frank, 1950; Frankel, 1970; Gingerich, 1971; Roberts, 1974a; 1974b; Robinson, 1946; Scott, 1955; Steinhardt, 1958; Tattersall, 1973; Taylor, 1986; Wilson, 1920; 1921).

Several lines of argument have been presented in support of the proposition that the condyles do not function as fulcra and have usually been based on one of two assertions: (1) The resultant masticatory muscle force always passes through the bite point during biting or chewing (Fig. 5–21); therefore, it is unnecessary to have force acting along the mandibular condyle to satisfy conditions of static equilibrium. (2) The tissues of the TMJ are unsuited to withstand reaction force; therefore, the mandibular condyles cannot act as fulcra if their tissues are not capable of bearing stress. Many studies have indicated, however, that the resultant masticatory muscle force does not always pass through the bite point (Hylander, 1975; 1978; Smith, 1978). Moreover, other studies have demonstrated that the tissues of the TMJ are capable of dissipating considerable joint reaction force (Hylander, 1975). Therefore, there is little evidence to support either of the above assertions regarding nonlever action of the mandible (Hylander, 1975; Picq, 1987).

Although most researchers agree that the mandible functions as a lever, there have been a number of disagreements over methods of analysis and the modeling of mandibular function. Until recently these disagreements fell within the context of the following three questions: (1) How does one go about analyzing moments acting on the mandible? (2) What type of lever best describes the way the mandible functions? (3) In what projection is the mandible best analyzed?

Analysis of Moments

Most researchers, when attempting a biomechanical analysis of the mammalian mandible, have analyzed moments about the load-bearing portion (or center) (Crompton, 1969; Davis, 1955; Smith, 1959; Turnbull, 1970). This is a useful procedure when analyzing muscle and bite-force moments because it eliminates the need to consider the moments associated

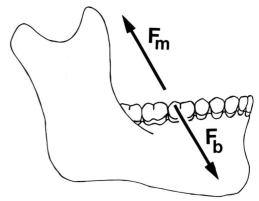

FIGURE 5–21. Nonlever action of the mandible. The resultant muscle force of the jaw elevators (Fm) passes through the bite point. All of the muscle force acting on the mandible results in an equal and opposite reaction force along the bite point (Fb). To maintain static equilibrium under these conditions, it is unnecessary to have any reaction force acting along the condyle. (Redrawn from Hylander, W.L.: Mandibular function and TMJ loading. *In* Carlson, D.S., McNamara, J.A., and Ribbens, K.A. (Eds.): Developmental Aspects of Temporomandibular Joint Disorders. Monograph 16: Craniofacial Growth Series. Center for Human Growth and Development, University of Michigan, Ann Arbor, MI, 1985.)

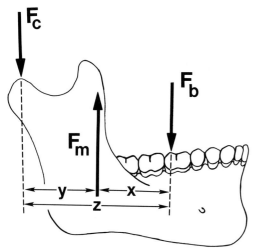

FIGURE 5–20. The human mandible functioning as a lever during biting along the first molar. Only the vertical components of the muscle and reaction forces are included in this figure. The resultant muscle force of the jaw elevators (Fm) is located posterior to the bite point. In order to maintain static equilibrium under these conditions, the muscle force is divided into reaction force along the bite point (Fb) and reaction force along the two mandibular condyles (Fc). For a given amount of muscle force, Fb can be determined by analyzing moments about Fc (i.e., Fb = (Fm)(y)/z). Fc can be determined by analyzing moments about Fm (or Fb) (i.e., Fc = (Fb)(x)/y or Fc = (Fm)(x)/z). (Redrawn from Hylander, W.L.: Mandibular function and TMJ loading. *In* Carlson, D.S., McNamara, J.A., and Ribbens, K.A. (Eds.): Developmental Aspects of Temporomandibular Joint Disorders. Monograph 16: Craniofacial Growth Series. Center for Human Growth and Development, University of Michigan, Ann Arbor, MI, 1985.)

with condylar reaction forces. Alternatively, moments can also be analyzed about the bite point or the resultant muscle force. This eliminates the need to consider moments associated with the bite force or the resultant muscle force, respectively. Although some researchers insist that moments be analyzed about the instantaneous axis of rotation of the mandible (Grant, 1973; Moss, 1959), this procedure makes the analysis slightly more complicated because none of the muscle-force or reaction-force moments can be ignored (Hylander, 1975; Stern, 1974). Moments can be analyzed about any point, of course, since by definition the summation of moments about any point is equal to zero under conditions of static equilibrium. Ordinarily, however, it is more convenient to analyze moments about either the bite, muscle, or condylar reaction forces.

Human Mandible: What Type of Lever?

In an attempt to model mandibular function, many researchers have argued about whether the mammalian jaw functions as a Class III, Class II, or as a modified Class I bent lever (Davis, 1955; Turnbull, 1970). Usually the mandible of humans is thought to function as a Class III lever (DuBrul, 1988), but this concept is overly simplistic because it implies that the various external forces acting on the mandible lie within the same plane. Moreover, an analysis of moments acting on the mandible is not dependent upon making this distinction, and such a classification gives little (if any) insight into how the mammalian jaw works.

Projections of Analysis

The mammalian mandible has usually been analyzed solely in the lateral projection. Whereas this procedure is particularly appropriate for an analysis of incisal and bilateral molar biting, it does not provide a complete analysis of reaction force along each TMJ during unilateral mastication or biting. For example, if we assume that the muscles on the ipsilateral side of the human jaw are slightly more active than those on the contralateral side during the power stroke of mastication, as some studies have suggested (Møller, 1966; 1974), the resultant muscle force must be located toward the ipsilateral side of the midsagittal plane (Fig. 5–22). For this system to be in equilibrium under these conditions, a compressive reaction force must be acting on the contralateral condyle.

A better approach to modeling the biomechanics of the mandible is to do a three-dimensional analysis of the magnitude and direction of all muscle and reaction forces (Anderson, 1988; Nelson, 1986; Osborn, 1985; Smith, 1986). This, however, is beyond the scope of this chapter. Following Smith (1978), a simplified analysis of forces and moments in both the lateral and frontal projection will be performed on the basis of the assumption that all muscle and reaction forces are essentially vertical and parallel to one another. Although it is doubtful whether such conditions ever exist, particularly during unilateral mastication, this analysis provides some interesting insights into patterns of reaction force along the ipsilateral and contralateral TMJs.

To analyze TMJ reaction force during unilateral biting, moments are first taken about the bite force in the lateral projection in order to solve for total condylar reaction force (Fig. 5–20). Before doing so, it is necessary to assign a relative value to the total muscle force applied (the combined ipsilateral and contralateral muscle force). After calculating the relative total condylar reaction force, this force is subtracted from the total muscle force to solve for the magnitude of the bite force (Fig. 5–20).

The next step involves analyzing moments in the frontal projection. First, moments are taken about the ipsilateral condyle to solve for the amount of force along the contralateral condyle

(or vice versa) (Fig. 5–23). Although the total relative bite and muscle force is already known from the analysis of moments in the lateral projection, to proceed with the frontal-projection analysis, the ratio of the ipsilateral to contralateral muscle force must be estimated so that the resultant muscle force can be positioned. If this ratio is 1.0 (equal force from both sides), the resultant muscle force is in the midline. If the ratio is greater than one (i.e., if the ipsilateral muscle force is larger), the resultant muscle force lies to the left of the midline for biting on the left side. Once its position is determined and the calculation of the contralateral condylar reaction force is made, the ipsilateral condylar reaction force is solved for by simply subtracting the contralateral condylar reaction force from the total condylar reaction force.

Using this method of analysis, the calculation of human TMJ reaction force with a constant total amount of muscle and bite force during isometric biting along the first molar indicates that although total condylar reaction force does not vary, the amount of ipsilateral and contra-

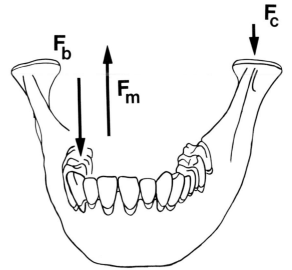

FIGURE 5–22. Forces acting along the mandible in the frontal projection. Only the vertical components of the muscle and reaction forces are included in this figure. The jaw elevators on the chewing side are generating slightly more force than the elevators on the nonchewing side. Under these conditions the resultant muscle force (F_m) is located along the ipsilateral side of the midline. F_b is the bite force and F_c is the condylar reaction force along the nonchewing side (Hylander, 1975). (Redrawn from Hylander, W.L.: Mandibular function and TMJ loading. *In* Carlson, D.S., McNamara, J.A., and Ribbens, K.A. (Eds.): Developmental Aspects of Temporomandibular Joint Disorders. Monograph 16: Craniofacial Growth Series. Center for Human Growth and Development, University of Michigan, Ann Arbor, MI, 1985.)

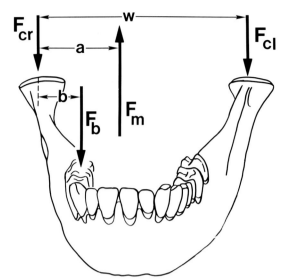

FIGURE 5–23. Forces acting along the mandible in the frontal projection (after Smith, 1978). Only the vertical components of the muscle and reaction forces are included in this figure. Fm is the resultant muscle force. Fb is the bite force; Fcl and Fcr are the condylar reaction forces along the left and right condyles, respectively. Fcl can be determined by taking moments about Fcr (i.e., Fcl = [(Fm)(a) − (Fb)(b)]/w). For a given amount of Fm, Fb and Fc (total condylar reaction force) are determined by analyzing moments in the lateral projection (Fig. 5–20). Fcr can be determined by analyzing moments about Fcl, Fb, or Fm. The easiest way, however, is to simply subtract Fcl from Fc (i.e., Fcr = Fc − Fcl). (Redrawn from Hylander, W.L.: Mandibular function and TMJ loading. *In* Carlson, D.S., McNamara, J.A., and Ribbens, K.A. (Eds.): Developmental Aspects of Temporomandibular Joint Disorders. Monograph 16: Craniofacial Growth Series. Center for Human Growth and Development, University of Michigan, Ann Arbor, MI, 1985.)

lateral condylar reaction force varies as a function of the relative amount of muscle force from the ipsilateral and contralateral sides (Fig. 5–24). If the ipsilateral muscle force is four times larger than the contralateral muscle force (an unlikely occurrence), the ipsilateral condyle experiences about seven times more force than does the contralateral condyle. If the ipsilateral muscle force is two times larger than the contralateral muscle force (a likely occurrence), the ipsilateral condylar force is about 1.4 times larger than the contralateral condylar reaction force. If the ipsilateral muscle force is 1.5 times larger than the contralateral muscle force (another likely occurrence), the condylar forces are reversed so that now the force on the contralateral condyle is about 1.4 times larger than the force on the ipsilateral condyle. When the ipsilateral muscle force is equal to the contralateral muscle force, the contralateral condylar force is about four times larger than the ipsilateral condylar force. Finally, when the contra-

lateral muscle force becomes larger than the ipsilateral muscle force (an unlikely occurrence), the ipsilateral condyle becomes unloaded or actually experiences tension.

This analysis demonstrates that differential loading of the mandibular condyles during isometric biting (and mastication) is highly dependent on slight shifts in muscle recruitment patterns (see Picq [1983] for a similar analysis). Recent work in both macaques (Hylander, 1983) and humans (Hylander, unpublished data) indicates that the ratio of ipsilateral to contralateral muscle force often varies as a function of the mechanical properties of the food. As macaques or humans engage in more powerful masticatory power strokes, most subjects tend to recruit relatively greater amounts of contralateral muscle force. For example, when macaque monkeys chew pieces of apple with no attached skin, the ipsilateral masseter tends to generate about three times more force than the contralateral masseter. When they chew primarily apple skin, the ipsilateral masseter force is about 1.5 times larger than the contralateral masseter (Hylander, unpublished data).

These results, coupled with the theoretical analysis presented in Figure 5–24, suggest that differential loading along the ipsilateral and contralateral TMJ during the power stroke of mastication may vary according to the mechanical properties of the food eaten. Moreover, as indicated in Figure 5–24, a slight shift in the ratio of the ipsilateral to contralateral muscle force can result in marked differences in TMJ loading patterns. The contralateral TMJ may be loaded more than the ipsilateral TMJ under some conditions, while the reverse may prevail under other conditions.

Experiments on macaques also indicate that under very limited and restricted conditions (e.g., powerful isometric biting along M_3), the ipsilateral TMJ is either unloaded or is loaded in tension (Hylander, 1979a). Although this can be demonstrated mathematically from either a three-dimensional analysis or from an analysis in both the lateral and frontal projections, it can be more easily visualized if the muscle and reaction forces acting along the mandible are analyzed in the occlusal projection (Druzinsky, 1979; Greaves, 1978).

The macaque mandible is supported at three points during unilateral biting along the left first molar: the left and right mandibular condyles and the left first molar. These three points form what Greaves (1978) has referred to as the triangle of support (LR1 in Fig. 5–25). Triangles of support during biting along the left second

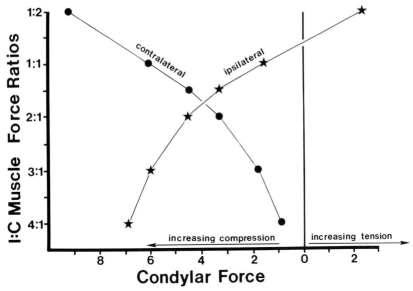

FIGURE 5–24. Plot of relative ipsilateral condylar reaction force values (stars) and contralateral condylar reaction force values (circles) during isometric biting along the first molar for various ipsilateral/contralateral (I:C) muscle force ratios. The total muscle force is held constant although the ratio of the ipsilateral muscle force relative to the contralateral muscle force varies. The ratio 4:1 indicates that the ipsilateral muscle force is four times larger than the contralateral muscle force. The ratio 1:1 indicates that the ipsilateral and contralateral muscle force values are identical. (Redrawn from Hylander, W.L.: Mandibular function and TMJ loading. *In* Carlson, D.S., McNamara, J.A., and Ribbens, K.A. (Eds.): Developmental Aspects of Temporomandibular Joint Disorders. Monograph 16: Craniofacial Growth Series. Center for Human Growth and Development, University of Michigan, Ann Arbor, MI, 1985.)

and third molars are LR2 and LR3, respectively.

The point 1:1 in Figure 5–25 is the position of the resultant elevator muscle force when equal amounts of muscle force are contributed from the ipsilateral and contralateral sides. The direction of the force along this point is toward the reader and, as a first-approximation, is perpendicular to the plane of the paper. When the ipsilateral muscle force is either two or three times larger than the contralateral muscle force, the resultant muscle force is located at points 2:1 or 3:1, respectively. When the position of the resultant adductor muscle force lies at 1:1 during biting along the left first molar, all points within the triangle of support (LR1) experience compression, i.e., a force directed away from the reader and into the plane of the paper. If the resultant muscle force is positioned at 2:1 or 3:1 during biting along the first, second, or third molar, a similar situation prevails. In contrast, when the muscle force is positioned at 1.25:1 during biting along the third molar, the ipsilateral (left) condyle is unloaded. Only the third molar and the contralateral condyle need be loaded in compression to achieve static equilibrium at this time. Finally, a very different situation prevails when the

position of the resultant muscle force lies outside the triangle of support during biting along the third molar, i.e., at 1:1. Under these conditions the contralateral condyle and the third molar are loaded in compression, but there is a tendency for the condyle (and disc) on the ipsilateral side to lift off the articular eminence because the resultant muscle force causes the mandible to rotate about an axis defined by the line R_3.

Differential Loading Within the Temporomandibular Joint

In humans, the stress-bearing portion of the TMJ is located along the articular surfaces of the articular eminence of the temporal bone and the mandibular condyle. There is considerable evidence, however, that reaction forces within this articular region are not always equally distributed. The evidence for differential loading within the human TMJ initially came from studies on patterns of remodeling and on pathological changes. For example, Moffett (1964) showed that the lateral aspect of the human TMJ remodels differently than the medial aspect. Although these remodeling patterns do not necessarily indicate the nature of the

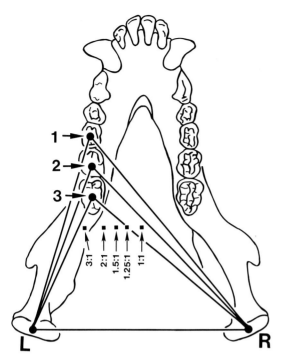

FIGURE 5–25. Occlusal view of a macaque monkey mandible. LR1, LR2, and LR3 are "triangles of support" during biting (Greaves, 1978) along the left molars 1, 2, and 3, respectively. The position of the resultant muscle force is indicated by the solid squares for various ipsilateral–contralateral–side recruitment patterns. For example, when the ipsilateral–side muscle force is two times larger than the contralateral–side muscle force, the resultant muscle force is located at 2:1. (Redrawn from Hylander, W.L.: Mandibular function and TMJ loading. *In* Carlson, D.S., McNamara, J.A., and Ribbens, K.A. (Eds.): Developmental Aspects of Temporomandibular Joint Disorders. Monograph 16: Craniofacial Growth Series. Center for Human Growth and Development, University of Michigan, Ann Arbor, MI, 1985.)

loading pattern, they do suggest possible differences in mechanical loading patterns within the TMJ.

A number of studies on degenerative changes in the human TMJ also suggest differential loading within the joint. For example, Oberg (1971) noted that the majority of articular disc perforations are found along the lateral aspect of the TMJ. As pathological changes in joints are often related to local mechanical factors, these data indicate that the lateral aspect of the human TMJ experiences more stress, i.e., more wear and tear, than the medial aspect. Finally, the distribution of glycosaminoglycans in the articular tissues of the human TMJ also indicates that the lateral aspect of the joint may experience more stress than the medial aspect (Kopp, 1976; 1978).

There are at least three possible reasons why the lateral aspect of the TMJ experiences more

chewing stress than its medial aspect. One is related to mandibular distortions that occur due to powerful muscle and reaction forces (Hylander, 1979a). The mandibular corpus of primates is twisted during the power stroke of mastication and during isometric biting. This twisting, which results in eversion of the lower border of the mandible and inversion of the coronoid process, causes the lateral part of the mandibular condyle to be pressed more vigorously against the articular eminence than its medial part (Fig. 5–26A). This presumably can occur on both the ipsilateral and contralateral condyles.

Another reason for increased loading of the lateral aspect of the TMJ has been advanced by Mohl (1988), who suggested that because the lateral pole of the condyle lies in front of the transverse axis of rotation of the mandible and the medial pole lies behind this axis, the lateral

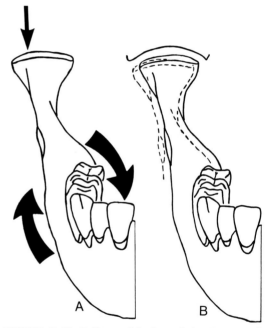

FIGURE 5–26. Differential loading of the TMJ. *A,* the mandibular corpus during mastication and biting is twisted about its long axis. The large arrows indicate the direction of twisting of the posterior half of the mandible. This pattern of twisting causes the lateral aspect of the TMJ (small arrow) to be loaded more than its medial aspect. *B,* the mandibular condyle and posterior slope of the articular eminence along the ipsilateral side during mastication. The disc is not included in drawing. The ipsilateral condyle is shifted laterally (dashed lines) during the opening stroke of mastication. This movement causes the medial aspect of the condyle and articular eminence to lose direct contact with one another. This in turn causes the lateral aspect of the TMJ to be loaded more than its medial aspect during mandibular closure as the condyle is moved back to its central position.

pole moves upward while the medial pole moves downward during the power stroke of mastication. These movements are thought to cause the lateral aspect of the mandibular condyle to be pressed against the articular eminence while the medial aspect of the condyle loses contact with the eminence.

The last and perhaps most important reason for differential loading within the TMJ is related to the mediolateral translation of the condyle relative to the articular eminence during unilateral mastication. As noted elsewhere in this chapter (see page 74), the ipsilateral condyle experiences a lateral shift (Bennett's movement) during the opening stroke of mastication. This is followed by a medial shift of the same condyle from this lateral position during the closing and power strokes. The medial shift is not only correlated with the occurrence of maximum masticatory force (and therefore maximum condylar reaction force), but it is also associated with the ipsilateral condyle being positioned somewhat more laterally relative to the articular eminence. This causes the lateral and central part of the condyle (and disc) to be pressed against the more lateral portion of the articular eminence (Fig. 5–26B), while at this time contact is reduced or lost between the medial half of the condyle, disc, and articular eminence.

Thus, throughout the early part of the power stroke, and on into the Phase I movement, the lateral aspect of the ipsilateral TMJ may experience more stress than its medial aspect due to the position of the condyle and disc relative to the articular eminence. When centric occlusion has been reached, the stress-bearing portion of the condyle and eminence will no longer have a steep medial-to-lateral gradient of increasing joint reaction force. Instead, the TMJ reaction force will be more evenly distributed along the condyle, disc, and eminence. Phase II movement probably does not result in significant differential loads within the TMJ simply because masticatory forces, and therefore condylar reaction forces, have declined considerably at this time.

Although the contralateral TMJ may frequently experience more overall stress than the ipsilateral TMJ during powerful chewing, as indicated earlier, presumably its articular surfaces will be more evenly loaded because the contralateral condyle does not experience a mediolateral type of movement that modifies the position of the articular components and thereby causes large stress concentrations. Instead, the contralateral condyle primarily rotates about a transverse axis and translates posteriorly down the articular eminence during the power stroke.

SUMMARY

The morphology of the bony elements, disc, and fibrous capsule of the temporomandibular joint (TMJ) have been described. This was followed by a detailed description of the attachment patterns and morphology of the temporalis, masseter, medial and lateral pterygoid, digastric, mylohyoid, geniohyoid, stylohyoid, and infrahyoid muscles. These two sections provided the background for an analysis of mandibular movements, jaw muscle function, and mandibular biomechanics.

The free and masticatory movements of the mandible also have been described. Emphasis was placed on movements of both the teeth and the mandibular condyles. Using anatomic and electromyographic data, the functional aspects of the various jaw muscles during mandibular movements also were considered. This was followed by an analysis of patterns of mandibular movement and jaw muscle function during both incision and mastication. In addition, the functional significance of condylar translation was discussed. Finally, following a simplified biomechanical analysis of the mandible in both frontal and lateral projections, the nature of TMJ reaction force during chewing and biting was analyzed. This analysis demonstrated that TMJ reaction forces often vary between the contralateral and ipsilateral sides during unilateral mastication. In many instances the ipsilateral TMJ is loaded more than the contralateral TMJ. The contralateral TMJ, however, may be loaded more than the ipsilateral TMJ during powerful chewing. Finally, differential loading appears to occur within the ipsilateral TMJ, with the lateral portion of this joint being loaded more than the medial portion.

ACKNOWLEDGMENTS: I thank Mr. Kirk Johnson for kindly reading and offering many suggestions on various drafts of this chapter. I also thank Drs. Kathleen Smith, Mary Maas, Richard Kay, Matt Ravosa, and Pascal Picq for their helpful comments.

REFERENCES

Ahlgren, J.: Mechanism of mastication: A quantitative cinematographic and electromyographic study of masticatory movements in children, with special reference to occlusion of the teeth. Acta Odontol. Scand. [Suppl. 44] 24:1–109, 1966.

Anderson, R. C., Van Buskirk, W. C., and Fontenot, M.

G.: Three-dimensional force analysis of the human mandible. J. Dent. Res. 67:359, 1988.

Belser, U. C., and Hannam, A. G.: The contribution of the deep fibers of the masseter muscle to selected tooth-clenching and chewing tasks. J. Prosthet. Dent. 56:629–635, 1986.

Bouvier, M., and Hylander, W. L.: The effect of dietary consistency on morphology of the mandibular condylar cartilage in young macaques (*Macaca mulatta*). In Dixon, A. D., and Sarnat, B. G. (Eds.): Factors and Mechanisms Influencing Bone Growth. New York, Liss, 1982.

Carlson, D. S.: Condylar translation and the function of the superficial masseter muscle in the rhesus monkey (*M. mulatta*). Am. J. Phys. Anthropol. 47:53–63, 1977.

Carlson, F. D., and Wilke, D. R.: Muscle Physiology. Englewood Cliffs, NJ, Prentice-Hall, 1974.

Carlsöö, S.: Nervous coordination and mechanical function of the mandibular elevators: An electromyographic study of the activity, and an anatomic analysis of the mechanics of the muscles. Acta Odontol. Scand. [Suppl. 11]. 10:1–132, 1952.

Crompton, A. W., Cook, P., Hiiemae, K., and Thexton, A. J.: Movement of the hyoid apparatus during chewing. Nature (Lond.). 258:69–70, 1975.

Crompton, A. W., and Hiiemae, K.: How mammalian molar teeth work. Discovery, Yale Peabody Museum 5:23–34, 1969.

Cuvier, G.: Leçons d'Anatomie Comparée, III. Paris, C. L. Duvernoy, 1805.

Davis, D. D.: Masticatory apparatus in the spectacled bear *Tremarctos ornatus*. Fieldiana: Zoology 37:25–46, 1955.

Davis, D. D.: The giant panda: A morphological study of evolutionary mechanisms. Fieldiana: Zoology Memoirs 3:1–339, 1964.

Druzinsky, R. E., and Greaves, W. S.: A model to explain the posterior limit of the bite point in reptiles. J. Morphol. 160:165–168, 1979.

DuBrul, E. L.: Oral Anatomy, 8th ed. St. Louis, Ishiyaku EuroAmerica, Inc., 1988.

Duterloo, H. S., and Jansen, H. W. B.: Chondrogenesis and osteogenesis in the mandibular condylar blastema. Trans. Eur. Orthod. Soc. 69:109–118, 1970.

Frank, L.: Muscular influence on occlusion as shown by x-rays of the condyle. Dent. Dig. 56:484–488, 1950.

Frankel, V. H., and Burstein, A. H.: Orthopaedic Biomechanics. Philadelphia, Lea & Febiger, 1970.

Gibbs, C. H.: Electromyographic activity during the motionless period of chewing. J. Prosthet. Dent. 34:35–40, 1975.

Gibbs, C. H., Mahan, P. E., Wilkinson, T. M., and Mauderli, A.: EMG activity of the superior belly of the lateral pterygoid muscle in relation to other jaw muscles. J. Prosthet. Dent. 51:691–702, 1983.

Gibbs, C. H., Messerman, T., Reswick, J. B., and Derda, H. J.: Functional movements of the mandible. J. Prosthet. Dent. 26:604–620, 1971.

Gibbs, C. H., Reswick, J. B., and Messerman, T.: Functional movements of the mandible. E.D.C. Report No. EDC 4-69-24. Cleveland, Case Western Reserve University, 1969.

Gingerich, P. D.: Functional significance of mandibular translation in vertebrate jaw mechanics. Postilla 152:1–10, 1971.

Graf, H.: Occlusal forces during function. In Rowe, N. H. (Ed.): Occlusion: Research in Form and Function. University of Michigan School of Dentistry and the Dental Research Institute, 1975.

Grant, P. D.: Biomechanical significance of the instantaneous center of rotation: The human temporomandibular joint. J. Biomech. 6:109–113, 1973.

Greaves, W. S.: The jaw lever system in ungulates: A new model. J. Zool. (Lond.). 184:271–285, 1978.

Griffin, C. J., and Sharpe, C. J.: The structure of the adult temporomandibular meniscus. Aust. Dent. J. 5:190–195, 1960.

Greenfield, B. E., and Wyke, B. D.: Electromyographic studies of some of the muscles of mastication. Br. Dent. J. 100:129–143, 1956.

Gysi, A.: Studies on the leverage problem of the mandible. Dent. Dig. 27:74–84, 144–150, 203–208, 1921.

Hannam, A. G., and Wood, W. W.: Medial pterygoid muscle activity during the closing and compressive phases of human mastication. Am. J. Phys. Anthropol. 55:359–367, 1981.

Harpman, J. A., and Woollard, H. A.: The tendon of the lateral pterygoid muscle. J. Anat. 73:112–115, 1938.

Hiiemae, K. M.: Mammalian mastication: A review of the activity of the jaw muscles and the movement they produce in chewing. In Joysey, K. A., and Butler, P. M. (Eds.): Development, Function and Evolution of Teeth. London, New York, and San Francisco, Academic Press, 1978.

Hiiemae, K. M., and Crompton, A. W.: Mastication, food transport, and swallowing. In Hildebrand, M., Bramble, D. M., Liem, K. F., and Wake, D. B. (Eds.): Functional Vertebrate Morphology. Cambridge, Harvard University Press, 1985.

Honée, G. L.: The anatomy of the lateral pterygoid muscle. Acta Morphol. Neerl. Scand. 10:331–340, 1972.

Hylander, W. L.: The human mandible: Lever or link? Am. J. Phys. Anthropol. 43:227–242, 1975.

Hylander, W. L.: Incisal bite force direction in humans and the functional significance of mammalian mandibular translation. Am. J. Phys. Anthropol. 48:1–7, 1978.

Hylander, W. L.: An experimental analysis of temporomandibular joint reaction force in macaques. Am. J. Phys. Anthropol. 51:443–456, 1979a.

Hylander, W. L.: Functional anatomy of the temporomandibular joint. In Sarnat, B. G., and Laskin, D. (Eds.): The Temporomandibular Joint: A Biologic Basis for Clinical Practice, 3rd ed. Springfield, IL, Charles C Thomas, 1979b.

Hylander, W. L.: Mechanical properties of food and recruitment of masseter force. J. Dent. Res. 62:1150, 1983.

Hylander, W. L.: Mandibular function and biomechanical stress and scaling. Am. Zool. 25:315–330, 1985a.

Hylander, W. L.: Mandibular function and TMJ loading. In Carlson, D. S., McNamara, J. A., and Ribbens, K. A. (Eds.): Developmental Aspects of Temporomandibular Joint Disorders. Monograph #16. Craniofacial Growth Series. Center for Human Growth and Development, University of Michigan, Ann Arbor, MI, 1985b.

Hylander, W. L., and Johnson, K. R.: Temporalis and masseter function in humans and macaques during incision. Int. J. Primatol. 6:289–322, 1985c.

Hylander, W. L., Johnson, K. R., and Crompton, A. W.: Loading patterns and jaw movements during mastication in *Macaca fascicularis*: A bone-strain, electromyographic and cineradiographic analysis. Am. J. Phys. Anthropol. 72:287–314, 1987.

Jankelson, B., Hoffman, G. M., and Hendron, J. A.: Physiology of the stomatognathic system. J. Am. Dent. Assoc. 46:375–386, 1953.

Kay, R. F., and Hiiemae, K. M.: Jaw movement and tooth use in recent and fossil primates. Am. J. Phys. Anthropol. 40:227–256, 1974.

Kopp, S.: Topographical distribution of sulphated glycosaminoglycans in human temporomandibular joint disks. J. Oral Pathol. 5:265–276, 1976.

Kopp, S.: Topographical distribution of sulfated glycosaminoglycans in the surface layers of the human temporo-mandibular joint. J. Oral. Pathol. 7:283–294, 1978.

Latif, A.: An electromyographic study of the temporalis muscle in normal persons during selected positions and movements of the mandible. Am. J. Orthod. 43:577–591, 1957.

Lipke, D. P., Gay, T., Gross, B. D., and Yaeger, J. A.: An electromyographic study of the human lateral ptery-goid muscle. J. Dent. Res. 56B:230, 1977.

McNamara, J. A., Jr.: The independent functions of the two heads of the lateral pterygoid muscle. Am. J. Anat. 138:197–205, 1973.

Merlini, L., and Palla, S.: The relationship between con-dylar rotation and anterior translation in healthy and clicking temporomandibular joints. Schweiz. Monatsschr. Zahnmed. 98:1191–1199, 1988.

Meyenberg, M., Kubik, S., and Palla, S.: Relationships of the muscles of mastication to the articular disc of the temporomandibular joint. Helv. Odont. Acta 30:1–20, 1986.

Mills, J. R. E.: Ideal dental occlusion in the primates. Dent. Pract. Bristol. 6:47–61, 1955.

Mills, J. R. E.: The relationship between tooth patterns and jaw movements in the hominoidea. In Joysey, K. A., and Butler, P. M. (Eds.): Development, Function and Evolution of Teeth. London, New York, and San Fran-cisco, Academic Press, 1978.

Moffett, B. C., Johnson, L. C., McCabe, J. B., and Askew, H. C.: Articular remodeling in the adult human tempo-romandibular joint. Am. J. Anat. 115:119–142, 1964.

Mohl, N. D.: The temporomandibular joint. In Mohl, N. D., Zarb, G. A., Carlsson, G. E., and Rugh, J. D. (Eds.): A Textbook of Occlusion. (Chicago, Quintessence Pub-lishing Co., Inc., 1988.

Møller, E.: The chewing apparatus: An electromyographic study of the action of the muscles of mastication and its correlation to facial morphology. Acta Physiol. Scand. [Suppl. 280] 69: 1966.

Møller, E.: Action of the muscles of mastication. In Kawa-mura, Y. (Ed.): Frontiers of Oral Physiology. Basel, Karger, 1974.

Moritz, T. H., and Ewer, R.: Der Ansatz des Musculus pterygoideus lateralis am Kiefergelenk des Menschen. Dtsch. Zahnärztl. Z. 42:680–685, 1987.

Moss, M.: Functional anatomy of the temporomandibular joint. In Schwartz, L. (Ed.): Disorders of the Temporo-mandibular Joint: Diagnosis, Management, Relation to Occlusion of Teeth. Philadelphia, W. B. Saunders, 1959.

Nelson, G. J.: Three-dimensional computer modeling of human mandibular biomechanics, Ph.D. thesis, Univer-sity of British Columbia, 1986.

Nevakari, K.: An analysis of the mandibular movement from rest to occlusal position: A roentgenographic-ceph-alometric investigation. Acta Odontol. Scand. [Suppl. 19] 14:1–129, 1956.

Oberg, T., Carlsson, G. E., and Fajers, C. M.: The temporomandibular joint. A morphologic study on a human autopsy material. Acta Odontol. Scand. 29:349–384, 1971.

Osborn, J. W., and Baragar, F. A.: Predicted pattern of human muscle activity during clenching derived from a computer assisted model: Symmetric vertical bite forces. J. Biomech. 18:599–612, 1985.

Picq, P. G., Plavcan, J. M., and Hylander, W. L.: Non-lever action of the mandible: The return of the hydra. Am. J. Phys. Anthropol. 74:305–307, 1987.

Picq, P. G.: L'articulation temporo-mandibulaire des hom-inidés fossiles: Anatomie comparée, biomécanique, évo-lution, biométrie. Mém. Sc. Terre Univ. Curie Paris 83–17, 1–183, 1983.

Posselt, U.: Physiology of occlusion and rehabilitation. Oxford and Edinburgh, Blackwell Scientific Publications, 1968.

Pruzansky, S.: The application of electromyography to dental research. J. Am. Dent. Assoc. 44:49–68, 1952.

Rack, P. M. H., and Westbury, D. R.: The short range stiffness of active mammalian muscle and its effect on mechanical properties. J. Physiol. 240:331–350, 1974.

Ramfjord, S. P., and Ash, M. M.: Occlusion. Philadelphia, W. B. Saunders, 1971.

Rees, L.: The structure and function of the mandibular joint. Br. Dent. J. 96:125–133, 1954.

Roberts, D.: The etiology of the temporomandibular joint dysfunction syndrome. Am. J. Orthod. 66:498–515, 1974a.

Roberts, D., and Tattersall, I.: Skull form and the mechan-ics of mandibular elevation in mammals. Novitates (American Museum of Natural History), No. 2536, 1974b, pp. 1–9.

Robinson, M.: The temporomandibular joint: Theory of reflex controlled nonlever action of the mandible. J. Am. Dent. Assoc. 33:1260–1271. 1946.

Ryder, S. A.: On the mechanical genesis of tooth forms. Proc. Acad. Nat. Sci. Philad., 79:45–80, 1878.

Savelle, W. P. M.: Some aspects of the morphology of the human temporomandibular joint capsule. Acta Anat. 131:292–296, 1988.

Schumacher, G. H.: Funktionelle morphologie der kau-muskulatur. Jena, Gustav Fischer Verlag, 1961.

Scott, J. H.: A contribution to the study of mandibular joint function. Br. Dent. J. 94:345–349, 1955.

Sheppard, I. M.: Incisive and related movements of the mandible. J. Prosthet. Dent. 14:898–906, 1964.

Sicher, H.: Functional anatomy of the temporomandibular joint. In Sarnat, B. G. (Ed.): The Temporomandibular Joint, 2nd ed. Springfield, IL. Charles C Thomas, 1964.

Smith, D. M., McLachlan, K. R., and McCall, W. D. Jr.: A numerical model of temporomandibular joint loading. J. Dent. Res. 65:1046–1051, 1986.

Smith, J. M., and Savage, R. J. G.: The mechanics of mammalian jaws. School Sci. Rev. 141:289–301, 1959.

Smith, R. J.: Mandibular biomechanics and temporoman-dibular joint function in primates. Am. J. Phys. Anthro-pol. 49:341–349, 1978.

Smith, R. J.: Comparative functional morphology of maxi-mum mandibular opening (gape) in primates. In Chivers, D. J., Wood, B. A., and Bilsborough, A. (Eds.): Food Acquisition and Processing in Primates, New York, Plenum Press, 1984.

Smith, R. J.: Functions of condylar translation in human mandibular movement. Am. J. Orthod. 88:191–202, 1985.

Steinhardt, G.: Anatomy and function of the temporoman-dibular joint. Int. Dent. J. 8:155–156, 1958.

Stern, J. T.: Biomechanical significance of the instantaneous center of rotation: The human temporomandibular joint. J. Biomech. 7:109, 1974.

Stohler, C. S., Ashton-Miller, J. A., and Carlson, D.S: The effects of pain from the mandibular joint and muscles on masticatory motor behavior in man. Arch. Oral. Biol. 33:175–182, 1988.

Stohler, C. S., Yamada, Y., and Ash, M. M. Jr.: Non-linear amplification of electromyographic signals with particular application to human chewing. Arch. Oral. Biol. 30:217–219, 1985a.

Stohler, C. S., Yamada, Y., and Ash, M. M. Jr.: Antago-nistic muscle stiffness and associated reflex behavior in the pain-dysfunctional state. Helv. Odont. Acta 29:13–20, 1985b.

Tattersall, I.: Cranial anatomy of Archeolemurinae (Lemuroidea, Primates). Anthropological Papers of the American Museum of Natural History 52:1–110, 1973.

Taylor, R. M. S.: Nonlever action of the mandible. Am. J. Phys. Anthropol. 70:417–421, 1986.

Turnbull, W. D.: Mammalian masticatory apparatus. Fieldiana: Geology 18:1–356, 1970.

Van der Linden, E. J., Burdi, A. R., and de Jongh, H. J.: Critical periods in the prenatal morphogenesis of the human lateral pterygoid muscle, the mandibular condyle, the articular disk, and medial articular capsule. Am. J. Orthod. Dentofac. Orthop. 91:22–28, 1987.

Vitti, M., and Basmajian, J. V.: Integrated actions of masticatory muscles: Simultaneous EMG from eight intramuscular electrodes. Anat. Rec. 187:173–189. 1977.

Weijs, W. A., Korfage, J. A. M., and Langenbach, G. J.: The functional significance of the position of the centre of rotation for jaw opening and closing in the rabbit. J. Anat. 162:133–148, 1989.

Widmalm, S. E., Lillie, J. H., and Ash, M. M. Jr.: Anatomical and electromyographical studies of the lateral pterygoid muscle. J. Oral Rehabil. 14:429–446, 1987.

Wilkinson, T. M.: The relationship between the disk and the lateral pterygoid muscle in the human temporomandibular joint. J. Prosthet. Dent. 60:715–724, 1988.

Wilkinson, T. M., and Maryniuk, G. A.: Sequential sagittal dissections of the temporomandibular joint {abstr}. J. Dent. Res. 62:655, 1983.

Wilson, G. H.: The anatomy and physics of the temporomandibular joint. J. Natl. Dent. Assoc. 7:414–420, 1920.

Wilson, G. H.: The anatomy and physics of the temporomandibular joint. J. Natl. Dent. Assoc. 8:236–241, 1921.

Winnberg, A., and Pancherz, H.: Head posture and masticatory muscle function. Eur. J. Orthod. 5:209–217, 1983.

Wood, W. W.: Medial pterygoid muscle activity during chewing and clenching. J. Prosthet. Dent. 55:615–621, 1986a.

Wood, W. W., Takada, K., and Hannam, A. G.: The electromyographic activity of the inferior part of the human lateral pterygoid muscle during clenching and chewing. Arch. Oral. Biol. 31:245–253, 1986b.

Yeager, J. A.: Mandibular path in the grinding phase of masticiation—A review. J. Prosthet. Dent. 39:569–573, 1978.

6

REMODELING*

MURRAY C. MEIKLE, B.D.S., M.S.D., PH.D., F.D.S.R.C.S.

INTRODUCTION

Metabolic studies have shown that maintenance of the structure and function of connective tissues requires the continual synthesis and
degradation of cellular and extracellular macromolecules. The dynamics of these normal
processes of turnover concern events at a molecular level and do not involve any change in
the histological or ultrastructural appearance of
the tissue. This distinguishes turnover from
remodeling. Remodeling is a process of biological adaptation to altered environmental circumstances; it changes the structure or morphology
of the tissue concerned. There are many different types and causes of remodeling activity
associated with the skeleton. Bones do not
enlarge by the simple addition of bone to their
external surfaces, and structural remodeling is
an essential adjustment mechanism for maintaining the shape, proportions, and relation-

ships of a bone during its growth (Enlow, 1963)
(see Chapter 4).

Articular remodeling has been defined by
Moffett (1966) as the morphological adaptation
of joints in response to biomechanical stress.
The response of each of the articulations in the
craniofacial complex depends upon the type of
articular tissue present. With the exception of
the temporomandibular joints (TMJs) and the
synchondroses of the cranial base, all the articulations of the craniofacial complex are fibrous
joints. These are very responsive to biomechanical stress. Indeed, the ease with which fibrous
joints can be remodeled by mechanical means
is the fundamental biological event on which
orthodontic treatment is based. In contrast, the
articular surfaces of the TMJ have undergone
morphological adaptation to minimize the effects of the biomechanical stresses originating
from mandibular function. The presence of condylar cartilage, the fibrocartilaginous articular
tissue, and the articular disc enable the TMJ to
withstand compression and loading better than
fibrous joints, an ability related to the physical
properties of the cartilage matrix.

---

*See Chapters 4, 5, 11, 13, 22, 24, and 26.

93

CHONDROGENESIS IN THE TEMPOROMANDIBULAR JOINT AND THE ROLE OF BIOMECHANICAL STRESS

The articular surfaces of the TMJ, in common with the sternoclavicular and acromioclavicular joints, are derived from membrane bone formation and not, like all other synovial joints, from the primary cartilaginous skeleton. Consequently, it has been necessary for the articular surfaces of the mandible and temporal bone to undergo morphological change to resist the accumulative effects of the biomechanical stresses originating from the functional movements of the joint. Failure to do so results in premature degenerative change in the fibrous tissue of the articular zone, as well as resorptive remodeling of the subarticular bone. This morphological adaptation takes two forms, both of which can be regarded as a remodeling response and both necessitating the intervention of chondrogenesis.

Structure of the Cartilage Matrix

The extracellular matrix of cartilage is a randomly oriented meshwork of type II collagen fibers (Fig. 6–1) embedded in a gel of proteoglycans and water. It is the presence of water in conjunction with the collagen and proteoglycans that imparts to cartilage its characteristic toughness and resilience. *Proteoglycan* (protein-polysaccharide) is the name given to those macromolecules of connective tissue composed of a central core of protein to which carbohydrate side chains (glycosaminoglycans) are attached. *Glycosaminoglycans* (mucopolysaccharides), of which chondroitin sulfate is the predominant representative in cartilage, do not exist as free polysaccharides in the extracellular matrix, but rather are always covalently linked to protein.

The function of the collagen fibers is to resist tension. Compression is resisted principally by the gel of proteoglycans and water, although the collagen fiber network does help resist compressive stresses by limiting displacement of the gel. Such physical properties bestow on cartilage the ability to grow under conditions of compressive stress, so that cartilage is found in bones subject to compression of both gravitational and functional origin. Thus, the epiphyseal plate is ideally suited to being the pacemaker of long bone growth, while the presence of condylar cartilage is essential to prevent resorption and facilitate growth in a region of

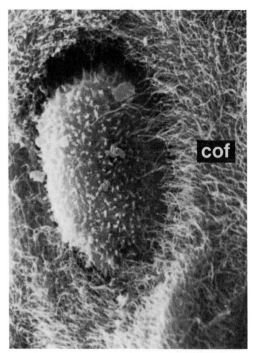

FIGURE 6–1. Scanning electron micrograph of a condylar cartilage cell in the early stage of undergoing hypertrophy. Note the dense network of type II collagen fibrils (cof) in the extracellular matrix. Noncollagenous material such as the proteoglycans are removed during processing. Bar measures 4 μm.

the mandible subjected to compressive stresses arising from function. This has an important bearing on the future remodeling characteristics of the TMJ.

Biomechanical Stress and Differentiation of Condylar Cartilage

Although the mandible is a membrane bone, its development is complicated by the formation of three secondary cartilages, one being the condylar cartilage. In the rat, for example, the condylar blastema appears at 17 days postconception within the mandibular blastema (Bhaskar, 1953). Duterloo (1969) observed that at 18 days postconception, the perichondrium covering the condylar blastema is continuous with the periosteum covering the bony sheath of the mandible. Because the chondroblasts of the condylar cartilage do not divide once they have differentiated from the proliferative zone (Blackwood, 1966), the only potential source of cells able to maintain growth of the mandible in this region is the cellular layer of the covering periosteum. Furthermore, transplantation studies have shown that once the TMJ has been transferred into a nonfunctional environment,

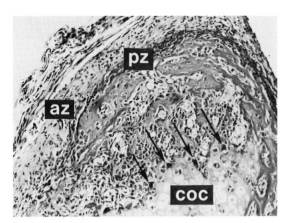

FIGURE 6–2. A coronal section through the condyle seven days after intracerebral transplantation of the mandibular joint into a littermate at one week of age. The section illustrates the spread of osteogenesis from the direction of the proliferative zone (pz). The arrows indicate chondroclasts eroding the cartilage. Condylar cartilage (coc). Articular zone (az). (Hematoxylin-eosin; original magnification × 200.)

chondrogenesis ceases and the cells of the proliferative zone differentiate into osteoblasts (Duterloo, 1967; Koski, 1963; 1964; 1965; Meikle, 1973a; 1973b) (Figs. 6–2 and 6–3). This indicates that the cells of the proliferative zone are multipotential and can produce either a cartilaginous or osseous matrix, depending upon the environmental circumstances.

There is, therefore, persuasive evidence for regarding the articular and proliferative zones of the condyle as being modified fibrous and cellular periosteum, respectively. The change from the normal osteogenic function of the

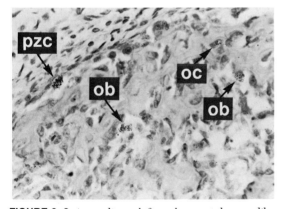

FIGURE 6–3. Autoradiograph from the seven-day mandibular joint transplant shown in Figure 6–2. The transplant was labeled with H³-thymidine before transplantation. The section illustrates one labeled cell (pzc) within the proliferative zone and two labeled osteoblasts (ob) and an osteocyte (oc) in the adjacent region of osteogenesis. Before transplantation, the labeled cells are confined to the proliferative zone. (Hematoxylin-eosin; original magnification × 500.)

cellular periosteum to one of chondrogenesis results from the evolutionary development of an articular condylar process in the mandible of mammals and, as a consequence, the altered functional demands placed upon the periosteum covering the articular surfaces. Indeed, only by regarding condylar cartilage as the product of periosteal chondrogenesis can the differences in structure and kinetics that exist between condylar cartilage and the epiphyseal plate of a long bone be adequately explained.

There are many situations in which connective tissues adapt to changing biomechanical circumstances. The example with the greatest relevance concerns the work of Murray (1963) who described the development of secondary cartilage in a number of articulations in the skull of the embryonic chick. The cartilage always developed in membrane bones, but only at articulations that were mobile or were at relevant developmental stages when the anatomy of the musculature could be expected to set up conditions of strain. Moreover, in grafted and paralyzed embryos (Murray, 1965), the cartilage did not form, and cells that normally would have formed cartilage instead produced bone. In a review of cellular differentiation in skeletal tissue, Hall (1970) pointed out that the common initiating factors in evoking osteogenesis and chondrogenesis are the degree of vascularity of the tissues and either the presence or absence of biomechanical stress. In vitro experimentation has shown that hypoxia enhances osteogenesis, and anoxia enhances chondrogenesis (Bassett, 1962; 1964; Goldhaber, 1963). This suggests that biomechanical stress may facilitate chondrogenesis by producing ischemia. Such an explanation accounts for the presence of cartilage at both the mandibular condyle and the articular surfaces of the temporal bone, the stimulus for differentiation being provided by extrinsic biomechanical stress originating from the functional activity of the TMJ (Meikle, 1973a; 1973b).

Biomechanical Stress and Chondrogenesis in the Articular Zone

Because the articular surfaces of the bones in the TMJ are derived from the periosteum, the outer layer, or fibrous periosteum, becomes what is normally referred to as the *articular zone*. During postnatal life, remodeling activity occurs in the fibrous connective tissue of this zone taking the form of a gradual metaplasia of the fibrous tissue into fibrocartilage (Fig. 6–4).

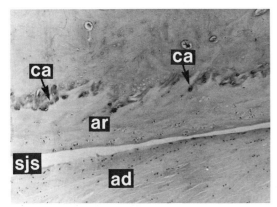

FIGURE 6–4. The articular eminence in an adult rhesus monkey. The appearance of cartilage cells (ca) within the articular tissue (ar) has transformed the fibrous tissue into fibrocartilage. Arrows indicate hypertrophic cells in the proliferative zone, the first sign of progressive remodeling. Articular disc (ad), superior joint compartment (sjs). (Hematoxylin-eosin; original magnification × 75.)

Ultrastructural studies in rodents have shown that at birth the articular tissue is composed of a highly cellular fibrous connective tissue covered by a layer of surface cells (Appleton, 1975; Meikle, 1975; Silva, 1967; 1969). These cells, which may be regarded as forming a synovial lining, have disappeared by two to four weeks. With age, the articular tissue undergoes a progressive reduction in cellularity until eventually the only remnants of the original cell population are a few cells bearing morphological characteristics of both chondrocytes and fibroblasts (Meikle, 1975; Silva, 1967), the tissue having become transformed into fibrocartilage (Fig. 6–4). The appearance of these cells in the articular tissue covering the condyle and other areas of the joint subject to compressive stress represents an attempt to increase the load-bearing capacity of the tissues.

The existence of similar cartilage or chondroid cells in the articular tissue of the TMJ of middle-aged and elderly humans has also been reported (Blackwood, 1966a; MacAlister, 1954; Moffett, 1962). Wright (1974), however, in a study of the human TMJ from birth to 21 years, did not observe cartilage cells in either the articular tissue or the disc. Autoradiographic studies of the mandibular condyle in rodents suggest that the cells of the articular tissue are renewed independently of the proliferative zone (Blackwood, 1966b; Gilhuus-Moe, 1969). This evidence, taken in conjunction with the morphological criteria, makes it likely that these cartilage cells originate by modulation from articular zone fibroblasts. Since the two most important extracellular macromolecules synthe-

sized by connective tissue cells are collagen and proteoglycan, it would not require a particularly profound alteration in biosynthetic activity on the part of a fibroblast to change from producing a predominantly collagenous matrix to one with a greater proportion of proteoglycan.

REMODELING OF THE HUMAN TEMPOROMANDIBULAR JOINT

Although the earliest concept of articular remodeling was advanced by Ogston (1875, 1878) more than a century ago, there has always been a tendency to regard joints as unchanging, inert structures. The articular cartilage, like the underlying bone, has the ability to adapt to alterations in the mechanical equilibrium of the skeleton, even in the adult. Ogston (1875) believed that the articular cartilage of a long bone was continually renewing itself from a central focus of growth. He observed that growth occurred outward from the joint surface to compensate for wear and tear, as well as inward, where it added to the subchondral bone through endochondral osteogenesis. This view has since been confirmed experimentally through the autoradiographic studies of Mankin (1962), in which the injection of H^3-thymidine into the knee joint of rabbits demonstrated the presence of a central zone of proliferative cells in the femoral articular cartilage.

Classification of Articular Remodeling

Articular remodeling in human synovial joints has been classified by Johnson (1959) into three categories: progressive, regressive, and peripheral or circumferential. Progressive remodeling results from a proliferation of articular cartilage followed by its mineralization and eventual osteogenic replacement. Johnson (1959) calculated that progressive remodeling added 3 mm of new bone to the femoral head between the ages of 30 and 60 years. Regressive remodeling results from osteoclastic resorption of the subchondral bone with subsequent filling of the cavities by mesenchymal tissue and its replacement by cartilage, bone, or both. Peripheral remodeling occurs at the margin of the articular cartilage and is a combination of progressive remodeling and periosteal deposition.

Changes in the Temporomandibular Joint

The morphological changes associated with articular remodeling in the human TMJ have been studied by Moffett (1964) and Blackwood (1959; 1966a). All three types of remodeling activity described by Johnson (1959) have been identified and showed the following distribution trends: progressive remodeling on the anterior part of the condyle, medial part of the articular eminence, and the roof of the glenoid fossa; regressive remodeling on the posterior part of the condyle and lateral part of the articular eminence; and peripheral remodeling mainly at the anterior articular margin of the condyle. The degree of remodeling activity did not show any correlation with age, but there was a high correlation between the number of missing teeth and the amount and extent of the remodeling. All the joints examined revealed remodeling activity in some part of the joint.

Progressive Remodeling

The earliest changes that can be observed histologically both at the condyle and the articular eminence, are hypertrophy of the cells of the proliferative zone accompanied by increased production of extracellular matrix (Fig. 6–5). This newly formed cartilaginous tissue becomes mineralized and eventually resorbed and replaced by bone (Fig. 6–6), although some islands of mineralized cartilage matrix may remain unreabsorbed. These changes take place without any apparent alteration in the structure of the articular zone.

Regressive Remodeling

In regressive remodeling, the first observable change is resorption of the subarticular bone

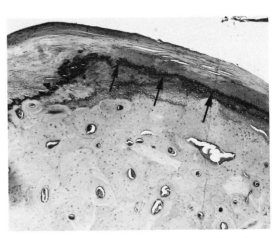

FIGURE 6–6. Progressive remodeling on the lateral part of the condyle in a 61-year-old male. The calcified zone has advanced toward the articular surface (*arrows*) and the tissue deep to it is being replaced by bone. (Frontal section, hematoxylin-eosin; original magnification × 25.) (From Moffett, B. C., Johnson, L. C., McCabe, J. B., and Askew, H. C.: Articular remodeling of the adult temporomandibular joint. Am. J. Anat. 155:119–142, 1964.)

and adjacent cartilage by osteoclasts (Fig. 6–7). It is likely that the osteoclasts involved in this phase of regressive remodeling are formed by the fusion of circulating osteoclast precursor cells having their origin in the bone marrow. Initially, the resorption cavity is filled by vascular mesenchymal tissue, but eventually this is replaced by fibrocartilage, bone, or both. Although the tissue of the articular zone re-

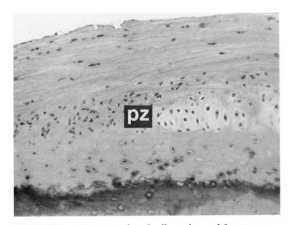

FIGURE 6–5. Hypertrophy of cells in the proliferative zone (pz) of the mandibular condyle in an adult human. This represents the earliest change observable histologically in progressive remodeling. (Hematoxylin-eosin; original magnification × 200). (From Blackwood, H. J. J.: Cellular remodeling in articular tissue. J. Dent. Res. 45:480–489, 1966.)

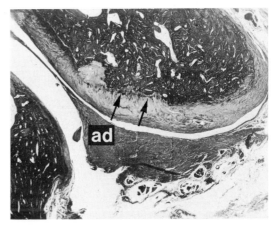

FIGURE 6–7. Regressive remodeling, lateral part of articular eminence, embalmed cadaver, age unknown. The resorption defect (outlined by *arrows*) in the subchondral bone represents an early stage in regressive remodeling. It is located just posterior to the crest of the eminence in a loaded area where the articular disc (ad) has become thinned almost to a perforation. (Sagittal section, hematoxylin-eosin; original magnification × 10). (From Moffett, B. C., Johnson, L. C., McCabe, J. B., and Askew, H. C.: Articular remodeling of the adult temporomandibular joint. Am. J. Anat. 115:119–142, 1964.)

mains intact, the net effect of regressive remodeling is to reduce the vertical dimension of the underlying bone.

In the majority of cases, both progressive and regressive remodeling are proceeding simultaneously in different parts of the same joint, and often where the articular disc has been perforated, progressive and regressive remodeling can be seen occurring on opposing articular surfaces (Figs. 6–8 and 6–9).

Peripheral Remodeling

The characteristic feature of peripheral remodeling is that the cellular activity originates from the proliferative zone. This gives rise to an outgrowth of cartilage at the anterior border of the condyle immediately above the insertion of the lateral pterygoid muscle. This cartilaginous outgrowth eventually becomes mineralized and replaced by bone to produce an osteophytic lipping of the articular contour (Figs. 6–8 and 6–9).

Articular Remodeling in Young Adults

The largest series of young adult human TMJs (20 to 36 years) available to date has been collected by Solberg (1985). Deviation in form (DIF), presence of arthrosis, changes in size and shape of the condyle, and disc displacement were evaluated in 95 TMJs obtained at autopsy. This material is particularly important because

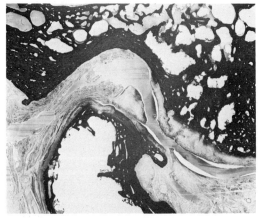

FIGURE 6–8. The TMJ from an 81-year-old-male with a perforated disc. This joint is well within the category of osteoarthritis. The severest changes are opposite the perforation of the disc. Progressive and circumferential remodeling has occurred on the anterior part of the condyle and regressive remodeling on the crest of the eminence (see Fig. 6–9). (Sagittal section, hematoxylin-eosin; original magnification × 5.)

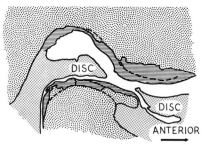

ARTICULAR REMODELING
SAGITTAL TRACING 68 D-1

FIGURE 6–9. Tracing of section shown in Figure 6–8. The dotted lines on the condyle and temporal bone represent the contours of their subchondral plates before remodeling. The new contours at the junction between bone (stippled) and articular tissue (horizontal stripe) result in a flattened, enlarged condyle and a partially resorbed articular eminence. (From Moffett, B. C., Johnson, L. C., McCabe, J. B., and Askew, H. C.: Articular remodeling of the adult temporomandibular joint. Am. J. Anat. *115*:119–142, 1964.)

young adults comprise the largest population of individuals presenting with TMJ problems. A remarkable finding was that only 13 per cent (12/95) showed no intracapsular changes, while 39 per cent (37/95) displayed mild to extreme DIF, with condylar changes being the most marked. Disc displacement was found in 12 per cent (11/95), and was more common in females. Morphological variation was documented in a further histological investigation of 33 condyles from this series (Lubsen, 1985). The proliferative zone was absent in 13 condyles and showed regional variability in an additional 18. Condylar cartilage was hypertrophic in ten and hyperplastic in nine. Remodeling of the subarticular bone was observed in nine condyles. It is clear from this material that remodeling changes are common in young adult TMJs.

Articular Remodeling and Osteoarthritis

Articular remodeling gradually merges into degenerative arthritis, and because all the adaptive mechanisms characteristic of remodeling are active in the osteoarthritic joint, it is difficult to make the distinction, histologically, between what can be regarded as a normally aged joint and one that has become pathologically involved (see Chapters 11, 22, and 24). Nevertheless, a useful criterion has been suggested by Moffett (1964) and is related to the integrity of the articular tissue. Moffett defined remodeling as being those changes associated with a proliferative response in the articular tissue, and considered that osteoarthritis represented those changes associated with the breakdown of the articular tissue: fibrillation, fissuring, eburnation, and cystic alterations.

EXPERIMENTAL REMODELING OF THE NONHUMAN TEMPOROMANDIBULAR JOINT

The effects of external mechanical stress in nonhuman primates have provided valuable information regarding the susceptibility of the craniofacial articulations to experimentally induced remodeling activity. The principal objective of such work has been to determine the extent to which articular remodeling can be utilized clinically in the correction of skeletal malocclusion. As one might anticipate from the preceding discussion concerning adaptation, the TMJs have been found to be less responsive to mechanical stress than either the periodontal or craniofacial sutures (for reviews, see Moffett, 1971; 1973).

Anterior Displacement of the Mandible in Primates

Irrespective of whether it was brought about by a biteplate (Baume, 1961; Breitner, 1940; 1941; Stockli, 1971) or Class II intermaxillary elastics (Adams, 1972; Norwick, 1969), anterior displacement of the mandible in young rhesus monkeys produces changes in the TMJs. In addition to the deposition of bone in the temporal fossa, condylar growth appears to be directed more posteriorly than normal, and the shape of the condyle becomes less rounded. Furthermore, comparisons of mandibular growth between experimental and control groups utilizing cephalometric radiography (Elgoyhen, 1972) and histology (McNamara, 1979; 1982) show significant increases in both the rate and amount of growth at the condyle, although these investigators found that such increases occurred only during the first three months of the experimental period. These data should be interpreted with caution, however, given the inaccuracies of cephalometric radiography. Moreover, the conclusions derived from the histological material were based on measurements of the thickness of the condylar cartilage, and in 1982 McNamara emphasized the wide variability in cartilage width within control and experimental groups. This brings into question the validity of using cartilage thickness for estimating growth changes, given the number of sections available from each condyle and the

practical need to select just a few for morphometric analysis. Furthermore, it could be argued that an increase in the thickness of the condylar cartilage might have resulted from a decrease in endochondral osteogenesis rather than an increase in cell proliferation or cartilage matrix formation. It also seems from the methodology section in these studies that the investigators knew a priori which were experimental and control condyles when the measurements were made. The importance of carrying out morphometric analyses blind is further considered in a later section.

The same force producing anterior mandibular displacement applied to adult monkeys (Hiniker, 1966; Meikle, 1970) does not produce any recognizable alteration in the activity of the slight amount of condylar cartilage that is usually still present and the condyle does not show evidence of articular remodeling. However, where it is compressed forcibly forward against the eminence by Class II intermaxillary elastics, the fibrocartilaginous tissue of that part of the eminence subjected to maximal articular compression undergoes a metaplastic transformation into a tissue resembling hyaline cartilage (Fig. 6–10). Again, this is presumably a functional adaptation to increase the load-bearing capacity of the articular tissue. If the compressive force is of sufficient magnitude it may initiate localized regressive remodeling and resorption of the subchondral bone (Fig. 6–11).

These changes provide experimental support for the concept that the remodeling seen in human TMJs represents a biological response to increased or altered articular loading.

Posterior Displacement of the Mandible in Primates

Changes in the TMJ produced by distal displacement of the mandible (Adams, 1969; Joho, 1973; Ramfjord, 1966) are similar in both young and adult monkeys and represent localized articular remodeling. Condylar growth does not appear to be directed more anteriorly, and the remodeling activity takes the form of bone resorption at the anterior surface of the postglenoid tubercle and posterior surface of the condyle (Fig. 6–12). It is of interest that similar changes were observed in the TMJs of monkeys in which extraoral cervical traction has been applied to the dentomaxillary complex (Sproule, 1968). Janzen (1965) created distal displacement of the mandible by an experimental situation similar to that which occurs clinically when a chin cup is used in the correction of Class III

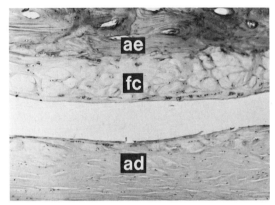

FIGURE 6–10. The articular eminence (ae) from an adult monkey following the application of Class II intermaxillary elastics. Note metaplasia of the fibrocartilaginous tissue (fc) into a tissue resembling hyaline cartilage. The superficial layers of the articular disc (ad) are similarly affected. (Hematoxylin-eosin; original magnification × 75.)

malocclusion. The mandibles in three young rhesus monkeys were transfixed by a Kirschner wire and a continually acting retraction force was applied. Changes similar to those previously described were noted but, in addition, bone deposition on the anterior surface of the condyle was observed. The findings also suggested that the condyle did not attain its full growth potential.

In a study conducted by Meikle (1970), a young adult monkey that showed histologically recognizable condylar growth received unilateral Class II and Class III intermaxillary elastics simultaneously. The condyle exposed to anterior displacement by the Class II force showed posteriorly directed endochondral osteogenesis as well as increased periosteal deposition at the

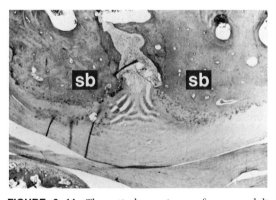

FIGURE 6–11. The articular eminence from an adult monkey after application of Class II intermaxillary elastics. The breakdown of the subarticular bone (sb) and the appearance of tissue resembling hyaline cartilage at the entrance of the defect have resulted from the effects of excessive compressive stress. (Hematoxylin-eosin; original magnification × 30.)

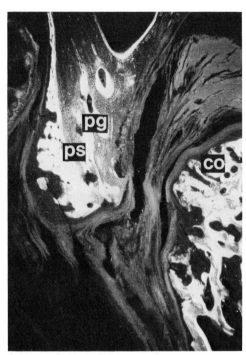

FIGURE 6–12. The postglenoid tubercle (pg) in an adult monkey, Class III side. Tetracycline was administered to the animal during the experimental period. Resorptive remodeling of the condyle (co) has occurred, while progressive remodeling, or deposition has taken place on the posterior surface (ps) of the postglenoid tubercle (pg). (Unstained ground section, ultraviolet illumination; original magnification × 15.)

posterior border of the condyloid process. In contrast, the condyle exposed to distal displacement by the Class III force demonstrated resorptive remodeling on both the condyle and the anterior surface of the postglenoid tubercle, accompanied by the compensatory deposition of bone along the posterior surface of the tubercle (note the histological appearance of these joints in Figs. 6–12 and 6–13). If continued long enough, these remodeling changes would have had the effect of producing a new articular surface and contour to the condyle.

Milwaukee Brace

To understand the influence of the Milwaukee brace on the dentofacial complex during the correction of scoliosis of the spine in man, the effect of a modified appliance on the TMJ in growing rhesus monkeys was evaluated cephalometrically and histologically by Cutler (1972) who found that although the brace appeared to reduce cellular activity, the TMJs showed little sign of articular remodeling. It was also concluded that the fibrous articular

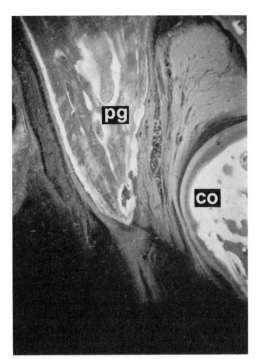

FIGURE 6–13. The postglenoid tubercle (pg) in the same adult monkey in Figure 6–12, Class II side. The contrast between the two joints is extreme. Note the uptake of tetracycline in the condyle (co), indicative of active mineralization and endochondral osteogenesis. The remodeling characteristics of the postglenoid tubercle are normal. (Unstained ground section, ultraviolet illumination; original magnification × 15.)

tissue was better adapted to withstand compressive stress than had been anticipated. No significant changes in the articular tissue covering the condyle and articular eminence were observed. The monkeys exhibited more than normal resorption of the postglenoid tubercle. This remodeling change is similar to that described by Adams (1969) and Meikle (1970) following the application of Class III intermaxillary elastics to the mandible. Cutler (1972) also noted that while condylar growth was retarded by the brace, following its removal growth initially was resumed at an accelerated rate.

Influence of Biomechanical Stress on Cellular Activity in the Proliferative Zone

The work of Melcher (1971) and the findings of transplantation studies in which H³-thymidine was used as a cellular label (Duterloo, 1967; Meikle, 1973a,b) have shown that cell division within the proliferative zone of the condyle can occur independently of any extrin-

sic functional factors. Nevertheless, there is evidence indicating that the cellular activity of the proliferative zone can be altered by external biomechanical stress of a functional origin (Blackwood, 1966a; Charlier, 1968; 1969; Folke, 1966; Moffett, 1964). Folke (1966) evaluated the effect of distal displacement of the mandible on the proliferative zone in adult rats utilizing tritiated H³-thymidine autoradiography to monitor alterations in cellular activity. The study concluded that cell division within the proliferative zone can be stimulated, even in the adult, in response to alterations in mandibular position. Further studies have suggested that mandibular hyperpropulsion (anterior displacement) in young rats can bring about additional growth of condylar cartilage by increasing the rate of cell division in the proliferative zone (Charlier, 1968; 1969; Petrovic, 1977; 1981).

Over the past few years attempts to duplicate these results using both fixed and removable anterior mandibular displacement devices were unsuccessful (Tewson, 1988; Tonge, 1982). Use of both biochemical methods and H³-thymidine autoradiography did not detect significant differences in radioactive indices for the anterior, middle, and posterior regions of the condyle in one month-old rats after 14 days of displacement (Tewson, 1988). Degroote (1984) also failed to detect an increase in the number of H³-thymidine-labeled cells in the proliferative zone of experimental condyles from one month-old rats subjected to full- and part-time anterior mandibular displacement for 28 days. Indeed, all the parameters measured by Degroote (1984) indicated that mandibular hyperpropulsion resulted in slowed condylar and mandibular growth compared to controls.

Animal experiments are frequently cited in the orthodontic literature as evidence that functional appliances can stimulate mandibular growth, but most are flawed by inadequacies in methodology and inconsistencies in the interpretation of data. For example, one of the methodological problems associated with the studies of Petrovic (1977, 1981) has been consistent failure to relate the incorporation of H³-thymidine into proliferative zone cells to the total cell population or any other parameter of condylar size to obtain a radioactive index. Merely counting the number of labeled cells in a series of autoradiographs is quite unsatisfactory for quantifying differences between experimental and control groups. Furthermore, it is important in morphometric studies of this type to have the autoradiographs coded by an independent assessor and counted blind to avoid subjective bias. One must conclude, therefore, that at the present time there is insufficient scientific evidence to support the hypothesis that functional mandibular displacement can significantly stimulate condylar growth. The major obstacle to a rational discussion of the available evidence, however, is that in the minds of some clinicians the theory of mandibular growth stimulation has achieved the status of a proven theory. In other words, instead of being a testable scientific hypothesis it has become an ideology.

CELLULAR AND MOLECULAR BASIS FOR TEMPOROMANDIBULAR JOINT REMODELING

Direct evidence for the biochemical mechanisms and cellular interactions mediating articular remodeling is not currently available for the TMJ. Nevertheless, it is possible by drawing on the findings of other areas of research, particularly into arthritic diseases, to make some educated guesses as to the mechanisms

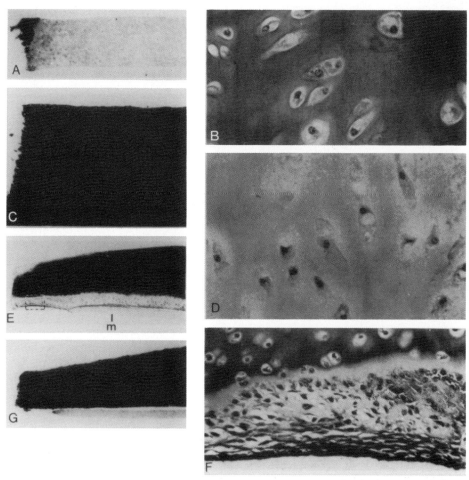

FIGURE 6–14. Effect of porcine synovial factor on bovine nasal and pig articular cartilage. *A,* Vertical section of explant of bovine nasal cartilage after eight days culture. Metachromasia is absent except in one corner where the cells are dead. (Toluidine blue; magnification × 20.) *B,* Horizontal section of a similar explant showing viable chondrocytes. (Celestine blue, Carazzi's hematoxylin, and van Gieson; magnification × 250.) *C,* Same as *A,* but cultured in control medium. There is no loss of metachromasia. (Toluidine blue; magnification × 20.) *D,* Same as *B,* but cultured in control medium. (Staining was the same as in *B* and shows viable chondrocytes; magnification × 250.) *E,* Porcine articular cartilage after 10 days culture. Note the peripheral loss of metachromasia. m, Millipore filter (Toluidine blue; magnification × 20.). *F,* Another section of the same explant (approximately within the area marked by the broken line in *E*) showing early breakdown of collagen. The chondrocytes are undergoing a fibroblastic transformation. (Celestine blue, Carazzi's hematoxylin, and van Gieson's stain; magnification × 188.) *G,* Paired explant of *A* grown in control medium. There is no loss of metachromasia. (Toluidine blue; magnification × 20.) (Reprinted by permission from Dingle, J. T., Saklatvala, J., Hembry, R. M., et al.: A cartilage catabolic factor from synovium. Biochem. J. *184:*177–180, 1979. Copyright 1979 The Biochemical Society, London.)

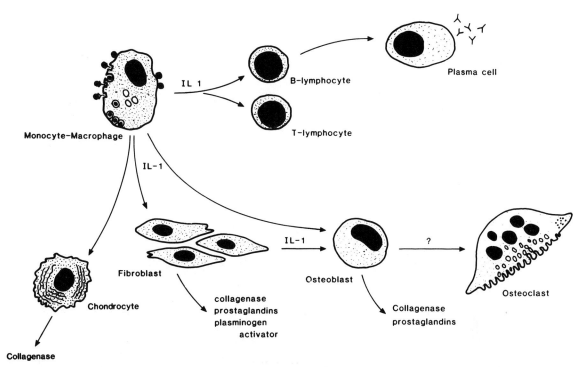

FIGURE 6–15. Summary of possible pathways whereby IL-1 could mediate signals between cells of relevance to TMJ remodeling and arthritis. Fibroblasts and osteoblasts can also produce IL-1 that might explain how tissue destruction in the TMJ can take place in the virtual absence of inflammatory cells. The action of IL-1 on its target cells is modified by other polypeptides such as the tumor necrosis factors, interferons, and growth factors (fibroblast growth factors, platelet-derived growth factor, transforming growth factors α and β).

involved. Connective tissue degradation in rheumatoid arthritis and other joint diseases is often attributed to the direct action of proteolytic enzymes. Neutrophils, which are abundant in rheumatoid synovial fluid, produce collagenase, elastase, and cathepsins; macrophages and synovial fibroblasts also produce a variety of metalloproteinases that can degrade the structural proteins of most connective tissues. It is now clear from in vitro evidence that has accumulated over the past decade, however, that chondrocytes, fibroblasts, and bone cells may contribute to the destruction of their own extracellular matrices. In other words, they can be induced to self-destruct.

In 1977 Fell reported that coculture of pig synovial tissue and articular cartilage in the same dish resulted in cartilage resorption; this suggested that the pig synovium had produced a factor that caused the chondrocytes to degrade their matrix (Fig. 6–14). The factor, which was called catabolin (Dingle, 1979) turned out to be interleukin-1 (IL-1).

The cytokine IL-1 and the functionally related tumor necrosis factors (TNFs) are polypeptides that act as early mediators of inflammation and immunity (Dinarello, 1985; Le, 1987). IL-1 exists in two distinct molecular forms, IL-1α (pI5) and IL-1β (pI7). The predominant molecular species produced by activated monocytes is IL-1β, the mRNA coding for this molecule being about 10 times more abundant than for IL-1α. Cultured human keratinocytes, on the other hand, contain 2 to 4 times more IL-1α mRNA than IL-1β mRNA.

The tumor necrosis factors TNFα and TNFβ (also called lymphotoxin) are products of activated monocytes and lymphocytes, respectively. Although originally defined by their cytotoxic action against certain transplanted tumors and neoplastic cell lines, the TNFs are also potent immunoregulatory molecules sharing multiple overlapping biological activities with IL-1 (Le, 1987). There is also evidence that lymphocyte derived interferon-γ (IFN-γ) modulates a broad range of biological activities associated with IL-1 and TNF. IFN-γ induces HLA-DR expression on mouse macrophages, human monocytes, vascular endothelial cells, and dermal fibroblasts. Furthermore, IFN-γ enhances IL-1 production by endothelial cells, TNF-receptor expression on several murine and human cell lines, and TNFα and TNFβ production by human peripheral blood mononuclear cells (Le, 1987).

In addition to their effects on the immune system, IL-1 and the TNFs are potent stimulators of connective tissue degradation in vitro. Both stimulate prostaglandin E_2 and collagenase production by fibroblasts, chondrocytes, and osteoblasts, as well as bone and cartilage resorption. Indeed, IL-1 is the most potent bone resorbing agent known. These data suggest that tissue destruction in joint diseases is mediated, at least in part, by these cytokines (Meikle, 1986), and there have been several reports of IL-1 in synovial fluid. Some of the intracellular interactions mediated by IL-1 are shown in Figure 6–15.

Clearly, the intercellular interactions mediated by IL-1 and other immunoregulatory cytokines during joint diseases are complex. However, both IL-1 and TNF have been shown by in vitro methods to have the potential to initiate the sequence of events leading to the loss of articular tissue and bone and cartilage resorption that are characteristic features of TMJ remodeling. Whether they do so in vitro can now be assessed using antibodies and molecular probes to cytokines and enzymes such as collagenase.

CLINICAL IMPLICATIONS

The finding that the TMJs can be remodeled by mechanical means has inevitably raised the question as to whether such alterations can be utilized clinically to correct skeletal discrepancies between the mandible and maxilla. The most satisfactory way to approach this somewhat controversial question is to consider the role of the condyle in the total growth of the mandible.

The significance of the condyle was highly exaggerated in the traditional concept of mandibular growth. This view was perhaps best summarized by the statement that ". . . mandible growth is solely controlled by the growth that takes place at the top of the condyle" (Charles, 1925). Early ideas concerning mandibular growth largely were based on decalcified histological material, and undoubtedly were influenced by the presence of cartilage in the condyle bearing a superficial resemblance to the epiphyseal cartilage of a long bone. Charles' conclusions were derived from a study of the mandible of the human fetus, a stage of development in which the wedge of condylar cartilage is most impressive. Only through the use of vital staining (Manson, 1968; Turpin, 1968) and implant techniques (Sarnat, 1956) have the extent and significance of the growth and remodeling changes in the other parts of the mandible been appreciated. Furthermore, attempts to establish the quantitative contribution of the condyle to the overall growth of the mandible through condylectomy studies have shown that the condyle makes only a localized contribution to the enlargement of the vertical ramus (Meikle, 1973b; Pimenidis, 1972; Sarnat, 1951; 1971a; 1971b).

If one accepts that the role of the condyle in mandibular growth is localized, then the addition of several layers of cells to the condyle (Charlier, 1969; Folke, 1966) is unlikely to increase the length of the mandible sufficiently to affect maxillomandibular relationships, despite claims to the contrary. The same can be said of the remodeling changes produced by experimental mandibular displacement in monkeys. Many investigators have made a clinical evaluation of the effects of anterior mandibular displacement on the growth of the condyle (Björk, 1951; Freunthaller, 1967; Jakobsson, 1967; Marschner, 1966; Softley, 1953). Nevertheless, to date, no convincing clinical study has been reported showing a significant alteration in mandibular growth as a result of orthodontic treatment, irrespective of the method used, which could not be explained on the basis of normal growth, individual variation, or both. One must conclude, therefore, that orthodontic appliances that produce anterior displacement of the mandible do not influence condylar growth by an amount that could be considered of clinical significance. Such appliances may initiate localized articular remodeling of the type described in the TMJ of rhesus monkeys and, indeed, may alter the cell division within the proliferative zone of the condyle. Any treatment plan that is dependent on increasing condylar growth to achieve its clinical objective, however, is biologically unsound.

Post hoc deductions abound in the clinical literature, but it is a fallacy to assume that because the mandible grew during the wearing of a functional appliance that the two events are necessarily related. Mandibles also grow during headgear treatment. Are we to draw the same conclusions? Given the ability of cartilage to withstand the effects of compressive stress, a similar cautionary note should be voiced concerning the efficacy of appliances such as the chin cup in restraining the forward growth of the mandible during the treatment of skeletal Class III malocclusion.

There is insufficient data to make many valid conclusions concerning the dental causes of remodeling in the TMJ. It is, however, known from animal experimentation that the adaptive changes in the TMJ are insignificant compared to the remodeling activity in the periodontium and compensatory movement that takes place in the teeth. Such findings indicate ". . . the need to adapt the occlusion to the joints rather than hoping for the joints to adapt to the occlusion" (Hiniker, 1966). Extremes of mandibular movement acting over many years produce significant remodeling changes in the joint. Moffett (1964) and Blackwood (1966a) found that the amount of remodeling activity was correlated with the number of missing teeth, and specimens showing osteoarthritic changes were frequently edentulous. Such findings indicate the need for replacement and restoration of the vertical dimension of the dentition following tooth loss.

SUMMARY

The articular surfaces of the temporomandibular joint (TMJ) are derived from membrane bones. During development and growth, they undergo morphological adaptation to resist the biomechanical stresses arising from mandibular function. This functional adaptation necessitates the intervention of chondrogenesis, which enables the joint to withstand the effects of compression and loading, an ability related to the physical properties of the cartilage matrix. Nevertheless, the TMJ retains the ability to adapt to alterations in the mechanical equilibrium of the joint, regardless of the cessation of skeletal growth. The contours of the joint continue to change throughout the lifespan as a result of articular remodeling. Three types of articular remodeling have been described in the human TMJ: progressive, regressive, and peripheral or circumferential. It is the ability of the cells of the proliferative zone to respond to alterations in biomechanical stress that is responsible for initiating the remodeling changes that take place. Eventually, however, with age and the diminishing proliferative capacity of the cell population, articular remodeling merges gradually into degenerative arthritis.

While experimental studies on animals indicate that remodeling activity can be initiated in the TMJ by functional displacement of the mandible, caution must be expressed in extrapolating such findings to the clinical situation as a rational basis for the treatment of skeletal malocclusion.

REFERENCES

Adams, C. D.: The effects of continuous posterior mandibular forces [class III] on the temporomandibular joint and the dentofacial skeleton of the *Macaca mulatta*. Unpublished dissertation. Seattle, University of Washington, 1969.

Adams, C. D., Meikle, M. C., Norwick, K. W., and Turpin, D. L.: Dentofacial remodeling produced by intermaxillary forces in *Macaca mulatta*. Arch. Oral Biol. *17*:1519–1535, 1972.

Appleton, J.: The ultrastructure of the articular tissue of the mandibular condyle in the rat. Arch. Oral Biol. *20*:823–826, 1975.

Bassett, C. A. L.: Current concepts of bone formation. J. Bone Joint Surg. [Am.]. *44*:1217–1244, 1962.

Bassett, C. A. L.: Environmental and cellular factors regulating osteogenesis. *In* Frost, H. M. (Ed.): Bone Biodynamics. Boston, Little, Brown, & Co., 1964, pp. 233–244.

Baume, L. J., and Derichsweiler, H.: Is the condylar growth centre responsive to orthodontic therapy? An experimental study in *Macaca mulatta*. Oral Surg. *14*:347–362, 1961.

Bhaskar, S. N.: Growth of the rat mandible from 13 days after insemination to 30 days after birth. Am. J. Anat. *92*:1–53, 1953.

Björk, A.: The principle of the Andresen method of orthodontic treatment. Am. J. Orthod. *37*:437–458, 1951.

Blackwood, H. J. J.: Development, growth and pathology of the mandibular condyle. Unpublished dissertation. Belfast, Queen's University, 1959.

Blackwood, H. J. J.: Cellular remodeling in articular tissue. J. Dent. Res. [Suppl.]. *45*:480–489, 1966a.

Blackwood, H. J. J.: Growth of the mandibular condyle of the rat studied with tritiated thymidine. Arch. Oral. Biol. *11*:403–500, 1966b.

Breitner, C.: Bone changes resulting from experimental orthodontic treatment. Am. J. Orthod. *26*:521–547, 1940.

Breitner, C.: Further investigations of bone changes resulting from experimental orthodontic treatment. Am. J. Orthod. *27*:605–632, 1941.

Charles, S. W.: The temporomandibular joint and its influence on the growth of the mandible. Br. Dent. J. *46*:845–855, 1925.

Charlier, J. P., Petrovic, A., and Hermann-Stutzmann, J.: Déterminisme de la croissance mandibulaire. Effets de l'hyperpropulsion de l'hormone somatotrope sur la croissance condylienne de jeune rats. Orthod. Fr. *39*:567–579, 1968.

Charlier, J. P., Petrovic, A., and Hermann-Stutzmann, J.: Effect of mandibular hyperpropulsion on the prechondroblastic zone of young rat condyle. Am. J. Orthod. *55*:71–74, 1969.

Cutler, B. S., Hassig, F. H., and Turpin, D. L.: Dentofacial changes produced during and after use of a modified Milwaukee brace on *Macaca mulatta*. Am. J. Orthod. *61*:115–137, 1972.

Degroote, C. N.: Alterability of mandibular condylar growth in the young rat and its implications. Published Monograph. Catholic University of Louvain, Belgium, 1984.

Dinarello, C. A.: An update on human interleukin-1 from molecular biology to clinical relevance. J. Clin. Immunol. *5*:287–297, 1985.

Dingle, J. T., Saklatvala, J., Hembry, R., et al.: A cartilage catabolic factor from synovium. Biochem. J. *184*:177–180, 1979.

Duterloo, H. S.: In vivo implantation of the mandibular

condyle of the rat. Published dissertation. Nijmegan, The Netherlands, University of Nijmegan, 1967.

Duterloo, H. S., and Jansen, H. W. B.: Chondrogenesis and osteogenesis in the mandibular condylar blastema. Trans. Eur. Orthod. Soc. 109–118, 1969.

Elgoyhen, J. C., Moyers, R. E., McNamara, J. A., and Riolo, M. L.: Craniofacial adaptation to protrusive function in young rhesus monkeys. Am. J. Orthod. 62:469–480, 1972.

Enlow, D. H.: Principles of Bone Remodeling. Springfield, IL, Charles C Thomas, 1963.

Fell, H. B., and Jubb, R. N.: The effect of synovial tissue on the breakdown of articular cartilage in organ culture. Arthritis Rheum. 20:1359–1371, 1977.

Folke, L. E. A., and Stallard, R. E.: Condylar adaptation to a change in intermaxillary relationship. J. Peridont. Res. 1:79–89, 1966.

Freunthaller, P.: Cephalometric observations in Class II division 1 malocclusion treated with the monobloc. Angle Orthod. 37:18–25, 1967.

Gilhuus-Moe, O.: Fractures of the Mandibular Condyle in the Growth Period. Norwegian Monographs on Medical Sciences. Oslo, Universitatsforloget, 1969.

Goldhaber, P.: Some chemical factors influencing bone resorption in tissue culture. Publ. Am. Assoc. Adv. Sci. 75:609–636, 1963.

Hall, B. K.: Cellular differentiation in skeletal tissue. Biol. Rev. 45:455–484, 1970.

Hiniker, J. J., and Ramfjord, S. P.: Anterior displacement of the mandible in adult rhesus monkeys. J. Prosthet. Dent. 16:503–512, 1966.

Jakobsson, S. O.: Cephalometric evaluation of treatment effects on class II division 1 malocclusion. Am. J. Orthod. 53:446–457, 1967.

Janzen, E. K., and Bluher, J. A.: The cephalometric, anatomic and histological changes in Macaca mulatta after application of a continuous-acting retraction force on the mandible. Am. J. Orthod. 51:823–855, 1965.

Johnson, L. C.: Kinetics of osteoarthritis. Lab. Invest. 8:1223–1238, 1959.

Joho, J. P.: The effects of extraoral lowpull traction to the mandibular dentition of Macaca mulatta. Am. J. Orthod. 64:555–577, 1973.

Koski, K., and Makinen, L.: Growth potential of transplanted components of the mandibular ramus of the rat. I. Suom. Hammaslaak. Toim. 59:296–308, 1963.

Koski, K., and Mason, K. E.: Growth potential of transplanted components of the mandibular ramus of the rat. II. Suom. Hammaslaak. Toim. 60:209–218, 1964.

Koski, K., and Rönning, O.: Growth potential of transplanted components of the mandibular ramus of the rat. III. Suom. Hammaslaak. Toim. 61:292–297, 1965.

Le, J., and Vilcek, J.: Tumour necrosis factor and interleukin-1: Cytokines with multiple overlapping biological activities. Lab. Invest. 56:234–248, 1987.

Lubsen, C. C., Hansson, T. L. and Nordström, B. B.: Histomorphometric analysis of cartilage and subchondral bone in mandibular condyles of young human adults at autopsy. Arch. Oral Biol. 30:129–136, 1985.

MacAlister, A. D.: A microscopic survey of the human temporomandibular joint. N. Z. Dent. J. 50:161–172, 1954.

Mankin, H. J.: Localization of tritiated thymidine in articular cartilage of rabbits. I. Growth in immature cartilage. J. Bone Joint Surg. [Am.]. 44:682–698, 1962.

Manson, J. D.: A Comparative Study of the Postnatal Growth of the Mandible. London, Henry Kimpton, 1968.

Marschner, J. F., and Harris, J. E.: Mandibular growth and class II treatment. Angle Orthod. 36:89–93, 1966.

McNamara, J. A., and Carlson, D. S.: Quantitative analysis of temporomandibular joint adaptation to protrusive function. Am. J. Orthod. 76:593–611, 1979.

McNamara, J. A., Hinton, R. J., and Hoffman, D. L.: Histologic analysis of temporomandibular joint adaptation to protrusive function in young adult rhesus monkeys (Macaca mulatta). Am. J. Orthod. 82:228–298, 1982.

Meikle, M. C.: The effect of a class II intermaxillary force on the dentofacial complex in the adult Macaca mulatta monkey. Am. J. Orthod. 58:323–340, 1970.

Meikle, M. C.: In vivo transplantation of the mandibular joint of the rat: An autoradiographic investigation into cellular changes at the condyle. Arch. Oral Biol. 18:1011–1020, 1973a.

Meikle, M. C.: The role of the condyle in the postnatal growth of the mandible. Am. J. Orthod. 64:50–62, 1973b.

Meikle, M. C.: The role of cartilage in the growth of bone with special reference to the mandible of the rat. Unpublished dissertation. Cambridge, University of Cambridge, 1975.

Meikle, M. C., Heath, J. K., and Reynolds, J. J.: Advances in understanding cell interactions in tissue resorption. Relevance to the pathogenesis of periodontal diseases and a new hypothesis. J. Oral Pathol. 15:239–250, 1986.

Melcher, A. H.: Behaviour of cells of condylar cartilage of foetal mouse mandible maintained in vitro. Arch. Oral Biol. 16:1379–1391, 1971.

Moffett, B. C.: The temporomandibular joint. In Sharry, J. J. (Ed.): Complete Dental Prosthodontics. New York, McGraw, 1962.

Moffett, B. C.: The morphogenesis of the temporomandibular joint. Am. J. Orthod. 52:401–415, 1966.

Moffett, B. C.: Remodeling of the craniofacial articulations by various orthodontic appliances in rhesus monkeys. Trans. Eur. Orthod. Soc. 207–216, 1971.

Moffett, B. C.: Remodeling of the craniofacial skeleton produced by orthodontic forces. In Zingeser, M. R. (Ed.): Symposia of the Fourth International Congress of Primatology. Basel, Karger, 1973, vol. 3, pp. 180–190.

Moffett, B. C., Johnson, L. C., McCabe, J. B., and Askew, H. C.: Articular remodeling of the adult temporomandibular joint. Am. J. Anat. 115:119–142, 1964.

Murray, P. D. F.: Adventitious (secondary) cartilage in the chick embryo and the development of certain bones and articulations in the chick skull. Aust. J. Zool. 11:360–430, 1963.

Murray, P. D. F., and Smiles, M.: Factors in the evocation of adventitious (secondary) cartilage in the chick embryo. Aust. J. Zool. 13:351–381, 1965.

Norwick, K. W.: The effect of reciprocal intermaxillary forces (class II) on the growing dentofacial complex in the Macaca mulatta. Unpublished dissertation. Seattle, University of Washington, 1969.

Ogston, A.: Articular cartilage. J. Anat. 10:49–74, 1875.

Ogston, A.: On the growth and maintenance of the articular ends of bones. J. Anat. 12:503–517, 1878.

Petrovic, A., and Stutzmann, J.: Further investigations into the functioning of the peripheral comparator of the servo system in the control of the condylar cartilage growth rate and the lengthening of the jaw. In McNamara, J. A. (Ed.): The Biology of Occlusal Development. Monograph No. 7. Craniofacial Growth Series. Center for Human Growth and Development, Ann Arbor, MI, 1977, pp 255–291.

Petrovic, A. G., Stutzmann, J., and Gasson, N.: The final length of the mandible: Is it genetically predetermined? In Carlson, D. S. (Ed.): Craniofacial Biology. Monograph No. 10. Craniofacial Growth Series. Center for Human Growth and Development, Ann Arbor, MI, 1981, pp. 105–126.

Pimenidis, M. Z., and Gianelly, A. A.: The effects of early

postnatal condylectomy on the growth of the mandible. Am. J. Orthod. *62*:42–47, 1972.

Ramfjord, S. P., and Hiniker, J. J.: Distal displacement of the mandible in adult rhesus monkeys. J. Prosthet. Dent. *16*:491–502, 1966.

Sarnat, B. G.: Growth pattern of the mandible: Some reflections. Am. J. Orthod. Dentof. Orthop. *90*:221–223, 1986.

Sarnat, B. G., and Engel, M. B.: A serial study of mandibular growth after removal of the condyle in *Macaca rhesus* monkey. Plast. Reconstr. Surg. *7*:364–380, 1951.

Sarnat, B. G., and Muchnic, H.: Facial skeletal changes after mandibular condylectomy in growing and adult monkeys. Am. J. Orthod. *60*:33–45, 1971a.

Sarnat, B. G., and Muchnic, H.: Facial skeletal changes after mandibular condylectomy in the adult monkey. J. Anat. *108*:323–338, 1971b.

Sarnat, B. G., and Robinson, I. B.: Surgery of the mandible: Some clinical and experimental considerations. Plast. Reconstr. Surg. *17*:27–57, 1956.

Silva, D. G.: Further ultrastructural studies on the temporomandibular joint of the guinea pig. J. Ultrastruct. Res. *26*:148–162, 1969.

Silva, D. G., and Hart, J. A. L.: Ultrastructural observations on the mandibular condyle of the guinea pig. J. Ultrastruct. Res. *20*:227–243, 1967.

Softley, J.: Cephalometric changes in seven post-normal cases treated by the Andresen method. Dent. Rec. *73*:485–494, 1953.

Solberg, W. K., Hansson, T. L., and Nordstrom, B. B.: The temporomandibular joint in young adults at autopsy: A morphometric classification and evaluation. J. Oral Rehab. *12*:303–321, 1985.

Sproule, M. R.: Dentofacial changes produced by extra-oral cervical traction to the maxilla of the *Macaca mulatta*. Unpublished dissertation. Seattle, University of Washington, 1968.

Stockli, P. W., and Willert, H. G.: Tissue reactions in the temporomandibular joint resulting from anterior displacement of the mandible in the monkey. Am. J. Orthod. *60*:142–155, 1971.

Tewson, D. H. T. K., Heath, J. K., and Meikle, M. C.: Biochemical and autoradiographic evidence that anterior mandibular displacement in the young growing rat does not stimulate cell proliferation or matrix formation at the mandibular condyle. Arch. Oral Biol. *33*:99–107, 1988.

Tonge, E. A., Heath, J. K., and Meikle, M. C.: Anterior mandibular displacement and condylar growth. An experimental study in the rat. Am. J. Orthod. *82*:277–287, 1982.

Turpin, D. L.: Growth and remodeling of the mandible in the *Macaca mulatta* monkey. Am. J. Orthod. *54*:251–271, 1968.

Wright, D. M., and Moffett, B. C.: The postnatal development of the human temporomandibular joint. Am. J. Anat. *141*:235–250, 1974.

7

NEUROPHYSIOLOGY*

ARTHUR T. STOREY, D.D.S., M.S., PH.D.

INTRODUCTION

Even a casual survey of the commonly accepted signs and symptoms of temporomandibular disorders (TMD) would justify classifying them as neurological disorders. Dentists are inclined to ignore sensory input other than pain from the temporomandibular joint (TMJ). A painful joint brings the patient to the dentist's office and brings this sensation to the clinician's attention (see Chapter 8). There is considerable evidence, however, that other conscious and unconscious sensations arise in the TMJ, sensory input that may play a significant role in the health of the stomatognathic system. TMJ receptors contribute to the position sense of the mandible and the detection and discrimination of objects between opposing teeth. The structural and functional characteristics of TMJ receptors suggest that they also play a role in protection of the TMJ, the dentition, and the airway; in determination of posture of the mandible and the tongue; and in the modulation of mandibular movement. In this chapter, the

neurology of the TMJ is addressed from a neuroanatomical, electrophysiological, and psychophysical perspective.

ANATOMY

Sensory Innervation

Gross Innervation

The primate TMJ is innervated by the mandibular division of the trigeminal nerve (Fig. 7–1). The joint capsule is innervated mainly by the auriculotemporal nerve, most densely in the posterior and lateral aspects. As in other joints of the body, the TMJ also receives innervation from nerves supplying adjacent muscles, namely the masseter and posterior temporalis. The anterior part of the capsule is sparsely innervated by small twigs of the auriculotemporal, posterior deep temporal, and masseter nerves. The medial part of the capsule is served by twigs from both the masseter and auriculotemporal nerves. In the human TMJ this muscle-nerve contribution is unexpectedly small;

---

*See Chapters 5, 8, 19, 21, and 25.

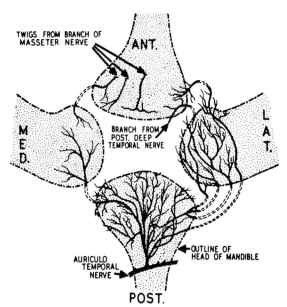

TWIGS FROM BRANCH OF MASSETER NERVE

ANT.

BRANCH FROM POST. DEEP TEMPORAL NERVE

MED.

LAT.

AURICULO TEMPORAL NERVE

OUTLINE OF HEAD OF MANDIBLE

POST.

FIGURE 7–1. Innervation of the human temporomandibular joint capsule (after Thilander, 1961). The richest innervation is provided by twigs of the auriculotemporal nerve to the lateral and posterior parts of the capsule. The anterior part of the capsule is sparsely innervated by twigs from the anterior deep temporal and masseter nerves. (From Storey, A. T.: Sensory functions of the temporomandibular joint. Can. Dent. Assoc. 34:294–300, 1968.)

the apparent absence of any innervation from the nerve of the intimately associated lateral pterygoid muscle is surprising.

While common in other joints, there appears to be no cutaneous contribution to the TMJ innervation (Larsson, 1964). According to Thilander (1961) the temporomandibular (lateral) ligament of the TMJ is innervated by the same nerves supplying the lateral aspect of the capsule. Some uncertainty has been raised by Savalle (1988) regarding the regular occurrence of the lateral ligament; in dissections of 16 postmortem human specimens Savelle found a true ligament in only three. The innervation of the other accessory ligaments appears not to have been investigated.

The articular surfaces of the joint and the disc, except for their peripheral borders, are not innervated. There is also no documentation of a synovial innervation. While the posterior attachment of the disc is frequently claimed to be richly innervated (the postulated origin of pain in patients with anteromedial displacements of the disc) such an innervation has not been carefully explored. Zenker (1956) cursorily refers to a rich medullated and nonmedullated innervation in the vicinity of the arteries. On the basis of innervation of joints elsewhere one would expect the cortical bone of the eminence

and the condyle not to be innervated (in contrast to the cancellous bone). More extensive reviews of the gross innervation of the TMJ in humans have been reported in the literature (Griffin, 1975; Klineberg, 1971; Thilander, 1961).

The major sensory input from the healthy TMJ is from the lateral and dorsal aspects of the capsule. In the absence of any receptors in the articulating surfaces of the joint it seems unlikely that there is any capability for monitoring loading across the joint surfaces. In joints with displaced discs there is the potential for painful stimulation arising from interposition of the posterior attachment between the condyle and eminence. However, pain cannot originate from intact articular surfaces. The apparent paucity of an interactive innervation from adjacent muscles and overlying skin is puzzling.

Receptor Innervation

Most mammalian TMJs contain three types of receptors common to other diarthrodial joints, namely (1) unencapsulated spray type endings, which have been called Ruffini receptors when located within the joint capsule and Golgi-tendon endings (organs) when located in the ligaments, (2) encapsulated Vater-Pacini corpuscles, and (3) free nerve endings (Fig. 7–2). These receptors have been assigned various names and numbers, but their identity is usually obvious. The various designations for the receptors appear in Table 7–1.

Free nerve endings, with their associated plexi, are found in large numbers throughout the innervated regions of the TMJ. The Ruffini endings, the predominant organized endings, are found in modest numbers in the posterior and posterolateral aspects of the capsule. Golgi-tendon endings are found occasionally in the temporomandibular ligament; the Vater-Pacini corpuscles are sparsely distributed throughout the same region. Fibers, 9 to 12 microns in diameter, supply the Vater-Pacini corpuscles, and fibers of 13 to 17 microns supply the Golgi-tendon endings.

In the human TMJ, the smallest nerve fibers (< 5 microns) predominate; fibers larger than 10 microns are rare (Thilander, 1961). Speculation on the roles of the various TMJ receptors (Table 7–2) ignores their numerical distribution. Both myelinated and unmyelinated small-sized fibers could be sympathetic postganglionic fibers running to the joint. Although such a contribution would be expected on the basis of studies on the knee joint (Ekholm, 1964), this has not been examined in the TMJ.

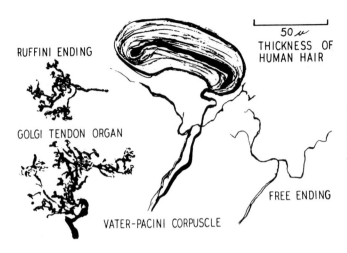

RUFFINI ENDING

GOLGI TENDON ORGAN

VATER-PACINI CORPUSCLE

50 μ
THICKNESS OF
HUMAN HAIR

FREE ENDING

FIGURE 7–2. Receptors of the human temporomandibular joint capsule (after Thilander, 1961). (From Storey, A. T.: Sensory functions of the temporomandibular joint. Can. Dent. Assoc. 34:294–300, 1968.)

Receptor Functions

The functions of the Ruffini and Vater-Pacinian endings have been inferred from the discharge characteristics of histologically identified receptors in the knee joint of the cat (Boyd, 1954; Grigg, 1985). While the specific functions of each TMJ receptor have not been specified, their collective role in perceiving pain, mandibular position, and objects between the teeth has been documented (see section on psychophysics). While pain is not the normal sensory experience of the TMJ, it is the sensation most likely to attract attention to the TMJ innervation. Free endings in the ligaments and capsule, posterior attachment, periosteum, and cancellous bone are the pain transducers. Since the stress-bearing tissues, i.e., articular surfaces, disc, and compact bone are not innervated, pressure on these tissues cannot give rise to pain. While the long discredited Costen's syndrome (Costen, 1934) was attributed to condylar impingement on the auriculotemporal nerve, Costen (1959) also attributed pain from the TMJ

to excitation of pain endings in the joint capsule and in the posterior attachment of the disc (see Chapters 1 and 18). The capsule and posterior attachment are still considered the most probable sites of pain, although Frost (1968) associates pain in other joints with hypersensitive synovia, irregular joint surfaces, expansile bone lesions and stiffening of the soft tissues of the joint. Endogenous chemical substances released in inflammation, such as histamine, bradykinin, and 5-hydroxytryptamine, may initiate or potentiate the joint pain.

Central Projection

Until recently the central projections of the TMJ receptors have been studied rarely, and only by electrical recording (see section on central termination of primary afferents). The use of chemical labels tracking central axoplasmic flow from the TMJ supports these physiological observations. Although TMJ receptors might be expected to have cell bodies in the

TABLE 7–1. Receptors of the Temporomandibular Joint*

INVESTIGATOR (SPECIES)	TYPE			
Thilander, 1961 (human)	Vater-Pacini corpuscle	Ruffini ending	Golgi tendon organ	Free ending
Franks, 1965 (rat, guinea pig, rabbit, cat)	Encapsulated ending	Compound "nonencapsulated" ending		Free nerve ending
Greenfield, 1966 (cat)	Type II	Type I	Type III	Type IV
Kawamura, 1967 (cat)		Golgi Mazzoni ending		
Keller, 1968 (monkey)	Paciniform ending	Ruffini ending	Golgi ending	Free ending
Griffin, 1975 (human)	Encapsulated mechanoreceptor		Golgi tendon ending	

*Classification of receptors of the temporomandibular joint according to various investigators. Receptors of the same type are listed vertically. (From Dubner, R., Sessle, B. J., and Storey, A. T.: The Neural Basis of Oral and Facial Function. New York, Plenum, 1978, p 161.)

TABLE 7–2. Temporomandibular Receptors and Their Inferred Reflex Roles*

ANATOMICAL DESIGNATION	FUNCTIONAL DESIGNATION	REFLEX ROLE
Ruffini ending	Static mechanoreceptor	Posture
Vater-Pacini corpuscle	Dynamic mechanoreceptor	Movement accelerator
Golgi tendon ending	Static mechanoreceptor	Protection (ligament)
Free ending	Pain receptor	Protection (joint)

*After Thilander (1961), Greenfield (1966), and Wyke (1967). (From Storey, A. T.: Reflex functions of the temporomandibular joint. J. Prosthet. Dent. 30:830–837, 1973.)

mesencephalic nucleus (as is commonly stated in the anatomical literature), both anatomical and physiological studies have shown conclusively that their cell bodies are located in the trigeminal ganglion. Romfh (1979) injected horseradish peroxidase into the TMJ of eight adult cats; these injections did not label any neurons of the mesencephalic nucleus. Capra (1987) has described the terminal distribution of these first order afferents using this technique. Terminals were found in greatest numbers in the dorsal part of the main sensory nucleus and subnucleus oralis, the same regions of projection as found by electrophysiological means (see section on central termination of primary afferents). Axon terminals were also found in the medullary dorsal horn, supporting the physiological evidence for a modulatory role in subnucleus caudalis (Broton, 1988).

Autonomic Innervation

Although an autonomic innervation is known for other joints in the body (Ekholm, 1964; Levine, 1984), this has not been rigorously established for the TMJ. Based on the observation of fibers entering the adventitia of vessels of the joint, Thilander (1961) speculated that the auriculotemporal branch ". . . is accompanied by a number of autonomic fibers." Schmid (1964) reported autonomic nerve fibers entering the medial aspect of the TMJ capsule of human infants, speculating that the sympathetic fibers originate in the sympathetic plexus of the internal maxillary artery and parasympathetic fibers in the lesser petrosal nerve. The small-sized myelinated and unmyelinated fibers seen in cross-sectional analysis of TMJ nerves could be sympathetic postganglionic fibers as well as pain afferents.

The studies of Levine (1984, 1985) indicate an interaction between sympathetic efferents and substance P-containing afferents in limb joints and suggest a nervous system contribution to the pathophysiology of rheumatoid ar-

thritis. Widenfalk (1988) injected wheat germ agglutinin-conjugated horseradish peroxidase into the elbow joint of adult rats and found labeled neurons in the ganglia of the ipsilateral sympathetic trunk. While sympathetic nerve fibers have been traced into various motor and sensory nerves in the face of the rat (Frost, 1968), a TMJ projection has yet to be reported.

In summary, while a sympathetic innervation of the TMJ would be expected from documented autonomic innervation of other joints in the body, this has yet to be rigorously documented for the TMJ. Because of a proposed neuropathological role in arthritis, an autonomic innervation of the TMJ needs confirmation.

PHYSIOLOGY

Sensory Function

Primary Afferents

Electrophysiological studies of TMJ receptors have provided useful information on the possible functions of the receptors subserved by the larger nerve fibers. What functions do these TMJ receptors serve? Studies of other joints have designated the Ruffini ending as a length of strain energy density ending (Grigg, 1985), the Golgi-tendon ending as a tension receptor, and the Vater-Pacini corpuscle as a pressure-transducing ending (Boyd, 1954). While free nerve endings have traditionally been assigned the role of sensing pain, some respond to several kinds of stimuli and may convey other information besides pain (see Chapter 8). The cornea, for example, which is innervated only by free endings, may perceive sensations of touch, warm, cold, and pressure as well as pain. Since some mammals do not have any organized TMJ receptors, it is likely that TMJ free nerve endings may serve other functions besides that of mediating pain.

The way in which a receptor discharges gives an indication of the type of information it could be relaying. Electrodes can record the discharges of single neurons (sensory units) from either their axons or cell bodies when these neurons are excited by stimulation of TMJ receptors (type usually unknown). The responses of three types of units recorded by Kawamura (1974) from the cat TMJ are illustrated in Figure 7–3. The upper traces are of action potentials recorded from single sensory units in the auriculotemporal nerve. The lower traces indicate movement of the isolated condyle containing the receptor. The figurines under the lower traces indicate the relative position of the condyle to the fossa. Trace A illustrates a rapidly adapting unit that fires only when the condyle is rotated through a specific angle. Traces B and C record the activity of slowly adapting receptors that continue to fire while the condyle is in a specific position.

In a study of sensory units in the trigeminal ganglion of rabbits, Lund (1981) identified 11 limited-range TMJ receptors from a total population of 1500 neurons. Three of the receptors were similar to the rapidly adapting unit A of Kawamura (1974) while the other eight were like Kawamura's units B and C. All the units were silent when the jaw was in the resting position and all fired preferentially on either opening or closing and were extremely sensitive to velocity. The slowly adapting receptors demonstrated marked hysteresis. Figure 7–4A illustrates the discharge characteristics of a TMJ receptor in the anterolateral region of the capsule on caudal displacement of the ipsilateral condyle. Figure 7–4B records the receptors' frequency of discharge at specific angular displacements to activation at three different velocities; the receptor fires at a higher frequency and for a longer period at higher stimulus velocities. As shown for other receptors, e.g. periodontal, the adaptation characteristics of a receptor are dependent on the intensity of stimulation. Of 10 units which fired on joint movement, only one could be classified as a limit receptor.

These findings of Lund (1981) are in agreement with the earlier work of Kawamura (1967), showing a preference for discharge in either an opening or closing direction. Butler (1977) found that all rapidly adapting units were active only on opening and fired throughout the full range of that jaw movement. Slowly adapting units discharged on both opening and closing.

It seems probable that rapidly adapting TMJ receptors convey some information relative to movement of the mandible whereas slowly adapting units convey information relative to the position of the mandible. Because of the technical difficulties of recording such units and at the same time identifying the specific receptor from which the discharges are arising, it is impossible to assign unequivocally any of these patterns to a specific TMJ receptor. On the basis of recordings from joints elsewhere in the

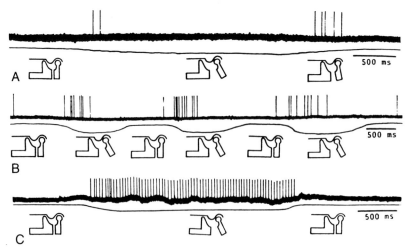

FIGURE 7–3. Action potential discharges in single nerve fibers of the auriculotemporal nerve innervating the temporomandibular joint of a cat. Upper traces are the oscilloscope record of these discharges at varying degrees of mouth opening indicated by the lower traces and in the figurines. Downward movement of the lower traces is in an opening direction. The condyle and adjacent mandibular ramus have been severed from the mandible to avoid excitation of muscle receptors. (From Kawamura, Y., and Abe, K.: Role of sensory information from temporomandibular joint. Bull. Tokyo Med. Dent. Univ. *21*:78–82, 1974.)

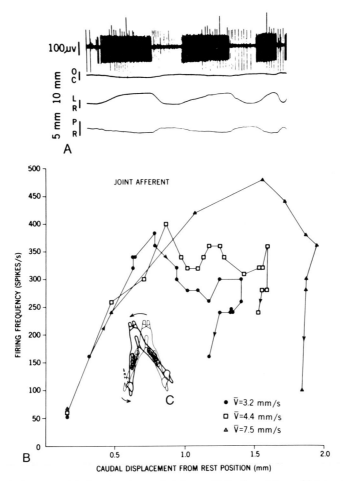

FIGURE 7–4. *A*, Action potentials (top trace) recorded from a TMJ afferent in a rabbit (medium-size spike) on three retrusive movements of the ipsilateral condyle consequent to passive displacement of the mandible to the left (see figurine in *C*). Lower traces record jaw movement in the vertical (open-close), mediolateral (left-right), and anteroposterior (protrusive-retrusive) directions. Calibration markers are depicted for spike amplitude (μV) and jaw displacement (mm). *B*, Firing frequency of the temporomandibular joint afferent in *A* with caudal displacement of the ipsilateral condyle at three velocities. The TMJ receptor fires more rapidly and longer at higher velocity (From Lund, J. P., and Matthews, B.: Responses of temporomandibular joint afferents recorded in the Gasserian ganglion of the rabbit to passive movements of the mandible. *In* Kawamura, Y., and Dubner, R. (Eds.): Oral-Facial Sensory and Motor Functions. Chicago, Quintessence, 1981.)

body, however, the TMJ receptors have been assigned the functional designations given in Table 7–2.

Since Ruffini endings and Golgi-tendon endings are slowly adapting receptors elsewhere in the body, they were designated static mechanoreceptors. Because the free nerve ending has been associated with pain, it was designated a pain receptor. It is tempting to continue this line of thought one step further and attribute the discharge in trace *A* in Figure 7–3 to a Vater-Pacini corpuscle, and the discharges in traces *B* and *C* to Ruffini endings or Golgi-tendon endings. One further assumption is made in assigning reflex roles to these recep-

tors. The Ruffini ending becomes the receptor for posture, the Vater-Pacini corpuscle for regulation of movement, and the Golgi-tendon ending and free endings for protection of the muscles and joint from damage. While Golgi endings were once regarded as high-threshold receptors, they may be excited by low-energy stimulation (Houk, 1967; Matthews, 1972). Do Golgi endings in the TMJ have similar thresholds? If so, they are unlikely to be silent during movement and, like the free endings, serve other functions than protection of the joint. Since small-sized fibers (Group III and IV) are the dominant population in the nerves of the human TMJ (Thilander, 1961; Klineberg, 1971) free endings, like those in other tissues, must serve mechanoreceptive as well as nociceptive functions.

Distension of the joint capsule changes the threshold of the joint receptors. Ferrell (1986) raised intra-articular pressure of the cat's knee joints by injection of liquid paraffin resulting in an increased discharge of low-threshold joint receptors served by 5 to 10 μ fibers. Figure 7–5 illustrates the effect of increased intra-articulator pressure at varying angles of the knee joint on the discharge of a single receptor recorded in the median articular nerve. Pressure within swollen joints changes the sensory input—possibly mechanoreceptive as well as nociceptive.

Small unit activity of joint receptors is increased by inflammation. Coggeshall (1983) demonstrated that the activity of small myelinated and unmyelinated fibers (Group III and IV afferent units) is increased in the medial articular nerve of the cat's knee joint at rest and during passive movements following experimental induction of inflammation within the joint. In both fiber groups, non-noxious passive movement of the knee considerably increased the number and frequency of discharging units originating in the inflamed joint; there was an increase of 60 per cent in the number of both Group III and IV units firing.

Schaible (1985) artificially induced arthritis in the knee joint of cats by intracapsular injection of a 4 per cent aqueous suspension of kaolin and lowered the threshold of firing of many Group III and IV afferent units, making them active at rest and increasing their responsiveness more readily to normally innocuous joint movements. Schaible speculated that this increased firing in posture and normal movements leads to a powerful activation of nociceptive pathways and induces reflexes counteracting excess movement, thus preventing joint damage.

Location of Cell Bodies of Primary Afferents

Although the cell bodies of primary afferents from TMJ receptors might be expected to be in the trigeminal mesencephalic nucleus, several studies have clearly demonstrated that the cell bodies are not located in the mesencephalic nucleus (Butler, 1977; Cody, 1972; Kawamura, 1967). The electrical stimulation of TMJ afferents does not evoke any electrical response in this nucleus. Lund (1981) recorded discharges originating in TMJ receptors of the rabbit in the trigeminal ganglion. This concurs with the axoplasmic tracer study of Romfh (1979) that localized the cell bodies of TMJ afferents in the caudolateral portion of the ganglion.

Central Termination of Primary Afferents

Kawamura (1967) and Butler (1977) have recorded evoked electrical activity in the sensory nuclear complex of the trigeminal nerve of the cat on passive opening and closing of the mandible. In Kawamura's study (1967), muscle input was eliminated by separating the jaw muscles from their attachments to the mandible and sectioning of the condylar neck so that movement was limited to the condyle. Kawamura (1967) recorded 13 units in the chief sensory and spinal trigeminal sensory nuclei. Butler (1977) recorded 122 units within the region designated as the supratrigeminal nucleus (located between the chief sensory and motor

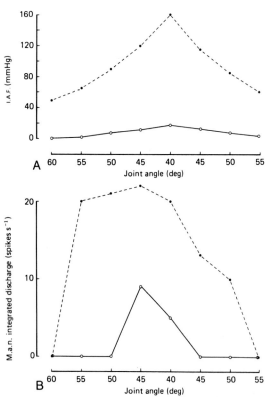

FIGURE 7–5. Discharge frequency (spikes per second) at specific joint angles *(B)* of a knee joint afferent (in a dog) recorded in the medial articular nerve before (solid line) and after (dotted line) infusion of 7.5 ml of liquid paraffin into the joint. Intra-articular pressure *(A)* recorded in mm Hg. At the optimal joint angle (45 degrees) the frequency of discharge increased by 13 spikes per second with an increase in intra-articular pressure of 142 mm Hg (From Ferrell, W. R., Nade, S., and Newbold, P. J.: The interrelation of neural discharge, intra-articular pressure, and joint angle in the knee of the dog. J. Physiol. 373:353–365, 1986.)

trigeminal nuclei). Since the means used to discriminate central terminals of first order afferents from the cell bodies of second order afferents were not used in these experiments, one can assume that unit discharges were from the cell bodies because of the greater ease in recording from this part of a neuron. More recently Broton (1988) demonstrated that TMJ afferents (in the cat) excited by electrical, mechanical, and chemical stimulation converge with facial skin and intraoral afferents onto the trigeminal subnucleus caudalis (see Chapter 8 for full discussion and significance). This convergence of inputs from several regions characterizes the trigeminal innervation in general.

Central Projections

The projection of TMJ afferents beyond the trigeminal sensory nuclei has not been explored. On the basis of homology with pathways activated at spinal levels by joint movements (Gardner, 1967; Skoglund, 1973), one would expect activation of multiple paths, some relaying through the thalamus to the cerebral cortex and others relaying to the cerebellum.

Motor Function

Reflexes of Temporomandibular Joint Origin

While some of the discharges of TMJ receptors are relayed to the cortex to be perceived as position of the mandible in space or to contribute to identification and discrimination of objects between the teeth (see section on psychophysics), other discharges initiate or modulate mandibular reflexes. Several studies (Clark, 1974; Greenfield, 1966; Kawamura, 1967) have demonstrated that isolated inputs from the TMJs of the cat can alter the ongoing activity of mandibular muscles or the motor neurons innervating them. Kawamura's study (1967) demonstrates the inhibition and facilitation effects of isolated TMJ receptors on jaw-closing motor neurons. The single unit recordings (upper trace) in Figure 7–6A and B are from the trigeminal motor nucleus in the region of the masseter motor neurons. Mandibular rotation (lower traces in A and B) in a closing direction (trace A) inhibited the masseteric discharge, while mandibular rotation in an opening direction (trace B) facilitated the discharge. What is striking is the similarity in patterns of motor neuron excitation and inhibition to those initiated by levator muscle spindles. TMJ receptors and muscle spindles functionally paral-

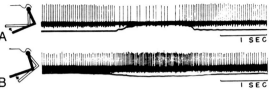

FIGURE 7–6. Inhibition *(A)* and facilitation *(B)* of a tonically firing masseter motor neuron (top traces) by temporomandibular joint receptors in the ipsilateral isolated condyle of a cat on movement (lower trace) in a closing direction *(A)* and an opening direction *(B)* as depicted in the figurines. The motor neuron action potentials were recorded extracellularly by means of an electrode stereotaxically positioned in the trigeminal motor nucleus (From Kawamura, Y., Majima, T., and Kato, I.: Physiologic role of deep mechanoreceptor in temporomandibular joint capsule. J. Osaka Dent. Univ. 7:63–76, 1967.)

lel each other in regulating jaw posture and movement.

Reflexes Protecting the Temporomandibular Joint

Receptors within the TMJ can give rise to reflexes protecting the joint from damage. Such reflexes come into play to restrict extreme opening movements, such as yawning, and to prevent subluxation of the condyle. In instances of inflammation of the joint, reflexes would be expected to spare the joint both in posture and during movement. There is evidence for such reflexes. Posselt (1965), in a study of border movements of the mandible recorded in the median plane, demonstrated that maximal opening could be increased with anesthesia of receptors in the capsule of the TMJ. Klineberg (1971) reported that both jaw-opening and jaw-closing reflexes are produced by electrical stimulation of the nerves supplying the joint. Shwaluk (1971) and Kawamura (1974), on the other hand, have been able to evoke only jaw-opening reflexes. Ferrell (1986) demonstrated that nerve endings of the cat knee joint will fire at intracapsular pressures greater than 10 to 13 mm Hg; elevated intracapsular pressures, increasing the discharge of TMJ receptors, would be expected to limit jaw movement and range of motion.

Although the receptors in joints do not monitor loading, it now seems likely that joint afferents are sensitive to muscle tension (Skoglund, 1973). Millar (1973) and Grigg (1975) have shown that activation of the muscles acting at the elbow and knee joints of the cat increases the number and the frequency of discharges of the joint receptors even though the joint angle is fixed. Millar (1979) and Tracey (1980) have produced experimental evidence for convergence of analogous information from limb joints and muscles. As Kawamura (1976) has contended, "We must always consider sensory functions of muscles, tendon and joint, and periodontal ligament all together." Receptors in muscles and joints must be regarded as complementary components of a single afferent system rather than as two separate systems.

The suggestion has frequently been made that there is an ideal location for the condyles when the teeth are in full intercuspation. This has sometimes been referred to as the centered position, and radiographic techniques have been advocated to define it. The neurophysiological significance of centering, however, is obscure. What TMJ receptors would be responsible for monitoring centricity? Are there other functional parameters that make more sense? Loading and stability are more probable physiological parameters.

When the condyles and discs translate bilaterally in protrusive biting and contralaterally in working side biting, the joint is unquestionably loaded (Hylander, 1979). Force and electromyographic data indicate that the biting force and elevator muscle activity are attenuated bilaterally in protrusive biting and unilaterally (on the contralateral side) in working side biting (Storey, 1985a). These responses are the consequences of negative feedback secondary to jaw position and bite location. Negative feedback from the teeth can be interpreted as protecting the teeth from excessive loading, but the same suppression of biting force could be seen to protect the TMJs. Since the joints have no receptors that can monitor loading, those of the periodontal ligaments and jaw muscles must serve this function. Again receptors in two anatomically discrete parts of the jaw system must be regarded as complementary components of a single afferent system. More evidence is accumulating that receptors in the TMJ, the periodontal ligament, and the jaw muscles do not initiate and regulate jaw functions in isolation. Reflexes of exclusive TMJ receptor origin are probably the result of painful stimulation.

Reference was made earlier, in the section on primary afferents, to the effects of inflammation on joint receptors served by myelinated and unmyelinated small fibers (Groups III and IV). Schaible (1985) speculated that the increased activity of these receptors, both in posture and movement, will induce reflexes limiting joint movement and thereby prevent further damage to the joint.

Learned Reflexes Protecting the Teeth

Learned reflexes resulting in mandibular deviation to avoid occlusal interferences have been espoused by some and refuted by others. This controversy is compounded by perpetuation of the myth that the teeth rarely come into contact in mastication (Dubner, 1978). There are a number of variables, including magnitude of the occlusal force, threshold of the receptors, frequency of occlusal contact, crown-root ratio, mandibular position, segment of arch loaded, and central modulation that can determine whether an interference will be reflexly avoided (Storey, 1985b).

When avoidance of occlusal interferences occurs, what is the signal that warns of approaching contact with the occlusal interferences? Does it arise from receptors in mucosa, skin, muscle, or the TMJ? Periodontal receptors cannot be implicated since the avoidance needs to occur before tooth contact. Receptors in mucosa and skin would be unlikely to give precise information as to the position of the mandible nearing contact with the offending tooth. The muscle spindle has a constantly changing threshold (due to gamma biasing) and would appear to be a poor candidate for position sense. TMJ receptors could serve this function well, although receptors in muscle and possibly the skin overlying the joints may also participate. The sequence of postulated events is illustrated in Figure 7–7. Since Schaerer (1967) demonstrated that balancing side interferences can lead to reflexes resulting in mandibular deviation, one can identify the balancing interference as the unconditioned stimulus for mandibular

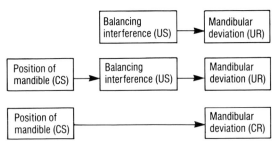

FIGURE 7–7. The postulated learning sequence for avoidance of a balancing-side occlusal interference. A balancing-side interference, unconditioned stimulus (US) gives rise to mandibular deviation, unconditioned reflex (UR) in an unlearned reflex. Repeated contact on the interference (US) coupled with sensory input indicating position of the mandible, conditioned stimulus (CS) eventually leads to mandibular deviation, conditioned response (CR) without contact on the interference. Temporomandibular joint receptors probably give origin to the CS. (From Storey, A. T.: Reflex functions of the temporomandibular joint. J. Prosthet. Dent. 30:830–837, 1973.)

deviation (Storey, 1976). Some other neural input monitoring position of the mandible before contact on the balancing interference, led to this neutral neural input, designated the conditioned stimulus, and initiated mandibular deviation without contact on the balancing interference.

Posture of the Mandible and Tongue

Muscle spindles have frequently been assigned the responsibility for reflex determination of postural position of the mandible. Do the joint receptors play any role in mandibular posture? Thilander (1961) and Ransjö (1963) have shown that the ability to perceive mandibular position is severely disrupted with anesthetization of the TMJs. An unpublished student project conducted by Posselt at the Royal Dental School in Malmö, Sweden demonstrated that infiltration of the TMJ with a local anesthetic agent also resulted in altered postural position.

Reference was made earlier to a study by Kawamura (1967) (Fig. 7–6 and in the section on reflexes of TMJ origin) demonstrating the effects of TMJ receptors on masseter motor neurons. Maintaining the mandible in an open position resulted in an increased discharge of these motor neurons. Since the altered firing of the tonically discharging masseter motor neuron is sustained, the evidence suggests that the TMJ receptors could be playing a role in the regulation of posture. While TMJ afferents would appear to contribute to the reflex determination of posture of the mandible, muscle receptors and receptors monitoring the airway are the primary determinants (Storey, 1988).

Lowe (1978) has shown that TMJ receptors also play a role in tongue posture. Figure 7–8 shows the effects of various degrees of mouth opening on the activity of the genioglossus muscle, a protractor of the tongue. With the teeth in occlusion (0 degree), the genioglossus muscle in the cat is silent; at 21 degrees of opening the genioglossus shows activity in a few motor units; at openings of 42 and 63 degrees, the amount of genioglossus activity is further increased. Infiltration with a local anesthetic agent into both TMJ capsules reversibly abolished the genioglossus reflex activation. While TMJ receptors have been proposed as the origin of the conditioned stimulus for reflex avoidance of occlusal interferences (Fig. 7–7), Lowe (1978) has proven them to be the origin of the conditioned stimulus for the genioglossus reflex. Presumably the unconditioned stimuli for this protective reflex of the pharyngeal airway would be receptors monitoring the adequacy of ventilation.

Intercuspal Position of the Mandible

Reflexes regulating intercuspal position, like postural position, may be initiated from the dentition, from the TMJ, and from receptors monitoring adequacy of the pharyngeal airway. Normally the best intercuspation of the teeth dictates the position of the joints: the TMJs dance to the tune of the teeth. In cases of inflammation of the joint, however, the hierarchy may be reversed; the joints may dictate intercuspal position. The resultant inflammation lowers the threshold of TMJ receptors in the capsule and initiates protective reflexes guarding against further damage to the joint.

Modulation of Movement

Evidence has been presented previously that TMJ receptors initiate unlearned and possibly learned reflexes to protect the teeth, the joints, and the airway. TMJ receptors may also regulate ongoing movement of the mandible, as suggested by Wyke (1967) in studies using the cat. Klineberg (1980) studied the effects of unilateral and bilateral anesthesia of the TMJ capsule on intraborder chewing movements in five adult human subjects. Jaw movement was monitored with a Kinesiograph (Myo-tronics Research, Inc., Seattle, Washington). The areas within the functional envelopes of 15 subjects were measured before and after local anesthesia. As a consequence of the anesthesia, the length and width of the functional envelope increased. According to Klineberg (1980), the anesthetic was restricted to the lateral and posterior aspects of the TMJ capsule; spread to adjacent muscles was unlikely. Bilateral anesthesia resulted in a greater increase in size and variation in form. Envelope size increased by nearly 25 per cent on unilateral anesthesia and by 40 per cent on bilateral anesthesia. These results suggest that articular mechanoreceptors continuously contribute to the reflex regulation of jaw movement. For a more extensive review of central processes underlying these protective reflexes of TMJ origin, see Chapter 8.

PSYCHOPHYSICS

Mandibular Position Sense

Some insight into the role of human TMJ receptors can be gained from altered perception

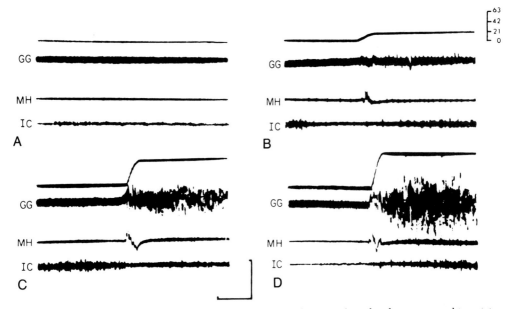

FIGURE 7–8. The effects of various degrees of mouth opening (top traces) on the electromyographic activity of the genioglossus (GG), mylohyoid (MH), and inferior constrictor (IC) muscles in a cat. Genioglossus muscle activity, which was minimal at jaw closure *(A)*, apparent at an opening of 21 degrees *(B)* and marked at 42 degrees *(C)* and 63 degrees *(D)*, was reversibly abolished by infiltration of both TMJs with local anesthetic. Reference markers are for time (seconds) and EMG amplitude (millivolts). (Reprinted with permission from Lowe, A. A.: Mandibular joint control of genioglossus muscle activity in the cat and monkey *(Mucaca mulatta).* Arch. Oral Biol. 23:787–793, 1978. Copyright 1978, Pergamon Press.)

of mandibular position and of the presence and size of objects held between the teeth on reversible or permanent loss of the jaw innervation. There is evidence both for and against TMJ receptors playing a significant role in the conscious perception of mandibular position. To identify the receptors signaling mandibular position, Thilander (1961) instructed 10 normal adult human subjects to duplicate an arbitrary position between postural position and maximal opening. The subjects were asked to duplicate this position 10 times, and on each occasion the distance between the incisors was measured. The difference between the highest and lowest measurements for the 10 duplicated positions was used as a measure of the accuracy of duplicating the original position. Mean range for the 10 normal adult subjects was 3.2 mm. When the sensory input from one or both joints was blocked with a local anesthetic, the subjects found it more difficult to assume the original position. The mean range increased to 9.4 mm with block of one joint. This increase was statistically significant; the individual measurements no longer clustered around the original position. Anesthetization of the contralateral joint did not further impair the perception of mandibular position.

Thilander (1961), Larsson (1964), and Öwall (1978) found a significant impairment of their

subjects' ability to replicate an arbitrary jaw position between postural position and wide open after infiltration of a local anesthetic around the joint capsule. These investigators concluded that human TMJ receptors contributed to the sense of mandibular position. On the other hand, Broekhuijsen (1983), in a study of position sense in human subjects following bilateral injection of a local anesthetic agent ventrally and dorsally in both mandibular joint capsules, found that subjects could precisely match a series of interincisal gauges with an error of only 1.0 to 1.5 mm compared to controls. This task is not the same, however, as that in the experiment of Thilander (1961); it has elements common to the task of interdental size discrimination that clearly has a significant sensory component originating in the jaw muscles (see section on interdental size discrimination). Differences could also be due to the technique of anesthetic infiltration.

Lindauer (1985) reported that injection of a local anesthetic agent into the lower compartment of the TMJ (rather than the capsule) in subjects did not affect their ability to replicate jaw position. Lindauer concluded that TMJ receptors were not involved. These findings could also be due to sparing of either cutaneous receptors or receptors in the pterygomandibular ligament with intra-articular injections. Thilan-

der (1961) and Larsson (1964) ruled out a cutaneous contribution to mandibular position
sense, however, by testing the effects of cutaneous and subcutaneous injections in their control subjects; position sense was not affected.
The same receptors found in the TMJ capsule
are found also in the temporomandibular ligament (Thilander, 1961). If these receptors were
spared by the intra-articular injection, their
activity could account for the unimpaired position sense in Lindauer's study (1985). Receptors
in the ligaments of the knee joint of the cat and
monkey have been shown to be spared by a
local anesthetic agent injected into the joint
space (Clark, 1979).

In the studies of both Öwall (1978) and Lindauer (1985) the greatest replication ability was
found near the intercuspal position and wide
opening. This finding is not supported by the
study of Van Willigen (1983) who found that
reproduction of joint position was independent
of jaw opening. While the receptors of many
joints of the body, such as the knee, wrist, and
elbow, tend not to fire in the middle range of
movement, those of the digits do. While Abe
(1974) found few brain stem units firing in the
middle of the TMJ's range of motion in the cat,
Lund (1981) found many middle range TMJ
units firing in the trigeminal ganglion of the
rabbit. Not only are there joint differences, but
also specie differences in patterns of TMJ innervation.

A study by Larsson (1964) sheds light on
another interesting facet of the TMJ's contribution to mandibular position sense. These
investigators discovered that replication difficulties after unilateral intracapsular injections
of an anesthetic agent were eliminated by pressure over the contralateral unanesthetized joint.
This improvement in mandibular position sense
does not occur unless there is impairment in
contralateral joint sensibility. This effect is also
found with sensory impairment due to TMJ
disease (Ransjö, 1963). Larsson (1964) speculated that the pressure over the intact joint
increases the firing rate of active receptors, and
recruits silent receptors, restoring the critical
excitatory state essential for identifying joint
position. If the hypothesis of Larsson (1964) is
correct, position is not signaled by a specific
population of joint receptors precisely tuned to
exact joint angles, but by a critical mass of
receptors. Muscles acting on a joint may increase this critical mass. Millar (1973) and Grigg
(1975) have shown that activation of the muscles
acting at the elbow and knee joints of the cat
increases the number and frequency of dis-

charges from the joint receptors even though
the joint angle is fixed. No joint has a tighter
mechanical couple than the lateral pterygoid
onto the capsule of the TMJ. It seems likely
that this muscle would have a profound effect
on the discharge of receptors in the TMJ capsule. This is worthy of investigation.

Christensen's (1975) study questions the primacy of the TMJ receptors in position sense of
the mandible. A local anesthetic agent was
injected bilaterally into the lateral pterygoid
muscles in nine normal subjects and, as with
capsular injections, replication of jaw position
was significantly impaired. The addition of unilateral intracapsular anesthesia in six of the
subjects, two hours later, did not impair replication ability further. It seems unlikely that the
results were due to uncoupling of a direct
mechanical effect of the lateral pterygoid muscle
on the capsule since protrusive and lateral
movements of the mandible were not affected
in any of the subjects. Because joints receive
their blood supply from muscles surrounding
the joint, it is possible that the anesthetic agent
might have been carried by this vascular supply
into the joint capsule. Since position sensibility
is not abolished by both lateral pterygoid and
joint anesthesia, other sensory inputs must be
contributing as well. Levator muscle receptors
would seem likely candidates. Excitation of
muscle receptors within the jaw muscles by
vibration has been shown by Hellsing (1978) to
create illusions of movement and impairment
of position sense. The vibration-induced illusion
of altered jaw position in Hellsing's study remained after bilateral intracapsular injection of
a local anesthetic agent.

Further insight into jaw position sense has
come from studies of subjects under treatment
for TMD and subjects with induced jaw muscle
fatigue. Ransjö (1963) determined the range of
mandibular position in 25 patients with TMJ
disorders due to severe malocclusion and reduced vertical dimension and in 19 patients
with TMJ disorders due to masticatory muscle
dysfunction. Ranges were computed before and
after treatment. The pretreatment range was
high in the malocclusion group and normal in
the muscle dysfunction group. The malocclusion group had a statistically significant reduction in the range of position after treatment.
There was no change, however, in the muscle
dysfunction group. The authors concluded that
severe malocclusions provoked changes in the
joints, which in turn impaired the joint receptors. Muscle dysfunction, on the other hand,
did not affect the sensory innervation. When

derangement of the TMJ is accompanied by inflammation, the threshold of the small fiber receptors is lowered (see section on primary afferents), triggering reflexes that otherwise would not occur. Reflexes protecting the TMJ are elicited from an inflamed capsule and ligaments in the same way that reflexes protecting the teeth are elicited from receptors in inflamed periodontal ligament and pulp.

Christensen (1976) examined the mandibular position sense in nine normal subjects after 20 minutes of either active lowering or raising and lowering a load of 1.6 gm hung from the mandible. In five of the nine subjects who developed fatigue, the mean mandibular replication ability dropped from 1.3 to 3.7 mm. Christensen attributed the distorted position sense to derangement of muscle or tendon receptor function.

All the studies on selective impairment of either muscle or joint sensibility suggest a shared rather than an exclusive role in position sense. Convergence of presumptive afferents serving position sense from the elbow joint of the cat with afferents from muscle and skin in the dorsal column nuclei (Millar, 1979; Tracey, 1980) supports the concept of a modality rather than a regional priority. High-threshold muscle, joint, and skin afferents converge in the trigeminal nucleus of the spinal tract in a similar modality pattern (see Chapter 8).

Size Threshold

The exquisite ability to perceive about .01 mm objects between the teeth could intuitively be thought to be a function of receptors in the periodontium excited by small axial displacements of the teeth on closing. Siirilä (1963) attributed the perception of size to receptors around the teeth even though the data suggest that other receptors are involved. In the sample of 36 young adults, Siirilä found that 12 detected foil of 8 μ, and all but three detected foil of 30 μ. There was no significant difference in thickness thresholds for the incisors and molars, suggesting that periodontal receptors were not responsible (biting forces would have to be measured to confirm this conclusion). When both upper and lower antagonistic teeth were anesthetized, the range of detection thresholds was 30 to 180 μ; 27 of the subjects could detect foil of 90 μ. As the authors state, ". . . the desensitizing effect of local anesthesia on tactile sensibility is surprisingly slight." It did not occur to these investigators that receptors elsewhere might be involved. One would not expect

only receptors in the skin of the first and second digits to convey information about the size of an object held between them.

Caffesse (1973) examined the possibility of TMJ receptors contributing to size thresholds. Detection thresholds between first molars free of restorations in 15 subjects were determined using aluminum foil before and after bilateral injection of a local anesthetic into both TMJ capsules. Thresholds were significantly increased from a mean of 16 to 32 μ in 60 per cent of the subjects, indicating that TMJ receptors can contribute to size threshold determination. In a study in which interdental size thresholds were determined before and during chewing (Öwall, 1974), tactile sensibility was found to be decreased 60 times during mastication. Although the threshold testing procedure was different in the two circumstances (static versus dynamic), the grosser capability in function suggests that the responsible receptor input is inhibited during chewing.

Interdental Size Discrimination

The receptors primarily involved in interdental size discrimination are not the periodontal receptors, but muscle and TMJ receptors. Discriminatory ability between unanesthetized vital incisors was found by Kawamura (1960) to be from 200 to 300 μ (using wires 500 to 5000 μ in diameter) and by Riis (1970) to be 14 μ (using plastic strips of 12.5, 25, 50, and 100 μ). Kawamura (1960) found discrimination equally good between natural incisors and natural molars. Size discrimination between natural incisors and denture incisors (Manly, 1952), and between maxillary and mandibular denture teeth (Kawamura, 1960), were not significantly different from size discriminations between natural teeth. Anesthetizing incisors decreased the discriminating ability from 14 to 40 μ (Riis, 1970). Clearly, size discrimination studies do not measure tactile sensibility of the teeth as is often inferred.

Siirilä (1972) attempted to define the relative contribution of masticatory muscle and TMJ receptors to size discrimination. A reference thickness tested between the incisors was compared to thinner, thicker, and equally thick test pieces in 17 dentulous and six complete denture subjects. The test pieces used were special sliding calipers, blades of a gap measurer, and strips of tinfoil. For seven dentulous patients, bilateral intracapsular injections of a local anesthetic were used to block TMJ receptors. These investigators found that the discrimination of differences in thickness between the teeth was not altered by anesthetization of both TMJs. It would appear that sensory information from muscles must be mainly responsible for discrimination of size between the teeth.

Several investigators have examined the effect of jaw position on size discrimination. While Kawamura (1960) and Ringel (1967) have shown improved discrimination at larger mouth openings, Broekhuijsen (1983) demonstrated worsened discrimination at large openings. Siirilä (1972) demonstrated improved discrimination at small jaw openings. One would intuitively expect the best discrimination near occlusal contact, where the need for the task is greatest. These differences may be due to differences in experimental techniques or uncontrolled variables. For example, the effects of biting force or translation of the condyle have not been examined.

SUMMARY

The human TMJ is primarily innervated by twigs of the auriculotemporal nerve and collaterals of nerves innervating adjacent muscles. The capsule is most richly innervated in its lateral and dorsal aspects; articular surfaces are not innervated. The innervation of the joint ligaments, synovium, and posterior attachment is poorly documented.

The receptors of the TMJ are the same as receptors found in other joints. Specialized endings are comparatively rare. Nonspecialized endings predominate. Earlier views that these endings are exclusively pain endings need to be revised. Unlike many other joint receptors, TMJ receptors fire throughout the range of jaw movement. The sensitivity of joint mechanoreceptors is increased by inflammation and elevated with increases in intracapsular pressure, presumably potentiating the reflexes regulating mandibular position and movement.

Cell bodies of the primary TMJ afferents are in the trigeminal ganglia and not in the mesencephalic nucleus as would be expected.

Since joint and muscle sensory inputs have been shown to be interactive elsewhere in the body, this can be anticipated for the TMJ. TMJ afferents do modulate the activity of the jaw muscles. Jaw muscle activity probably affects the sensitivity of the TMJ receptors.

While TMJ receptors are sited so as to protect the TMJ from capsular and posterior attachment damage, they cannot protect the joint against unfavorable loading. This function is probably served by periodontal and muscle receptors.

TMJ receptors must function in parallel and interact with receptors of the periodontal ligament and jaw muscles in the initiation and modulation of simple and complex jaw reflexes. TMJ receptors may also serve as the conditioned stimulus for reflexes protecting the teeth, the joints, and the airway.

Mandibular position sense, interdental size threshold, and interdental size discrimination are the result of a mixture of inputs from the TMJ, the jaw muscles, and the periodontium. The afferent mix responsible for these perceptual tasks varies with the task. Malocclusion, muscle fatigue, and internal derangements can distort these perceptual tasks.

Receptors in different sites may serve parallel roles. This redundancy may compensate for loss of input from one site. A *crucial mass* of receptors may be more important than a *crucial mix*.

REFERENCES

Abe, K.: A role of sensory information from the temporomandibular joint. Jap. J. Oral Biol. 16:117–128, 1974.

Boyd, I. A.: The histological structure of the receptors in the knee joint of the cat correlated with their physiological response. J. Physiol. 124:476–488, 1954.

Broekhuijsen, M. L., and Van Willigen, J. D.: Factors influencing jaw position sense in man. Arch. Oral Biol. 28:387–391, 1983.

Broton, J. G., Hu, J. W., and Sessle, B. J.: Effects of temporomandibular joint stimulation on nociceptive and nonnociceptive neurons of the cat's trigeminal subnucleus caudalis (medullary dorsal horn). J. Neurophysiol. 59:1575–1589, 1988.

Butler, W. B.: An analysis of brain stem responses to temporomandibular joint rotation in the cat. Master's Thesis. Ann Arbor, The University of Michigan, 1977.

Caffesse, P. G., Carraro, J. J., and Albano, E. A.: Influence of temporomandibular joint receptors on tactile occlusal perception. J. Periodont. Res. 8:400–403, 1973.

Capra, N. F.: Localization and central projections of primary afferent neurons that innervate the temporomandibular joint in cats. Somatosens. Res. 4:201–213, 1987.

Christensen, L. V.: Mandibular kinesthesia in fatigue of human jaw muscles. Scand. J. Dent. Res. 84:320–326, 1976.

Christensen, L. V., and Troest, T.: Clinical kinesthetic experiments on the lateral pterygoid muscle and temporomandibular joint in man. Scand. J. Dent. Res. 83:238–244, 1975.

Clark, F. J., Horch, K. W., Bach, S. M., and Larson, G. F.: Contributions of cutaneous and joint receptors to static knee-position sense in man. J. Neurophysiol. 42:877–888, 1979.

Clark, R. K. F., and Wyke, B. D.: Contributions of temporomandibular articular mechanoreceptors to the control of mandibular posture: an experimental study. J. Dent. 2:121–129, 1974.

Cody, F. W. J., Lee, R. W. H., and Taylor, A.: A functional analysis of the components of the mesencephalic nucleus of the fifth nerve in the cat. J. Physiol. 226:249–261, 1972.

Coggeshall, R. E., Park Hong, K. A. H., Langford, L. A., et al.: Discharge characteristics of fine medial articular afferents at rest and during passive movements of inflamed knee joints. Brain Res. 272:158–188, 1983.

Costen, J. B.: A syndrome of ear and sinus symptoms dependent upon disturbed function of the temporomandibular joint. Otol. Rhinol. Laryngol. 43:1–15, 1934.

Costen, J. B.: Outline of the mandibular joint syndrome. Laryngoscope 69:408–414, 1959.

Dubner, R., Sessle, B. J., and Storey, A. T.: The Neural Basis of Oral and Facial Function. New York, Plenum Press, 1978.

Ekholm, J., and Skoglund, S.: Autonomic contributions to myelinated fibres in peripheral nerves. Acta Morph. Neerl. Scand. 6:55–63, 1964.

Ferrell, W. R., Nade, S., and Newbold, P. J.: The interrelation of neural discharge, intra-articular pressure, and joint angle in the knee of the dog. J. Physiol. 373:353–365, 1986.

Franks, A. S.: De beheersing van de bewegingen in het kaakgewricht; onderzoekingen naar de innervatie van het gewricht en van de m. pterygoideus lateralis. Nederl. T. Tandheelk. 72:605–619, 1965.

Frost, H. M.: Musculoskeletal pain. In Alling, C. C.: Facial Pain. Philadelphia, Lea & Febiger, 1968.

Gardner, E.: Spinal cord and brain stem pathways for afferents from joints. In De Reuck, A. V. S., and Knight, J. (Eds.): Ciba Foundation Symposium on Myotatic Kinesthetic and Vestibular Mechanisms, 1967, pp 56–76.

Greenfield, B. E., and Wyke, B.: Reflex innervation of the temporomandibular joint. Nature 211:940–941, 1966.

Griffin, C. J., and Harris, R.: Innervation of the temporomandibular joint. Aust. Dent. J. 20:78–85, 1975.

Grigg, P.: Mechanical factors influencing response of joint afferent neurons from cat knee. J. Neurophysiol. 38:1473–1484, 1975.

Grigg, P., and Hoffman, A. H.: Ruffini mechanoreceptors in isolated joint capsule: responses correlated with strain energy density. Somatosens. Res. 2:149–162, 1985.

Hellsing, G.: Distortion of mandibular kinesthesia induced by vibration of human jaw muscles. Scand. J. Dent. Res. 86:486–494, 1978.

Houk, J., and Henneman, E.: Responses of Golgi tendon organs to active contractions of the soleus muscle of the cat. J. Neurophysiol. 30:466–481, 1967.

Hylander, W. L.: An experimental analysis of temporomandibular joint reaction force in macaques. Am. J. Phys. Anthrop. 51:433–456, 1979.

Johansson, K., Arvidsson, J., and Thomander, L.: Sympathetic nerve fibers in peripheral sensory and motor nerves in the face of the rat. Auton. Nerv. Syst. 23:83–86, 1988.

Kawamura, Y.: Discussion. In Anderson, D. J., and Matthews, B. (Eds.): Mastication. Bristol, John Wright, 1976.

Kawamura, Y., and Abe, K.: Role of sensory information from temporomandibular joint. Bull. Tokyo Med. Dent. Univ. 21:78–82, 1974.

Kawamura, Y., Majima, T., and Kato, I.: Physiologic role of deep mechanoreceptor in temporomandibular joint capsule. J. Osaka Dent. Univ. 7:63–76, 1967.

Kawamura, Y., and Watanabe, M.: Studies on oral sensory thresholds. Med. J. Osaka Univ. 10:291–301, 1960.

Keller, J. H., and Moffett, B. C. Jr.: Nerve endings in the temporomandibular joint of the Rhesus macaque. Anat. Rec. 160:587–594, 1968.

Klineberg, I.: Structure and function of temporomandibular joint innervation. Ann. R. Coll. Surg. Engl. 49:268–288, 1971.

Klineberg, I.: Influences of temporomandibular articular mechanoreceptors on functional jaw movements. J. Oral Rehabil. 7:307–317, 1980.

Klineberg, I., and Lillie, J.: Regional nerve block of the temporomandibular joint capsule. A technique for clinical research and differential diagnosis. J. Dent. Res. 59:1930–1935, 1980.

Larsson, L. E., and Thilander, B.: Mandibular positioning. The effect of pressure on the joint capsule. Acta Neurol. Scand. 40:131–143, 1964.

Levine, J. D., Clark, R., Devor, M., et al.: Intraneuronal substance P contributes to the severity of experimental arthritis. Science 226:547–549, 1984.

Levine, J. D., Collier, D. H., Basbaum, A. J., et al.: Hypothesis: The nervous system may contribute to the pathophysiology of rheumatoid arthritis. J. Rheumatol. 12:406–411, 1985.

Lindauer, S. J., and Gay, T.: Jaw position sensitivity as a function of degree of opening. J. Dent. Res. 64, Special Issue, Abstract #811, 1985, p 265.

Lowe, A. A.: Mandibular joint control of genioglossus muscle activity in the cat and monkey (Macaca mulatta). Arch. Oral Biol. 23:787–793, 1978.

Lund, J. P., and Matthews, B.: Responses of temporomandibular joint afferents recorded in the Gasserian ganglion of the rabbit to passive movements of the mandible. In Kawamura, Y., and Dubner, R. (Eds.): Oral-Facial Sensory and Motor Functions. Chicago, Quintessence, 1981.

Manly, R. S., Pfaffman, C., Lathrop, D. D., and Keyser, J.: Oral sensory thresholds of persons with natural and artificial dentitions. J. Dent. Res. 31:305–312, 1952.

Matthews, P. B. C.: Mammalian Muscle Receptors and their Central Actions. London, Arnold, 1972.

Millar, J.: Joint afferent fibres responding to muscle stretch, vibration and contraction. Brain Res. 63:380–383, 1973.

Millar, J.: Convergence of joint, cutaneous and muscle afferents onto cuneate neurons in the cat. Brain Res. 175:347–350, 1979.

Öwall, B.: Interocclusal perception with anesthetized and unanaesthetized TM-joints. Swed. Dent. J. 2:199–208, 1978.

Öwall, B., and Møller, E.: Oral tactile sensibility during biting and chewing. Odontol. Rev. 25:327–346, 1974.

Posselt, U., and Thilander, B.: Influence of the innervation of the temporomandibular joint capsule on mandibular border movements. Acta Odont. Scand. 23:601–613, 1965.

Ransjö, T. K., and Thilander, B.: Perception of mandibular position in cases of temporomandibular joint disorders. Odont. Tijdschr. 71:134–144, 1963.

Riis, D., and Giddon, D. B.: Interdental discrimination of small thickness differences. J. Prosthet. Dent. 24:324–334, 1970.

Ringel, R. L., Saxman, J. H., and Brooks, A. R.: Oral perception: II. Mandibular kinesthesia. J. Speech Hear. Res. 10:637–641, 1967.

Romfh, J. H., Capra, N. F., and Gatipon, G. B.: Trigeminal nerve and temporomandibular joint of the cat: A horseradish peroxidase study. Exper. Neurol. 65:99–106, 1979.

Savalle, W. P. M.: Some aspects of the morphology of the human temporomandibular joint capsule. Acta Anat. 131:292–296, 1988.

Schaerer, P., Stallard, R., and Zander, H. A.: Occlusal interferences and mastication: An electromyographic study. J. Prosthet. Dent. 17:438–449, 1967.

Schaible, H. G., and Schmidt, R. F.: Effects of an experimental arthritis on the sensory properties of fine articular afferent units. J. Neurophysiol. 54:1109–1122, 1985.

Schmid, F.: On the nerve distribution of the temporomandibular joint capsule. Oral Surg. 28:63–65, 1964.

Shwaluk, S.: Initiation of reflex activity from the temporomandibular joint of the cat. J. Dent. Res. 50:1641–1646, 1971.

Siirilä, H. S., and Laine, P.: The tactile sensibility of the periodontium to slight axial loadings of the teeth. Acta Odontol. Scand. *21*:415–426, 1963.

Siirilä, H. S., and Laine, P.: Sensory thresholds in discriminating differences in thickness between the teeth by different degrees of mouth opening. Proc. Finn. Dent. Soc. *68*:134–139, 1972.

Skoglund, S.: Joint receptors and kinaesthesis. *In* Iggo, A. (Ed.): Handbook of Sensory Physiology, Vol. 2, Somatosensory System. Berlin, Springer-Verlag, 1973.

Storey, A. T.: Sensory functions of the temporomandibular joint. J. Can. Dent. Assoc. *34*:294–300, 1968.

Storey, A. T.: Reflex functions of the temporomandibular joint. J. Prosthet. Dent. *30*:830–837, 1973.

Storey, A. T.: Temporomandibular joint receptors. *In* Anderson, D. J., and Matthews, B. (Eds.): Mastication. Bristol, Wright, 1976.

Storey, A. T.: The neurophysiology of temporomandibular disorders. *In* Carlson, D. S., McNamara, J. A., and Ribbens, K. A. (Eds.): Developmental Aspects of Temporomandibular Joint Disorders. Ann Arbor, MI, Center for Human Growth and Development, 1985a.

Storey, A. T.: The neurobiology of occlusion. *In* Johnston, L. E. (Ed.): New Vistas in Orthodontics. Philadelphia, Lea & Febiger, 1985b.

Storey, A. T.: Maturation of the orofacial musculature. *In* Moyers, R. E. (Ed.): Handbook of Orthodontics. Chicago, Year Book Medical, 1988.

Thilander, B.: Innervation of the temporo-mandibular joint capsule in man. Trans. R. Sch. Dent. Stockholm and Umeå *7*:9–67, 1961.

Tracey, D. J.: The projection of joint receptors to the cuneate nucleus in the cat. J. Physiol. (Lond.). *305*:433–449, 1980.

Van Willigen, J. D., and Broekhuijsen, M. L.: On the self perception of jaw positions in man. Arch. Oral Biol. *28*:117–122, 1983.

Widenfalk, B., Elfvin, L. G., and Wiberg, M.: Origin of sympathetic and sensory innervation of the elbow joint in the rat: A retrograde axonal tracing study with wheat germ agglutinin conjugated horseradish peroxidase. Comp. Neurol. *271*:313–318, 1988.

Wyke, B.: The neurology of joints. Ann. R. Coll. Surg. Engl. *41*:25–49, 1967.

Zenker, W.: Das retroarticuläre plastische Polster des Kiefergelenkes Kiefergelenkes und seine mechanische Bedeutung. Zeitsch. Anat. Entwickl. *119*:375–388, 1956.

8

NEUROBIOLOGY OF FACIAL AND DENTAL PAIN*

BARRY J. SESSLE, B.D.S., M.D.S., B.Sc., Ph.D.

INTRODUCTION

PERIPHERAL SENSORY MECHANISMS

BRAIN STEM RELAY MECHANISMS

THALAMOCORTICAL MECHANISMS

RELATED REFLEX AND BEHAVIORAL RESPONSES

MECHANISMS OF MODULATION OF NOCICEPTIVE TRANSMISSION AND PAIN CONTROL

Modulation by Peripheral Afferent Stimulation or Damage
SENSORY STIMULATION
INFLAMMATION
DEAFFERENTATION

Modulation by Central Neural Pathways

SUMMARY

INTRODUCTION

Some of the most common acute pains in the body occur in the orofacial region, such as pain accompanying acute pathological states in the teeth and associated structures. Moreover, the face, mouth, and jaws represent frequent sites of chronic and referred pains. The mechanisms underlying acute pain, and chronic pain in particular, still have not been completely clarified. Likewise, the processes that account for the effectiveness of the various therapeutic procedures presently in use for controlling orofacial pain have not yet been fully delineated. This gap in knowledge is partly a reflection of the multidimensional nature of pain, since pain is now conceptualized as a complex, multifactorial experience encompassing sensory-discriminative, affective (emotional), cognitive, and motivational dimensions (Fields, 1987; Sessle, 1987; Wall, 1984). Fortunately, advances in the neurobiology of pain in the last few years have unraveled some of the mysteries of acute and chronic orofacial pain, and have contributed to an improved understanding of both the basis of orofacial pain and its control.

---

*See Chapters 5, 7, 9, 11, 19–22, and 25.

PERIPHERAL SENSORY MECHANISMS

Free nerve endings in the face and mouth provide the peripheral structural basis for pain. Many of these free nerve endings act as nociceptors; that is, they are the receptors that respond to noxious orofacial stimuli, providing sensory-discriminative information about the quality, intensity, location, and duration of the noxious stimulus. Free nerve endings have long been recognized in virtually all orofacial tissues including skin, oral mucosa, temporomandibular joint (TMJ), periodontium, tooth pulp, periosteum, and muscles. They are associated with slow-conducting, small-diameter, myelinated (A-delta) afferent fibers or even slower conducting unmyelinated (C) afferent fibers that convey the neural information from the nociceptors into the brain stem sensory nuclear complex of the fifth (V) cranial nerve (Dubner, 1978). The larger, faster conducting afferent fibers (A-beta) carry tactile and proprioceptive information from more complex receptors into the brain stem.

Most of our information about the properties of these nociceptive afferent inputs into the central nervous system (CNS) comes from several studies in the orofacial region, particularly of facial skin and tooth pulp afferents, as well as from numerous studies of afferents supplying

124

viscera or cutaneous muscle or articular tissues of the limbs. While the proportion of A-delta to C fiber nociceptive afferents may vary between these different tissues, they show basically the same properties. The area of skin, mucosa, or deep tissue from which a nociceptive afferent fiber (or central neuron) and its associated nociceptors can be excited by a threshold stimulus is called the receptive field of the fiber (or neuron). In the case of a nociceptive afferent fiber, the threshold for its excitation from its receptive field is very high, in the noxious range.

In the facial skin of cats and monkeys, three major classes of nociceptive afferents have been described and invoked as providing the input to the brain that is necessary for pain perception (Dubner, 1983; 1985; Hu, 1988). These three classes are (1) the A-delta mechanothermal nociceptive afferents that respond to intense thermal and mechanical stimuli; (2) C polymodal nociceptive afferents, which are excited by strong mechanical, thermal, and chemical stimuli; and (3) high-threshold mechanoreceptive afferents most of which conduct in the A-delta range, although some have been reported in the A-beta and C ranges. This last class responds best to intense mechanical stimuli, but sometimes may also respond to noxious heat after sensitization, that is, if the threshold of the nociceptors is lowered by chemical agents or repeated noxious stimuli.

The sensitivity of all classes of nociceptive afferents actually increases following mild injury and this increase is thought to be a major factor in producing hyperalgesia, such as the increased sensitivity of the skin after sunburn. Chemical mediators are involved in this heightened sensitivity, and indeed underlie much of the responsivity of the nociceptive afferents to the different forms of noxious stimuli. Thus, the afferent endings are acting as sensors of the chemical environment in which they are located. While the precise mechanisms whereby chemical agents participate in the peripheral transduction of pain are not clear, there appear to be three classes of chemical agents involved (Fields, 1987; Lynn, 1984; Yaksh, 1982). Some activate small-diameter, high-threshold afferents and produce pain when they are applied locally; examples are histamine, bradykinin, serotonin (5-HT), and potassium (Fig. 8–1). Others, such as the prostaglandins, facilitate the pain evoked by chemical and physical stimuli, but are relatively ineffective in evoking pain themselves.

In addition, there are those chemicals, such

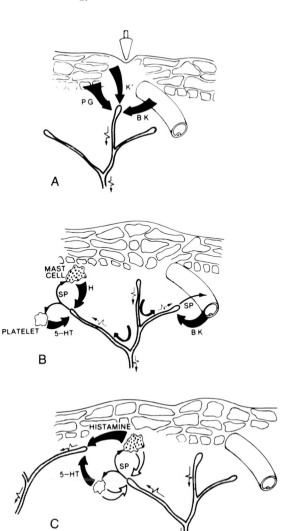

FIGURE 8–1. Mechanisms involved in activation of the peripheral endings of nociceptive afferents and in sensitization and spread in the afferents. *A,* A noxious stimulus, such as intense pressure, causes cell damage and release of potassium (K) and the synthesis of substances such as the prostaglandins (PG) and bradykinin (BK); PG enhances the sensitivity of the endings to BK and other substances. *B,* Indirect activation of the afferents may occur. Action potentials generated in the stimulated endings of an afferent travel not only toward the CNS, but also into collaterals in which they bring about substance P (SP) release in other endings of the afferent. SP produces vasodilation, edema, and release of histamine (H) and serotonin (5-HT) from cells. *C,* The rise in H and 5-HT levels in the peripheral tissues sensitizes the endings of other nearby nociceptive afferents, and results in hyperalgesia or tenderness. (From Fields, H. L.: Pain. New York, McGraw-Hill, 1987.)

as substance P, whose release at nerve endings in peripheral tissues as a result of tissue damage appears to increase capillary permeability and result in extravasation and the release into the tissue of agents that elicit pain and increase small afferent fiber activity. Substance P not only causes the generation of orthodromic nerve impulses that are conducted by afferent fibers toward the CNS, but also produces impulses that are conducted back along collaterals of the afferents toward the periphery where additional substance P is released at the afferent endings (Fig. 8–1). The release of agents such as substance P is associated with the peripheral spread and tenderness of an injury, and coincides with the local synthesis of certain prostanoids that facilitate the algesic activity of these agents as well as sensitize the receptors to physical stimuli such as repeated thermal stimulation.

As previously mentioned, most knowledge of the properties of these afferents and chemical mediators in the orofacial region comes from studies of pulp afferents and limited investigations of facial cutaneous afferents. No detailed studies of the TMJ or masticatory muscle nociceptive afferents appear to have been carried out that are analogous to those on afferents supplying limb joints and muscles (Guilbaud, 1988; Mense, 1986), although it is known that small diameter afferent innervation is abundant in the TMJ and masticatory muscles (Dubner, 1978). We can assume that they show properties comparable to those found for nociceptors in deep tissues of the limb such as innervation by A-delta and C fiber afferents; sensitivity to extreme mechanical stimuli, algesic chemicals and inflammatory conditions; and reduced responsiveness in the presence of anti-inflammatory agents such as aspirin (Fields, 1987; Guilbaud, 1988; Lynn, 1984; Mense, 1986; Schaible, 1987).

With respect to dental tissues, little study has been directed at periodontal afferents, although a small sample of A-delta periodontal afferents has been examined and reported to have properties suggestive of an involvement in nociceptive mechanisms (Mei, 1977). The innervation and central pathways of the tooth pulp have evoked much more research. A detailed consideration is beyond the scope of this chapter, but extensive, recent reviews are available (Byers, 1984; Dubner, 1978; Narhi, 1985; Olgart, 1985; Sessle, 1987). Nerves entering the pulp arborize and form the subodontoblastic plexus, which gives rise to fibers that may pass into the overlying odontoblast layer and sometimes into the dentinal tubules. Currently there are three major theories of how stimuli delivered to the enamel or dentin can activate pulpal nerve fibers: (1) activation of the intradentinal extensions of the pulpal nerves, (2) a hydrodynamic mechanism within the dentinal tubules and pulp, and (3) a transduction mechanism involving the odontoblast or its dentinal process. Current evidence favors the hydrodynamic mechanism, although research has not ruled out the other two possibilities completely.

The nerves that enter the dental pulp are mainly small myelinated (A-delta) and unmyelinated (C) nerve fibers that contain a number of neuropeptides and other neurochemicals implicated in several functions including pain. This range of small fibers is comparable with those afferents in the rest of the body that are associated with nociception. Consequently, these observations, coupled with clinical observations suggesting that pain may be the only sensation experienced from the pulp, have been taken as evidence in support of the view that the sensibility of the pulp is exclusively related to nociception. Not all A-delta and C fibers elsewhere in the body, however, are involved in nociception. Some are implicated in tactile and warm and cold sensibilities. Many of the unmyelinated fibers also may not be nociceptive *afferents* but autonomic *efferents*, which may regulate both the microcirculation of the pulp and the activity of other pulpal nerve fibers.

Furthermore, the small fibers distributed within the pulp may be sensitive to a wide range of stimuli, including possibly non-noxious stimuli, and may be associated with parent fibers of larger diameter outside the pulp. These features are not inconsistent with a role in non-noxious sensory functions. Finally, other findings on the central pathways and behavioral (perceptual and reflex) responses that can be elicited by pulp stimulation also strongly suggest that not all responses evoked by tooth pulp stimuli may be related to pain (Byers, 1984; Dubner, 1978; Sessle, 1987).

BRAIN STEM RELAY MECHANISMS

Neural information from facial and oral tissues is carried by the trigeminal nerve (V) predominantly through the gasserian or semilunar ganglion, where the primary afferent cell bodies are located, and then into the brain stem where the first synaptic relay of the information occurs. Here the nerve fibers may ascend or descend in the spinal tract before entering the V sensory nuclear complex to activate second-order neurons (Fig. 8–2). The sensory complex can be subdivided into the main (principal) sensory nucleus and the spinal tract nucleus. The latter comprises three subnuclei, the most caudal of which, subnucleus caudalis, extends into the

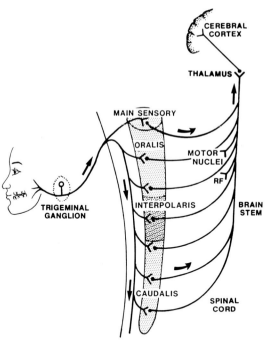

FIGURE 8–2. Major pathway for transmission of sensory information from the face and mouth. The primary afferents project via the trigeminal ganglion to second-order neurons in the trigeminal brain stem sensory complex. These neurons may project to neurons in higher levels of the CNS such as in the thalamus or cerebral cortex or in brain stem regions such as the cranial nerve motor nuclei or reticular formation (RF). (From Sessle, B. J.: Recent developments in pain research: Central mechanisms of orofacial pain and its control. J. Endodont. *12*:435–441, 1986. Copyright by the American Association of Endodontists.)

cervical spinal cord and merges with the spinal dorsal horn (Fig. 8–2).

Neurons in each subdivision of the complex have axons that may project directly to the thalamus and are thereby crucial elements underlying perceptual, cognitive, emotional, and motivational responses to orofacial stimuli. Many neurons, however, may project indirectly to the higher levels of the brain involved in these functions via connections with adjacent brain stem regions such as the reticular formation. Some also may project to the spinal cord or other subnuclei of the complex. Furthermore, by virtue of their connections with the cranial nerve motor nuclei, many neurons within or adjacent to the complex may also serve as reflex interneurons in the numerous reflex responses that can be evoked by orofacial stimuli (Dubner, 1978).

Studies of the afferent input to these second-order neurons have involved electrophysiological approaches, as well as anatomical techniques that utilize degeneration or labeling of afferent nerves by means of autoradiography, immuno-

histochemistry, and enzymes such as horseradish peroxidase (HRP). These studies have shown that cutaneous nociceptive afferents as well as tooth pulp and small-diameter muscle afferents terminate in laminae I and II, and V and VI of subnucleus caudalis (Gobel, 1981; 1982; Ishidori, 1986; Jacquin, 1986; Johnson, 1987; Nishimori, 1986). In contrast, low-threshold, mechanosensitive primary afferents, which are primarily large-diameter and rapidly conducting axons (A-beta), terminate in the laminae III to VI of caudalis, as well as in more rostral parts of the V brain stem complex. These input patterns to caudalis are consistent with the electrophysiologically documented laminar location and responses to low- or high-threshold afferent inputs of the neurons.

Anatomical studies have also provided information on the morphology and other related features of the different neurons in caudalis or more rostral V nuclei (Dubner, 1983; Gobel, 1981; 1982; Jacquin, 1986; Sessle, 1987). The caudalis neurons projecting out of the nucleus to various sites are found mainly in laminae I and III to VI of caudalis. In lamina II, the so-called substantia gelatinosa (SG), several morphologically distinct cell types have been described. Some of these SG neurons receive low-threshold peripheral afferent inputs, whereas others receive nociceptive inputs. Inputs from higher brain centers involved in somatosensory modulation are also especially apparent in the SG (Basbaum, 1985; Dubner, 1983; Fields, 1987; Gobel, 1981; 1982). Because the axons of most of the SG neurons arborize locally within the V complex, the SG represents a crucial interneuronal system underlying the powerful sensory and descending modulation of somatosensory transmission that occurs in subnucleus caudalis and more rostral components of the V complex.

The more rostral parts of the V sensory nuclear complex, in particular the main sensory nucleus and the subnucleus oralis of the spinal tract nucleus, classically have been viewed as the major relay sites of orofacial tactile information to higher centers, although it is now clear that tactile information also relays through caudalis. Caudalis has also been considered to be the principal brain stem relay site of orofacial nociceptive information, and this view is supported by several lines of evidence.

There are relevant clinical observations that the V tractotomy procedure, which has been used for the relief of trigeminal neuralgia in humans, produces a profound orofacial analgesia and thermanesthesia, with much less complete loss of tactile sensibility (Dubner, 1978; Kerr, 1979). This clinical finding suggests that the tractotomy is interfering with the relay of nociceptive information through subnucleus caudalis since it transects the V spinal tract near the level of its rostral pole. However, some recent observations in animals and humans suggest that such a tractotomy-induced analgesic effect is not necessarily seen with all orofacial pain, such as from the teeth (see further on). Nonetheless, further support for a crucial role in pain of subnucleus caudalis also comes from anatomical studies that have shown that small diameter axons in the V spinal tract, presumed to represent nociceptive primary afferents, terminate primarily in the subnucleus caudalis. There are also the parallels in structure previously mentioned, and projection sites (Gobel, 1981) between caudalis and the spinal cord dorsal horn that are the well-documented integral components of the spinal nociceptive mechanism.

These input patterns to caudalis are consistent with recent electrophysiological evidence of the lamina location and response properties to low- or higher-threshold afferent inputs to caudalis neurons. On the basis of their response properties to cutaneous (facial) stimuli, neurons have been found in the subnucleus caudalis of anesthetized, decerebrate, or unanesthetized animals that respond to noxious stimuli (Dubner, 1983; 1985; Sessle, 1987). Consistent with analogous neurons found in the spinal dorsal horn, the V nociceptive neurons have been classified into two main groups: the wide dynamic range (WDR) neurons that are excited by non-noxious, tactile stimuli as well as by noxious stimuli, and nociceptive-specific (NS) neurons that respond exclusively to noxious stimuli such as pinch and heat (Fig. 8–3). These pain-transmission neurons are concentrated in laminae I and II and V and VI of subnucleus caudalis, as they are in the spinal dorsal horn. In addition to these cutaneous nociceptive neurons, low-threshold mechanoreceptive (LTM) neurons comprise the third major group of caudalis neurons. They do not respond to noxious cutaneous stimuli, although some are excited by electrical stimulation of the tooth pulp, but are activated by light tactile stimuli applied to a restricted region (the so-called mechanoreceptive field) of skin, mucosa, or teeth. These LTM neurons are localized mainly in laminae III and IV of caudalis. They have properties comparable to the principal neuron type reported in the rostral V brain stem nuclei and are considered essential for the relay of orofacial

touch, although there may be differences between the rostral and caudal LTM neurons in their ability to transmit precise information related to a tactile stimulus.

The neurochemical mechanisms underlying nociceptive transmission in the V brain stem complex have recently been investigated. Neuropeptides have been discovered in the complex that may represent the neurotransmitter(s) underlying the excitatory nociceptive transmission process. An important role for the polypeptide substance P in pain pathways has been suggested from iontophoretic, electrophysiological, and immunocytochemical studies (Basbaum, 1985; Dubner, 1983; Sessle, 1987). Substance P is found in small-diameter afferents (the spectrum of afferents carrying nociceptive information) of nerves supplying the skin and tooth pulp, and in their ganglion cell bodies. Moreover, as mentioned previously, it has also been implicated in peripheral injury and inflammation. It is also concentrated in endings in the superficial and deep laminae of caudalis and the spinal dorsal horn where the nociceptive neurons predominate. When substance P is applied iontophoretically within these laminae, it is especially effective in exciting these neurons. Several other endogenous neurochemicals, however, such as amino acids and somatostatin, have also been implicated in the excitatory processes underlying nociceptive transmission. Moreover, the internal neuronal circuitry in caudalis and other brain areas involved in pain transmission and its control also contain other substances thought to be more involved with suppression of nociceptive transmission; examples are enkephalin, dynorphin, and 5-HT.

The caudalis neurons that project out of the nucleus occur mainly in laminae I and III to VI of caudalis. In common with the projections of other neurons in the V complex, the nociceptive output neurons relay the nociceptive information that they receive to several areas (Fig. 8–2). Much of the information is relayed directly or indirectly to higher brain centers in the thalamus and then to the cerebral cortex. These areas are involved in perception as well as in emotional and motivational reactions to the noxious stimulus. Subnucleus caudalis, however, is not functioning simply as a straight-through brain stem relay station of nociceptive information from the periphery to higher brain centers and local reflex centers. The relay of the information can be regulated (see page 137). Moreover, some neurons project to other subdivisions of the V brain stem sensory nuclear complex and thus may themselves be capable

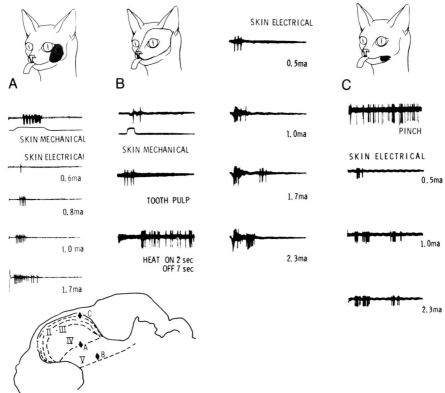

FIGURE 8–3. Characteristics of the major types of neurons in the trigeminal brain stem sensory complex of the cat. *A,* The responses of a low-threshold mechanoreceptive neuron to light mechanical (tactile) stimulation and electrical stimuli (at different current intensities) applied to its mechanoreceptive field outlined in black. *B,* Example of a wide dynamic-range neuron activated by mechanical and noxious heat stimuli applied to its outlined mechanoreceptive field as well as by electrical stimulation of the tooth pulp and facial skin. The early discharges to the skin electrical stimuli are thought to reflect activation of the neuron by inputs to the neuron from fast-conducting tactile afferents, and the later burst of discharges elicited only by the high-intensity electrical stimuli may reflect inputs from slow-conducting nociceptive afferents. *C,* Responses of a nociceptive-specific neuron to pinch or electrical stimuli applied to its localized mandibular mechanoreceptive field. The discharges evoked by the electrical stimuli are thought to reflect input from slow-conducting nociceptive afferents. These three neurons were located in V subnucleus caudalis (shown in cross-section): *A* in lamina IV, *B* in lamina V, and *C* in lamina I. The time durations of the traces are *A,* 50 ms, *B,* 100 ms, and *C,* 200 ms except for the pinch and heat traces (10s).

of regulating the flow of sensory information through these parts (Greenwood, 1976; Hu, 1981; Young, 1972).

Because many caudalis WDR and NS neurons can be excited only by localized natural stimulation of cutaneous or mucosal tissues, they have properties consistent with a role in the detection, discrimination, and localization of superficial noxious stimuli. The activity of these neurons during behavioral tasks that require monkeys to discriminate noxious facial thermal stimuli indeed indicate that they code specific neural information essential for these tasks and for detection of stimulus quality, intensity, and location (Dubner, 1985; Hoffman, 1981). Nonetheless, many WDR and NS neurons classified on the basis of their cutaneous (or mucosal) mechanoreceptive field properties can also be

excited by other types of peripheral afferent inputs. For example, a proportion of the neurons in caudalis that respond to cutaneous (or mucosal) stimulation can also be excited by electrical or natural (thermal) stimulation of the tooth pulp (Hu, 1984).

Of particular interest are findings (Amano, 1986; Broton, 1988) that activation of afferents supplying jaw and tongue muscles and the TMJ by electrical stimuli, noxious mechanical stimuli, and by algesic chemical stimuli such as hypertonic saline and bradykinin, also excites many of the WDR and NS neurons (Fig. 8–4). These excitatory effects are consistent with the demonstrated excitatory effects of these stimuli on nociceptive afferents supplying joint and muscle, and explain how damage to the TMJ and masticatory muscles can be signaled and

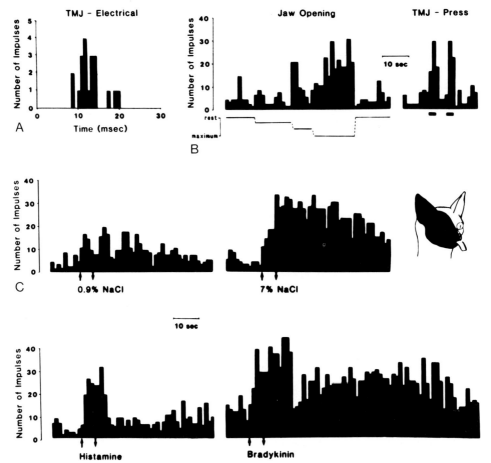

FIGURE 8–4. Responses of a nociceptive-specific neuron in the cat's V subnucleus caudalis to TMJ stimuli. The neuron could be activated by noxious pinching and heating of all the ipsilateral facial skin (outlined in black) as well as by electrical stimulation of the TMJ *(A)* and by heavy pressure applied to the TMJ capsule and by extreme jaw opening *(B)*. Note that in C the injection into the TMJ of the algesic chemicals hypertonic saline, histamine, and bradykinin produced a sustained increase in activity of the neuron (compared with isotonic saline). Arrows indicate time of chemical application. (From Broton, J. G., Hu, J. W., and Sessle, B. J.: Effects of temporomandibular joint stimulation on nociceptive and non-nociceptive neurons of the cat's trigeminal subnucleus caudalis (medullary dorsal horn). J. Neurophysiol. 59:1575–1589, 1988.)

relayed through the brain. These inputs from deep structures are particularly directed at those caudalis cells functionally identified on the basis of their cutaneous and mucosal receptive field properties as nociceptive neurons (i.e. WDR and NS), and very few neurons appear to be exclusively activated by these deep inputs. These findings are also consistent with observations that nearly all the V brain stem neurons excited by electrical and natural (thermal) stimulation of the tooth pulp, as well as most of the spinal dorsal horn neurons receiving muscle, joint, or visceral inputs, are WDR and NS nociceptive neurons with cutaneous afferent inputs.

A large proportion (50 to 60 per cent) of nociceptive neurons in caudalis indeed show extensive convergence from skin, mucosal, vis-

ceral (laryngeal), TMJ, jaw and tongue muscle, tooth pulp, and even neck afferents (Sessle, 1986), and from cutaneous and dural vessel afferents (Davis, 1988; Strassman, 1986). On the basis of these and similar observations of a spatial organization of afferent inputs in the spinal somatosensory system (Cervero, 1985; Dubner, 1983; Fields, 1987; Willis, 1985), it has been proposed that this mechanism may explain the poor localization of deep noxious stimuli, such as in TMJ or myofascial pain (Amano, 1986; Sessle, 1986). Moreover, this extensive convergence may also underlie the spread and referral of pain that are frequently seen in many craniofacial and intraoral pain conditions and headache.

Many of these convergent afferent inputs can only be demonstrated with electrical stimuli.

Natural (pinch, tactile, chemical) stimulation does not evoke responses in the neurons from sites supplied by these afferents. This observation has led to the proposal (Sessle, 1986) that these hard-wired, yet relatively ineffective, convergent connections may provide a basis for central V neural plasticity. These so-called long-range afferent inputs and relatively ineffective synapses (Wall, 1986) also have been implicated in the development of certain chronic pain conditions and in pathophysiological situations such as inflammation where their unmasking may contribute to the spread and referral of pain.

While the foregoing discussion focuses on nociceptive mechanisms in subnucleus caudalis because this subdivision appears to be particularly important for pain, other subdivisions of the V brainstem nuclear complex may also have nociceptive functions. Lesions in or adjacent to caudalis do not necessarily eliminate completely all orofacial nociceptive reflex or behavioral responses, whereas rostral lesions may interfere with pain behavior evoked by noxious thermal or mechanical stimuli applied to facial or intraoral tissues (Greenwood, 1976; Pickoff-Matuk, 1986; Vyklicky, 1977; Young, 1984). Nociceptive neurons with properties comparable to those in caudalis have also been found in the rostral parts of the V brain stem nuclear complex (Azerad, 1982; Hayashi, 1984).

In addition, a number of studies have shown that electrical stimulation of the tooth pulp is particularly effective in exciting neurons in the subnuclei oralis and interpolaris and the main sensory nucleus, regions traditionally associated with the relay of information concerning touch (Azerad, 1982; Hayashi, 1984; Hu, 1984; Nord, 1976; Sessle, 1976). Few of these studies, however, have used a natural pulp stimulus such as thermal stimulation. Because electrical stimulation is an unnatural stimulus, and so may reveal long-range afferent inputs that might have little if any role in normal function, the functional significance of the pulp afferent input to the rostral V nuclei is unclear (Hu, 1984). It may prove to be involved in the localization and discrimination of pulpal stimuli, but conceivably could also be involved in referred pain mechanisms, in some sensory experience(s) other than pain, or in reflex responses to pulpal stimuli. The relative importance of the rostral and caudal components of the V brain stem complex in orofacial pain, and tooth pulp pain in particular, is a major issue to be clarified by future research.

THALAMOCORTICAL MECHANISMS

The so-called thalamic ventrobasal complex, posterior group, and medial thalamic areas all receive nociceptive inputs from relays in the V brain stem complex and spinal cord, and all have been implicated in various aspects of pain transmission (Albe-Fessard, 1985; Dubner, 1978; Fields, 1987; Willis, 1985; Yokota, 1987). The precise functional role in pain of each region, however, is still unclear. WDR and NS neurons have been found in all three regions, and tooth pulp-activated neurons also occur in these regions. The properties of these neurons are generally similar to those described for comparable neurons in the subthalamic relays such as subnucleus caudalis. Whereas most studies describe WDR and NS neurons scattered throughout the ventrobasal complex proper, some have reported that WDR and NS neurons receiving V or spinal nociceptive information occur in a shell region surrounding the ventrobasal complex (Willis, 1985; Yokota, 1987).

In general, it is currently believed that those nociceptive neurons of the lateral thalamus that are associated with the ventrobasal complex, and possibly the posterior group, have properties (localized receptive field and somatotopic organization) and connections with the overlying somatosensory cerebral cortex indicative of a role in the sensory-discriminative dimension of pain. In contrast, those neurons in the medial nuclei appear to have properties and connectivity suggestive of a role more in the affective-motivational aspects of pain (Fig. 8–5).

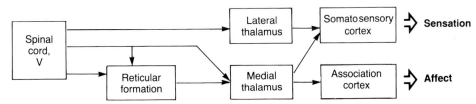

FIGURE 8–5. Diagrammatic representation of the major somatosensory pathways that contribute to pain. (From Fields, H. L.: Pain. New York, McGraw-Hill, 1987, 354 pp.)

The cerebral cortex receives a projection from the thalamus, but its role in pain is not clear. Some somatosensory cortical neurons have recently been found that can be excited by noxious cutaneous or tooth pulp stimuli (Albe-Fessard, 1985; Dubner, 1978; Fields, 1987; Willis, 1985). In view of the crucial role that the somatosensory cerebral cortex plays in general sensory perception, it seems highly probable that it is also involved in pain perception, localization, and the modulation of nociceptive transmission. The somatosensory cortex and other parts of the forebrain have also been implicated in other aspects of the pain experience, including those related to motivation, emotion, and pain memory, but the nature of their involvement in pain still requires much further investigation.

RELATED REFLEX AND BEHAVIORAL RESPONSES

Recent investigation has focused not only on the mechanisms involved in the relay of V nociceptive information to higher brain centers, but also on processes involved in other nociceptive responses to noxious orofacial stimuli in humans and experimental animals (Dubner, 1978; Mason, 1985; Sessle, 1987). The jaw-opening reflex (JOR) can be recorded in the digastric muscle of animals and has served as a frequent model of nociceptive reflexes, particularly when elicited by stimulation of the tooth pulp, a presumed source of exclusively nociceptive afferents. Recent use has also been made of V nerve or pulp-evoked cerebral potentials (Chapman, 1979; Dong, 1987) and operant conditioning and avoidance paradigms utilizing noxious facial heat (Dubner, 1985; Hoffman, 1981; Pickoff-Matuk, 1986) or stimulation of the tooth pulp (Nord, 1977; Vyklicky, 1977; Young, 1984). These approaches have been applied to investigations of various modulatory influences on nociceptive transmission. Single neuron recording in the V brain stem complex of awake monkeys trained to discriminate between, and escape from, noxious facial thermal stimuli (Dubner, 1985; Hoffman, 1981) and tooth pulp stimulation (Nord, 1977) have also been used to delineate more clearly the roles of the various neuronal types in nociception and its control.

The silent period in the jaw-closing musculature that is a component of the JOR has elicited considerable interest in the last 20 years. Like the JOR, the silent period can also be evoked by a variety of noxious and less intense stimuli applied not only to virtually all orofacial tissues but also to noncranial tissues (Dubner, 1978; Mason, 1985; Sessle, 1987). This inhibitory effect in the jaw-closing muscles is puzzling when trying to place it in the perspective of the concepts of TMJ and myofascial pain dysfunction (MPD) that are based on jaw muscle hyperactivity resulting from peripheral inputs (occlusion, muscle, TMJ) (see Chapters 5, 19–21, 25). Indeed, the seemingly countless documentations of a silent period induced by these peripheral inputs, and the lack of any substantive and sustained increase in jaw-closing muscle activity reflexly induced by orofacial stimuli, have led some authors to discard almost completely the possibility that orofacial stimuli can reflexly induce increased jaw-closing activity.

A limiting factor in these previous investigations, however, may have been the form or duration of the stimulus used to evoke reflex effects and the artificial, experimental conditions under which the silent period has been evoked. It is now clear that in certain situations intense orofacial stimuli can evoke increases in jaw-closing muscle activity that may be sustained. For example, heavy occlusal pressure on a tooth has been shown to produce considerable and maintained increases in masticatory muscle activity in subprimates (Lund, 1971) and primates (Sessle, 1982). Moreover, Broton (1988) demonstrated that algesic chemical stimuli applied to the TMJ reflexly induce sustained increases in masticatory muscle activity in cats.

These effects are comparable to the increased activity of some V brain stem neurons induced by these TMJ or analogous muscle stimuli. Since some of these neurons may project to brain stem motor nuclei, such as the V motor nucleus that contains the motoneurons supplying the jaw muscles, these neurons might be involved in the reflex pathways and mechanisms responsible for sustained increases in muscle activity. It is conceivable that this may then increase the activity of muscle nociceptors, thereby producing muscle tenderness and spread and referral of pain (Fields, 1987). Such findings are also consistent with concepts of TMJ and MPD, which claim that reflexly induced muscle hyperactivity is an important feature of these conditions, although this has to be proven.

MECHANISMS OF MODULATION OF NOCICEPTIVE TRANSMISSION AND PAIN CONTROL

With the crucial elements in V nociceptive transmission now identified, this research knowledge then allows us to see how the transmission processes can be regulated. Several factors account for the recent focus on the modulatory mechanisms underlying the control of orofacial pain. These include the discovery and documentation of substantial populations of nociceptive neurons in the brain stem and spinal cord, findings of endogenous pain-suppressive neurochemical mechanisms, and the demonstrated therapeutic effectiveness of peripheral stimulation procedures such as acupuncture and transcutaneous electrical nerve stimulation (TENS). An additional factor has been the research interest generated by the gate control theory of pain (Melzack, 1965). While this theory has undergone some revision in the last 25 years (Fields, 1987; Wall, 1984), it has provided a conceptual framework of possible mechanisms that can modulate nociceptive transmission in the CNS, initially by way of sensory interactions between large diameter and small diameter afferent inputs to the CNS and secondly by descending controls from higher brain centers.

Recent studies have documented that the V brain stem complex and thalamic regions are not simply acting as relay stations: they are subject to modulation. Modification at thalamic and cortical neuronal levels occurs, but the modification of ascending somatosensory messages appears to be largely a reflection of changes occurring earlier in the V pathway, namely, in the brain stem. Therefore, most studies of the central mechanisms of orofacial pain control have concentrated on the V brain stem sensory nuclei. The intricate organization of each subdivision of the V brain stem complex and the variety of inputs and interconnections of each underlie numerous interactions between the various inputs derived from several orofacial sites and brain regions. These interactions may involve not only the process of excitatory synaptic transmission, which would favor facilitation and enhancement of the nociceptive signals, but also may involve inhibitory processes that act to suppress nociceptive transmission.

Modulation by Peripheral Afferent Stimulation or Damage

The activity and response properties of neurons in the V brain stem complex are not rigidly linked to the orofacial stimulus parameters evoking the neurons' activities, but can be modified by other incoming afferent inputs from the periphery or central brain regions. They can be influenced by alterations to the peripheral afferent inputs to the complex that may result from inflammation or trauma. These alterations may be reflected in either an enhanced sensory input, as in direct stimulation of peripheral nerves and in inflammation, or a decreased input, as may occur through nerve damage resulting in deafferentation.

Sensory Stimulation

Investigations on sensory stimulation primarily have centered on two approaches. The first involves the documentation of the efficacy of therapeutic procedures such as acupuncture and TENS in suppressing orofacial reflexes, brain-evoked potentials, or perceptual responses in humans and laboratory animals. These studies mainly have used electrical stimulation of the tooth pulp as the presumed noxious stimulus evoking the response. The second approach has examined the suppressive effects of either of these procedures or other sensory stimuli on central nociceptive neuronal responses. Acupuncture and TENS may inhibit, for example, the pulp-evoked JOR and also raise the threshold of pulp-evoked sensations (Dubner, 1978; Sessle, 1987). Acupuncture may also suppress brain stem neuronal activity, and the responses of single V brain stem neurons evoked by small-diameter afferent inputs excited by tooth pulp or noxious facial stimuli can be suppressed by non-noxious stimuli (e.g., vibratory or tactile) that excite large afferent nerve fibers (Sessle, 1981; 1987). These documented interactions between small-fiber and large-fiber afferent inputs provide evidence supportive of a basic tenet of the gate control theory of pain, namely sensory interaction.

Responses evoked by muscle or TMJ stimuli, as well as by skin or pulp stimuli, can also be suppressed, even by stimuli applied to sites as remote as the limbs (Cadden, 1985; Sessle, 1976; 1981). In addition, small-fiber afferent inputs may also inhibit neuronal responses to other small-fiber afferent inputs; that is, pain inhibits pain. For example, the excitatory responses of WDR neurons in subnucleus caudalis to noxious stimulation of their orofacial receptive field can be inhibited by noxious stimulation of other, widespread regions of the body (Dickenson, 1983).

This concept of so-called diffuse, noxious inhibitory controls involves a central pathway or loop and could conceivably underlie the analgesic efficacy of some forms of TENS and acupuncture. The extent to which the effectiveness of acupuncture and TENS can be explained by segmental mechanisms or by recruitment of descending influences from higher brain regions, however, is still not clear. Also unclear is the relative contribution made by presynaptic and postsynaptic inhibitory mechanisms to afferent-induced suppression (Sessle, 1987). The neurochemical basis for the suppressive effects also requires more study. Some, but not all, of these effects have been reported to be partly reversible by the opiate antagonist naloxone. This implies that endogenous opiate-related mechanisms may be, at least in part, involved in accordance with some views on acupuncture- or TENS-induced analgesia of spinal nociception (Melzack, 1984; Woolf, 1984). Other neurotransmitters have also been identified, however, as likely candidates involved in the afferent-induced effects in the V system. These include 5-HT, noradrenalin, and GABA (Basbaum, 1985; Chan, 1979; Lovick, 1983; Salt, 1983).

Inflammation

Trauma and inflammation are also associated with alterations in the activity of V brain stem neurons. As previously pointed out, peripheral phenomena related to the release and spread of neurochemical substances (such as histamine and kinins) have long been thought to underlie the spread of pain from the site of injury and the subsequent inflammation in adjacent tissues. This results in the activation and heightened sensitivity of the peripheral endings of nociceptive afferents in a now extensive region of peripheral tissue involved in the inflammatory process. Recent studies in which peripheral phenomena have been experimentally bypassed, however, have shown expansions in receptive fields and heightened excitability of central neurons in nociceptive pathways (Guilbaud, 1988; Wall, 1986) that can be explained by an opening up or central strengthening of the convergent afferent inputs to the neurons that were mentioned previously (Fig. 8–6). In the rat V system, for example, Hu (1988) noted that the injection of an inflammatory agent into the deep masseter muscle can enhance the responses of WDR and NS neurons of subnucleus caudalis to stimuli applied to their cutaneous mechanoreceptive field. This altered state outside their natural receptive field, as in

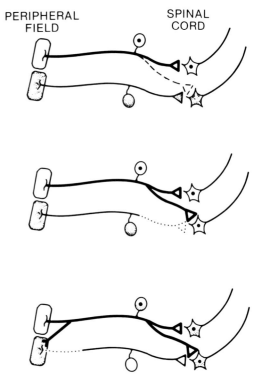

PERIPHERAL FIELD   SPINAL CORD

FIGURE 8–6. Examples of possible factors involved in plasticity of afferent inputs to the CNS. The top diagram shows the normal central connectivity of two primary afferent inputs, each innervating a defined peripheral field on the left. Note that one of these afferent inputs has some central connectivity (dashed line) that is normally ineffective and that each of the two CNS neurons on the right normally only responds to stimulation of the input from its own peripheral field. The middle diagram shows the possible consequence of an injury or interruption (dotted line) to the central processes of one of these primary afferent inputs. The formerly ineffective central connection of the other primary afferent input becomes effective, so that both CNS neurons now only respond to stimulation of the innervated (unstippled) peripheral field. The lowest diagram illustrates the possible effect of an injury or interruption (dotted line) of the peripheral processes of one of the primary afferent inputs. Changes may occur in the CNS neurons that are comparable to those outlined in the middle diagram, but in addition, the peripheral processes of the undamaged primary afferent may sprout into the injured or denervated peripheral field. As a result, both CNS neurons would respond to stimulation of both peripheral fields. (From Fields, H. L.: Pain. New York, McGraw-Hill, 1987.)

muscle, also may be associated with an expansion of the mechanoreceptive field of the neurons.

While these effects may occur in minutes, it is conceivable that long-standing trauma or inflammation may also induce changes in the neurochemicals such as substance P that are found within primary afferent nerve fibers. These changes may be reflected in alterations in the neurochemistry and neurophysiology of the central as well as peripheral terminals of the afferents. Of particular note are findings that either the systemic or local application of capsaicin, the active ingredient of hot pepper, preferentially destroys small-diameter fibers, especially the C fibers. This destruction is associated with depletion of substance P in the afferents and in their terminals in the CNS (Lynn, 1987; McMahon, 1986). Since this may lead to physiological changes in nociceptive pathways, a considerable amount of study is presently being devoted to the neurochemical and associated morphological and physiological changes that can occur in these pathways after experimental manipulation of afferent inputs into the CNS.

Deafferentation

Deafferentation refers to either the partial or total loss of a sensory nerve supply to a particular body region. The recently mentioned preferential destruction of small fibers by capsaicin is an example. Other examples of deafferentation are phantom limb, dental extraction, and transection of dental nerves during oral surgical procedures. The central convergent phenomena mentioned in the last section also seem to be involved in the deafferentation-induced changes that can occur in somatosensory pathways. The relevance of these alterations to this discussion is that they are thought to be involved in processes underlying the development of chronic pain. Several clinical conditions manifesting chronic pain have been linked to deafferentation, such as causalgia, sensory neuropathies, postherpetic neuralgia, phantom limb (and tooth) pain, and perhaps so-called atypical facial pain. Indeed, many are designated as deafferentation pain syndromes (Kerr, 1979; Sunderland, 1978; Tasker, 1984).

Deafferentation may be associated with morphological, neurochemical, and physiological changes in the spinal somatosensory system in adult animals, and these alterations are especially prominent in neonatal animals (Kaas, 1983; Wall, 1986). In the V system, selective cutaneous deafferentation of whiskers, for example, leads to morphological and physiological changes at all levels of the neonatal V somatosensory system (Kaas, 1983; Killackey, 1987). Degenerative-like morphological changes can be induced in afferent endings in the brain stem and in neurons of the adult cat's V spinal tract nucleus by a selective deafferentation of only part of the V afferent input to the brain, such as the tooth pulp (Gobel, 1984; Johnson, 1987),

and can be enhanced by neurochemical alterations in these pathways (Sugimoto, 1987). The endodontic procedure also produces changes in the functional properties of V brain stem LTM neurons (Hu, 1986a; 1989).

Pulp deafferentation in adult cats can lead to a statistically significant increase in the incidences of V brain stem neurons in subnucleus oralis, with an extensive receptive field, spontaneous activity, or responsiveness only to tap stimuli applied to widespread regions of the face and mouth (Fig. 8–7). There may also be a disruption in the fine detail of the representation of the face and mouth within the V brain stem complex. The effects of a single pulp deafferentation procedure, however, are reversible (Fig. 8–7) and they are less effective on LTM and nociceptive neurons in subnucleus caudalis (Hu, 1986a; 1989). A previous report (Black, 1974) that dental or more extensive V deafferentations produce hyperexcitability in the caudal components of the V complex was not confirmed in these recent studies using pulp deafferentation.

The natural deafferentation process related to the shedding of the primary dentition has

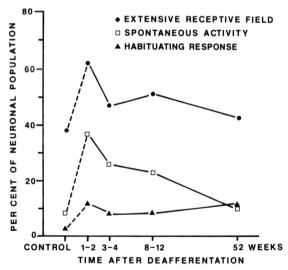

FIGURE 8–7. Effects of tooth pulp deafferentation on properties of brain stem neurons in the cat's V subnucleus oralis. Endodontic removal of coronal pulps of posterior ipsilateral teeth produced, at 1 to 2 weeks postoperatively, statistically significant increases in the incidence of oralis neurons showing an extensive mechanoreceptive field involving two or three V divisions, spontaneous activity (i.e. tonic firing unrelated to a defined peripheral stimulus), and habituating responsivity to orofacial tactile stimuli and sensitivity only to brisk tap stimuli. After this postoperative period, the incidences gradually returned to control levels obtained in normal (nondeafferented) cats. (From Sessle, B. J.: The neurobiology of facial and dental pain: Present knowledge, future directions. J. Dent. Res. 66:962–981, 1987.)

not been shown to be associated with comparable central changes in physiological properties of neurons in oralis and caudalis of kittens (Hu, 1987; 1989), although degenerative terminals have been described in the V brain stem complex at the mixed dentition stage (Johnson, 1987). It is possible that the maturing V brain stem system is inherently more resistant to changes than that in the adult and so the sequential shedding of the deciduous teeth and eruption of the permanent dentition produce no central functional alterations. Alternatively, the central endings of the deciduous pulp afferents may not undergo the extensive degenerative changes seen in the adult after pulp deafferentation. It is also possible that the permanent tooth is mainly supplied by collaterals of the same afferent fibers that supplied its predecessor or other orofacial tissues, and that as a result of this, the neural degeneration associated with the shedding of the deciduous tooth may be primarily limited to the peripheral portion of the deciduous dental afferents (Hu, 1987; Sessle, 1987).

The mechanisms underlying the central alterations induced by deafferentation are still not completely clear. The most likely explanations are either sprouting of collaterals of non-affected afferents in the periphery or in the brain, or the unmasking or disinhibition of the existing but ineffective synapses that were mentioned earlier (Fig. 8–6). Recent research in the spinal somatosensory system has especially invoked the long-range convergent afferents that are normally ineffective and that can be shown to exist only with electrical stimuli. They become strengthened or sensitive to natural stimuli after deafferentation. These types of convergent afferents were described earlier in relation to inflammation and to the referral and spread of pain. Data are consistent with the view that some of the existing convergent afferent connections demonstrated in V brain stem neurons may be involved in the changes that occur in these neurons as a consequence of deafferentation (Hu, 1986a). Because deafferentation interferes with the flow of neurochemicals as well as nerve impulses in the damaged axons, so-called neurotrophic factors also may be involved in these mechanisms. Mention has already been made of the neurochemical changes that can occur not only at the peripheral, but also at central endings of primary afferents after deafferentation.

The nucleus raphe magnus in the brain stem is normally a source in the CNS of powerful modulation of V somatosensory transmission. A change in its efficacy in inducing inhibition of V brain stem neurons might explain the apparent increase in neuronal excitability that occurs after pulp deafferentation and that is reflected in, for example, an extensive receptive field size and spontaneous activity. The central changes, however, do not appear to involve a change in central inhibition from the nucleus raphe magnus (Hu, 1986b) since raphe stimulation is just as effective a source of inhibition in pulp-deafferented cats as it is in normal animals.

Despite these uncertainties about the precise mechanisms underlying the effects of deafferentation, one very important feature that these various studies do highlight is the plasticity of the somatosensory systems. The adult V brain stem region, for example, is not hard wired, but rather it is remarkably plastic and sensitive to even relatively minor sensory alterations in the oral cavity. These deafferentation-induced changes are of considerable interest in terms of CNS development, neuroplasticity, and regenerative phenomena. They also are of potential significance in the etiology of certain pain states.

Sensory alterations induced by nerve trauma have been considered to be possible factors that may initiate events leading in some cases to chronic pain states such as painful sensory neuropathies, trigeminal neuralgia, atypical facial pain, and TMJ and MPD conditions. While extensive deafferentations (V sensory root section) may lead to pain behavior (Black, 1974), pulp-deafferented animals show no behavior indicative of pain, and the effects of a single deafferentation procedure are reversible (Hu, 1986a; 1989; Sessle, 1985). Moreover, the effects of this deafferentation appear to be more prominent in subnucleus oralis than in caudalis which, as previously pointed out, is usually considered the essential brain stem relay of V nociceptive information.

Nonetheless, although such considerations caution against jumping to a conclusion causally linking pain specifically with dental deafferentation, the accumulating data of the central consequences of deafferentation at the very least indicate that dentists should place greater emphasis on the dental history of patients with chronic pain in view of the possible association of oral trauma and deafferentation with changes in central somatosensory neurons. A more conservative approach in dental procedures that inflict damage to orofacial tissues might also be argued since central neural changes, perhaps of an irreversible nature, could possibly ensue.

Deafferentation per se may not be the only

factor precipitating these alterations in the CNS. As pointed out earlier, the activity of nociceptive afferents might also be altered by the application of either substances or procedures associated with heightened pain sensitivity, such as algesic chemicals, injury to peripheral tissues, and nerve transection leading to neuroma formation (Devor, 1984; Dubner, 1983; Olgart, 1985; Yaksh, 1982). In addition, modification of the activity of spinal nociceptive afferents (Roberts, 1986) and afferents supplying the tooth pulp (Edwall, 1971; Matthews, 1976; Olgart, 1985) can be produced by sympathetic efferent stimulation and might be related to a number of causalgic and other pain conditions in which the sympathetic nervous system appears to be integrally involved (Janig, 1985; Roberts, 1986). It is thus possible that other factors that ultimately lead to an alteration in the afferent input to the brain might result in CNS changes that subsequently result in the development of certain chronic pain states.

Finally, it should be reemphasized that although it is possible that the primary initiating factor in many of these chronic pain conditions may be mainly of a peripheral nature, central mechanisms are undoubtedly also involved. The preceding pages have reviewed some of the central neural consequences of peripheral damage or inflammation. Briefly consider one clinical example where central changes subsequent to peripheral alterations conceivably could be crucial to the development of pain. In trigeminal neuralgia, King (1967), Dubner (1978), Fromm (1989), and others have drawn attention to the signs and symptoms of the disorder that suggest the involvement of factors related to central summation, convergence, and inhibition. The WDR neurons, in particular, recently have been singled out (Dubner, 1987; Fromm, 1989; Sessle, 1987) because these three properties are a feature of these particular neurons that are crucially important in the encoding of noxious stimuli. They alone, of the three general classes of central mechanosensitive neurons (LTM, WDR, NS), receive, in addition to nociceptive afferent inputs, inputs from large-diameter afferents that are activated by tactile stimuli of the form that precipitate a trigeminal neuralgia attack. Future studies aimed at examining further the central consequences of peripheral nerve lesions or alterations, plus factors that influence the central processing of nociceptive information, particularly in the brain stem, should be very helpful in clarifying the mechanisms underlying the chronic orofacial pain states.

Modulation by Central Neural Pathways

Nociceptive transmission can be modulated by intrinsic brain mechanisms. These findings have borne out one of the major features of the gate control theory of pain, the concept of descending central controls (Melzack, 1965). Neurons involved in transmission of pain can be modulated not only by stimulation or alteration of afferent inputs into the CNS, but also by influences exerted by neural pathways intrinsic to the CNS. Many of these pathways emanate from higher brain centers involved in cognition and in motivational and emotional behaviors. The output of V nociceptive neurons in the brain stem can be considerably suppressed, for example, by stimulation of brain sites such as those in the midbrain periaqueductal gray matter (PAG), and the nucleus raphe magnus (NRM) in the lower brain stem (Fig. 8–8). This intrinsic brain system is involved in emotional and motivational functions and other complex behaviors. It might also be brought into operation by peripheral stimuli related to diffuse noxious inhibitory controls, TENS, and acupuncture.

Stimulation of this system produces analgesia and also suppression of reflex and other behavioral responses to noxious stimuli (Basbaum, 1984; Fields, 1987). It may be implied, but still needs to be proven, that the sustained increase in masticatory muscle activity reflexly induced by orofacial stimuli can be suppressed by such mechanisms. Also of note is the current therapeutic use of stimulation of this descending system in humans suffering from severe chronic pain such as that associated with terminal cancer.

Several studies have documented inhibitory influences exerted by the PAG and NRM on V nociceptive neurons in the brain stem. Such effects probably contribute to the suppression of the nociceptive reflex and behavioral responses since many of these neurons serve as interneurons in these responses (Dubner, 1983; Sessle, 1987). The analgesic effects may also involve suppression of nociceptive neurons at higher levels of the pain transmission process, for example in the thalamus or cortex.

One or more neurochemicals are involved in these suppressive effects. Enkephalin, noradrenalin-, and 5-HT-containing terminals have been described within subnucleus caudalis. Many of these neurochemicals originate from the raphe and other brain stem sites and thus have been implicated in the modulatory influences exerted by these loci on caudalis neurons

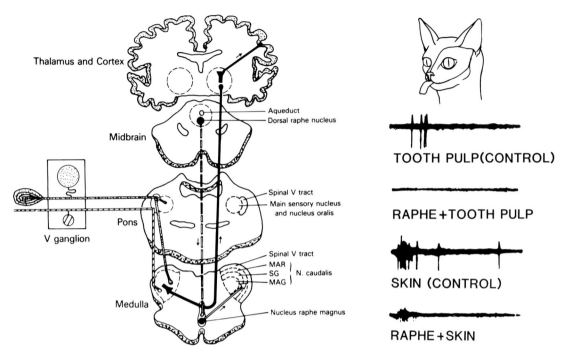

TOOTH PULP(CONTROL)

RAPHE+TOOTH PULP

SKIN (CONTROL)

RAPHE+SKIN

FIGURE 8–8. Effects of a descending modulatory pathway on the responses of a nociceptive neuron recorded in V subnucleus caudalis in the cat. Caudalis nociceptive neurons projecting to higher brain centers may receive both fast-conducting, large-fiber input (stippled path) and slower-conducting, small-fiber input (cross-hatched path), i.e. wide dynamic range neurons, or only the latter input, i.e. nociceptive-specific neurons. The responses to these inputs of both types of neurons can be suppressed by activation of the descending pathway involving the dorsal raphe nucleus in the PAG and the NRM in the medulla. Note on the right that the responses of a wide dynamic range neuron to tooth pulp or noxious facial skin stimuli can be extremely depressed by stimulation of the raphe system. Time duration of each record is 100 ms.

(Basbaum, 1985; Dubner, 1983). Nonetheless, some of these suppressive influences may also involve neurochemicals existing within cells of the neural circuitry that is intrinsic to the V spinal tract nucleus, such as the substantia gelatinosa (SG) of subnucleus caudalis. As mentioned earlier, SG is composed of local interneurons containing these substances and other neurochemicals, such as the inhibitory neurotransmitter GABA. The SG neurons are thought to exert powerful modulatory influences over the pain transmission neurons occurring in the other laminae of subnucleus caudalis (Basbaum, 1985; Dubner, 1983; Sessle, 1987).

These same local or segmental circuits and neurochemicals may be brought into operation by other descending influences as well as by therapeutic procedures used in the relief of pain. For example, because some of these endogenous chemicals are pharmacologically and structurally related to the opiates, it is not surprising that the action of narcotic analgesics, such as morphine and fentanyl, has been linked to such systems, and therapeutic procedures that involve skin, muscle, or nerve stimulation to produce analgesia (TENS and acupuncture)

also may operate in part by exciting pathways to the brain that ultimately lead to activation of the endogenous analgesic systems. An improved understanding of the neurochemistry and circuitry of the V complex and the spinal cord dorsal horn holds promise of the development of even better analgesic drugs and therapies to relieve pain.

Stimulation of other regions, such as the cerebral cortex, is less effective in suppressing the V nociceptive neurons, although cortical stimulation does have a profound influence on neurons excited by non-noxious stimuli (Darian-Smith, 1966; Sessle, 1981). Comparable findings have been reported for modulation of spinal transmission processes of pain and touch. Thus there appear to be preferential inhibitory actions of the raphe system on nociceptive transmission and of cerebral cortical stimulation on tactile transmission. Nonetheless, the effects of stimulation of even the raphe system are not specific for nociceptive transmission. The responses of many of the LTM neurons to tactile orofacial stimuli can also be suppressed by raphe stimulation (Hayashi, 1984; Sessle, 1981). Moreover, the raphe system has been shown to be just one of many descending pathways that can modulate nociceptive transmission. For example, others have been demonstrated in the brain stem reticular formation and parts of the thalamus. Some of these pathways may have a role in facilitating rather than in suppressing nociceptive transmission and so account for the enhancement of pain that may occur in conditions associated with, for instance, stress and anxiety.

These mechanisms may be involved in changes that occur in the nociceptive response properties of caudalis neurons in association with different behavioral contingencies an animal may be carrying out (Dubner, 1985). Such effects at the very first synaptic relay in V pain pathways may contribute to the well-recognized effects that motivation, anxiety, attention, or distraction may have on pain. They are also indicative of the involvement of multiple descending and segmental influences on V nociceptive transmission. Related studies in behaving monkeys also indicate that some caudalis nociceptive neurons can exhibit activity during a behavioral task (associated with discrimination of a noxious facial stimulus) that is unrelated to the parameters of the noxious stimulus and pain discrimination. These task-related neuronal activities may reflect the animal's evaluation of behaviorally important sensory signals that the animal must detect or discriminate so as to perform the task successfully (Dubner, 1985).

These various findings indicate that there are multiple descending influences that can affect orofacial nociceptive transmission by utilizing several neurochemical mechanisms. Knowledge of their suppressive effects on nociceptive transmission has expanded our understanding of pain mechanisms and has provided a more scientific rationale for developing better pain control procedures. A number of important therapeutic modalities may exert their analgesic effects by acting through these descending control systems. Finally, the existence of these descending systems exemplifies the multidimensional nature of pain and underscores the role that central neural influences as well as peripheral factors may play in influencing pain. Such knowledge is important in view of the increasing credence given in chronic orofacial pain conditions to so-called psychological factors related to stress, motivation, emotion, and depression.

SUMMARY

This chapter outlines recent advances in our knowledge of the central neural mechanisms underlying orofacial pain, including pain from the temporomandibular joint and masticatory muscles. The review first points out that pain is now conceptualized as a multifactorial experience that can be modified by cognitive, emotional, and motivational influences, and then focuses on recent research data that have identified peripheral neural processes and crucial neural elements in the brain concerned with the sensory-discriminative aspect of orofacial pain. Recent studies have also documented central neural pathways and mechanisms involved in the modulatory influences on orofacial pain transmission. In addition to providing explanations of how pain may be transmitted and controlled, these recent findings have also provided insights into how particular orofacial pain problems may occur, and possible mechanisms that may underlie problems such as spread and referral of pain. The neuroplasticity of the adult as well as neonatal trigeminal somatosensory system is also emphasized since its expression in conditions associated with inflammation and deafferentation, in particular, may be involved in several chronic orofacial pain states.

REFERENCES

Albe-Fessard, D., Berkley, K. J., Kruger, L., et al.: Diencephalic mechanisms of pain sensation. Brain Res. Rev. 9:217–296, 1985.

Amano, N., Hu, J. W., and Sessle, B. J.: Responses of neurons in feline trigeminal subnucleus caudalis (medullary dorsal horn) to cutaneous, intraoral, and muscle afferent stimuli. J. Neurophysiol. 55:227–243, 1986.

Azerad, J., Woda, A., and Albe-Fessard, D.: Physiological properties of neurons in different parts of the cat trigeminal sensory complex. Brain Res. 246:7–21, 1982.

Basbaum, A. I.: Functional analysis of the cytochemistry of the spinal dorsal horn. Advances in Pain Research and Therapy, vol. 9. New York, Raven, 1985, pp. 149–175.

Basbaum, A. I., and Fields, H. L.: Endogenous pain control systems: Brainstem spinal pathways and endorphin circuitry. Ann. Rev. Neurosci. 7:309–338, 1984.

Black, R. G.: A laboratory model for trigeminal neuralgia. Adv. Neurol. 4:651–659, 1974.

Broton, J. G., Hu, J. W., and Sessle, B. J.: Effects of temporomandibular joint stimulation on nociceptive and nonnociceptive neurons of the cat's trigeminal subnucleus caudalis (medullary dorsal horn). J. Neurophysiol. 59:1575–1589, 1988.

Broton, J. G., and Sessle, B. J.: Reflex excitation of masticatory muscles induced by algesic chemicals applied to the temporomandibular joint of the cat. Arch. Oral Biol. 33:741–747, 1988.

Byers, M. R.: Dental sensory receptors. Int. Rev. Neurobiol. 25:39–94, 1984.

Cadden, S. W.: The digastric reflex-evoked by tooth-pulp stimulation in the cat and its modulation by stimuli applied to the limbs. Brain Res. 336:33–43, 1985.

Cervero, F.: Visceral nociception: Peripheral and central

aspects of visceral nociceptive systems. Philos. Trans. R. Soc. Lond. [Biol.]. *308*:325–337, 1985.

Chan, S. H. H., and Yip, M. K.: Central neurotransmitter systems in the morphine suppression of jaw-opening reflex in rabbits: The cholinergic system. Exp. Neurol. *63*:201–210, 1979.

Chapman, C. R., Chen, A. C. N., and Harkins, S. W.: Brain evoked potentials as correlates of laboratory pain: A review and perspective. *In* Bonica, J. J., Liebeskind, J. C., and Albe-Tessard, D. G. (Eds.): Advances in Pain Research and Therapy, vol. 3. New York, Raven, 1979, pp. 791–803.

Darian-Smith, I.: Neural mechanisms of facial sensation. Int. Rev. Neurobiol. *9*:301–395, 1966.

Davis, K. D., and Dostrovsky, J. O.: Responses of feline trigeminal spinal tract nucleus neurons to stimulation of the middle meningeal artery and sagittal sinus. J. Neurophysiol. *59*:648–666, 1988.

Devor, M.: The pathophysiology and anatomy of damaged nerve. *In* Wall, P. D., and Melzack, R. (Eds.): Textbook of Pain. London, Churchill Livingstone, 1984, pp. 49–64.

Dickenson, A. H., and Le Bars, D.: Diffuse noxious inhibitory controls (DNIC) involve trigeminothalamic and spinothalamic neurones in the rat. Exp. Brain Res. *49*:174–180, 1983.

Dong, W. K., Kawakami, Y., and Chudler, E. H.: Non-invasive assessment of peripheral and central neural injury by cerebral evoked potentials. *In* Pubols, L. M., and Sessle, B. J. (Eds.): Effects of Injury on Trigeminal and Spinal Somatosensory Systems. New York, Liss, 1987, pp. 339–346.

Dubner, R.: Recent advances in our understanding of pain. *In* Klineberg, I., and Sessle, B. (Eds.): Oro-Facial Pain and Neuromuscular Dysfunction: Mechanisms and Clinical Correlates. Oxford, Pergamon, 1985, pp. 3–19.

Dubner, R., and Bennett, G. J.: Spinal and trigeminal mechanisms of nociception. Annu. Rev. Neurosci. *6*:381–418, 1983.

Dubner, R., Sessle, B. J., and Storey, A. T.: The Neural Basis of Oral and Facial Function. New York, Plenum, 1978.

Dubner, R., Sharav, Y., Gracely, R. H., and Price, P. D.: Idiopathic trigeminal neuralgia: Sensory features and pain mechanisms. Pain *31*:23–33, 1987.

Edwall, L., and Scott, D.: Influence of changes in micro-circulation on the excitability of the sensory unit in the tooth of the cat. Acta. Physiol. Scand. *82*:555–566, 1971.

Fields, H. L.: Pain. New York, McGraw-Hill, 1987.

Fromm, G. H., and Sessle, B. J.: Trigeminal Neuralgia: Current Concepts Regarding Pathogenesis & Treatment. Stoneham, MA, Butterworths, 1990.

Gobel, S.: An electron microscopic analysis of the trans-synaptic effects of peripheral nerve injury subsequent to tooth pulp extirpations on neurons in laminae I and II of the medullary dorsal horn. J. Neurosci. *4*:2281–2290, 1984.

Gobel, S., Bennett, G. J., Allen, B., et al.: Synaptic connectivity of substantia gelatinosa neurons with reference to potential termination sites of descending axons. *In* Sjolund, B., and Bjorkland, A. (Eds.): Brain Stem Control of Spinal Mechanisms. New York, Elsevier/North Holland, 1982.

Gobel, S., Hockfield, S., and Ruda, M. A.: Anatomical similarities between medullary and spinal dorsal horns. *In* Kawamura, Y., and Dubner, R. (Eds.): Oral-Facial Sensory and Motor Functions. Tokyo, Quintessence, 1981, pp. 211–223.

Greenwood, L. F., and Sessle, B. J.: Inputs to trigeminal brain stem neurones from facial, oral, tooth pulp and pharyngolaryngeal tissues: II. Role of trigeminal nucleus caudalis in modulating responses to innocuous and noxious stimuli. Brain Res. *117*:227–238, 1976.

Guilbaud, G.: Peripheral and central electrophysiological mechanisms of joint and muscle pain. *In* Dubner, R., Gebhart, G. F., and Bond, M. R. (Eds.): Proceedings of the Vth World Congress on Pain. Amsterdam, Elsevier, 1988, pp. 201–215.

Hayashi, H., Sumino, R., and Sessle, B. J.: Functional organization of trigeminal subnucleus interpolaris: Nociceptive and innocuous afferent inputs, projections to thalamus, cerebellum, and spinal cord, and descending modulation from periaqueductal gray. J. Neurophysiol. *51*:890–905, 1984.

Hoffman, D. S., Dubner, R., Hayes, R. L., and Medline, T. P.: Neuronal activity in medullary dorsal horn of awake monkeys trained in a thermal discrimination task. 1. Responses to innocuous and noxious thermal stimuli. J. Neurophysiol. *46*:409–427, 1981.

Hu, J. W., Broton, J. G., Lenz, Y., et al.: Brainstem effects of naturally occurring dental deafferentation in kittens. *In* Pubols, L. M., and Sessle, B. J. (Eds.): Effects of Injury on Trigeminal and Spinal Somatosensory Systems. New York, 1987, Liss, pp. 189–196,

Hu, J. W., Chen, X., and Sessle, B. J.: Effects of diffuse noxious stimuli and inflammatory agents on trigeminal medullary dorsal horn nociceptive neurones in the rat. Neuroscience Abstracts *14*:563, 1988.

Hu, J. W., Dostrovsky, J., Lenz, Y., et al.: Tooth pulp deafferentation is associated with functional alterations in the properties of neurons in the trigeminal spinal tract nucleus. J. Neurophysiol. *56*:1650 1668, 1986a.

Hu, J. W., Dostrovsky, J. O., and Sessle, B. J.: Functional properties of neurons in subnucleus caudalis of the cat. I. Responses to oral-facial noxious and non-noxius stimuli and projections to thalamus and subnucleus oralis. J. Neurophysiol. *45*:173–192, 1981.

Hu, J. W., and Sessle, B. J.: Comparison of response of cutaneous nociceptive and nonnociceptive brain stem neurons in trigeminal subnucleus caudalis (medullary dorsal horn) and subnucleus oralis to natural and electrical stimulation of tooth pulp. J. Neurophysiol. *52*:39–53, 1984.

Hu, J. W., and Sessle, B. J.: Properties of functionally identified nociceptive and nonnociceptive facial primary afferents and presynaptic excitability changes induced in their brainstem endings by raphe and orofacial stimuli in cats. Exp. Neurol. *101*:385–399, 1988.

Hu, J. W., and Sessle, B. J.: Effects of tooth pulp deafferentation on nociceptive and non-nociceptive neurons of the feline trigeminal subnucleus caudalis (medullary dorsal horn). J. Neurophysiol. *61*:1197–1206, 1989.

Hu, J. W., Sessle, B. J., Dostrovsky, J. O., and Lenz, Y.: Effects of nucleus raphe magnus stimulation on jaw-opening reflex and trigeminal brainstem neurone responses in normal and tooth pulp-deafferented cats. Pain *27*:349–360, 1986b.

Ishidori, H., Nishimori, T., Shigenaga, Y., et al.: Representation of upper and lower primary teeth in the trigeminal sensory nuclear complex in young dog. Brain Res. *370*:153–158, 1986.

Janig, W.: Causalgia and reflex sympathetic dystrophy: In which way is the sympathetic nervous system involved? Trends in Neuroscience *8*:471–477, 1985.

Jacquin, M. F., Renehan, W. E., Mooney, R. D., and Rhoades, R. W.: Structure-function relationships in rat medullary and cervical dorsal horn. I. Trigeminal primary afferents. J. Neurophysiol. *55*:1153–1186, 1986.

Johnson, L. R., Westrum, L. E., Henry, M. A., and

Canfield, R. C.: Transganglionic degeneration following dental lesions. *In* Pubols, L. M., and Sessle, B. J. (Eds.): Effects of Injury on Trigeminal and Spinal Somatosensory Systems. New York, Liss, 1987, pp. 151–158.

Kaas, J. H., Merzenich, M. M., and Killackey, H. P.: The reorganization of somatosensory cortex following peripheral nerve damage in adult and developing mammals. Annu. Rev. Neurosci. 6:325–356, 1983.

Kerr, F. W. L.: Craniofacial neuralgias. Advances in Pain Research and Therapy, vol. 3. New York, Raven, 1979, pp. 283–295.

Killackey, H. P.: Three phases in the vulnerability of the somatosensory system to peripheral nerve damage. *In* Pubols, L. M., and Sessle, B. J. (Eds.): Effects of Injury on Trigeminal and Spinal Somatosensory Systems. New York, Liss, 1987, pp. 363–370.

King, R. B.: Evidence for a central etiology of tic douloureux. J. Neurosurg. 26 (Suppl.): 175–180, 1967.

Lovick, T. A., and Wolstencroft, J. H.: Actions of GABA, glycine, methionine-enkephalin and B-endorphin compared with electrical stimulation of nucleus raphe magnus on responses evoked by tooth pulp stimulation in the medial reticular formation in the cat. Pain 15:131–144, 1983.

Lund, J. P., McLachlan, R. S., and Dellow, P. G.: A lateral jaw movement reflex. Exp. Neurol. 31:189–199, 1971.

Lynn, B.: The detection of injury and tissue damage. *In* Wall, P. D., and Melzack, R. (Eds): Textbook of Pain. London, Churchill Livingstone, 1984, pp. 19–33.

Lynn, B., Pini, A., and Baranowski, R.: Injury of somatosensory afferents by capsaicin: Selectivity and failure to regenerate. *In* Pubols, L. M., and Sessle, B. J. (Eds.): Effects of Injury on Trigeminal and Spinal Somatosensory Systems. New York, Liss, 1987, pp. 115–124.

Mason, P., Strassman, A., and Maciewicz, R.: Is the jaw-opening reflex a valid model of pain? Brain Res. Rev. 10:137–146, 1985.

Matthews, B.: Effects of sympathetic stimulation on the response of intradental nerves to chemical stimulation of dentin. Advances in Pain Research and Therapy. New York, Raven, 1976, pp. 195–203.

McMahon, S. B., and Fitzgerald, M.: Plasticity without degeneration: Changes in sensory processing after capsaicin treatment. *In* Goldberger, M. E., Gorio, A., and Murray, M. (Eds.): Development and Plasticity of the Mammalian Spinal Cord. Padova, Liviana Press, 1986, pp. 121–130.

Mei, N., Hartmann, F., and Aubert, M.: Periodontal mechanoreceptors involved in pain. *In* Anderson, D. J., and Matthews, B. (Eds.): Pain in the Trigeminal Region. Amsterdam, Elsevier/North Holland, 1977, pp. 103–110.

Melzack, R.: Acupuncture and related forms of folk medicine. *In* Wall, P. D., and Melzack, R. (Eds.): Textbook of Pain. London, Churchill Livingstone, 1984, pp. 691–700.

Melzack, R., and Wall, P. D.: Pain mechanisms: A new theory. Science 150:971–978, 1965.

Mense, S.: Slowly conducting afferent fibers from deep tissues: Neurobiological properties and central nervous actions. *In* Ottoson, D. (Ed.): Progress in Sensory Physiology 6. Berlin, Springer-Verlag, 1986, pp. 140–219.

Narhi, M. V. O.: The characteristics of intradental sensory units and their responses to stimulation. J. Dent. Res. 64:564–571, 1985.

Nishimori, T., Sera, M., Suemune, S., et al.: The distribution of muscle primary afferents from the masseter nerve to the trigeminal sensory nuclei. Brain Res. 372:375–381, 1986.

Nord, S. G.: Responses of neurons in rostral and caudal trigeminal nuclei to tooth pulp stimulation. Brain Res. Bull. 1:489–492, 1976.

Nord, S. G., and Ross, G. S.: Behavioral and neurophysiological correlates of dental pulp stimulation in the monkey. *In* Anderson, D. J., and Matthews, B. (Eds.): Pain in the Trigeminal Region. Amsterdam, Elsevier/North Holland, 1977, pp. 259–270.

Olgart, L. M.: The role of local factors in dentin and pulp in intradental pain mechanisms. J. Dent. Res. 64:572–578, 1985.

Pickoff-Matuk, J. F., Rosenfeld, J. P., and Broton, J. G.: Lesions of the mid-spinal trigeminal complex are effective in producing perioral thermal hypoalgesia. Brain Res. 382:291–298, 1986.

Roberts, W. J.: A hypothesis on the physiological basis for causalgia and related pain. Pain 24:297–312, 1986.

Salt, T. E., and Hill, R. G.: Neurotransmitter candidates of somatosensory primary afferent fibres. Neuroscience 10:1083–1103, 1983.

Schaible, H.-G., Schmidt, R. F., and Willis, W. D.: Spinal mechanisms in arthritic pain: Enhancement of response of tract neurons in the course of inflammation. *In* Schmidt, R. F., Schaible, H.-G. and Vahle-Hinz, C. (Eds.): Fine Afferent Nerve Fibers and Pain. Weinheim, FRG, Verlagsgesellschaft, 1987, pp. 399–410.

Sessle, B. J.: Dental deafferentation can lead to the development of chronic pain. *In* Klineberg, I., and Sessle, B. (Eds.): Oro-Facial Pain and Neuromuscular Dysfunction: Mechanisms and Clinical Correlates. Oxford, Pergamon, 1985, pp. 115–129.

Sessle, B. J.: The neurobiology of facial and dental pain: Present knowledge, future directions. J. Dent. Res. 66:962–981, 1987.

Sessle, B. J., and Greenwood, L. F.: Inputs to trigeminal brain stem neurones from facial, oral, tooth pulp and pharyngolaryngeal tissues: I. Responses to innocuous and noxious stimuli. Brain Res. 117:211–226, 1976.

Sessle, B. J., and Gurza, S. C.: Jaw movement-related activity and reflexly induced changes in the lateral pterygoid muscle of the monkey *Macaca fascicularis*. Arch. Oral Biol. 27:167–173, 1982.

Sessle, B. J., Hu, J. W., Amano, N., and Zhong, G.: Convergence of cutaneous, tooth pulp, visceral, neck and muscle afferents onto nociceptive and non-nociceptive neurones in trigeminal subnucleus caudalis (medullary dorsal horn) and its implications for referred pain. Pain 27:219–235, 1986.

Sessle, B. J., Hu, J. W., Dubner, R., and Lucier, G. E.: Functional properties of neurons in trigeminal subnucleus caudalis of the cat. II. Modulation of responses to noxious and non-noxious stimuli by periaqueductal gray, nucleus raphe magnus, cerebral cortex and afferent influences, and effect of naloxone. J. Neurophysiol. 45:193–207, 1981.

Strassman, A., Mason, P., Moskowitz, M., and Maciewicz, R.: Response of medullary trigeminal neurons to electrical stimulation of the dura. Brain Res. 379:242–250, 1986.

Sugimoto, T.: Effects of chemical convulsants on chronic transsynaptic destruction of medullary dorsal horn neurones following inferior alveolar neurectomy in adult rats. *In* Pubols, L. M., and Sessle, B. J. (Eds.): Effects of Injury on Trigeminal and Spinal Somatosensory Systems. New York, Liss, 1987, pp. 167–174.

Sunderland, S.: Nerves and Nerve Injuries, 2nd ed. Edinburgh, Churchill Livingstone, 1978, 1046 pp.

Tasker, R. R.: Deafferentation. *In* Wall, P. D., and Melzack, R. (Eds.): Textbook of Pain. London, Churchill Livingstone, 1984, pp. 119–132.

Vyklicky, L., Keller, O., Jastreboff, P., et al.: Spinal trigeminal tractotomy and nociceptive reactions evoked by tooth pulp stimulation in the cat. J. Physiol. (Paris) 73:379–386, 1977.

Wall, P. D.: Changes in adult spinal cord induced by changes in the periphery. In Goldberger, M. E., Gorio, A., and Murray, M. (Eds.): Development and Plasticity of the Mammalian Spinal Cord. Padova, Liviana Press, 1986, pp. 101–110.

Wall, P. D., and Melzack, R.: Textbook of Pain. London, Churchill Livingstone, 1984.

Willis, W. D.: The Pain System. The Neural Basis of Nociceptive Transmission in the Mammalian Nervous System. Basel, Karger, 1985.

Woolf, C. J.: Transcutaneous and implanted nerve stimulation. In Wall, P. D., and Melzack, R. (Eds.): Textbook of Pain. London, Churchill Livingstone, 1984, pp. 679–690.

Yaksh, T. L., and Hammond, D. L.: Peripheral and central substrates involved in rostral transmission of nociceptive information. Pain 13:1–85, 1982.

Yokota, T. Koyama, N., and Nishikawa, Y.: Nociceptive neurons in the shell region of the ventrobasal complex of the thalamus. In Pubols, L. M., and Sessle, B. J. (Eds.): Effects of Injury on Trigeminal and Spinal Somatosensory Systems. New York, Liss, 1987, pp. 305–312.

Young, R. F., and King, R. B.: Excitability changes in trigeminal primary afferent fibers in response to noxious and nonnoxious stimuli. J. Neurophysiol. 35:87–95, 1972.

Young, R. F., and Perryman, K. M.: Pathways for orofacial pain sensation in the trigeminal brain-stem nuclear complex of the macaque monkey. J. Neurosurg. 61:563–568, 1984.

PATHOPHYSIOLOGY OF THE MASTICATORY MUSCLES*

ROBERT YEMM, B.D.S., B.Sc., Ph.D., F.D.S.R.C.S. (Ed)

INTRODUCTION

Dysfunction of the masticatory muscles, myofascial pain dysfunction (MPD) syndrome, is relatively common (Helkimo, 1974). The frequency with which those with symptoms seek assistance is, however, somewhat variable. The condition is characterized by pain and tenderness in the jaw muscles, usually unilaterally, and by altered movement, sometimes restricted and sometimes involving deviation of the midline of the chin on mouth opening. In this movement alteration, jaw muscles are behaving abnormally. Indeed, they are the primary site of the pathology (Schwartz, 1968).

In contrast to earlier views that temporomandibular joint (TMJ) pathology was the central feature, with its associated effects, such as condylar displacement and nerve compression (Costen, 1934) (see Chapters 1 and 18), it is now regarded as a less common cause of mandibular pain and dysfunction (Schwartz, 1968) and the original associations have been entirely discredited (Zimmermann, 1951). Although pain is commonly described by the patient as being widespread and including the joint region, this is a consequence of referral from neighboring sites (Kellgren, 1937). In addition, tenderness in the joint region may be a consequence of pathology in the lateral pterygoid muscle, because of the insertion of this muscle into the condyle and joint capsule.

The hypothesis of a muscle origin for the altered jaw behavior and pain necessitates further consideration of possible mechanisms.

ORIGIN OF MUSCLE PAIN

Two explanations have been suggested to account for the occurrence of masticatory muscle pain, tenderness, and limitation of jaw movement: a muscle, or a localized zone of a muscle, has become spastic or has become injured.

Muscle Spasm

Muscle spasm is defined as a state of continuous activity, with the consequence of a maintained contractile force. This is difficult to envisage. A condition of muscle fiber hyperexcitability would be needed to maintain the contraction, or a continued excitatory input would be required from the muscle's motor neurons. Neither situation appears to exist,

---

*See Chapters 5, 11, 18–21, 23, and 26.

since continuous activity has not been detectable using electromyographic (EMG) techniques (Franks, 1965; Lund, 1989; Møller, 1971). Supporting this finding is the observation that in patients with dysfunction involving limited opening, there is an abnormal level of muscle activity only when opening is attempted, and especially when the limit of movement is approached (Schwartz, 1968; Stohler, 1985; Yemm, unpublished data), but that at rest the level of activity is not obviously different from the situation in a normal subject, or in the patient's contralateral, usually symptom-free, muscles (Yemm, 1971).

Muscle Injury

An alternative to the spasm theory is that the jaw muscle has been injured or damaged. This is known to be possible under experimental circumstances in animals (Christensen, 1967), with development of an initial inflammatory state, followed by a healing process that eventually entails fibrous tissue formation at the injury site. This experimental response results from temporary exposure of the muscle to high levels of tension during stimulated contraction.

Masticatory dysfunction is associated with jaw muscle hyperactivity (Laskin, 1969; Sherman, 1985). This has been verified by sleep laboratory and home monitoring studies. The association also has been tested experimentally, by observing the effects of voluntary hyperactivity by human subjects (Christensen, 1971). Not only did this result in a prolonged period of facial pain, with many of the characteristics of that experienced by patients with dysfunction, but also there was an increase in muscle tissue fluid pressure, of much longer duration than could be attributed to the biochemical consequences of the hyperactivity itself. The inference is that an inflammatory reaction, similar to that observed in the animal experiments described above, follows the hyperactivity, with the tissue fluid pressure increase being a measure of the associated edema from increased vascular permeability. Indirect evidence in support of such a hypothesis is that, at least in the acute phase of dysfunction, it is possible to detect an increase in skin surface temperature corresponding in distribution to a tender area in the masseter muscle, which is not seen contralaterally over a clinically normal muscle (Berry, 1974b; Kopp, 1981).

Underlying Pathology: Tentative Conclusions

Although the evidence is incomplete, and essentially indirect, the best explanation available would appear to be that a high level of muscle activity results in localized damage, that an inflammatory reaction occurs, and that this produces pain and altered muscle behavior. The damage itself has been shown in animal experiments (Christensen, 1967) to be associated with the connective tissue components of the muscle. This may account for the relationship between muscle pain and certain types of clicking in the TMJ on opening and closing the mouth; the connective tissue components of the lateral pterygoid muscle are closely associated with the joint capsule, and thus with disc function. For instance, damage to the anterior fibers of the joint capsule into which the lateral pterygoid muscle is inserted, could diminish forces coordinating the forward movement of disc and condyle during mouth opening. This would perhaps account for the rapid uncoordinated movements of the disc in relation to the other joint components, which are thought to be the origin of the transient or inconsistent clicking in MPD patients.

An alternative to the muscle damage hypothesis is that periods of maintained activity result in muscle fatigue, and with it pain, resulting from ischemia (or reduced blood flow) during contraction and accumulation of muscle metabolites. While discomfort from muscle fatigue is undoubtedly possible, the duration of the symptoms is too great to be accounted for in this way, as is clearly indicated by subjects' experiences following voluntary hyperactivity (Christensen, 1971).

In essence, the hypothesis of muscle damage, pain, and altered function can be regarded as being analogous to the situation arising when limb and other body muscles become painful following unaccustomed physical exertion, with the dysfunction far outlasting the period of exercise. This analogy suggests the possibility that it is unaccustomed muscle activity that is relevant, and requires consideration of the possibility that this is a common factor in the etiology of masticatory dysfunction.

JAW MUSCLE HYPERACTIVITY

Hyperactivity of jaw muscles could arise in two ways—in association with a functional activity, such that more muscle involvement than normal occurs, and in association with abnormal jaw activity.

Variation in Muscle Activity During Normal Oral Function

The primary jaw muscle functions during chewing, swallowing, and speech are brought about by patterns of muscle activity that are characteristic of the individual, despite general similarities between human subjects (Ahlgren, 1966; Møller, 1966). An important factor in determining the actual muscle utilization is the form of the dental occlusion. Sudden iatrogenic or experimental alterations of the occlusion result in major changes in both the level and distribution of activity within the jaw muscle complex (Shiau, 1989). However, the reverse also appears to be true; in the absence of such alterations, each individual develops a stable behavior pattern, albeit characteristic of that individual (Ahlgren, 1966). In terms of a theoretical normal or average for the human subject, any individual is likely to exhibit higher than normal functional activity in some parts of the masticatory system and lower than normal in others. For that individual, however, such a pattern can be regarded as normal, and it is against this habitual and accustomed level of muscle activity that changes have to be judged.

It has been suggested that there can be gradual adaptive changes in muscle activity patterns associated with progressive changes in dental occlusion (Ahlgren, 1966). For instance, such changes obviously must occur during development of the occlusion in early years, and subsequently with occlusal modification, by attrition for example. Similarly, it is likely that sudden changes in the distribution of muscle activity may become necessary when rapid and extensive intraoral change occurs. For instance when gross occlusal modification takes place as a consequence of tooth loss or restoration. The existence of a muscle activity norm for the individual, which depends upon gradual adaptation of inherent muscle capability to suit local circumstances (dental occlusion and diet in particular), but which is susceptible to disturbance by changes in dental occlusion characteristics, could account for the clinical observations regarding the relationship between occlusion and dysfunction. However, no firm relationship has been defined between existing dental malocclusion and the occurrence of dysfunction (Droukas, 1985; Thomson, 1971). Although many patients with dysfunction exhibit malocclusion, other subjects with equally severe defects func-

tion adequately without suffering signs and symptoms. In these instances of slowly evolving occlusal changes, it must be that an adaptive pattern of muscle activity has arisen; one that is normal, stable, and tolerable for that individual.

It is often possible to determine a relationship between an occlusal change and the onset of dysfunction, even if the change was in theory an iatrogenic attempt at improvement of the occlusion (Moulton, 1968). In such cases, the individual's normal, stable, and tolerable muscle activity has been disrupted, necessitating adoption of a new pattern, which, even if the overall activity level is reduced, requires increases in activity of a localized nature. An example would be the greater mandibular protrusion in function following loss of posterior teeth, requiring increased lateral pterygoid muscle activity.

Increased Muscle Activity Associated with Abnormal Mandibular Function

There are two circumstances in which high levels of parafunctional muscle activity have been shown to occur. One is in nocturnal tooth grinding (bruxism) and the other is in daytime tooth clenching.

Bruxism

Forceful tooth clenching and grinding during sleep is not uncommon. The forces produced are very high, as is apparent from the volume of the sound produced, which is difficult to simulate voluntarily. In the past, such activity has been attributed to interferences in the dental occlusion leading to stimulation of intraoral receptors and resulting in reflex jaw-closing muscle activity (Ramfjord, 1961). This mechanism seems unlikely, however, since the principal effect of tooth stimulation is inhibition of the jaw-closing muscles, not excitation. Although there have been reports of an excitatory effect of stimulation of intraoral receptors, such as those of the periodontal ligament, these reports may be due to an experimental artifact (Matthews, 1988). The alternative explanation is that the excitation producing the bruxism is of central nervous system origin, and is associated with certain phases of sleep in which not only jaw but also body movements are concentrated (Pollmann, 1974; Reding, 1968). Furthermore, and of some significance, there is the observation that the tendency to nocturnal bruxism varies. For instance, a relationship has been demonstrated between the daytime stress experience of the individual and nocturnal activity (Rugh, 1979). In general, daytime stress or worry is followed by higher levels of nocturnal jaw muscle activity.

Daytime Tooth Clenching

Environmental stress leads to increases in skeletal muscle activity (Benson, 1961; Shipman, 1970) and this also occurs in the jaw-closing muscles (Perry, 1960; Yemm, 1968; 1969a). It is difficult to make comparisons of the responses of different subjects, because the electromyographic methods used are subject to intersubject variation. It has been shown in several laboratories that patients with masticatory dysfunction respond to experimental stress with either more prolonged or greater increases in tension than do control subjects (Johnson, 1972; Rugh, 1987; Thomas, 1973; Yemm, 1969b). In addition, one study (Yemm, 1969b) showed that at least some of these patients exhibited an abnormally protracted response even after resolution of the clinical condition. This indicated that the abnormal response is not simply a result of the clinical condition.

The mechanism resulting in these increases in activity of jaw muscles is unclear. In animals stimulation of an area of the brain associated with responses to stress causes an increase in excitability of the motor neurons of jaw-closing muscles (Landgren, 1977).

Conclusions on the Role of Nonfunctional Muscle Activity

Some individuals are more susceptible to environmental stress, and respond by increased jaw muscle tension, either at night in the form of bruxism, or with daytime tooth clenching. There is no evidence to indicate whether those prone to bruxism are also susceptible to daytime clenching, but an experimental relationship has been demonstrated between the existence of dysfunction and the extent of the daytime response as described in the preceding section. In addition, some clinicians consider there is a link between bruxism and painful dysfunction in some MPD patients (Laskin, 1969; Ramfjord, 1961).

The susceptibility of the jaw-closing muscles to changes in activity as a response to stress also throws doubt upon the role of these muscles in producing so called anti-gravity activity (muscle tone), with a stabilizing role upon man-

dibular posture. The results of the experiments showing stress-related activity in these muscles are more consistent with the proposal that the ongoing activity often reported to be associated with the mandibular resting position is more likely to be a consequence of low levels of stress (for instance in experimental circumstances). The principal factor in determining rest position seems to depend on the development of an equilibrium between external forces such as gravity and internal forces developed by elasticity of muscles and other tissues (Yemm, 1969c; 1975; 1977a). The ease with which stress-induced increases in activity arise would not be predicted if an anti-gravity mechanism had to be overridden.

SUSCEPTIBILITY TO MUSCLE DAMAGE

Experimental evidence has already been identified that supports the contention that there is a relationship between muscle hyperactivity and signs and symptoms similar to those of masticatory dysfunction, together with indications that damage accompanies such voluntary hyperactivity (Christensen, 1971). These findings, and the clinical observations that they support, invite the question as to whether the jaw muscles are particularly susceptible to damage.

Histologically, the jaw-closing muscles have been shown to consist of a variety of muscle fiber types. This structural evidence has been interpreted as indicating a mixture of fiber properties, with varying degrees of fatigue sensitivity dependent upon speed of contraction (slow or fast twitch). Physiological examination shows them to be within the fast twitch category (Goldberg, 1977; Yemm, 1977b) and comparable to those of a small hand muscle (Milner-Brown, 1973). The variability of the histological picture instead may be an indication of the condition of the fibers. The degree of activity of a skeletal muscle influences its structure, including the contractile protein content and bulk (as in athletic training and fitness) (Maughan, 1983). In modern man, in a western society, masticatory muscles are used at a level grossly below the physiological capacity (Berry, 1974a), and are therefore likely to be unfit. Unfit or untrained muscle is relatively weak and is also more easily fatigued. However, it is unlikely that dysfunction arises as a result of a continuing state of fatigue, for a number of reasons. First, electromyographic recordings show the jaw muscles of patients with dysfunction to be no more active than those of normal subjects when the mandible is at rest (Lund, 1989). Second, it is not reasonable to consider that build up of metabolic products, or the presence of neuromuscular junction exhaustion, could exist for a protracted period, as do the symptoms of dysfunction, unless the musculature is continuously and permanently active, which it is not. Finally, voluntary hyperactivity experiments (Christensen, 1971) show pain symptoms to last for a matter of days in subjects who would not be expected to be indulging in continued hyperactivity, and in whom it would be expected that metabolic recovery would be rapid.

In summary, jaw muscles may be weak and unable to sustain a sudden increase in activity without physical damage to their structural components, with a more prolonged effect than fatigue. Furthermore, the hyperactivity may be localized within individual muscles, with the consequence that damage is confined to parts of the muscle rather than occurring in the whole organ. This, in fact, is what is most commonly seen in MPD patients.

CRITERIA FOR SUCCESSFUL TREATMENT: CLINICAL CONSIDERATIONS

The foregoing hypotheses regarding the role for muscle hyperactivity of various origins in initiating a process of muscle damage would indicate that a crucial component of treatment

should be to bring about a period of rest. Unless this is achieved, continuing activity would be likely to maintain or worsen the damage. The dysfunctional state may, to some extent, achieve this, at least as far as functional activity is concerned. For instance, the limitation of movement and the discomfort undoubtedly inhibit chewing. Many patients are worried by the condition, however, and this may constitute an additional stressful stimulus. In any case, daytime or nighttime hyperactivity causing or contributing to the onset of the condition may be maintained by the original source of stress.

It would be reasonable to expect that an improvement in the condition would need a withdrawal or at least a reduction in the stimulus, especially in respect to environmental stress-induced dysfunction. A further possibility is that, once a section of muscle is damaged, activity needs to be reduced to a sub-normal level for recovery by healing to be as rapid as possible.

Many forms of treatment have been reported to be successful. The success of some can clearly be explained on the basis of achievement of rest. These include biofeedback, relaxation training, treatment with tranquilizers or muscle relaxants, and counseling and reassurance, which diminish the effects of stress. The manner in which other forms of treatment such as bite appliance therapy and occlusal adjustment produce overall reduction in activity is less obvious, but it can be argued that this is exactly what they do. For example, any such modification of occlusion, whether temporary or permanent, results in altered patterns of mandibular move-

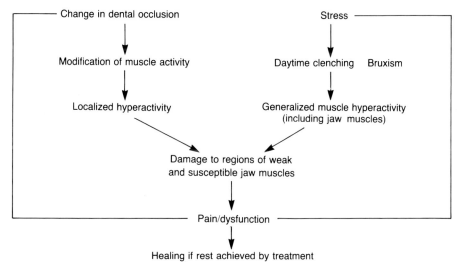

FIGURE 9–1. Diagrammatic representation of the overall hypothesis developed. Each arrow represents a supposed link; for some of these the clinical or experimental evidence for the connection is strong, in others it is more tentative.

ment by redistributing muscle activity levels. Furthermore, major disturbances of existing occlusion probably initially reduce functional activity because of the unfamiliarity of the occlusion. In support of this hypothesis, there is evidence that bite appliance therapy produces a reduced level of muscle activity (Clark, 1979) (see Chapter 21).

SUMMARY

An attempt has been made in this chapter to develop a working hypothesis that temporomandibular dysfunction is a condition in which there is reversible soft tissue damage, centered on muscle. Although it has been possible to cite experimental evidence to support the hypothesis, some at least has been circumstantial. As in many clinical and scientific fields, however, formulation of a hypothesis can be useful in identifying new experimental approaches as basis for further study. Figure 9–1 illustrates the component parts of the hypothesis presented.

To summarize the critical components of the current hypothesis, it is possible to pose the following questions: (1) Does muscle hyperactivity generate signs and symptoms identical with dysfunction? (2) Does hyperactivity actually precede the condition, and which of the three possible origins (functional, daytime clenching, bruxism) is relevant, and when? (3) What is the pathology? (4) Are current treatment methods appropriate and effective, and are there further possibilities to explore?

The first three of these questions are each answered to some degree in the preceding pages; however, for all, there is reasonable doubt remaining.

REFERENCES

Ahlgren, J.: Mechanism of mastication. A quantitative cinematographic and electromyographic study of masticatory movements in children, with special reference to occlusion of the teeth. Acta Odontol. Scand. 24(suppl.):44, 1966.
Benson, A. J., and Gedye, J. L.: Some supraspinal factors influencing generalized muscle activity. In Riker Symposium (no editor cited): Skeletal Muscle Spasm. Leicester, Ward and Wheeler, 1961, pp. 31–50.
Berry, D. C., and Poole, D. F.: Masticatory function and oral rehabilitation. J. Oral Rehabil., 1:191–205, 1974a.
Berry, D. C., and Yemm, R.: A further study of facial skin temperature in patients with mandibular dysfunction. J. Oral Rehabil. 1:255–264, 1974b.
Christensen, L. V.: Facial pain and internal pressure of masseter muscle in experimental bruxism in man. Arch. Oral Biol. 16:1021–1031, 1971.
Christensen, L. V., and Moesmann, G.: On the etiology, pathophysiology and physiology of muscular fibrositis due to hyperfunction: A discussion based on recent investigations. Tandlaegebladet 71:230–237, 1967.
Clark, G. T., Boemsterboer, P. L., Solberg, W. K., and Rugh, J. D.: Nocturnal electromyographic evaluation of myofascial pain dysfunction in patients undergoing occlusal splint therapy. J. Am. Dent. Assoc. 99:607–611, 1979.
Costen, J. B.: Syndrome of ear and sinus symptoms dependent upon disturbed function of the temporomandibular joint. Ann. Otol. Rhinol. Laryngol. 43:1–15, 1934.
Droukas, B., Lindee, C., and Carlsson, G. E.: Occlusion and mandibular dysfunction: A clinical study of patients referred for functional disturbances of the masticatory system. J. Prosthet. Dent. 53:402–406, 1985.
Franks, A. S.: Masticatory muscle hyperactivity and temporomandibular joint dysfunction. J. Prosthet. Dent. 15:1122–1131, 1965.
Goldberg, L. J., and Derfler, B.: Relationship among recruitment order, spike amplitude, and twitch tension of single motor units in human masseter muscle. J. Neurophysiol. 40:879–890, 1977.
Helkimo, M. L.: Studies on function and dysfunction of the masticatory system. II. Index for anamnestic and clinical dysfunction and occlusal state. Swed. Dent. J. 67:101–121, 1974.
Johnson, D. L., Shipman, W. G., and Laskin, D. M.: Physiologic responses to stressful stimuli in patients with myofascial pain dysfunction syndrome. International Association for Dental Research, 50th General Session, Abstract 191, 1972, p. 96.
Kellgren, J. H.: Observations on referred pain arising from muscle. Clin. Sci. 3:175–190, 1937.
Kopp, S., and Haraldson, T.: Skin surface temperature over the temporomandibular joint and masseter muscle in patients with mandibular dysfunction. Gothenburg, Sweden, Gothenburg University, Department of Stomatognathic Physiology. Report no. 37, 1981.
Landgren, S., and Olsson, K.A.: The effect of electrical stimulation in the defense attack area of the hypothalamus on the monosynaptic jaw closing and disynaptic jaw opening reflexes in the cat. In Anderson, D. J., and Matthews, B. (Eds.): Pain in the Trigeminal Region. Amsterdam, North Holland Biomedical Press, Elsevier, 1977, pp. 385–394.
Laskin, D. M.: Etiology of the pain-dysfunction syndrome. J. Am. Dent. Assoc. 79:141–153, 1969.
Lund, J. P., Widmer, C. G., and Schwartz, G.: What is the link between myofascial pain and dysfunction? In van Steenburghe, D., and De Laat, A. (Eds.): Electromyography of Jaw Reflexes in Man. Leuven, Leuven University Press, 1989.
Matthews, B., Yemm, R., and Cadden, S. W.: An artifact of signal averaging. J. Dent. Res. 67:206, 1988.
Maughan, R. J., Watson, J. S., and Weir, J.: Relationship between muscle strength and muscle cross-sectional area in male sprinters and endurance runners. Eur. J. Applied Physiol. 50:309–318, 1983.
Milner-Brown, H. S., Stein, R. B., and Yemm, R.: The orderly recruitment of human motor units during voluntary isometric contractions. J. Physiol. 230:359–370, 1973.
Møller, E.: The chewing apparatus. Acta Physiol. Scand. 69(suppl.):280, 1966.
Møller, E., Sheik-Ol-Eslam, A., and Lous, I.: Deliberate relaxation of the temporal and masseter muscles in subjects with functional disorders of the chewing apparatus. Scand. J. Dent. Res. 79:478–482, 1971.
Moulton, R. E.: Emotional factors in non-organic temporomandibular joint pain. In Schwartz, L., and Chayes,

C. M. (Eds.): Facial Pain and Mandibular Dysfunction. Philadelphia, W. B. Saunders, 1968, pp. 318–334.

Perry, H. T., Lammie, G. A., Main, J., and Teuscher, G. W.: Occlusion in a stress situation. J. Am. Dent. Assoc. 60:626–633, 1960.

Pollmann, L., Hildebrandt, G., and Janke, H. S.: Activity of masticatory muscles and sleep studies. ZWR, 84:692–694, 1975.

Ramfjord, S. P.: Bruxism, a clinical and electromyographic study. J. Am. Dent. Assoc. 62:21–44, 1961.

Reding, G. R., Zepelin, H., Robinson, J. E., et al.: Nocturnal teeth grinding: All night physiologic studies. J. Dent. Res. 47:786–797, 1968.

Rugh, J. D., and Solberg, W. K.: Psychological implications in temporomandibular pain and dysfunction. In Zarb, G. A., and Carlsson, G. E. (Eds.): Temporomandibular Joint: Function and Dysfunction. Copenhagen, Munksgaard, 1979, pp. 239–268.

Rugh, J. D., and Montgomery, G. T.: Physiological reactions of patients with TM disorders vs symptom-free controls on a physical stress task. J. Craniomandib. Disord. 1:243–250, 1987.

Schwartz, L.: The pain-dysfunction syndrome. In Schwartz, L., and Chayes, C.M. (Eds.): Facial Pain and Mandibular Dysfunction. Philadelphia, W.B. Saunders, 1968, pp. 140–155.

Sherman, R. A.: Relationships between jaw pain and jaw muscle contraction level: Underlying factors and treatment effectiveness. J. Prosthet. Dent. 54114–118, 1985.

Shiau, Y.-Y., and Ash, M. M.: Immediate and delayed effects of working interferences on EMG and jaw movement. In van Steenburghe, D., and De Laat, A. (Eds.): Electromyography of Jaw Reflexes in Man. Leuven, Leuven University Press, 1989.

Shipman, W. C., Heath, H. A., and Oken, D.: Response specificity among muscular and autonomic variables. Arch. Gen. Psychiatry, 23:369–374, 1970.

Stohler, C., Yamada, Y., and Ash, M.M.: Antagonistic muscle stiffness and associated reflex behaviour in the pain-dysfunction state. Helv. Odont. Acta 29:13–20, 1985.

Thomas, L. J., Tiber, N., and Schireson, S.: The effects of anxiety and frustration on muscular tension related to the temporomandibular joint syndrome. Oral Surg. 36:763–768, 1973.

Thomson, H.: Mandibular dysfunction syndrome. Br. Dent. J. 130:187–193, 1971.

Yemm, R.: Irrelevant muscle activity. Dent. Pract. Dent. Rec. 19:51–54, 1968.

Yemm, R.: Variations in the electrical activity of the human masseter muscle occurring in association with emotional stress. Arch. Oral Biol. 14:873–878, 1969a.

Yemm, R.: Temporomandibular dysfunction and masseter response to experimental stress. Br. Dent. J. 127:508–510, 1969b.

Yemm, R.: Comparison of the activity of left and right masseter muscles of normal individuals and patients with mandibular dysfunction during experimental stress. J. Dent. Res. 50:1320–1323, 1971.

Yemm, R.: The mandibular rest position: The roles of tissue elasticity and muscle activity. J. Dent. Assoc. S. Afr. 30:203–208, 1975.

Yemm, R.: The question of "resting" tonic activity of motor units in the masseter and temporal muscles in man. Arch. Oral Biol. 22:349–351, 1977a.

Yemm, R.: The orderly recruitment of motor units of the masseter and temporal muscles during voluntary isometric contraction in man. J. Physiol. 265:163–174, 1977b.

Yemm, R., and Berry, D. C.: Passive control in mandibular rest position. J. Prosthet Dent. 22:30–36, 1969c.

Zimmermann, A.A.: An evaluation of Costen's Syndrome from an anatomic point of view. In Sarnat, B.G. (Ed.): The Temporomandibular Joint. Springfield, IL, Charles C Thomas, 1951, pp. 82–110.

10

PATHOLOGICAL ASPECTS OF DEVELOPMENTAL, INFLAMMATORY, AND NEOPLASTIC DISEASE*

*J. PHILIP SAPP, D.D.S., M.S.,
and HENRY M. CHERRICK, D.D.S., M.S.D.*

INTRODUCTION

Diseases affecting the temporomandibular joint (TMJ) are primarily inflammatory and degenerative, with developmental, metabolic, and neoplastic conditions being of relatively rare occurrence. In the early stages of either metabolic or neoplastic conditions, the correct diagnosis is often missed and appropriate treatment is delayed. A familiarity with the features of these less common pathological conditions greatly increases the probability that they will be appropriately suspected and diagnosed when patients present with signs and symptoms of TMJ origin (see Chapters 3 on Morphogenesis and 5 on Functional Anatomy for the normal

structures that become altered during the following disease processes).

DEVELOPMENTAL ABNORMALITIES

Developmental abnormalities are either congenital or acquired postnatally. Congenital deformities may be genetically determined or due to prenatal injury. Postnatally acquired abnormalities usually result from trauma or nutritional deficiencies, while still others occur during the process of parturition (see Chapters 3, 12, 13, and 24).

Condylar Agenesis and Hypoplasia

Condylar agenesis is frequently associated with various syndromes of the head and neck

---

*See Chapters 3–5, 11–13, 16, 24, and 26.

(Gorlin, 1990; Kazanjian, 1938; 1956). When it occurs unilaterally, there is pronounced facial asymmetry. The resultant underdevelopment of the mandible causes a distortion and depression of that side of the face in which the condyle is missing (see Fig. 24–4). The postnatal deformity has been demonstrated experimentally in monkeys (Sarnat, 1971). Other defects that may be associated with condylar agenesis are macrostomia, absence of the external ear, microtia, absence of the internal ear, and absence of segments of the temporal bone (Kazanjian, 1939; Rushton, 1944; 1946). The dental abnormalities associated with agenesis of the condyle consist primarily of alterations in dental occlusion, caused not only by the deficiency in length of the mandibular body, but also by lack of vertical development of the ramus with a resultant reduced development of the face and alveolar processes and incomplete eruption of the teeth (Diamond, 1944). Bilateral condylar agenesis has been reported on multiple occasions and the clinical findings consist essentially of symmetrical severe underdevelopment of the mandible (Gilmour, 1926; Kazanjian, 1956; Prowler, 1954).

Condylar hypoplasia occurs far more frequently than does condylar agenesis. The defect resulting from underdevelopment of the mandibular condyle may be either congenital or acquired, and unilateral or bilateral. The acquired form of hypoplasia results from any incident, whether infectious, metabolic, or traumatic, that interferes with the growth site of the developing condyle. The most frequent cause is trauma to the condylar region in infants or young children (see Fig. 24–24) (Burke, 1961; Steinhauser, 1973). Other common causes are radiation therapy, infection, and rheumatoid arthritis in children (see Fig. 24–7) or young adults. A number of endocrine and vitamin deficiencies in experimental animals also have been reported to cause disturbances in growth and development of the mandibular condyles (see Chapters 12 and 13) (Collins, 1946; 1949; Frandsen, 1953; Levy, 1950; Weinmann, 1946). The possibility that such factors could play a significant role in the development of TMJ hypoplasia in humans has not been fully evaluated but appears to be of some clinical importance.

Facial deformity results when hypoplasia affects the condyle. The older the patient is at the time of the disturbance in growth, the less severe the facial deformity. Functionally, there is usually limitation of lateral excursion, and the mandibular midline shifts to the involved side during opening of the mouth, accentuating the deformity. Hypoplasia of the condyle nearly always produces a malocclusion.

As with condylar agenesis, condylar hypoplasia can also be associated with syndromes of the head and neck (see Chapter 12). Syndromes with condylar hypoplasia (and sometimes agenesis) include the following: mandibulofacial dysostosis (Gorlin, 1990); hemifacial microsomia (Kazanjian, 1956); oculoauriculovertebral syndrome (Goldenhar's syndrome) (Boudet, 1958; Mahneke, 1956); oculomandibulodyscephaly (Hallermann-Streiff syndrome) (Van Balan, 1961); Hurler's syndrome (Worth, 1966); and Morquio's disease, Hunter's syndrome, and ophthalmomandibulomelic dysplasia (Pillay, 1964).

Double Mandibular Condyle

The double mandibular condyle is an extremely rare condition first reported by Hrdlicka (1941). From an anthropological standpoint, on skeletal remains collected from various parts of the world, Hrdlicka described 12 examples. Subsequently, Schier (1948) and Stadnicki (1971) reported similar cases. The etiology of the double condyle may be either embryologic or traumatic (Thomason, 1986). One suggestion (Blackwood, 1957) is that it can be caused by the formation of a fibrous tissue septum in the condylar cartilage during early postnatal development and that the blood vessels found within the septum may rupture, impair ossification of the condyle, and thus cause the bifid appearance. Stadnicki (1971) suggested that trauma from obstetrical delivery was the cause of double condyle. In other instances, it may result from reattachment of a fractured, displaced condyle with regeneration of a new condyle on the residual stump. Poswillo (1972) and Sarnat (1971) have demonstrated this phenomenon following experimental condylectomy in monkeys.

The double mandibular condyle occurs predominantly as a unilateral anomaly and appears to be more common in females. When viewed anatomically, two condyles with only one mandibular neck are found. On occasion, double articular facets in the glenoid fossa that articulate with the two condyles have been found. When two condyles are present, the lateral condyle has most frequently been reported to be the larger.

Condylar Hyperplasia

It is sometimes difficult to differentiate clinically, radiographically, and microscopically between condylar hyperplasia and a benign neoplasm of bone (see Fig. 16–43). On occasion, an osteoma (Lyon, 1963), chondroma, or osteochondroma has been mistakenly reported as condylar hyperplasia. Thoma (1954), in differentiating between benign osseous neoplasms and hyperplasia, suggested that neoplasia is characterized by a lobulated enlargement, in contrast to the symmetrical enlargement of the condyle and a proportionate elongation of the entire condyloid process seen with hyperplasia. Since condylar hyperplasia is caused by stimulation of the growth site, with a resultant increase in the length of the condyloid process, it allows the relative proportions of the condyle to be preserved.

The etiology of condylar hyperplasia is unknown. It is at times associated with infections, such as those occurring in osteomyelitis of the subcondylar region or of the condyle itself. Other local factors associated with condylar hyperplasia are middle ear infection, abscess of the infratemporal fossa, and trauma. Although a hereditary etiology has also been mentioned when no local factors are present, the more frequent unilateral occurrence strongly suggests a local phenomenon (Gottlieb, 1951).

Clinical Features

The extent of the clinical features of condylar hyperplasia are determined by the age at which the abnormal stimulus begins to affect the growth of the condyle. According to Engel (1948), the development of the TMJ is completed by the age of 25 years. Growth activity is greatest during the fetal period and the early years of life, slowing considerably during the ages of 16 to 20 years. However, the potential for continued cartilaginous deposition, and therefore some form of condylar growth, persists throughout most of life, contrary to the situation in most other joints of the body.

When condylar hyperplasia starts early in life, the symmetry of the entire face may be affected. The elongation of the mandible on the affected side often produces a crossbite deformity in the child, with a resultant oblique attrition of the teeth. The function of the joint becomes impaired and there may be limited motion. The degree of limitation may be minimal if compensation also occurs in the glenoid fossa during this growth period. When hyperplasia occurs in the adult, lateral displacement and open bite are the frequent result. The open bite often is associated with an increase in the length of the clinical crowns of the teeth due to supraeruption.

Histopathological Findings

When hyperplasia occurs in young individuals, the architecture of the cells of the bone and cartilage may not be affected noticeably, as endochondral bone replacement of the hypertrophic cartilage keeps pace with chondrogenesis. When the hyperplasia occurs in much older individuals, only the proliferative and hypertrophic zones of the cartilage are mainly involved, while the articular zone remains remarkably intact (Oberg, 1962). Rushton (1944; 1946) has shown that hyperplasia of the condyle is probably caused by overactivity of the cartilage, which increases the thickness of the precartilaginous and cartilaginous layers. Rushton also demonstrated that the cartilage matrix was included in the bone trabeculae as far as 1 cm below the surface of the condyle. Flohr (1952) and Gruca (1926) have also demonstrated these histological findings.

ANKYLOSIS

Ankylosis is one of the most common sequelae following infection or trauma to the TMJ (see Chapters 13 and 24). By definition, ankylosis is chronic hypomobility or immobility of a usually moveable articulating structure. Ankylosis has been classified as being unilateral or bilateral; true (intra-articular) or false (extra-articular); fibrous or bony; and partial or complete. There is frequently an overlap between several types. True ankylosis is the more common type and is described either as fibrous or bony, but both of these are probably variations of the same process. False ankylosis is generally partial, fibrous, and unilateral (Kazanjian, 1938; Lyon, 1963).

Etiology

Ankylosis is almost always an acquired condition. A rare and often debated type of ankylosis is that referred to as infantile or congenital ankylosis. Currently, there has been only one documented case reported in the literature. The majority of cases suggested as being congenital ankylosis probably occur as a result of injuries to the TMJ during delivery (Burket, 1936). Trauma and infection are the most common predisposing factors. Topazian (1964), in reviewing the causes of ankylosis, reported that the incidence of trauma as an etiologic agent ranged from 26 to 75 per cent, whereas infection ranged from 44 to 88 per cent. The type and site of the trauma most likely to result in ankylosis have been subject to debate. Several investigators have suggested that crushing blows directly to the joint are more likely to cause ankylosis than are blows to the mandible in which the force is indirectly transmitted to the joint region (El-Mofty, 1972; Pizer, 1966; Topazian, 1964). Whether an actual fracture of the condyloid process is necessary to produce an ankylosis has also been debated. Several investigators suggest that fracture of at least the joint surface must occur, whereas others believe that a fracture is not necessary and that any trauma resulting in intra-articular bleeding is sufficient (El-Mofty, 1972; Stratigos, 1973).

Primary noninfectious and nontraumatic inflammatory conditions are also common causes of TMJ ankylosis. The most frequently encountered condition is rheumatoid arthritis, with the mandibular articulation involved in nearly half of the cases (Blackwood, 1957). In these instances, ankylosis is usually bilateral and of the fibrous variety. A less common primary noninfectious cause is Marie-Strümpell disease (ankylosing spondylitis), which affects the TMJ in four per cent of the cases (Maes, 1961; Resnick, 1974). Secondary noninfectious inflammatory changes resulting from radiation therapy directed through the joint at adjacent neoplasms, metastatic neoplasms, and Paget's disease have also been implicated in promoting ankylosis of the TMJ (Beekhuris, 1965; Lindsey, 1966; Sundell, 1966).

Of the primary infectious forms of inflammation, those of bacterial origin such as gonorrhea, tuberculosis, syphilis, scarlet fever, typhoid fever, and actinomycosis have been implicated in the development of ankylosis of the TMJ on rare occasion. Although inflammation of the TMJ arising from blood-borne infection is rare, it does occur (see Fig. 24–8) (Dagher, 1957; Keefer, 1937). Secondary infection of the mandibular joint may also occur by direct extension from adjacent regions of such conditions as otitis media, mastoiditis, osteomyelitis of the temporal bone, and infections of the parotid gland (Padgett, 1948; Topazian, 1964). The organism most frequently involved is the hemolytic Streptococcus.

The most common disorders causing false ankylosis are of muscle, nerve, and psychogenic origin, or those involving bone impingement (see Fig. 24–25), fibrous adhesions, and tumors (Miller, 1975). The conditions in the surrounding muscle that can cause false ankylosis are primarily from infection or myositis ossificans of the elevator muscles of mastication. Neurogenic disorders such as brain tumors, bulbar paralysis, and cerebral vascular accidents, can cause a flaccid paralysis of the masticatory muscles, resulting in an indirect type of immobility (see Chapter 26). A psychoneurotic type of ankylosis, termed hysterical trismus, also has been described, with fright as the most common cause (Stolzenberg, 1953). Rowe (1966) reported a case of false ankylosis occurring as a secondary complication of dystrophic epidermolysis bullosa. The primary defect was the formation of fibrous scar bands from the healing bulla of the overlying skin (Rowe, 1957; Rhymes, 1963). Temporomandibular changes have also been reported in patients with psoriasis and calcium pyrophosphate dehydrate arthropathy (Lundberg, 1967; Pritzker, 1976). Similarly, complications of scar formation in the overlying tissues following radiation and surgery, along with extracapsular impingement from exostosis of adjacent bones, frequently result in false ankylosis. A fracture that depresses the zygomatic arch will also produce this entity. Neoplastic diseases of the surrounding tissues, whether benign or malignant, can also cause false ankylosis.

Histopathological Findings

The tissue changes in true ankylosis vary with the severity of the precipitating factors and their duration. In mild and early cases, the findings will be subtle, with focal, scant infiltrates of lymphocytes and plasma cells within the existing normal soft tissues, along with a slight increase in the percentage of fibroblasts and dense collagen bundles. The early bony changes will also be subtle, with the fatty marrow exhibiting a mild chronic inflammatory cell infiltrate and some replacement of the fat cells with fibroblasts. In both tissues there will be varying degrees of increased vascularity. The gradual replacement of normal tissues with fibrous tissue, as occurs in chronic situations, usually is not associated with pain or other symptoms.

In those instances in which the onset and course are more acute, both the tissue changes and the associated symptoms are quite different. If the precipitating factor is either sudden and traumatic or an acute suppurative infection resulting in the loss of normal structures, there will be a great deal of granulation tissue formed and focal accumulations of acute inflammatory cells, predominantly neutrophils and diffuse infiltrates of lymphocytes, plasma cells, and macrophages, in the surrounding tissues. As the inflammation subsides, any tissues that were acutely inflamed will be replaced with dense fibrous tissue that will mature even further to scar tissue. Therefore, the degree of ankylosis will be dependent upon the extent of the destruction during the active acute inflammatory phase before the onset of the healing (fibrous) phase. If this has been severe and prolonged, both articular surfaces, the intra-articular disc, and the synovium may first become replaced by a continuous proliferation of granulation tissue and later by dense fibrous tissue that can continue to contract and cause decreased mobility.

A common finding in bony ankylosis is complete destruction of the disc. Initial osseous changes primarily consist of a flattening of the articulation, with the glenoid fossa and articular eminence becoming less pronounced, and the condyloid process becoming enlarged (Miller, 1975). Blackwood (1963) reported this in two joints with fibrous ankylosis. The disc was missing completely and the entire joint space was filled with dense fibrous connective tissue that was indistinguishable from the periarticular capsular tissues. The condyle was partially infiltrated by the fibrous connective tissue. Laskin (1978) has also reported absence of the disc in ankylosis and proposed this as a significant etiologic factor.

If surgical intervention is not undertaken, calcification and ossification of the fibrous tissue within the joint may eventually develop. Ultimately, a bony fusion may take place between the articular surfaces so that the normal anatomical features are obscured by masses of dense bone. Depending upon the severity of the involvement, the fibrous or osseous tissues may

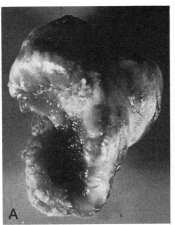
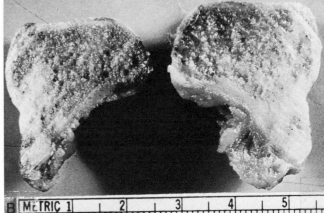
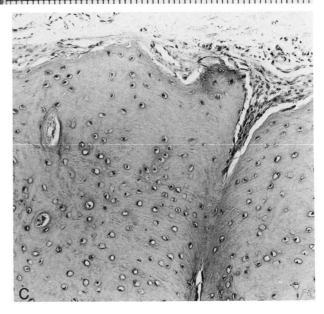

FIGURE 10–1. *A*, Gross appearance of surgical specimen of an osteoma appearing as a lobulated, circumscribed mass that distorts the symmetry of the condyle. *B*, Sagittal section of condyle exhibiting a uniform dense texture. (Photographs courtesy of B. G. Sarnat, M.D., D.D.S., Beverly Hills, CA). *C*, Microscopic appearance of the periphery illustrates the cellular periosteum and the thickened nodular layer of dense cortical bone with an increased osteocyte count (original magnification, × 100).

also involve the coronoid process, the glenoid fossa, and the zygomatic arch.

NEOPLASTIC DISEASES

In general, neoplastic processes are among the least common conditions arising in the TMJ. Some of the lesions with names indicating that they may be benign neoplasms are often not a neoplasm at all, but rather a mixed metaplastic and hyperplastic reaction. On even rarer occasions, a neoplasm of the TMJ may have metastasized to the joint from other parts of the body.

When true neoplasms have been found, they have been described as arising from within the bone and cartilage of the mandibular condyle, the articular fossa, the joint capsule, or the articular disc. Lesions of cartilage and bone origin are by far the most frequent.

Benign Tumors

Osteoma

The osteoma is the most common of the benign neoplasms involving the TMJ, occurring most often on the condyle. It is sometimes erroneously diagnosed as condylar hyperplasia and can readily be confused with this condition. An easy and obvious criterion to separate these two lesions is the appearance of a spherical and lobulated mass on the condyle (osteoma) rather than a uniform enlargement of the entire condyloid process (hyperplasia) (see Fig. 24–13). When an osteoma occurs within the condyle, however, the proportions are generally preserved (McNichol, 1946; Thoma, 1954; Worman, 1946). The microscopic features of both osteoma and condylar hyperplasia exhibit cancellous bone with a regular trabecular pattern and normal adipose marrow. Thus, it is usually difficult to differentiate these lesions without the aid of a radiograph or the benefit of a gross examination of the lesion at the time of surgery (Fig. 10–1 A, B, and C).

Chondroma, Osteochondroma, and Chondroblastoma

After the condyle develops, a form of cartilage remains just below the articular surface throughout life. Although this cartilage remains, benign tumors of cartilaginous origin are still rarely encountered. Pure chondromas of the condyle have been reported by Ivy (1927), Kanthak (1938), and Jokinen (1976). The osteo-

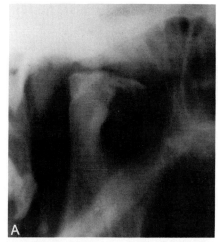
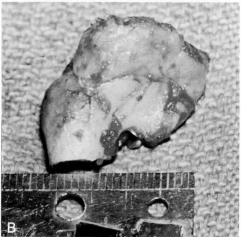

FIGURE 10–2. A, Radiographic and B, gross appearance of an osteochondroma of the condyle resembling an osteoma.

chondroma is the most common lesion and exhibits features of both osteoma and chondroma. Cases of osteochondroma of the condyle have been reported by Curtin (1959), Chaudhry (1961), and Ramon (1964).

The usual location of a chondroblastoma in the body is in the epiphyseal plate of the long bones. Because the mandibular condyle has a different arrangement of tissues, it is epiphyseal-like. A case was reported that arose extraosseously from the subarticular cartilage of the mandibular condyle (Spahr, 1982). Surprisingly, a patient with a chondroblastoma within the medullary bone of the condyle has been reported by Goodsell (1964).

Clinically, all the benign cartilaginous tumors produce symptoms similar to those of the osteoma. Osteochondroma, in particular, is very difficult to distinguish from osteoma because it has similar radiographic and gross features (Fig.

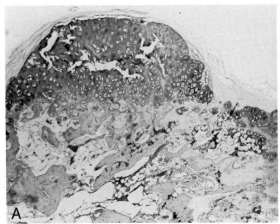
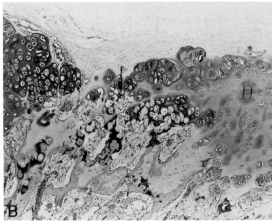

FIGURE 10–3. *A,* Microscopic appearance of a raised hypercellular nodule of cartilage on the surface of an osteochondroma of the condyle. The lack of cellularity of the outermost thin layer of connective tissue is indicative of the benign nature of the lesion (original magnification, × 25). *B,* Higher magnification of the zone of an osteochondroma containing whorled hypercellular cartilage intermingled with osteoid and bone. The more central regions of the lesion contain matured trabecular bone, loose connective tissue, and hematopoietic marrow (original magnification, × 40).

10–2 *A* and *B*). Microscopically, the osteochondroma is distinguished by its outer rim of active cartilage, overlying a zone of intermingled osteoid and bone. Centrally, mature trabeculae of bone and hematopoietic bone marrow are predominant (Fig. 10–3 *A* and *B*). Melarkey (1966) emphasized the potentially malignant nature of these benign cartilaginous tumors.

Giant Cell Tumor

The nature of giant cell lesions of bone is still unknown. A number of bone lesions will contain giant cell tissue as part of their histological makeup that are not giant cell tumors. These include cherubism, fibrous dysplasia, aneurysmal bone cyst, chrondroblastoma, villonodular synovitis, "brown tumor" of hyperparathyroidism, and peripheral giant cell granuloma. Some are somewhat innocuous to the extent that they do not require treatment, while others can be more destructive and persistent. Although the giant cell tumor is always a somewhat destructive lesion, its degree of aggressiveness will vary. The tumor is usually graded based on its histological appearance (Fig. 10–4 *A* and *B*). A low-grade lesion will have a high fibrous component with few giant cells, while the high-grade lesion will be very cellular, with a predominance of multinucleated cells, frequent mitotic figures, and relatively little fibrous tissue. There are usually foci of old extravasated

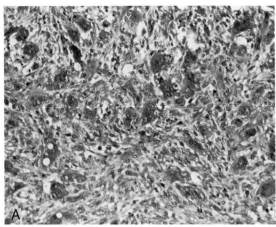
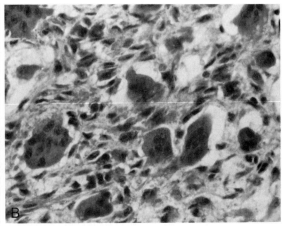

FIGURE 10–4. *A,* Low-power photomicrograph of a giant cell tumor showing the abundant multinucleated giant cells in a background of mononuclear cells (original magnification, × 250). *B,* High-power view shows the uniformity of the nuclei of both the multinucleated and the mononuclear cells indicative of a benign (low-grade) lesion (original magnification, × 900).

blood and associated hemosiderin pigment. Dispersed throughout the lesion are new trabeculae of osteoid or bone. The experience of the pathologist is important because the extent of treatment will vary considerably with the grade given.

There have been relatively few cases of giant cell tumor of the condyle reported. One has been said to be associated directly with a traumatic injury; in a second, there was suspicion of trauma (Hofer, 1952; Kochan, 1963). This association with trauma leaves considerable doubt that the lesion is a neoplasm in the true sense of the word. There is a growing consensus that except for the highest grade giant cell tumor, which may in reality represent an osteosarcoma, the presence of giant cell tissue in any lesion may be incidental or of a reactive nature.

Many lesions are known to heal after debulking and thorough curettage. Some even have been known to heal spontaneously or without surgical intervention. The giant cell lesions of hyperparathyroidism and some traumatic (hemorrhagic) bone cysts are such examples. There has, however, been one well-documented report (Mintz, 1981) of malignant giant cell tumor of the mandible in a middle-aged man who died from metastasis to the lungs. This case is sufficient to alert the clinician to the necessity of careful diagnosis and management of all giant cell lesions involving this bone.

Since the giant cell tumor has been reported infrequently in the mandibular condyle, the symptoms are not well understood. Clinically, the lesion presents as a swelling in the preauricular region, with pain as the primary complaint. Crepitus upon opening and closing the mouth also has been reported. Radiographically, the lesion may appear as either a unilocular or multilocular radiolucency with an indistinct border. The cortical bone is generally expanded and thin and may be completely eroded.

Synovial Chondromatosis

This condition is frequently referred to by several other names. The most common is synovial osteochrondromatosis, used especially when the cartilaginous nodules are calcified or contain bone. Synovial chrondrometaplasia, synovial chondrosis, and articular chondrosis are other synonyms. This relatively uncommon benign condition affects the joints in males more frequently than in females and is seen mainly in young and middle-aged patients. In general, the condition primarily occurs in monoarticular joints, most commonly involving the knee and only occasionally the TMJ. Electron microscopic study of tissue from an affected TMJ shows that the cartilaginous nodules are the result of transformation of the less-differentiated connective tissue cells into chondrocytes that form nodules of cartilage in the subintima of the synovium (Fig. 10–5 A and B). These nodules move to the intimal layer, becoming pedunculated. Some may even separate and float freely in the joint space (Fig. 10–5C) (de Bont, 1988). Although the etiology is still unknown, chronic trauma appears to be a common denominator. A recent experimental study utilizing monkeys has established a relationship between synovial chondromatosis and osteoarthritis (Helmy, 1989).

The clinical symptoms of synovial chondromatosis are pain, swelling, limitation of motion, and a snapping sound during jaw movement (Alling, 1963; Ballard, 1972; Kusen, 1969; Reinert, 1989; Schulte, 1969). The occasional clinical presentation as a preauricular mass has resulted in the need to separate the lesion from a parotid salivary gland tumor (Cannon, 1987). The clinical diagnosis is often based on the finding of faint radiopaque masses within the synovium or loose bodies confined within the joint capsule. The osseous destruction characteristic of malignant tumors is not present.

Microscopically, the lesion consists of fibrous tissue and synovium with areas of cartilaginous metaplasia and proliferation. The atypical cartilage cells may sometimes make it difficult to distinguish the lesion from a low-grade chondrosarcoma. Such changes are attributed to very active growth rather than malignant alteration. The appearance of the surrounding connective tissue provides reassurance of the benign nature of the lesion (Fig. 10–5 B).

A clinical correlation with the histological findings should be made before a definitive diagnosis is rendered, since the transformation of synovial chondromatosis to chondrosarcoma has been well documented in other joints (Mullins, 1965). The clinician should give careful consideration to whether there is an absence of radiographic evidence of the destructive changes seen with chondrosarcoma and also whether the lesion is both grossly and histologically confined to the synovial tissues within the joint capsule. It is capable of severe local destruction and erosion into the base of the brain (Sun, 1990).

Treatment of synovial chondromatosis consists of removal of the detached particles and excision of the affected synovial membrane.

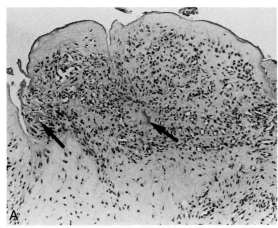

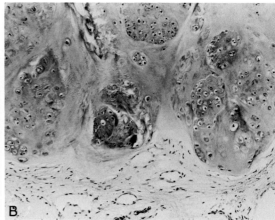

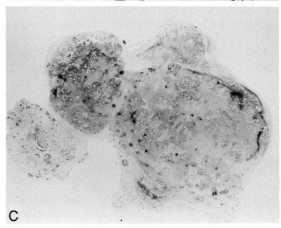

FIGURE 10–5. Synovial chondromatosis. *A*, Chronic synovitis of the TMJ exhibiting the initial stage of metaplasia of the connective tissue with the formation of cartilage nodules (arrows) (original magnification, × 100). *B*, Well-formed nodules of cartilage within the subintima of the synovium (original magnification, × 100). *C*, Unattached cartilage nodules removed from the joint space (original magnification, × 40).

Condylectomy is not necessary unless the condyle is directly affected or exhibits severe arthritic change (Blankestijn, 1985).

Hemangioma

Hemangiomas of soft tissues are common, but rare within bone. A number of cases of intraosseous hemangioma of the mandible have been reported, although only a few have been found within the condyle (Atkinson, 1988; Maclennan, 1958; Uotila, 1966). The most frequent clinical symptom of hemangioma of the mandibular joint is dull pain. This is increased by chewing or during excessive movement of the mandible. Usually, there is some limitation of motion and swelling. If the lesion is large, a bruit may be heard. Radiographically, the lesion may appear as circumscribed or as a fine, soap bubble radiolucency that is sometimes accompanied by a sunburst appearance. The radiographic appearance of this intraosseous vascular lesion can be similar to a number of other less critical ones.

Microscopically, the intraosseous hemangioma consists of numerous vascular spaces lined by a single layer of endothelial cells supported by a delicate fibrous connective tissue stroma and bony trabeculae (Fig. 10–6). The vascular spaces vary considerably in their size and shape, with numerous sinusoidal channels. Most of the spaces are packed with red blood cells.

Treatment of intraosseous hemangioma is difficult, often requiring ligation of the appropriate external carotid artery prior to resection. Halazonitis (1982) reported several cases in which merely ligating the ipsilateral external carotid artery resulted in the lesion undergoing regression and thus suggested that this approach should always be tried as a preliminary step, with a period of evaluation before the usual more aggressive surgical treatment of resection.

Miscellaneous Tumors

Isolated instances of other benign tumors in the TMJ have been reported. These are the myxoma, ossifying fibroma, and glomus tumor (Griffin, 1962; Thoma, 1947; 1954).

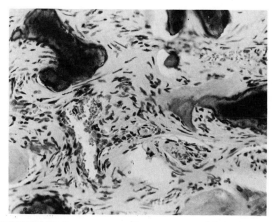

FIGURE 10–6. Intraosseous hemangioma exhibiting spicules of bone, loose cellular connective tissue, and multiple, irregularly shaped sinusoidal spaces containing red blood cells (original magnification, × 250).

Malignant Tumors

Malignant tumors of the TMJ are extremely uncommon and are usually a result of direct extension of neoplasms from the overlying epithelialized surfaces of either the skin or nasopharynx, or from within the parotid gland (Catone, 1990). Lesions arising within the TMJ do occur, however, and primarily consist of chondrosarcoma, synovial sarcoma, fibrosarcoma, and multiple myeloma. Another source of malignant lesions is the metastatic carcinoma from a remote site. In a recent thorough review of the literature of malignant lesions of the TMJ, cases of malignant schwannoma and malignant fibrous histiocytoma were added to the primary lesions, along with a large list of malignant salivary gland and squamous and transitional epithelial lesions that involved the TMJ either through direct extension or distant metastasis (Bravitz, 1990).

Chondrosarcoma

The chondrosarcoma is a rare tumor of the jaws, in general, but it is one of the most common primary malignant neoplasms within the TMJ. Chondrosarcomas have been classified into primary and secondary types. The primary lesion is thought to arise directly from previously normal bone, periosteum, or cartilage. The secondary type is thought to arise from pre-existent benign cartilaginous lesions and is found in an older age group.

The major clinical finding with chondrosarcoma is a symptomless, enlarging mass in the preauricular region that occurs in a short period of time. Pain is generally present in the later stages of the disease. Other reported symptoms are similar to those found in the myofascial pain-dysfunction syndrome (Gingrass, 1954; Lanier, 1971; Morris, 1987; Richter, 1974). Another reported symptom has been hearing loss due to pressure on the eustachian tube. The early radiographic features are widening of the TMJ space and an erosion of the glenoid fossa.

To make a microscopic diagnosis of chondrosarcoma, a knowledgeable interpretation of the appearance of the chondrocytes in the lesion is required. The morphology of the chondrocytes within chondroma or chondromatosis can also exhibit changes that can cause concern. A diagnosis of chondrosarcoma is made by evaluating the extent of the variation in the size of the cells and the presence of binucleated and bizarre, hyperchromatic nuclei in both the cartilaginous deposits and the surrounding connective tissue (Fig. 10–7 A). The absence of mitotic figures is of little diagnostic significance. Any calcification or ossification seen within chondrosarcoma is usually abnormal (Fig. 10–7 B) (Geschickter, 1949).

Synovial Sarcoma

Synovial sarcoma has been reported to occur within the TMJ (del Balso, 1982; Jonsson, 1948; Knutsson, 1948). The clinical signs of synovial sarcoma do not particularly differ from those of other malignant neoplasms of the joint. Symptoms primarily consist of severe pain upon mastication and tenderness upon palpation of the preauricular region.

The basic microscopic pattern of the synovial sarcoma consists of tissue spaces that are either slit-like clefts or well-defined, gland-like structures containing either serous or mucinous fluid. This pattern varies from tissue containing compact groups of oval or polygonal cells replacing the gland-like structures to tissue with papillary projections extending into the clefts and gland-like spaces. A common feature of this tumor is the reproduction of lining cells resembling secretory epithelial cells on a supporting stroma of compact tissue composed of elongated cells with small, dark-staining nuclei. The presence of two cell types and patterns (biphasic pattern) is considered characteristic of synovial sarcoma (Fig. 10–8). The tumor is locally invasive, destroying the joint, and capable of easily penetrating the blood vessels and causing early metastasis to the lungs and other organs. Thus, the five-year prognosis is usually not very good.

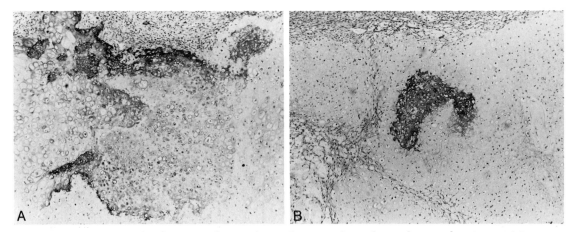

FIGURE 10–7. A, Chondrosarcoma showing the usual pattern of irregular cartilaginous deposits containing pleomorphic and hyperchromatic chondrocytes arranged in a haphazard pattern (original magnification, × 40). B, Well-differentiated chondrosarcoma with less cellular cartilage and containing central deposits of abnormal calcified bone. The surrounding connective tissue is excessively cellular, indicative of the malignant nature of the lesion (original magnification, × 40).

Fibrosarcoma

Fibrosarcoma of the TMJ is derived from either the capsule or the periosteum. The most characteristic clinical feature is extreme tenderness and pain during jaw motion (Thoma, 1948). Microscopically, the fibrosarcoma exhibits great variation. Some tumors are well differentiated (Grade I) and the cells closely resemble the normal fibroblasts found in the surrounding tissue. Others are poorly differentiated, with the cells exhibiting all the features of a bizarre neoplasm. The cells are usually spindle-shaped, with elongated nuclei, and the associated fibers are generally arranged in interlacing bands or fascicles (Fig. 10–9). Abnormal mitotic figures and cells exhibiting pleomorphic and hyperchromatic nuclei are frequently seen in the poorly differentiated (Grade III) tumors. The management and prognosis are the same as for a similar grade fibrosarcoma in other locations.

Multiple Myeloma

Multiple myeloma has been reported as occurring within the condyle as part of the usual widespread involvement throughout the skeleton. Radiographically, the lesions have been described as punched-out radiolucencies (Cohen, 1956; Hereb, 1984; Jaggers, 1978). Microscopically, the tumor consists of sheets of cells similar in appearance to normal plasma cells, with an absence of other inflammatory cells (Fig. 10–10). Frequently, eosinophilic, amorphous accumulations known as Russell

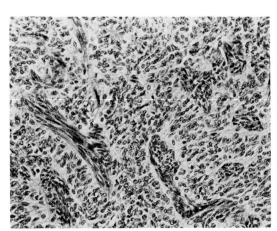

FIGURE 10–8. Synovial sarcoma exhibiting the biphasic pattern of rounded epitheloid cells and spindle-shaped hyperchromatic cells (original magnification, × 250).

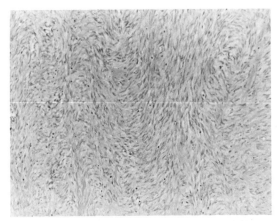

FIGURE 10–9. Well-differentiated fibrosarcoma exhibiting enlarged uniform fibroblasts in densely cellular fascicles with a herringbone pattern (original magnification, × 100).

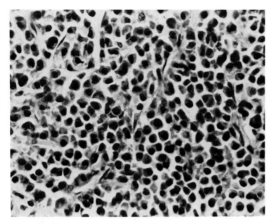

FIGURE 10–10. Multiple myeloma containing densely packed cells with eccentric hyperchromatic nuclei resembling normal plasma cells. There is an absence of background support tissue or inflammatory cells (original magnification, × 400).

bodies also are seen. In some lesions amyloid deposits may be present. The neoplastic plasma cells can be distinguished from their inflammatory counterparts by the use of immunohistochemistry to characterize the predominant protein component of the immunoglobulins being produced (Wright, 1981).

Metastatic Carcinoma

Metastatic tumors from the uterus and breast, as well as transitional cell carcinoma, metastatic adenocarcinoma, and malignant melanoma have been reported in the condyle (Blackwood, 1962; Bottomley, 1965; Cuttino, 1988; Rubin, 1989; Salman, 1954; Thoma, 1954; Webster, 1988) (see Fig. 25–2). The radiographic findings often may be negative, but when present, they frequently mimic osteomyelitis.

The early clinical signs and symptoms of the various malignancies of the TMJ generally are not specific and tend to resemble a typical case of TMJ dysfunction. If either adequate radiographs are not used or the patient does not respond to the usual treatments, the clinician should be alerted to the possibility that the initial diagnosis may not be correct. Asymmetry or swelling in the preauricular region, paresthesia and paresis, auditory changes, vertigo, and rapid changes in the occlusion, especially with a conspicuous absence of pain in the joint, should alert the clinician to the possibility of a malignant process (Bravitz, 1990).

MISCELLANEOUS DISEASES

The TMJ can be secondarily involved in patients with a variety of systemic diseases.

Osteitis deformans (Paget's disease) affects the maxilla much more frequently than the mandible, but when the mandible is involved, the condyle is occasionally affected, resulting in condylar enlargement. The clinical findings are limitation of movement and asymmetry of the face (Rushton, 1944). The microscopic findings are similar to those in other bones.

Acromegaly can be associated with enlargement of the condyle. The excessive condylar growth can lead to mandibular joint arthropathy and mandibular prognathism (see Fig. 24–16). The condylar growth often coincides with areas of new growth in other parts of the mandible (Kellgren, 1952; Korkhaus, 1933; Rushton, 1944).

Blackwood (1962) reported a case of renal rickets (secondary hyperparathyroidism) in which growth of both the condyle and mandible was impeded.

SUMMARY

Most pathological conditions that can arise in other joints of the body also afflict the temporomandibular joint (TMJ) or its component structures. Often the clinical symptoms do not correlate with the gross and microscopic findings.

Developmental abnormalities of the TMJ are frequently associated with syndromes affecting the head and neck. Of the anomalies affecting this joint, hyperplasia of the condyle is the most common proliferative condition. Clinically, radiographically, and often microscopically, it is difficult to differentiate condylar hyperplasia from a benign neoplasm. Condylar agenesis and hypoplasia, and the double mandibular condyle are generally diagnosed on the basis of clinical and radiographic findings.

Inflammatory disturbances, trauma, and ankylosis are the most common pathological entities affecting the TMJ. The diagnosis of these conditions is often made from the clinical findings supported by radiographic studies.

Neoplastic disturbances are the least common pathological conditions affecting the TMJ. Of the benign conditions, the osseous and cartilaginous neoplasms are the most common. Examples of most benign tumors occurring in bone have been reported in the TMJ. Although malignant neoplasms occur less frequently than benign neoplasms in the condyle, malignant tumors have been reported from all of the cell types native to the condyle and supporting tissues. Carcinomas from overlying epithelial structures and of metastatic origin have likewise been reported.

TMJ involvement with systemic diseases, such as osteitis deformans, gout, acromegaly, renal rickets, epidermolysis bullosa dystrophica, and psoriasis, occasionally occurs. When it does, it presents special diagnostic and therapeutic problems.

REFERENCES

Alling, C. C., Rawson, D. W., Staats, J., and Middleton, R. A.: Synovial chondromatosis of the temporomandibular joint. J. Oral Surg. 31:691–693, 1963.

Atkinson, J. J., Wolf, S., Anavi, Y., and Wesley, R.: Synovial hemangioma of the temporomandibular joint: Report of a case and review of the literature. J. Oral Maxillofac. Surg. 46:804–808, 1988.

Ballard, R., and Weiland, L. H.: Synovial chondromatosis of the temporomandibular joint. Cancer 30:791–795, 1972.

Beekhuris, G. J., and Harrington, E. B.: Trismus: Etiology and management of inability to open the mouth. Laryngoscope 75:1234–1258, 1965.

Blackwood, H. J.: The double-headed mandibular condyle. Am. J. Phys. Anthropol. 15:1–8, 1957.

Blackwood, H. J.: Intra-articular fibrous ankylosis of the temporomandibular joint. Oral Surg. 10:634–642, 1957.

Blackwood, H. J.: Disease of the mandibular joint in the child. In Oral Pathology in the Child. Proceedings of a Conference held at Royal College of Surgeons, June 29, 1962. New York, International Academy of Oral Pathology, 1962, pp. 64–74.

Blackwood, H. J.: Arthritis of the mandibular joint. Br. Dent. J. 115:317–326, 1963.

Blackwood, H. J.: Pathology of the temporomandibular joint. J. Am. Dent. Assoc. 79:118–124, 1969.

Blankestijn, J., Panders, A. K., Vermey, A., and Scherpbier, A. J. J.A.: Synovial chondromatosis of the temporomandibular joint. Cancer 55:479–485, 1985.

Bottomley, W. L.: Temporomandibular joint syndrome associated with cerebral neoplasms. Oral Surg. 20:550–555, 1965.

Boudet, M. C.: Anomalies oculaires congenitales et malformations: Craniofaciales. Assoc. Montpellier Med. 53:704–714, 1958.

Bravitz, J. B., and Chewning, L. C.: Malignant disease as temporomandibular joint dysfunction: Review of the literature and report of a case. J. Am. Dent. Assoc. 120:163–166, 1990.

Burke, P. H.: Case of acquired unilateral mandibular condylar hypoplasia. Proc. R. Soc. Med. 54:507–510, 1961.

Burket, L. W.: Congenital bony temporomandibular joint ankylosis and facial hemiatrophy. JAMA 106:1719–1722, 1936.

Cannon, C. R.: Osteochondrosis of the temporomandibular joint presenting as an apparent parotid mass. Ann. Otol. Rhinol. Laryngol. 96:330–332, 1987.

Catone, G. A., and Carlson, E. R.: Squamous cell carcinoma of the temporomandibular joint. J. Oral Maxillofac. Surg. 48:515–517, 1990.

Chaudhry, A. P., Robinovitch, M. R., Mitchell, D. F., and Vickers, R. A.: Chondrogenic tumors of the jaws. Am. J. Surg. 102:402–411, 1961.

Cohen, B. M., and Meyers, H. N.: Multiple myeloma involving the temporomandibular joint. Oral Surg. 9:1274–1280, 1956.

Collins, D. A., Becks, H., Simpson, M. E., and Evans, H. M.: Growth and transformation of the mandibular joint in the rat. II. Hypophysectomized female rats. Am. J. Orthod. Oral Surg. 32:443–446, 1946.

Collins, D. A., Becks, H., Simpson, M. E., and Evans, H. M.: The effects of thyroidectomy at birth. Oral Surg. 2:315–317, 1949.

Curtin, J. W., and Greeley, P. W.: Osteochondroma of the mandibular condyle. Plast. Reconstr. Surg. 24:511–521, 1959.

Cuttino, C. L., and Steadman, R. B.: Myofascial pain syndrome masking metastatic carcinoma. Va. Dent. J. 65:12–16, 1988.

Dagher, I. K., and MacDonald, J. J.: Ankylosis of the temporomandibular joint. Oral Surg. 10:1145–1155, 1957.

de Bont, L. G. M., Liem, R. S., and Boering, G.: Synovial chondromatosis of the temporomandibular joint: A light and electron microscopic study. Oral Surg. 66:593–598, 1988.

del Balso, A. M., Pyatt, R. S., Busch, R. S., et al.: Synovial cell sarcoma of the temporomandibular joint. Arch. Otolaryngol. 108:520–522, 1982.

Diamond, M.: The development of dental height. Am. J. Orthod. 30:589–592, 1944.

El-Mofty, S.: Ankylosis of the temporomandibular joint. Oral Surg. 33:650–660, 1972.

Engel, M. B., and Brodie, A. G.: Condylar growth and mandibular deformities. Oral Surg. 1:790–806, 1948.

Flohr, W.: Epiphysare Hyptrophie des Unterkiefers durch enchondrale Knochenapposition am Proccssus articularis. Dtsch. Zahnaertz. Z. 7:1235–1241, 1952.

Frandsen, A. M., Becks, H., Nelson, M. M., and Evans, H. M.: Growth and transformation of the mandibular joint in the rat. V. The effect of pantothenic acid deficiency from birth. Oral Surg. 6:892–897, 1953.

Geschickter, C. F., and Copeland, M. M.: Tumors of Bone. Philadelphia, J. B. Lippincott, 1949.

Gilmour, W. H.: An abnormal mandible. Br. Dent. J. 47:960–962, 1926.

Gingrass, R. P.: Chondrosarcoma of the mandibular joint: Report of case. J. Oral Surg. 12:61–63, 1954.

Goodsell, J. O., and Hubinger, H. L.: Benign chondroblastoma of the mandibular condyle. J. Oral Surg. 22:355–363, 1964.

Gorlin, R. J., Pindborg, J. J., and Cohen, M.: Syndromes of the Head and Neck, 3rd ed. New York, McGraw-Hill, 1990.

Gottlieb, O.: Hyperplasia of the mandibular condyle. J. Oral Surg. 9:118–135, 1951.

Griffin, C. J.: Glomus tumour in the bilaminar zone of the human temporomandibular meniscus. Aust. Dent. J. 7:377–380, 1962.

Gruca, A., and Meisels, E.: Asymmetry of the mandible from unilateral hypertrophy. Ann. Surg. 83:755–768, 1926.

Halazonitis, J. A., Kountouris, J., and Halazonitis, N. A.: Arteriovenous aneurysm of the mandible. Oral Surg. 53:454–457, 1982.

Helmy, E. S., Bays, R. A., and Sharawy, M. M.: Synovial chrondromatosis associated with experimental osteoarthritis in adult monkeys. J. Oral Maxillofac. Surg. 47:823–827, 1989.

Hereb, I., Gyenes, V., and Szabo, G.: Multiple myeloma involving the temporomandibular joint. Fogorv. Sz. 77:105–108, 1984.

Hofer, O.: Zur Klinik und Therapie der zentralen Riesenzellganulome der Kiefer Oest. Z. Stomatol. 49:324–328, 1952.

Hrdlicka, A.: Lower jaw: Double condyles. Am. J. Phys. Anthropol. 28:75–89, 1941.

Ivy, R. H.: Benign bony enlargement of the condylar process of the mandible. Ann. Surg. 85:27–30, 1927.

Jaggers, R. G., Helkimo, M., and Carlsson, G. E.: Multiple myeloma involving the temporomandibular joint. J. Oral Surg. 36:557–559, 1978.

Jokinen, K., Stenback, F., Palva, A., and Sutenen, S.: Benign cartilaginous tumor of the temporomandibular joint. J. Laryngol. Otol. 51:299–303, 1976.

Jonsson, G.: Points regarding synovial fibrosarcoma. Acta Radiol. [Diagn.] (Stockh.). 29:356–357, 1948.

Kanthak, F. F., and Harkins, H. N.: Unilateral hypertrophy of the mandibular condyle associated with chondroma. Surgery 4:898–907, 1938.

Kazanjian, V. H.: Ankylosis of the temporomandibular joint. Surg. Gynecol. Obstet. 67:333–348, 1938.

Kazanjian, V. H.: Congenital absence of the ramus of the mandible. J. Bone Joint Surg. 21:761–722, 1939.

Kazanjian, V. H.: Bilateral absence of the ascending rami of the mandible. Br. J. Plast. Surg. 9:77–82, 1956.

Keefer, C. S., and Spink, W. W.: Gonococcic arthritis: Pathogenesis, mechanism of recovery and treatment. JAMA 109:1448–1453, 1937.

Kellgren, J. H., Ball, J., and Tutton, G. H.: The articular and other limb changes in acromegaly: Clinical and pathological study of 25 cases. Q. J. Med. 21:405–424, 1952.

Knutsson, F.: Two synovial fibrosarcomas. Acta Radiol. [Diagn.] (Stockh.). 29:4–6, 1948.

Kochan, E. J.: Reparative giant cell granuloma. J. Oral Surg. 21:390–395, 1963.

Korkhaus, G.: Changes in form of jaws and in the position of teeth produced by acromegaly. Int. J. Orthod. 19:160–174, 1933.

Kusen, G. J.: Chondromatosis: Report of case. J. Oral Surg. 27:735–738, 1969.

Lanier, V. C., Rosenfeld, L., and Wilkenson, H. A.: Chondrosarcoma of the mandible. South Med. J. 64:711–714, 1971.

Laskin, D. M.: Role of the meniscus in the etiology of post-traumatic temporomandibular joint ankylosis. Int. J. Oral Surg. 7:340–345, 1978.

Levy, B. M.: The effect of pyridoxine deficiency on the jaws of mice. J. Dent. Res. 29:349–357, 1950.

Lindsey, J. S., Fulcher, C. L., Sazima, H. J., and Green, H. G.: Surgical management of ankylosis of the temporomandibular joint: Report of two cases. J. Oral Surg. 24:264–270, 1966.

Lundberg, M., and Ericson, S.: Changes in the temporomandibular joint in psoriasis arthopathica. Acta Derm. Venereol. (Stockh.). 47:354–358, 1967.

Lyon, L. Z., and Sarnat, B. G.: Limited opening of the mouth caused by enlarged coronoid processes. J. Am. Dent. Assoc. 67:644–650, 1963.

Maclennan, W. D.: Haemangioma of the mandibular condylar process. Br. Dent. J. 105:93–94, 1958.

Maes, H. J., and Dihlmann, W.: Befall der Temporomandibulargelenke bei der Spondylitis ankylopoetica. Fortchr. Roentgenstr. 109:513–516, 1961.

Mahneke, A.: Epibulbar dermoids. Acta Ophthalmol. (Kbh.). 34:412–420, 1956.

McNichol, J. W., and Roger, A. T.: An original method of correction of hypoplastic asymmetry of the mandible. Plast. Reconstr. Surg. 1:288–299, 1946.

Melarkey, D. W., Roffinela, J. P., and Kaplan, H.: Osteocartilaginous exostosis (osteochondroma) of the mandibular condyle. J. Oral Surg. 24:271–275, 1966.

Miller, G. A., Page, H. L., and Griffith, C. R.: Temporomandibular joint ankylosis: Review of the literature and report of two cases of bilateral involvement. Oral Surg. 33:792–803. 1975.

Mintz, G. A., Abrams, A. M., Carlsen, G. D., et al.: Primary malignant giant cell tumor of the mandible. Oral Surg. 51:164–171, 1981.

Morris, M. R., Clark, S. K., Porter, B. A., and Delbecq, R. J.: Chondrosarcoma of the temporomandibular joint. Head Neck Surg. 10:113–117, 1987.

Mullins, F., Berard, C. W., and Eisenberg, S. H.: Chondrosarcoma following synovial chondromatosis. Cancer 18:1180–1188, 1965.

Oberg, T., Fajers, C. M., Lyell, G., and Friberg, U.: Unilateral hyperplasia of the mandibular condylar process. A histological, microradiographic, and autoradiographic examination of one case. Acta Odontol. Scand. 20:485–504, 1962.

Padgett, E. C., Robinson, D. W., and Stephenson, K. L.: Ankylosis of the temporomandibular joint. Surgery 24:426–437, 1948.

Pillay, V. K., and Orth, M. C.: Ophthalmomandibulomelic dysplasia: An hereditary syndrome. J. Bone Joint Surg. (Am.). 46:858–862, 1964.

Pizer, M. E.: Ankylosis of the temporomandibular joint treated by subcondylar resection. Oral Surg. 21:706–708, 1966.

Poswillo, D. E.: The late effects of mandibular condylectomy. Oral Surg. 33:500–512, 1972.

Pritzker, K. P. H.: Pseudotumor of the temporomandibular joint: Destructive calcium pyrophosphate dehydrate arthropathy. J. Rheumatol. 3:70–81, 1976.

Prowler, J. R., and Glassman, S.: Agenesis of the mandibular condyles. Oral Surg. 7:133–139, 1954.

Ramon, Y., Lerner, M. A., and Leventon, G.: Osteochondroma of the mandibular condyle. Oral Surg. 17:16–21, 1964.

Reinert, S., and Hammer, U.: Synovial chrondromatosis of the temporomandibular joint: A differential diagnosis to parotid gland tumor. Laryngorhinootologie 68:216–220, 1989.

Resnick, D: Temporomandibular joint involvement in ankylosing spondylitis. Comparison with rheumatoid arthritis and psoriasis. Radiology 112:587–591, 1974.

Rhymes, R., Hardin, J. C., Metts, D., and Krantz, R.: Dystrophic epidermolysis bullosa: Extra-articular ankylosis treated with oral skin grafts: Report of case. J. Oral Surg. 21:63–67, 1963.

Richter, K. J., Freeman, N. S., and Quick, C.: Chondrosarcoma of the temporomandibular joint: Report of case. J. Oral Surg. 32:777–781, 1974.

Rowe, N. L., and Hislop, I. H.: Periostitis and osteomyelitis of the mandible in childhood. Br. Dent. J. 103:67–78, 1957.

Rowe, N. L., and Sowray, J. H.: Extra-articular ankylosis as a complication of dystrophic epidermolysis bullosa. Br. J. Oral Surg. 3:136–145, 1966.

Rubin, M. M., Jui, V., and Cozzi, G. M.: Metastatic carcinoma of the mandibular condyle presenting as temporomandibular joint syndrome. J. Oral Maxillofac. Surg. 47:507–510, 1989.

Rushton, M. A.: Growth at the mandibular condyle in relation to some deformities. Br. Dent. J. 76:57–68, 1944.

Rushton, M. A.: Unilateral hyperplasia of the mandibular condyle. Proc. R. Soc. Med. 39:431–442, 1946.

Salman, J., and Langel, I: Metastatic tumors of the oral cavity. J. Oral Surg. 7:1091–1107, 1954.

Sarnat, B. G., and Muchnic, H.: Facial skeletal changes after mandibular condylectomy in growing and adult monkeys. Am. J. Orthod. 60:33–45, 1971.

Schier, M. B. A.: The temporomandibular joint. A consideration of its probably functional and dysfunctional sequelae and report: Condyle-double head in a living person. Dent. Items Interest 70:779–787, 1948.

Schulte, W. C., and Rhyne, R. R.: Synovial chondromatosis of the temporomandibular joint. Oral Surg. 28:906–913, 1969.

Spahr, J., Elzay, R. P., Kay, S., and Frable, W. J.: Chrondroblastoma of the temporomandibular joint arising from articular cartilage. Oral Surg. 54:430–435, 1982.

Stadnicki, G.: Congenital double condyle of the mandible causing temporomandibular joint ankylosis: Report of case. J. Oral Surg. 29:208–211, 1971.

Steinhauser, E. W.: The treatment of ankylosis in children. Int. J. Oral Surg. 2:129–136, 1973.

Stolzenberg, J.: Case report on periodic hysterical trismus. Oral Surg. 6:453–454, 1953.

Stratigos, G. T.: Reconstruction of the temporomandibular joint by permanent fixation of silastic to the temporal bone. Trans. Congress. Int. Assoc. Oral Surg. 4:284–287, 1973.

Sun, S., Helmy, E., and Bays, R.: Synovial chondromatosis with intracranial extension. Oral Surg. 70:5–9, 1990.

Sundell, B.: Ankylosis of the temporomandibular joint. Ann. Chir. Gynaecol. Fenn. 55:118–123, 1966.

Thoma, K. H.: Tumors of the condyle and temporomandibular joint. Oral Surg. 7:1091–1107, 1954.

Thoma, K. H., Holland, D. J., Burrow, J. G., and Sleeper, E. J.: Fibrosarcoma of the mandibular joint. Oral Surg. 1:61–66, 1948.

Thoma, K. H., Holland, D. J., and Rounds, C. E.: Myxoma of the mandibular condyle treated by excision. Am. J. Orthod. Oral Surg. (Oral Surg. Sect.). 33:344–347, 1947.

Thomason, J. M., and Yusuf, H.: Traumatically induced bifid mandibular condyle: A report of two cases. Br. Dent. J. 161:291–293, 1986.

Topazian, R. G.: Etiology of ankylosis of the temporomandibular joint: Analysis of 44 cases. J. Oral Surg. 22:227–233, 1964.

Uotila, E., and Westerholm, N.: Hemangioma of the temporomandibular joint. Odontologisk Tidskrift (Göteborg) 74:202–206, 1966.

Van Balen, A. J. M.: Dyscephaly with microphthalmos, cataract and hypoplasia of the mandible. Ophthalmologica 141:53–63, 1961.

Webster, K.: Adenocarcinoma metastatic to the mandibular condyle. J. Cranio-Maxillofac. Surg. 16:230–232, 1988.

Weinmann, J. P., and Schour, I.: Rachitic changes in mandibular condyle of the rat. J. Dent. Res. 25:509–512, 1946.

Worman, H. G., Waldron, C. W., and Radiesch, D. F.: Osteoma of the mandibular condyle with deviation prognathic deformity. J. Oral Surg. 4:27–32, 1946.

Worth, H. M.: Hurler's syndrome. Oral Surg. 22:21–35, 1966.

Wright, B. A., Wysocki, G. P., and Bannerjee, D.: Diagnostic use of immunoperoxidase technique for plasma cell lesions of the jaws. Oral Surg. 52:615–622, 1981.

11

PATHOLOGICAL ASPECTS OF ARTHRITIDES AND DERANGEMENTS*

TORE L. HANSSON, D.D.S., ODONT. DR.

INTRODUCTION

ARTHRITIDES

Infectious

Traumatic

Inflammatory

RHEUMATOID
JUVENILE RHEUMATOID
ANKYLOSING SPONDYLITIS
PSORIATIC

Degenerative

Metabolic

INTRA-ARTICULAR DISC DERANGEMENTS

Anterior Displacement with Reduction (Clicking)

Anterior Displacement without Reduction (Locking)

RELATIONSHIPS BETWEEN DISC DERANGEMENTS AND DEGENERATIVE JOINT DISEASE

CLINICAL CONSIDERATIONS

SUMMARY

INTRODUCTION

Arthritis is a disease of various forms and obscure etiologies, most of which are systemic in origin. Many of the rheumatic diseases share, to a variable degree, immunological abnormalities and immune complex reactions, probably on the basis of the pathological changes (Arnett, 1989; Bennett, 1989; Grennan, 1984; Korst, 1982; MacLeod, 1984; Scully, 1982; Tegelberg, 1987c). Most forms also show overlapping clinical symptoms and the diagnosis is usually confirmed on the basis of generally accepted laboratory tests.

Arthritis of the temporomandibular joint (TMJ), however, is mostly local and degenerative, and seems to be dependent on the malfunction of the stomatognathic system. Other local forms include infectious and traumatic arthritis. The diagnosis is most often made from the history and particular combination of clinical signs and symptoms rather than on the basis of laboratory findings.

*See Chapters 6, 10, 16, 17, 19, 22–26.

The TMJ is also subject to derangements of the intra-articular disc. These derangements may be preceded by arthritic changes or may be a sequel to them. This chapter will consider the pathological aspects of the various arthritides and derangements that involve the TMJ.

ARTHRITIDES

Infectious

Infectious arthritis is uncommon in the TMJ. However, in the literature (Sarnat, 1991) it is mentioned as a possible consequence of such diseases as gonorrhea, syphilis, tuberculosis, typhoid fever, dysentery, pneumonia, influenza, scarlet fever, and measles. With the general decrease in the prevalence of these diseases it is more likely to be a consequence of local extension of infections from the middle ear, mastoid process, parotid gland, teeth, and mandible. There is also a risk of infectious arthritis when bacteria have entered the blood stream after injuries or as a result of traumatic penetration of the joint capsule.

165

Bacterial contamination leads to an inflammation of the synovial tissues. When the infection continues, the synovial membrane will be infiltrated by polymorphonuclear leucocytes and later replaced by granulation tissue (Jessop, 1973). With destruction of the synovial membrane, the joint compartment becomes the target of the bacteria. Pyogenic bacteria can cause complete destruction of the fibrocartilage and the bone if the process is not immediately interrupted (American Rheumatism Association, 1975; Worth, 1979). As a result, a fibrous or even a bony ankylosis can occur.

In young patients, infectious arthritis can result in underdevelopment of the mandibular condyle and extremely irregular condylar form (see Chapter 24). An asymmetry of the mandible generally also develops, with the chin point deviating to the affected side. Radiographic changes seen later in life may be the result of altered function resulting from long lasting overloading as well as from the effects of the disease itself.

Traumatic

Traumatic arthritis is the immediate intra-articular inflammatory response to injury of the joint tissues. The force directed toward the mandible may not necessarily cause a fracture, although clinically there still may be considerable deviation of the chin point, with partial to complete loss of tooth contact on the injured side. Most often the posteriorly or laterally directed forces result in a compression of the intra-articular soft tissues. The highly vascularized parts in the posterior aspect of the joint and at the periphery of the disc react with excessive bleeding. Tearing of the border between the disc and the loose soft tissue attachments can also occur. Inflammation develops rapidly. The increased vascular permeability results in edema, with mild to severe joint effusion. With the increased thickness of the loose soft tissues and the edema and hemorrhage, the intra-articular disc and condyle are displaced. The mandible is forced toward the contralateral side. The increased distance between the articulating components of the traumatized side is also the reason for the sudden loss of the ipsilateral tooth contact.

Besides the loss of tooth contact, deviation of the mandible in the intercuspal position and on opening, limitation of movement, and pain with attempted function are the characteristic signs and symptoms. The acute symptoms normally subside within a few days. Therefore, irreversible dental treatment, such as adjustment of the occlusal surfaces of the teeth, is absolutely contraindicated for the management of this problem, which is most often temporary.

Inflammatory

Rheumatoid

Rheumatoid arthritis (RA) is a chronic inflammatory systemic disease that involves primarily the peripheral joints. The disease is often associated with extra-articular features and appears to be mediated immunologically. An abnormal immunoglobulin is formed in the joint tissues and an auto-antibody to the abnormal immunoglobulin (rheumatoid factor) is produced in response. The immune complex formation then may lead to the activation of complement, inflammation, and synovial damage.

The overall prevalence of RA in developed countries is about three per cent, with a female to male ratio of 3:1. The age of onset of the disease is usually in the third and fourth decades. The age of onset follows a normal distribution curve, with no age group excluded. There may be a genetic predisposition (Carlsson, 1979; Tegelberg, 1987a).

The onset is often insidious, with increasing stiffness of the joints of the hands or feet that is usually worse in the morning. The disease progresses in a centripetal and symmetrical direction. Later in the course, the wrist, elbow, ankle, and knee joints are commonly involved. The disease may also start as an acute polyarthritis, with severe symptoms of weight loss, fever, profound fatigability, and malaise.

Extra-articular manifestations include: (1) subcutaneous nodules found at sites of pressure or friction in 20 to 25 per cent of patients; (2) osteoporosis, muscle weakness, and wasting occurring adjacent to inflamed joints and more diffusely as part of a systemic disturbance; (3) pleurisy or pleural effusions occurring in 25 per cent of men with RA; (4) asymptomatic pericarditis reported in 40 per cent of patients; (5) additional manifestations of valvular insufficiency and conduction disturbances; (6) peripheral neurological symptoms that may occur from potentially reversible entrapment neuropathies and cervical myelopathy caused by vasculitis; (7) anemia secondary to gastrointestinal blood loss from long-lasting treatment with analgesic anti-inflammatory drugs; and (8) Raynaud's phenomenon, which not only is a prodromal feature but also occurs throughout the course of the disease.

Articular manifestations include: (1) stiffness and joint pain, usually most severe in the morning and decreasing during the day; and (2) signs of articular inflammation, with swelling, warmth, erythema, and tenderness to palpation and symmetrical involvement of the small joints of the hands and the feet, the middle interphalangeal and metacarpophalangeal joints, the wrists, and subtalars. The large joints become involved later in the course of the disease. Although the cervical spine may be affected, the thoracic and lumbosacral parts of the spine are usually spared.

Joint pain causes an immediate reaction in the musculature. Limitation of motion occurs and, in the advanced stages of the disease, muscle contraction and ankylosis, with permanent joint deformity, are common. The most characteristic deformities of the hand are the enlarged knuckles, ulnar deviation, and the spindle shape of the fingers (Barnes, 1973a) (Fig. 11–1).

TMJ pain is relatively common, but is overshadowed by pain in other joints. There may be a restriction of condylar translation and an anterior opening of the bite. Severely restricted mouth opening rarely occurs. Severe destruction of the joints is seen in the more advanced stages of RA (Larheim, 1983; Tegelberg, 1987a). Recent studies (Tegelberg, 1987b; 1987c) indicate the close relationship between the involvement of the stomatognathic system and the severity of RA. The severity of TMJ involvement in RA is correlated with the concentration of serum acute phase reactants and with the

accepted rheumatic indices of Ritchie and Lee (Tegelberg, 1987c).

The histopathology of the TMJ in rheumatoid arthritis does not differ from that seen in other joints. The active stage of the disease is characterized by inflammation of the synovial tissues accompanied by an intense infiltration of lymphocytes and plasma cells. This infiltration results in destruction of the articular surfaces of the joint and resorption of the subarticular bone. The degree of inflammatory cell infiltration is dependent upon the severity and the stage of the disease. With severe deformity of the articular surfaces, fibrous ankylosis is often a final result. The ankylosis may be partial, involving only the lower joint compartment, or complete, with total destruction of the articular disc and union of the bony surfaces by fibrous or bony tissue.

The prevalence of radiographic findings in the TMJ varies in different patient groups (Åkerman, 1984; Syrjäneen, 1985). Fifty to 80 per cent show radiographic evidence of soft tissue swelling and periarticular demineralization. Progression to the deeper layer of cartilage and bone destruction result in narrowing of the joint spaces and the development of erosions. The findings are generally bilateral (Fig. 11–2).

Juvenile Rheumatoid

Juvenile rheumatoid arthritis (JRA) most likely is not a single disease but a group of disorders that cause crippling in young individuals. The prevalence of JRA is about 0.5 per 1000 children at risk and occurs predominantly in females. The term juvenile rheumatoid arthritis may be misleading as many forms of JRA are seronegative for IgM rheumatoid factor (Barnes, 1973b). The disease is clinically separate from adult RA. Some children, however, subsequently develop adult forms of such inflammatory arthritides as ankylosing spondylitis and seropositive rheumatoid disease.

There are several characteristic patterns of onset. The patient may develop an asymmetrical polyarticular arthritis. The knees, wrists, ankles, and neck are common sites of initial involvement, with only one or two joints being affected. Systemic manifestations are generally mild, but the articular involvement is often unremitting. Iridocyclitis is most likely to develop before six to eight years of age. In males with HLA-B27 antigen, an ankylosing spondylitis often develops during puberty. A high spiking fever and a severe toxic state (Still's disease) can be expected, especially among males. These children have splenomegaly, hep-

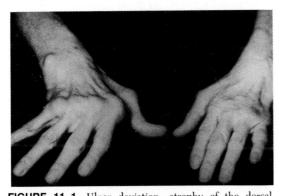

FIGURE 11–1. Ulnar deviation, atrophy of the dorsal musculature and subluxation, and extreme swelling of the metacarpophalangeal joints, particularly of the right hand, in a patient with advanced rheumatoid arthritis. (From Klinenberg, J. R.: The arthritides. In Sarnat, B. G., and Laskin, D. M.: The Temporomandibular Joint: A Biological Basis for Clinical Practice, 3rd ed. Springfield, IL, Charles C Thomas, 1980. Courtesy of the Arthritis Foundation, Atlanta, Georgia.)

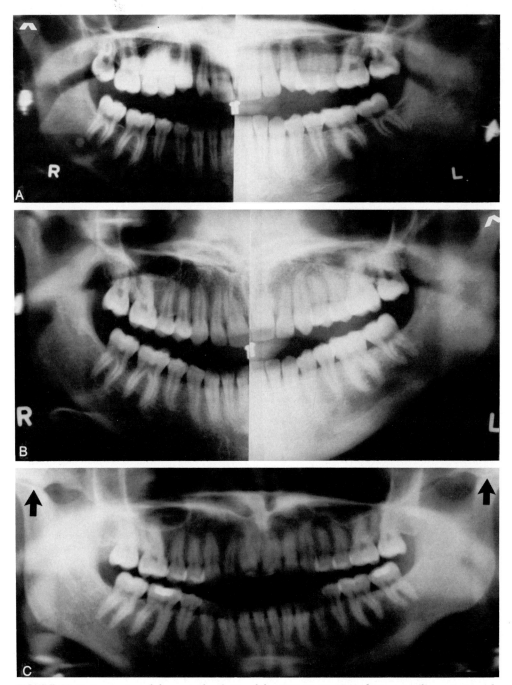

FIGURE 11–2. Progression of rheumatoid arthritis of the TMJs at 13, 15, and 22 years of age. *A,* Irregular condyles (arrow) at the age of 13 years. *B,* Flattening of the condyle (arrow) is seen on the left side at the age of 15 years. *C,* Bilateral flattening (arrow) is seen at the age of 22 years (see Fig. 24–7).

atosplenomegaly, pericarditis, lymphadenopathy, and a characteristic salmon-colored, morbilliform skin rash. Polyarthralgias usually precede the frank arthritis.

The first symptoms of TMJ involvement may be pain, tenderness on palpation, or crepitus. The symptoms are more noticeable in the morning upon awakening. Condylar growth is impaired and micrognathia develops (Larheim, 1981) (see Fig. 24–7). The combination of direct interference with condylar growth and restricted mandibular function results in the characteristic bird face deformity seen in these patients.

Bacterial infections should be considered in the differential diagnosis when a febrile child does not present with the salmon-colored, maculopapular rash. A viral polyarthritis also causes fever and rash, but this type of arthritis usually subsides within a few weeks. Disseminated malignancies may cause musculoskeletal pain in children and should be suspected if persistent bone pain is present. Joint involvement with rheumatic fever is less common than with JRA, and is associated with a migratory and more transient form of arthritis.

Ankylosing Spondylitis

Ankylosing spondylitis belongs to the group of disorders with overlapping clinical features and a common genetic predisposition—the seronegative arthropathies (Mason, 1973). It is characterized by: (1) an asymmetrical, inflammatory, seronegative oligoarthritis; (2) sacroiliitis/spondylitis; (3) peripheral arthritis with the tendency to develop inflammatory lesions in the attachments between tendon and bone; (4) anterior uveitis; (5) hereditary tendency; and (6) a high prevalence of HLA-B27 antigen (90 per cent) (Wenneberg, 1983). Environmental factors and a genetic susceptibility influence the pathogenesis.

The disease affects both sexes with a male to female ratio of 3:1. It is usually milder in females, however, and therefore less frequently diagnosed. The age of onset is usually in the second or third decades of life (Carter, 1980). The initial symptoms include low back pain and joint stiffness. The symptoms are worse in the morning. Pain in the hips, buttocks, and shoulder regions is also common. Arthritis is often seen concomitantly in such peripheral joints as the shoulder, hip, knee, foot, wrist, and fingers. The extra-articular manifestations are: (1) iritis or iridocyclitis, which may be the very first symptom, and (2) cardiac symptoms of aortic insufficiency or conduction defects.

The articular symptoms result from inflammation of the synovial tissue and insertions of ligaments and tendons, followed by ossification. Bony bridges fuse adjacent vertebral bodies. The back subsequently becomes fixed in extreme flexion, which limits chest expansion and thereby impairs respiration. The patient has a characteristic bent-over posture, a rigid spine, and an exaggerated dorsal kyphosis.

The TMJ usually is involved several years after the onset of the disease. TMJ pain and stiffness, with difficulty in mouth opening, are the most common symptoms. The involvement and the severity of the symptoms correlate with the general severity of the disease (Heir, 1983; Wenneberg, 1983).

In the beginning, osteoporosis and erosions of the spine are seen radiographically. In the advanced stage of the disease, sclerotic fusions between the vertebrae are recognized. Intervertebral ossification is described as a bamboo spine appearance (Boland, 1969).

Psoriatic

Psoriatic arthritis is a seronegative erosive arthritis seen in a low percentage of patients with longstanding cutaneous psoriasis (Mason, 1973). At the onset of the disease, fever and fatigue are common symptoms. The joint symptoms are mostly asymmetrical. They occur mainly in the distal interphalangeal joints. Females show a somewhat higher prevalence than males. Genetic factors appear to play a role in the etiology. HLA-B27 antigen is increased in patients with psoriatic arthritis.

Distinct patterns of psoriatic arthritis recognized are: (1) distal arthropathy of the interphalangeal joints of fingers and toes, with associated changes of the nails; (2) asymmetrical oligoarthritis of the joints of the hands and feet involved at random, ranging from solitary, red, swollen fingers and toes, to more severe forms of the disease with extensive bone resorption and telescoping digits; (3) a seronegative inflammatory polyarthritis that may be symmetrical and very difficult to distinguish from a seronegative RA; and (4) sacroiliitis and spondylitis, with symptoms of peripheral arthritis. HLA-B27 antigen is found mostly in these patients. The articular manifestations occasionally may be present before the skin lesions. Psoriatic arthritis often mimics the clinical symptoms of RA.

The extra-articular manifestations may include widespread scaling lesions over the extensor surfaces of the extremities. The scaling, however, may be limited only to the scalp. Changes in the nails, such as pitting, subungual hyperkeratosis, and horizontal ridging, are very common. An anterior uveitis also may be present.

The TMJs show a wide range of involvement from being symptom-free to exhibiting fibrous ankylosis (Little, 1987; Wood, 1983). When the TMJs are involved, pain, swelling, tenderness, restricted movement, and crepitation can be present. Patients with psoriatic arthritis frequently show condylar erosion radiographically.

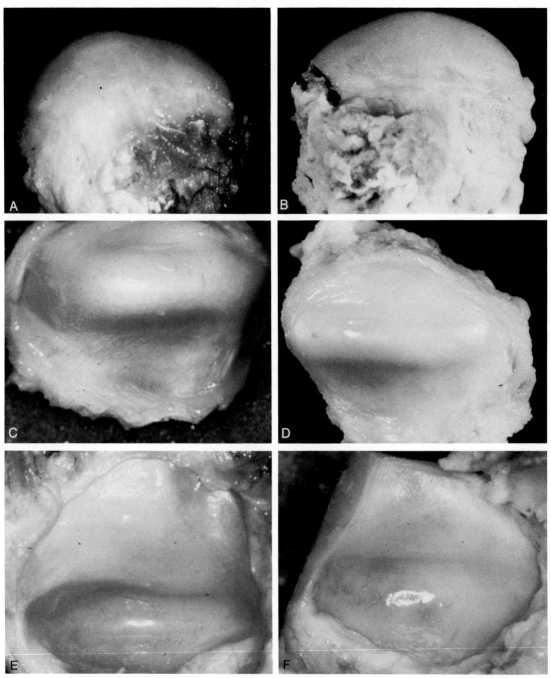

FIGURE 11–3. Normal TMJ components from an older individual and a young adult with an age difference of 40 years. *A,* Frontal view of a right normal condyle of a 65-year-old showing a smooth articulating surface. *B,* Frontal view of a left normal condyle of a 25-year-old showing a smooth articulating surface. *C,* Superior view of the right disc from condyle shown in A. *D,* Superior view of the disc from condyle shown in B. *E,* Inferior view of the right temporal component (articular fossa) associated with the condyle in A and the disc in C. *F,* Inferior view of the left temporal component (articular fossa) associated with the condyle in B and the disc in D. (A, C, E from Bean, L. K., Omnell, K. Å., and Öberg, T., Departments of Radiology and Stomatognathic Physiology, School of Dentistry, University of Lund, Malmö, Sweden. B, D, F from Solberg, W. K., and Hansson, T. L., Temporomandibular Joint Laboratory, UCLA Dental Research Institute, Los Angeles, California.)

However, in general, the radiographic changes in the TMJ are nonspecific. The severity of subjective symptoms in the TMJ seems to be linked to the severity and extent of the skin disorders (Könönen, 1986; 1987a; 1987b).

In the differential diagnosis the only real clinically diagnostic criterion is the presence of skin lesions. The absence of the rheumatoid factor and involvement of the distal interphalangeal joints distinguish the disease from RA. When symptoms are not diagnostic for either psoriatic arthritis or ankylosing spondylitis, a radiographic examination of the spine is essential.

Degenerative

Degenerative arthritis is the most common form involving the TMJ. Synonyms for this condition are arthrosis, degenerative joint disease, osteoarthritis, and osteoarthrosis. The term degenerative arthritis is clinically justified when interpreted as the overall description for the different events that take place in the joint from the initial symptom of pain until the complete deterioration of the joint components.

Degenerative arthritis is usually a local disease involving mostly one particular joint. It is most often the result of several years of adverse loading of the intra-articular tissues. Preceding the signs of inflammation and subsequent pain during movement are often symptoms of fatigue, stiffness, aching pain, and numbness in the surrounding muscles. The disease has never been shown to be purely age-dependent although its final stages are more prevalent in the age groups above 40 years (20 to 25 per cent) (Hansson, 1975). The etiology is multifactorial and systemic factors may predispose to the disease. Mechanical stress and trauma are the most probable etiological factors in degenerative arthritis of the TMJ (Hylander, 1979). Tooth loss, occlusal interferences, excessive forces of the muscles in bruxism, and morphological differences between the two congruous sides of the stomatognathic system are other factors ascribed to the contribution of adverse loading (Axelsson, 1987; Bezuur, 1988b; Hansson, 1979; Kobayashi, 1982; McCarroll, 1988; Mongini, 1972; Öberg, 1971; Randow, 1976; Richards, 1981; Solberg, 1985; 1986a; 1986b).

Under normal conditions, there is always an equilibrium between form and function. The articulating components of the TMJ (the condyle, the articular eminence, and the disc) are stable after growth is completed, i.e., during adult life. The equilibrium between form and function is maintained by remodeling (see Chapter 6). This remodeling maintains the relationship between the soft and the hard tissues without changing the contour of the joint components (Fig. 11–3). When loading conditions change so that particular regions of the articulating surfaces are exposed to additional forces or overloading, the remodeling activity increases in these particular areas. Changes develop as a result of an increase in the soft tissue thickness in the overloaded areas of the condyle and articular eminence originating from the undifferentiated mesenchymal cells (Figs. 11–4 to 11–7). Because there is no undifferentiated mesenchyme in the disc, it only adapts to the changes occurring in the other two components. The disc becomes thinner (Figs. 11–8 and 11–9), and with continuing overloading it may perforate in the adapted area. Concomitant changes, with surface deterioration, occur in the temporal component and later in the condyle, but not until all the undifferentiated mesenchymal cells are depleted in the previous adaptive process. At this stage, hard tissue changes also will become apparent (Hansson, 1977; Lubsen, 1985).

The initial stage of osteoarthrosis of the TMJ is the splitting of the fibrous connective tissue lining. However, this does not occur until all the potential of cartilage formation is depleted. Because of the elasticity of the fibrous connective tissue lining, this layer follows the new formation of the underlying fibrocartilage. An irregular contour of the condyle and the tem-

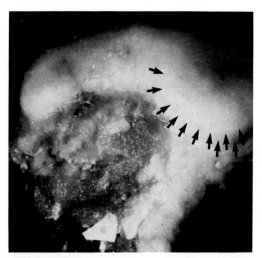

FIGURE 11–4. Extensive anterolateral soft tissue formation on left condyle of young person. (From Solberg, W. K., and Hansson, T. L., Temporomandibular Joint Laboratory, UCLA Dental Research Institute, Los Angeles, California.)

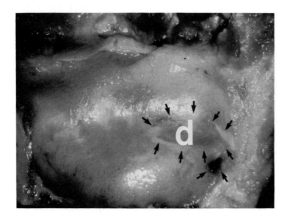

FIGURE 11–5. Soft tissue formation and deterioration in lateral aspect of the temporal component associated with the condyle of Figure 11–4. Arrows denote the soft tissue formation surrounding the deteriorated area in d.

FIGURE 11–6. The four tissue layers of the condyle and of the temporal component. (From Hansson, T. L., Honée, W., and Hesse, J.: Craniomandibulaire Dysfunctie. Samsom Stafleu, Alphen aan den Rijn/Brussel, 1985b.)

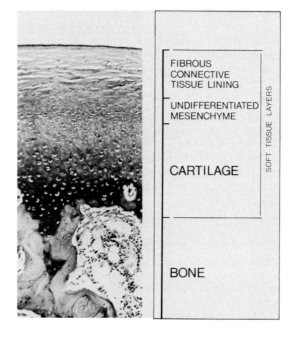

FIBROUS
CONNECTIVE
TISSUE LINING

UNDIFFERENTIATED
MESENCHYME

CARTILAGE

SOFT TISSUE LAYERS

BONE

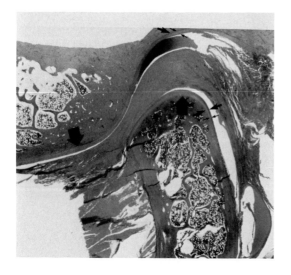

FIGURE 11–7. Sagittal section of a left TMJ. Note the difference in soft tissue thickness, being thicker on the superior part of the condyle and on the articular eminence (large arrows), and thinner posteriorly on the condyle (small arrows) and in the mandibular fossa.

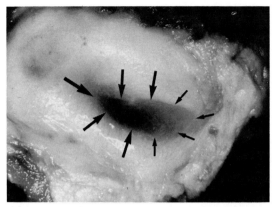

FIGURE 11–8. Superior view of the left disc associated with the condyle in Figure 11–4 and the temporal component in Figure 11–5. Note the very thin area laterally that is juxtaposed to the areas of changes in the other two components.

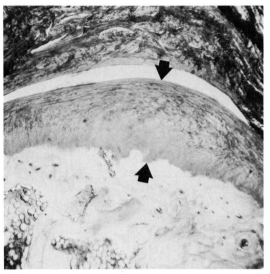

FIGURE 11–10. The irregular condylar contour (arrows) resulting from locally extensive cartilage formation. (From Lubsen, C. C., Hansson, T. L., Nordström, B. B., and Solberg, W. K.: Histomorphometric analysis of cartilage and subchondral bone in mandibular condyles of young human adults at autopsy. Arch. Oral Biol. 30:129–136, 1985.)

poral component is therefore often seen, but yet, the surface is smooth (Fig. 11–10). Before the fibrillation occurs, the fibrocartilage seems to make a final effort to produce new cartilage by cellular division (hyperplastic cartilage) (Fig. 11–11). At this stage an irregular border layer between the cartilage and subchondral bone is also recognized (Fig. 11–12). When finally the surface layer deteriorates, open lesions in the fibrocartilage in the form of vertical cracks are seen. Granulation tissue grows in to cover the exposed bone (Fig. 11–13).

If repair is not successful, the lesions grow deeper, with deterioration of the deep calcified cartilage and compact bone, and also infiltration of the spongy bone. At this stage perforation of the disc may develop in the juxtaposed area. The clinical sign of crepitation then occurs as a result of the rough surfaces of the condyle and

temporal component articulating against each other.

As the initial phases of degenerative arthritis take place in the soft tissue and not in the bone, the diagnosis is mostly established on the basis of the clinical criteria rather than on the radiographic findings. The inflammatory reaction is a response to the continuous traumatization of the synovial membrane by the irregular articulating surfaces during function. These changes also may be responsible for joint sounds. When clicking occurs at the same mandibular position during both opening and closing, the sound is most likely caused by a permanent local irregularity rather than a disc displacement.

When the changes reach the hard tissue, radiographic signs will confirm the deterioration of the joint surface. The clinical sign of TMJ crepitation will also confirm the diagnosis. At this stage of the disease flattening will be recognized in the temporal component as well as on the condyle (Fig. 11–14), which frequently forms osteophytes on the anterior surface. When the disc has been perforated, there no longer will be space between the temporal and condylar components when visualized by the tomographic radiograph (Hansson, 1983) (Fig. 11–15).

Local lesions of degenerative arthritis are much more prevalent than extensive lesions.

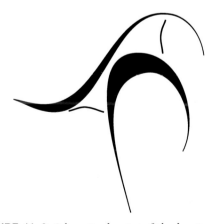

FIGURE 11–9. Schematic drawing of the location of the major increase in soft tissue change, which later is followed by deterioration and hard tissue changes.

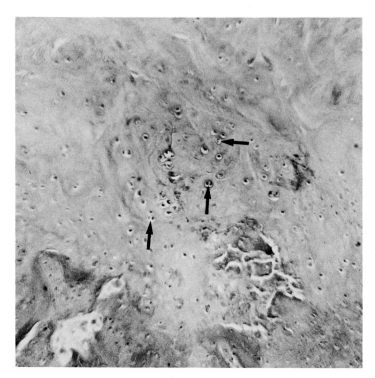

FIGURE 11–11. High magnification of hyperplastic cartilage showing active cellular division. (From Lubsen, C. C., Hansson, T. L., Nordström, B. B., and Solberg, W. K.: Histomorphometric analysis of cartilage and subchondral bone in mandibular condyles of young human adults at autopsy. Arch. Oral Biol. *30*:129–136, 1985.)

Autopsy studies have shown that the lateral part of the joint is more affected by loading than the central and medial parts (Lysell, 1977). This is probably the reason why improved masticatory and joint function can be restored despite the local irreversible changes. It also seems that undifferentiated mesenchymal cells from the areas adjacent to a condylar lesion may possess the potential for joint repair. New formation of hard tissue is often recognized in post-therapeutic radiographs, in combination with improved mandibular function (Fig. 11–16).

Metabolic

Gout (arthritis urica) and pseudogout (pyrophosphate arthropathy or chondrocalcinosis articularis) are the two types of metabolic arthritis (Carlsson, 1979; Currey, 1973). The former involves the deposition of crystals of urate in the joint tissues and the latter involves calcium pyrophosphate dihydrate. The increased amount of uric acid in the body is the result of an increase of purine production or the result of a deficiency in the excretion of uric acid in

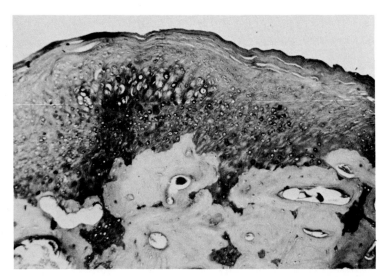

FIGURE 11–12. Hyperplastic cartilage covering the irregular layer of subchondral bone. (From Lubsen, C. C., Hansson, T. L., Nordström, B. B., and Solberg, W. K.: Histomorphometric analysis of cartilage and subchondral bone in mandibular condyles of young human adults at autopsy. Arch. Oral Biol. *30*:129–136, 1985.)

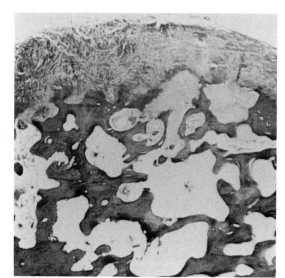

FIGURE 11–13. Complete deterioration of the soft tissue covering with vertical cracks, an open lesion into the spongy bone, and formation of granulation tissue.

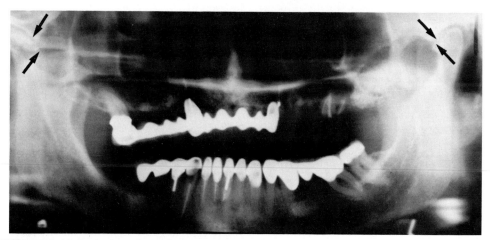

FIGURE 11–14. Panoramic radiograph showing bilateral degenerative joint disease. Flattening is seen in the temporal components as well as in the condyles (arrows).

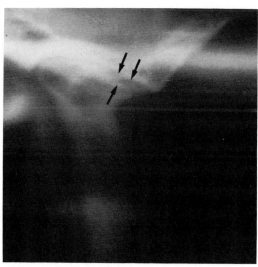

FIGURE 11–15. Tomogram of the right TMJ seen in Figure 11–14. In this lateral cut the flattening and osteophyte formation are clearer. Note the loss of the compact layers (arrows) as well as the narrrowed joint space.

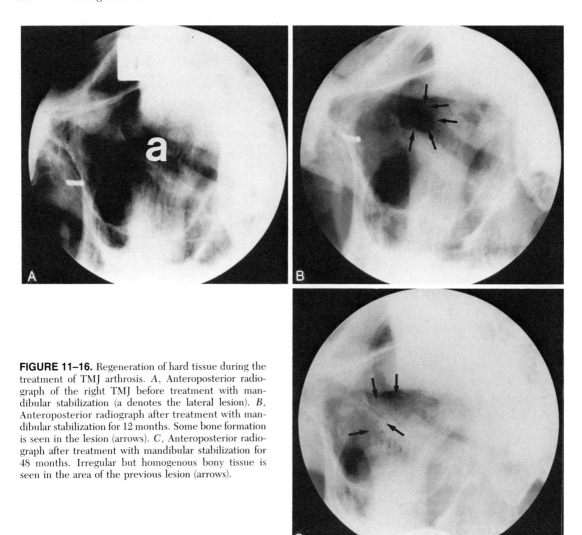

FIGURE 11–16. Regeneration of hard tissue during the treatment of TMJ arthrosis. *A,* Anteroposterior radiograph of the right TMJ before treatment with mandibular stabilization (a denotes the lateral lesion). *B,* Anteroposterior radiograph after treatment with mandibular stabilization for 12 months. Some bone formation is seen in the lesion (arrows). *C,* Anteroposterior radiograph after treatment with mandibular stabilization for 48 months. Irregular but homogenous bony tissue is seen in the area of the previous lesion (arrows).

the urine. Crystals of calcium pyrophosphate dihydrate may occur in hyperparathyroidism or diabetes mellitus. The deposited crystals are the cause of intra-articular inflammation (crystal synovitis).

The attack of pain is sudden and the joint is swollen, red, and tender. Analysis of the synovial fluid confirms the clinical diagnosis. Not until several years after the onset of the disease will radiographic signs of calcified areas in the disc and destruction of the hard tissues become apparent.

INTRA-ARTICULAR DISC DERANGEMENTS

The clinical features of intra-articular disc derangements have been thoroughly described

(Farrar, 1982) (see Chapters 16, 17, 23, and 24). They are divided into two groups: anterior displacement with reduction and anterior displacement without reduction.

Anterior Displacement with Reduction (Clicking)

In addition to TMJ pain at rest and during mandibular movements, there is also a distinct clicking sound of varying magnitude in the joint (see Fig. 19–4). The clicking may occur in any position during opening/closing of the mouth. It is most frequent, however, near maximum occlusion (stage I) or in the middle of opening/closing of the mouth (stage II) (Hansson, 1985a). The clicking is audible or palpable and, in contrast to sounds produced by an irregular articular surface, the position at which the open-

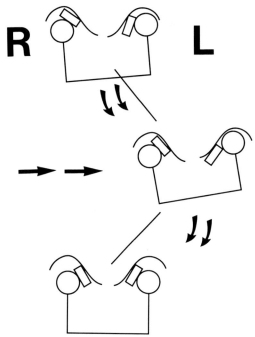

R **L**

FIGURE 11–17. Schematic frontal view illustration of condyle (○) and disc (▭) relationship during opening. Note anterior displacement with reduction on left side. Before clicking occurs the condylar movement on the left side is delayed, with mandibular deviation to the left (L). After clicking, the condyle-disc relationship is restored. Opening ends in a symmetrical mandibular position.

ing and closing click occurs is not identical. Before the clicking occurs, condylar movement is delayed, which results in a noticeable deviation of the mandible to the ipsilateral side during opening of the mouth (Fig. 11–17). After the clicking has occurred, however, the mouth opening is symmetrical when observed in the frontal plane. Depending on when the clicking

occurs during closing, there will be deviation of the equivalent movement.

When the disc is out of place, it is generally located anterior and medial to the condyle, with part of the retrodiscal tissue in the articular zone (Figs. 11–18 and 11–19). The clicking occurs when the condyle slips back in front of the posterior band of the disc and returns to its normal position. With continuous function, the condyle traumatizes the posterior loose tissue of the disc (bilaminar zone), or the junction between the disc and capsule, and inflammation occurs. Due to intra-articular swelling, the disc remains out of place. A vicious cycle is begun and it must be interrupted before tearing of the attachment or ligaments occurs.

Disc displacement with reduction may be caused by muscle incoordination, hyperlaxity of the capsule and ligaments, degenerative changes in the articulating surfaces, or a nonproportional relation between the sizes of the articulating components. A common etiological factor seems to be trauma.

Anterior Displacement without Reduction (Locking)

Two distinct forms of anterior displacement without reduction are clinically distinguishable, the acute form and the chronic form (Hansson, 1985b) (see Fig. 19–5). The acute form happens suddenly, although a history of clicking generally precedes the episode. The condition thus can be looked upon as a continuous process of wear and tear. The patient presents with acute pain due to an inflammatory response in the retrodiscal tissues. Mandibular movements are extremely painful. On opening of the mouth

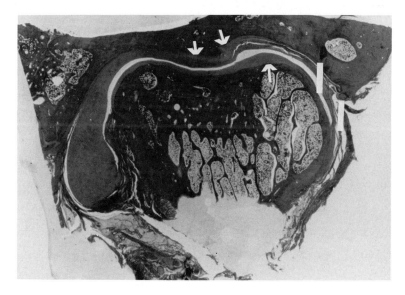

FIGURE 11–18. Coronal view of anteriorly and medially displaced left disc. Note large irregularities on the condyle and in the temporal component (arrows) as well as the medial extension of the lateral ligament (l). (From Solberg, W. K., and Hansson, T. L., Temporomandibular Joint Laboratory, UCLA Dental Research Institute, Los Angeles, California.)

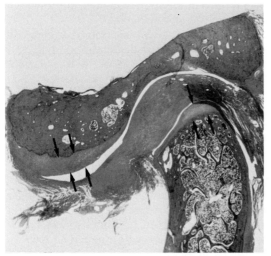

FIGURE 11–19. Anteriorly displaced left disc. Arrows denote soft tissue thickening on the condyle and of the temporal component. (From Solberg, W. K., and Hansson, T. L., Temporomandibular Joint Laboratory, UCLA Dental Research Institute, Los Angeles, California.)

(Fig. 11–20), as well as on protrusion (Fig. 11–21), the mandible deviates toward the affected side. Laterotrusion is possible toward the ipsilateral side, but reduced toward the contralateral side. The clinical findings are easy to comprehend as they all are the result of the articulating part of the disc being an impediment to intra-articular movement. The disc is

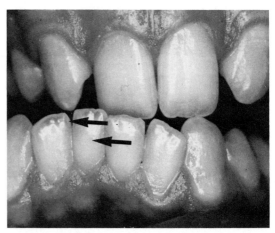

FIGURE 11–21. View of occlusion of patient in Figure 11–20 showing deviation of the midline toward the affected ipsilateral side on protrusion. Note relationship of upper and lower incisors. The right TMJ is involved.

caught in the anterior and medial part of the fossa (Figs. 11–18 and 11–22).

Anterior disc displacement without reduction is often the result of adverse loading of the TMJ causing failure of the retrodiscal tissue and the attachment of the disc to the lateral pole of the condyle. Another reason may be sudden trauma. In addition to the sudden stretching of the tissues that occurs, the acute inflammatory response, with edema of the loose disc tissue, causes anterior and medial displacement of the disc. This is true especially if originally there was hyperlaxity of the joint or if the injured

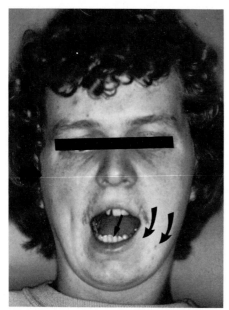

FIGURE 11–20. View of patient showing deviation to the side of disc displacement on opening. The right TMJ is involved.

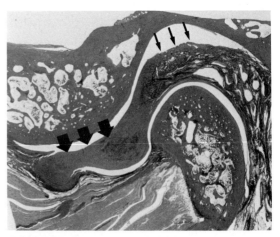

FIGURE 11–22. Anteriorly displaced disc. Small arrows denote the retrodiscal tissue stretched over the condyle superiorly, while the normal articulating part of the disc is locked in front of the condyle (large arrows). (From Solberg, W. K., and Hansson, T. L., Temporomandibular Joint Laboratory, UCLA Dental Research Institute, Los Angeles, California.)

disc was the intra-articular connection between a relatively small condyle and a normal-sized temporal component.

When there is a tearing of the loose retro-discal tissue, the displacement is most likely to remain permanent. When no tearing of the tissue is present, it is often possible to reposition the articulating part of the disc during the acute phase by manual traction of the condyle inferiorly and medially (Fig. 11–23). The procedure, however, can be extremely painful. If such manipulation is successful, a minor clicking sound usually is heard or felt by the operator when the disc slips back on the condyle. Following reduction, the mandibular opening movement is increased and no deviation occurs at the position of maximum opening of the mouth.

The chronic form of the anterior displacement without reduction presents the same clinical features as the acute form, except for the immediate excruciating pain. However, crepitation may occur if the posterior, loose retrodiscal tissue or the lateral attachment to the condyle is perforated. The deformed remnants of the disc remain as a permanent obstacle to mandibular movement.

RELATIONSHIPS BETWEEN DISC DERANGEMENTS AND DEGENERATIVE JOINT DISEASE

The results of autopsy studies (Åkerman, 1984; Axelsson, 1987; Öberg, 1971; Solberg, 1985) show that intra-articular changes in the TMJ are common in all age groups. Soft tissue changes from minor local elevations of the articulating surface to advanced degenerative changes with exposure of bone are seen. Thinned discs, with maintained biconcave form to completely deformed shapes, are also observed. Adaptation seems to be an ongoing process. Hence, the changes can be separated into either a stage of degeneration or a stage of regeneration.

Partial displacement of the disc is twice as common as total displacement in autopsy specimens (Solberg, 1985). Few studies report perforation of the posterior, loose retrodiscal tissue or perforation of the lateral attachment of the disc to the condyle. Perforation of the middle, dense part of the disc in sites juxtaposed to areas of recognized irregularity of the condyle, and to regions of the temporal component with degenerative changes, is common. Perforation is far less prevalent than displacement of the disc (Solberg, 1985).

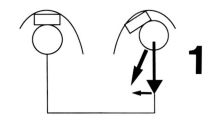

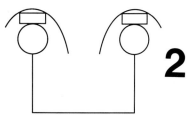

FIGURE 11–23. Schematic diagram showing traction on side with displaced disc (1). The condyle (O) is pushed inferiorly and medially to engage in the inferior biconcave surface of the disc (▭). Successful manipulation immediately restores the intra-articular relationship (2).

When displacement of the disc is present, adaptive changes are also visible in the condyle and in the temporal bone components. These local soft tissue changes precede the displacement of the disc and hence are a result of the previous changes.

The tissue changes in the condyle and the temporal component may decrease the intra-articular space. Through this reduction of space, the disc is exposed to the interfering deviations

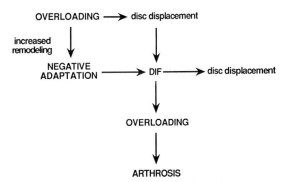

FIGURE 11–24. Schematic diagram of the probable development of TMJ arthrosis, denoting the relationship between derangements and degenerative joint disease (DIF = deviation in form).

in form during mandibular function. Therefore, it may be mechanically displaced by these juxtaposed irregularities. With time, the deteriorating changes reduce the elasticity of the retrodiscal tissues. The deformed articulating part of the disc then becomes located in the more spacious regions of the joint, anteriorly and medially, causing a locking.

With the variable tissue conditions and major discrepancies in size between the articulating components that exist, an initial displacement of the disc may also be the cause of a progressively increased loading of the other joint components. Under such circumstances, the displacement of the disc may precede the deviations in form (Fig. 11–24). When epidemiological data (Hansson, 1975) are taken into account, however, the incidence of TMJ sounds coincides with the prevalence of reported soft tissue irregularities.

CLINICAL CONSIDERATIONS

When pain is present, the primary task is to distinguish whether the pain is mainly arthrogenous or myogenous in origin (Hansson, 1980; 1988). TMJ clicking is common when the pain results from muscle incoordination and inflammation (Bezuur, 1988c). In the context of craniomandibular disorders, the muscular afflictions are definitely more prevalent than the established joint lesions (Naeije, 1986). The epidemiological data also support this concept when tenderness to palpation and the regions of described pain are considered.

The preliminary diagnosis of arthritis can often be confirmed with a screening radiograph (panoramic view), in which the total maxillomandibular relationship is seen. When bony changes have occurred, the arthritides are easily recognized as the radiograph reveals the established hard tissue changes in the posteroanterior diagonal section of the central and lateral parts of the joint (Habets, 1988). When no such alterations are visible, the joint problem may be caused by pure intra-articular soft tissue changes or inflammation in the surrounding muscles. When bilateral hard tissue changes are seen, and the clinical history has revealed symptoms in other joints of the body, a systemic disease must be suspected. Further medical examinations are then indicated.

Unilateral joint lesions, or a discrepancy between the magnitude, size, and extension of the hard tissue changes in the two joints, indicates that the changes have a functional basis.

Degenerative arthritis is to be expected when no symptoms have been reported in other joints. The clinical history, the analysis of the mandibular movements, and a correct evaluation of the presence of joint sounds differentiate the different stages of degenerative arthritis from the pure intra-articular disc derangements. No initial therapy should ever be started without a preliminary diagnosis.

SUMMARY

The pathological aspects of the arthritides and derangements involving the TMJ have been presented, with emphasis on clinical interpretation. The systemic diseases require assessment of the available data, medical consultation, and guidance. When more than one specialist is involved in the management of the disease, the most suitable or knowledgeable expert must be the leader. For treatment of degenerative arthritis or intra-articular disc derangements of the TMJ, the qualified dentist is appropriate. Research data on the biomechanics of the stomatognathic system support adverse loading of the system to be the main etiological factor in causing arthritis and disc derangements in the TMJ. Well-trained dentists can serve to diagnose the various conditions and participate in the team effort to manage and alleviate these sources of facial pain.

REFERENCES

Åkerman, S., Rohlin, M., and Kopp, S.: Bilateral degenerative changes and deviation in form of temporomandibular joints. An autopsy study of elderly individuals. Acta Odontol. Scand. 42:205–214, 1984.

The American Rheumatism Association, Section of the Arthritis Foundation AMA: Primer on the Rheumatic Diseases. In the Netherlands and Belgium: Gids voor de reumatologie, deel II. Nienhuis, R. L. F., Dequeker, J. V., de Blécourt, J. J. (Eds.): Bacteriële Arthritis. Leiden, Stafleu's Wetenschappelijke Uitgeversmaatschappij B. V., 1975, pp. 252–256.

Arnett, F. C.: Immunogenetics and rheumatic diseases. In McCarty, D. J. (Ed.): Arthritis and Allied Conditions. A Textbook of Rheumatology, 11th ed. Philadelphia, Lea & Febiger, 1989, pp. 453–464.

Axelsson, S., Fitins, D., Hellsing, G., and Holmlund, A.: Arthrotic changes and deviation in form of the temporomandibular joint—An autopsy study. Swed. Dent. J. 11:195–200, 1987.

Barnes, C. G.: Reumatoide arthritis. In Mason, M., and Currey, H. L. F. (Eds.): Klinische Reumatologie. (de Blécourt, J. J., van der Korst, J. K., Nienhuis, R. L. F.) Leiden, Stafleu's Wetenschappelijke Uitgeversmaatschappij B. V., 1973a, pp. 25–70.

Barnes, C. G.: Juvenile reumatoide arthritis. In Mason, M., and Currey, H. L. F. (Eds.): Klinische Reumatologie. (de Blécourt, J. J., van der Korst, J. K., Nienhuis,

R. L. F.) Leiden, Stafleu's Wetenschappelijke Uitgeversmaatschappij B. V., 1973b, pp. 71–80.

Bennett, J. C.: Etiology of rheumatic diseases. In Kelly, W. N., Harris, E. D. Jr., Ruddy, S., and Sledge, C. B., (Eds.): Textbook of Rheumatology, 3rd ed. Philadelphia, W. B. Saunders, 1989, pp. 138–147.

Bezuur, J. N., Habets, L. L. M. H., and Hansson, T. L.: The recognition of craniomandibular disorders—A comparison between clinical, tomographical and dental panoramic radiographical findings in thirty-one subjects. J. Oral Rehabil. 15:549–554, 1988a.

Bezuur, J. N., Habets, L. L. M. H., Jimenez Lopez, V., et al.: The recognition of craniomandibular disorders—A comparison between clinical and radiographic findings in eighty-nine subjects. J. Oral Rehabil. 15:215–221, 1988b.

Boland, E. W.: Ankylosing spondylitis. In Hollander, J. L. (Ed.): Arthritis and Allied Conditions, 7th ed. Philadelphia, Lea & Febiger, 1969, pp. 633–656.

Carlsson, G. E., Kopp, S., and Öberg, T.: Arthritis and allied diseases of the temporomandibular joint. In Zarb, G. A., and Carlsson, G. E. (Eds.): Temporomandibular Joint: Function and Dysfunction. Copenhagen, Munksgaard, 1979, pp. 269–320.

Carter, M. E.: Epidemiology. In Moll, J. M. H. (Ed.): Ankylosing Spondylitis. Edinburgh, Churchill-Livingstone, 1980, pp. 16–25.

Currey, H. L. F.: Jicht en chondrocalcinose. In Mason, M., and Currey, H. L. F. (Eds.): Klinische Reumatologie. (de Blécourt, J. J., van der Korst, J. K., Nienhuis, R. L. F.) Leiden, Stafleu's Wetenschappelijke Uitgeversmaatschappij, B. V., 1973, pp. 177–206.

Farrar, W. B., and McCarty Jr, W. L.: A Clinical Outline of Temporomandibular Joint Diagnosis and Treatment, 7th ed. Montgomery, Normandie Publications, 1982.

Grennan, D. M.: Rheumatology. London, Balliere's Concise Medical Textbooks, 1984, pp. 20–35.

Habets, L. L. M. H., Bezuur, J. N., Naeije, M., and Hansson, T. L.: The orthopantomogram, an aid in diagnosis of temporomandibular joint problems. II. The vertical symmetry. J. Oral Rehabil. 15:465–471, 1988.

Hansson, T.: Temporomandibular Joint Changes: Occurrence and Development. Thesis, University of Lund, Malmö, Sweden, 1977.

Hansson, T.: Craniomandibular disorders and sequencing their treatment. Aust. Prosthod. J. 2:9–15, 1988.

Hansson, T.: Infrared laser in the treatment of craniomandibular disorders arthrogenous pain. J. Prosthet. Dent. 61:614–617, 1989.

Hansson, T., and Nilner, M.: A study of the occurrence of symptoms of diseases of the temporomandibular joint, masticatory musculature and related structures. J. Oral Rehabil. 2:313–324, 1975.

Hansson, L. G., Hansson, T., and Petersson, A.: A Comparison between clinical and radiologic findings in 259 temporomandibular joint patients. J. Prosthet. Dent. 50:89–94, 1983.

Hansson, T., Honée, W., and Hesse, J.: Craniomandibulaire Dysfunctie. Samsom Stafleu, Alphen aan den Rijn/Brussel, 1985a, pp. 86–88.

Hansson, T., Honée, W., and Hesse, J.: Craniomandibulaire Dysfunctie. Samsom Stafleu, Alphen aan den Rijn/Brussel, 1985b, pp. 92–93.

Hansson, T., Solberg, W. K., Penn, M. K., and Öberg, T.: Anatomic study of the TMJs of young adults. A pilot investigation. J. Prosthet. Dent. 41:556–560, 1979.

Hansson, T., Wessman, C., and Öberg, T.: Säkrare diagnoser med ny teknik. Förslag till funktionsbedömning av käkleder och tuggmuskler. Tandläkartidning 72:1372–1374, 1980.

Heir, G. M., Berett, A., and Worth, D. A.: Diagnosis and management of TMJ involvement in ankylosing spondylitis. J. Craniomandib. Pract. 1:75–81, 1983.

Hylander, W. L.: An experimental analysis of temporomandibular joint reaction force in Macaques. Am. J. Phys. Anthropol. 51:433–456, 1979.

Jessop, J. D.: Infecties van gewrichten. In Mason, M., and Currey, H. L. F. (Eds.): Klinische Reumatologie (de Blécourt, J. J., van der Korst, J. K., Nienhuis, R. L. F.) Leiden, Stafleu's Wetenschappelijke Uitgeversmaatschappij B. V., 1973, pp. 207–215.

Kobayashi, Y.: Influences of occlusal interference on human body. J. Int. Coll. Dent. 13:56–64, 1982. (Jpn)

Könönen, M.: Craniomandibular disorders in psoriatic arthritis. Correlations between subjective symptoms, clinical signs and radiographic changes. Acta Odontol. Scand. 44:377–383, 1986.

Könönen, M.: Clinical signs of craniomandibular disorders in patients with psoriatic arthritis. Scand. J. Dent. Res. 95:340–346, 1987a.

Könönen, M.: Radiographic changes in the condyle of the temporomandibular joint in psoriatic arthritis. Acta Radiol. 28:185–188, 1987b.

Korst, J. K. V. D.: Gewrichtsziekten. Utrecht, Bohn, Scheltema & Holkema, 1982.

Larheim, T. A., and Haanes, H. R.: Micrognathia, TMJ changes and occlusion in juvenile rheumatoid arthritis of adolescents and adults. Scand. J. Res. 89:329–338, 1981.

Larheim, T. A., Storhaug, K., and Tveito, L.: Temporomandibular joint involvement and dental occlusion in a group of adults with rheumatoid arthritis. Acta Odont. Scand. 41:301–309, 1983.

Little, J. W.: Psoriatic arthritis of the TMJ. Oral Surg. 53:351–357, 1987.

Lubsen, C. C., Hansson, T. L., Nordström, B. B., and Solberg, W. K.: Histomorphometric analysis of cartilage and subchondral bone in mandibular condyles of young adults at autopsy. Arch. Oral Biol. 30:129–136, 1985.

Lysell, L.: Epidemiologisk röntgendiagnostisk undersökning av tänder, käkar och käkleder hos 67-åringar i Dalby. Thesis, University of Lund, Malmö, Sweden, 1977.

MacLeod, J.: Davidson's Principles and Practice of Medicine. Edinburgh, Churchill-Livingstone, 1984, pp. 551–590.

Mason, M.: Seronegatieve Gewrichtsaandoeningen. In Mason, M., and Currey, H. L. F. (Eds.): Klinische Reumatologie. (de Blécourt, J. J., van der Korst, J. K., Nienhuis, R. L. F.) Leiden, Stafleu's Wetenschappelijke Uitgeversmaatschappij B. V., 1973, pp. 81–112.

McCarroll, R. S.: Muscle Balance and Occlusion. Thesis. University of Amsterdam, Amsterdam, 1988.

Mongini, F.: Remodelling of the mandibular condyle in the adult and its relationship to the condition of the dental arches. Acta Anat. 82:437–453, 1972.

Naeije, M., and Hansson, T. L.: Electromyographic screening of myogenous and arthrogenous TMJ dysfunction patients. J. Oral Rehabil. 13:433–441, 1986.

Öberg, T., Carlsson, G. E., and Fajers, C. M.: The temporomandibular joint. A morphologic study on a human autopsy material. Acta Odontol. Scand. 29:349–384, 1971.

Randow, K., Carlsson, K., Edlund, J., and Öberg, T.: The effect of an occlusal interference on the masticatory system. Odontol. Rev. 27:245–256, 1976.

Richards, L. C., and Brown, T.: Dental attrition and degenerative arthritis of the temporomandibular joint. J. Oral Rehabil. 8:293–307, 1981.

Sarnat, B. G., and Laskin, D. M.: Surgery of the temporomandibular joint. In Sarnat, B. G., and Laskin, D. M. (Eds.): The Temporomandibular Joint, A Biological Basis for Clinical Practice, 4th ed. Philadelphia, W.B. Saunders, 1991.

Scully, C., and Cawson, R. A.: Medical Problems in Dentistry. Bristol, Wright PSG, 1982, pp. 405–417.

Solberg, W. K.: Temporomandibular disorders: clinical significance of TMJ changes. Br. Dent. J. 160:231–236, 1986a.

Solberg, W. K., Bibb, C. A., Nordström, B. B., and Hansson, T. L.: Malocclusion associated with temporomandibular joint changes in young adults at autopsy. Am. J. Orthod. 89:326–330, 1986b.

Solberg, W. K., Hansson, T. L., and Nordström, B.: The temporomandibular joint in young adults at autopsy: A morphologic classification and evaluation. J. Oral Rehabil. 12:303–321, 1985.

Syrjäneen, S. M.: The temporomandibular joint in rheumatoid arthritis. Acta Radiol. [Diagn.] 26:235–243, 1985.

Tegelberg, Å.: Temporomandibular Joint Involvement in Rheumatoid Arthritis, A clinical study. Thesis, University of Lund, Malmö, Sweden, 1987a.

Tegelberg, Å., and Kopp, S.: Subjective symptoms from the stomatognathic system in individuals with rheumatoid arthritis and osteoarthrosis. Swed. Dent. J. 11:11–22, 1987b.

Tegelberg, Å., Kopp, S., Huddenius, K., and Forssman, L.: Relationship between disorder in the stomatognathic system and general joint involvement in individuals with rheumatoid arthritis. Acta Odont. Scand. 45:1–8, 1987c.

Wenneberg, B.: Inflammatory Involvement of the Temporomandibular Joint. Diagnostic and Therapeutic Aspects and a Study of Individuals with Ankylosing Spondylitis. Thesis. Universities of Göteborg and Lund, Göteborg and Malmö, Sweden, 1983.

Wood, N., and Stankler, L.: Psoriatic arthritis of the TMJ. Br. Dent. J. 154:17–18, 1983.

Worth, H. M.: Radiology of the Temporomandibular Joint. In Zarb, G. A., and Carlsson, G. E. (Eds.): Temporomandibular Joint: Function and Dysfunction. Copenhagen, Munksgaard, 1979, pp. 321–372.

12

CONGENITAL AND DEVELOPMENTAL ANOMALIES*

*DAVID POSWILLO, C.B.E., D.D.S., D.Sc., M.Dнс, F.D.S., F.R.C.Pатн.,
and PAUL ROBINSON, B.D.S., M.B., B.S., F.D.S.R.C.S.*

INTRODUCTION

Congenital malformations of the temporo-mandibular joints (TMJs) have been known and recorded since the first drawings were scratched on rock walls by primitive cave dwellers. It

*See Chapters 1, 3, 4, 10, 13, 16, 24, and 26.

seems unlikely, however, that the relationship between the dysmorphology of the joints and the pattern of malformation was then known or understood. Nonetheless, the abnormal facies associated with those malformations that involved both temporomandibular structures and their close embryological companion and neigh-

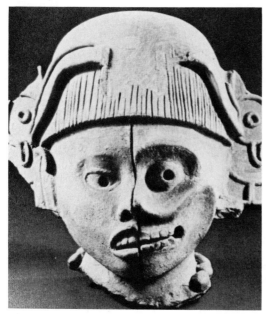

FIGURE 12–1. Photograph of pre-Colombian terra cotta decoration from a funerary urn showing facial characteristics of craniofacial microsomia.

bor, the ear, have been recorded by artists of early civilizations (Fig. 12–1). There is folklore suggesting that individuals with abnormal facies were regarded as superior beings. Possessed of normal intelligence and a strikingly different appearance, they were automatically set apart from, and above, the remainder of their tribe. This is not true in present civilizations.

In the past 25 years, there has been a steadily increasing amount of literature on the psychological importance of physical, especially facial, appearance. Macgregor (1970) referred to individuals with otomandibular deformities as the marginal or forgotten people with defects that, unlike many other physical handicaps, cannot be lost during conversation. The psychological problems increase as the child reaches puberty, an age when facial appearance is of great personal significance. Thus, the recognition, prevention and treatment of congenital malformations of the TMJ are matters of considerable significance not only to those born deformed but also to all those responsible for providing total health care.

Errors of Development

The embryological development of the TMJ has been described in detail in Chapter 3. There are, however, several significant aspects of morphogenesis that bear a special relationship to the mechanisms of abnormal development of the condyle and glenoid fossa. These are an essential introduction to the understanding of abnormal morphogenesis or teratogenesis.

The time sequence of morphodifferentiation bears an important relationship to the pathogenesis of malformation. The teratogen-sensitive period for most body structures begins at about day 20 of human embryonic development and concludes at about day 45. In comparison with synovial joints in other parts of the body, the TMJ develops late. When the knee, hip, and elbow joints all resemble their adult form, the morphodifferentiation of the TMJ has barely commenced. Moreover, whereas most human joints pursue a direct developmental course to adult form, the TMJ passes through stages in development that are reminiscent of patterns seen in the evolutionary development of the jaw. The expanded time sequence and the circuitous course of development of the jaw joint do not reduce the teratogen sensitivity of the developing structures. However, a long or complex sequence of developmental stages may enable a joint affected by teratogenic influences to catch up to its normal developmental stage before the full sequence of differentiation is switched off by the genetic program. The relative rarity of congenital anomalies of the TMJs in comparison with other human synovial joints suggests that the latter possibility may operate to the advantage of these, the most essential of human joints.

There are specific stages in the morphogenesis of the TMJs when the risk of malformation may be particularly high (see Chapter 3.) The first of these coincides with the development of the cartilaginous bar of Meckel's cartilage in the mandibular arch. This condensation occurs in mesenchyme that is derived, to a large degree, from cells that have migrated to the first visceral arch from the neural crest. In the branchial arch, these cells combine with preaxial mesoderm to provide the basis for the visceral arch cartilages. The migration and mixing of neural crest ectomesenchyme takes place at about day 20 in the human embryo. Any disturbance to the migration or mingling of the neural crest-derived cells may disturb the subsequent differentiation of the mandibular condyle. The pattern of development of the TMJs differs from that found in other joints where segmentation occurs in a continuous rudiment at the joint destined to become the hinge. Usually, the original cartilage model is eventually replaced by bone, except for the articular cartilage, which is incorporated into the joint. This pattern is not followed by the TMJ where the temporal and mandibular components arise separately rather than from one continuous cartilaginous predecessor.

Some time after the mingling of the neural crest-derived cells and the preaxial mesoderm cells of the first branchial arch, the Meckelian joint becomes incorporated in the development of the ear. About this time, several areas of membrane bone appear on the cranial side of the joint. This marks the second stage of joint formation, the origin of the glenoid fossa. It appears likely that the squamous temporal bone develops in tissue that has a large but different contribution from cells that also migrate, at a later stage, from the neural crest. Disturbance in this later migration could also disturb the normal patterns of development of the upper compartment of the TMJ.

During the morphogenesis of the TMJ, there is an important relationship between it and the developing auditory apparatus. There is a common region of origin for the TMJ and the structures of the middle and external ear. Not only do all these structures derive from mesenchymal tissues around the first branchial arch, but also, from about day 32 to 42 of development, they share a common blood supply from the stapedial arterial stem. This is a stopgap system of vascularization that assumes responsibility for the blood supply of structures developing in the first and second branchial arches after the closure of the first and second aortic arches and before the stapedial system is definitively annexed by the emerging external carotid artery in the neck (soon after day 40 of human development). The stapedial artery, which supplies the regions of the mandibular condyle and middle ear during this stage of development, finally disappears in the human between day 40 and 50 of prenatal life.

The initial association of the developing TMJ and middle and external ears explains the frequent combination of malformations of these parts. Developmental failure of any of these tissues, or failure of their blood supply, may result in associated malformations in neighboring parts derived from similar embryological antecedents.

Scope of Vulnerability in Development

While errors in morphogenesis account for a considerable proportion of TMJ developmental anomalies, they do not account for all. Dysmorphology may arise from events such as deformation by mechanical pressure acting in utero

after the TMJ is fully formed. Additionally, formed structures may be disrupted by physical, mechanical, or chemical influences before birth, and finally events may occur in utero that have a significant effect, short-term or long-term, on the normal patterns of postnatal growth and development.

There is, as yet, little clear evidence to explain dysplasia as it influences the growth and form of the condyle. Until more is known about the role of the condylar cartilage in growth of the mandible, little can be said about the factors that may delay or accelerate condylar growth. Yet significant dysplasias are readily identified and categorized. Future research in this area would profit from analysis of mechanisms that could have a profound effect on the rate of proliferation of the cells of the condylar cartilage both in utero and during subsequent growth and development.

Intrauterine Growth Failure

There has been much speculation on the effects of intrauterine growth retardation or failure on the development of the fetus as a whole; little attention has been given to effects on structures such as the TMJ although much is known about effects on contiguous structures such as the cerebral hemispheres.

Range of Abnormal Variations in Form

Anomalous development may vary from complete agenesis or induced absence of the condyle, unilaterally or bilaterally, to changes in size and shape seen in the growth dysplasias in which hyperplasia and hypertrophy have been implicated. While basic classic types of either condylar underdevelopment or overdevelopment have clearly been described, there also exist mixed forms in which neither the pathogenesis nor the ultimate description can be clarified. Such confusion exists particularly in bilateral craniofacial microsomia and variations in hemimandibular hyperplasia, where abnormal shortening of the mandible on the lesser or unaffected side and corresponding changes in the size and shape of the condyle exist. The extreme range is expressed in a case of hyperplasia of one condyle and either one or another of the hemimandibular overgrowth dysplasias on the other (Obwegeser, 1986). Another mixed anomaly is hemimandibular elongation on one side and hemimandibular hyperplasia on the other. Until such time as the pathogenetic mechanisms of such obscure developmental anomalies are resolved, it will be impossible to provide a correct biological description of the individual variations in form.

THE CONDYLE

Malformations

General Variations in Expression

Although the sources of individual variations in growth of the TMJ have not yet been completely identified, evidence is accumulating on the general patterns of growth of the face that lead to specific facial types. Gasson (1977) and Houston (1988) have described rotation patterns of the maxilla and mandible that influence the ultimate form and position of the skeletal components and hence the shape of the face. Within the range of normal variation considerable differences are found in the size and shape of the condyle, the depth and breadth of the glenoid fossa, and the prominence of the articular eminence. Even in many extreme variations of form such as prognathism or severe retrognathism, the morphology of the TMJ may be considered to be within normal limits. It is when these variations extend beyond the rather arbitrary range of normal variation, or can be grouped within a number of other markers to constitute a recognized malformation syndrome, that dysmorphogenesis of the TMJ can be established and cataloged.

Growth, in the broadest sense, is a composite of five developmental events: the origin of craniofacial tissues, mainly from the neural crest; the migration of committed craniofacial cells to their finite site in the embryo, that is the TMJ; the localization of these cells at these sites, chiefly in response to extracellular matrix products associated with the developing neuroepithelium; differentiation of cartilage and bone in response to epigenetic evocation from matrix products associated with embryonic epithelia; and morphogenesis of skeletal elements that appear to be preprogrammed but that can be molded into altered shapes by epigenetic influences during development. Given the countless opportunities for variation in regulation of all these processes in a three-dimensional developing organism modulated by a one-dimensional genetic code, it is not surprising to find variations in expression of TMJ morphology from complete absence to gross hypertrophy or hyperplasia.

Syndromic Patterns

A malformation syndrome exists when a group of signs and symptoms occur together and are considered characteristic of that particular abnormality. In the main, in establishing syndromic patterns of maldevelopment in the TMJ, the difficulty comes in assembling, logistically, multiple cases of rare disorders and making the fine distinction between coincidence and causal association. The problems are contributed to by genetic heterogeneity and the fact that some features of given syndromes are not invariably present. Recognition of TMJ syndromes is slow and probably far from complete. Because the identification of a syndrome cannot be considered complete until the cause is defined, syndromic patterns described in this section are limited to those that have explanations of either the causal mechanism or evidence of a Mendelian basis for the anomaly. They are grouped on the basis of the likely mechanism, in broad terms, for this arrangement may offer the clinician a significant understanding of the likely response of the problem to various types of clinical intervention.

Facial Microsomia (Craniofacial Microsomia, First or Second Arch Syndrome, Lateral Facial Dysplasia)

Facial asymmetry due to hypoplasia of tissues in the first and second branchial arch territory is the hallmark of this malformation. In about 70 per cent of cases, the principal abnormalities of ear and jaw are unilateral, while the remaining 30 per cent also show lesser deformities of the contralateral side (Ross, 1975). Facial microsomia occurs once in about 3500 live births, the sexes are equally affected, and there is no discernable genetic background. Most cases are sporadic, but familial trends have been noted. The most frequently involved structures are the TMJ, mandibular ramus, middle and external ear, zygoma, parotid gland, facial nerve, and masticatory muscles (Fig. 12–2).

The mandibular deformities involve the upper compartment of the TMJ, the condyle, and the ramus. Only occasionally is the body of the mandible anterior to the antegonial notch affected. The most severe cases show complete agenesis of the ramus and condyle (Fig. 12–2). Such severely affected mandibles grow less than normal, in particular when the muscles of mastication are rudimentary and function is thereby limited. In this way the asymmetry of the face becomes progressively worse as growth pro-

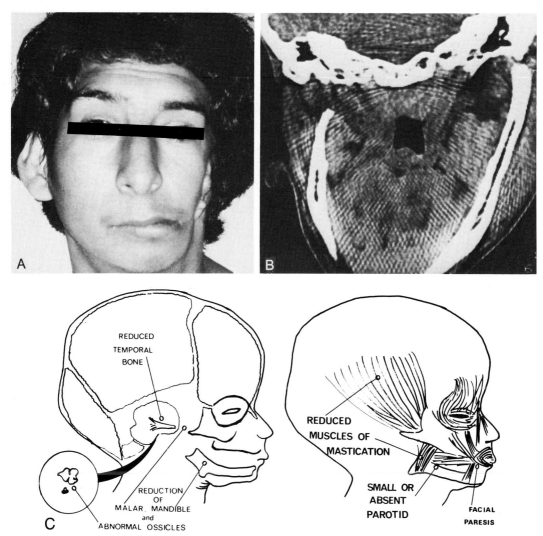

FIGURE 12–2. A, Photograph, B, computed tomography scan, and C, diagrams of spectrum of defects of severe unilateral facial microsomia.

ceeds. In the least severe cases, a normal condyle may be present in an abnormal fossa. Mildly affected subjects may show defects in the tympanic plate (posterior boundary of the fossa), ranging from a central window to a complete absence of that bone. Visible deformity in these mild cases may be limited to abnormalities of the external ear (microtia). A useful diagnostic radiologic feature is the lowering of the tegmen tympani often seen in facial microsomia (Phelps, 1983) (Fig. 12–3).

Between these extremes, variations in size and shape of the condyle and the glenoid fossa are seen (Lauritzen, 1985) (Fig. 12–4). These defects may be observed on one or both sides of the jaw. When bilateral they are invariably asymmetrical, an important point in the diagnosis of bilateral otomandibular deformity.

Poswillo (1973; 1974; 1975a) demonstrated on an animal model that unselected destruction of differentiating tissues in the vicinity of the ear and jaw by an expanding hematoma produced the characteristic defects of this anomaly. The causative event took place at the time of rapid differentiation of structures designed to form the functional matrix of the craniofacial complex. The disruptive effect on initial morphology and subsequent growth was first related to the degree of local destruction and second to the degree of catch-up differentiation in that brief interval before the end of genetically programmed morphogenesis. In minor cases, where the hemorrhage was small and localized close to the original site (at the anastomosis forming the stapedial artery stem), only minimal damage was done to the otomandibular structures (Fig. 12–5).

Minor defects were observed in the outer

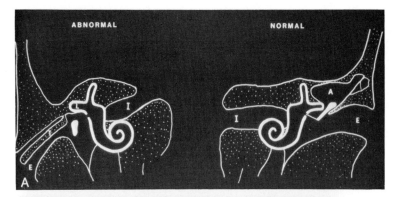

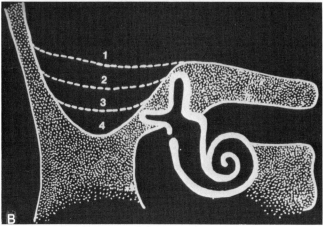

FIGURE 12–3. *A*, Diagram of middle ear defects of auditory canal and tegmen in facial microsomia compared with normal ear and *B*, variations in levels of severity of descent of the tegmen tympani in mild to severe facial microsomia.

and middle ear and condyloid process of the mandible, but the integrity of the principal growth determinant, the muscle-bone-periosteal matrix, was only slightly impaired. In severe cases, where the hematoma was extensive, vast tracts of tissue destined to form ramus and masticatory muscles were obliterated. The size of the hematoma delayed resorption of the debris and subsequent repair, with the result that severe damage was done to the ear, orbit, mandible, and the masticatory and facial musculature (Fig. 12–6).

Some patients with facial microsomia have malformations of other structures, notably vertebral anomalies, and cleft palate and cardiac defects. Some authors believe facial microsomia to be part of a spectrum of phenotypic expression that includes Goldenhar's syndrome.

Goldenhar's Syndrome (Oculoauriculovertebral Dysplasia)

The fundamental pattern of asymmetrical facial deformity seen in Goldenhar's syndrome is

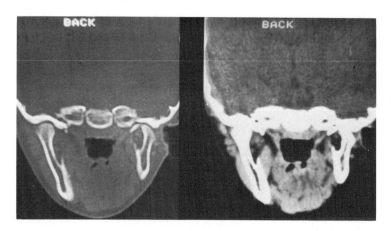

FIGURE 12–4. Computed tomography scan of normal and hypoplastic condyles in hemifacial microsomia.

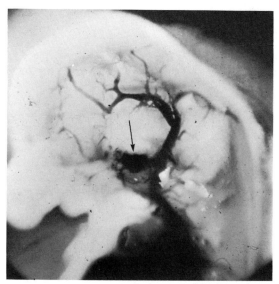

FIGURE 12–5. A facial hematoma (arrow) at site of origin of stapedial arterial stem in mouse model of facial microsomia on day 14 of development.

It seems likely that the pathogenesis of the facial deformity (including the TMJ) in Goldenhar's syndrome is similar to that in facial microsomia; the other defects remain unexplained. Overlap of phenotypical expression between Goldenhar's and the autosomal dominant, branchio-oto-renal syndrome has been described by Rollnick (1987), and various aberrant karyotypes have been noted in Goldenhar's syndrome (Herman, 1988). However, the pattern of sporadic occurrence and the discordance seen in monozygotic twins (Burck, 1983) point to a postgenetic event. In both facial microsomia and Goldenhar's syndrome, the impact of the deficiencies in facial tissues, in particular the masticatory apparatus, on growth and development of the facial skeleton is profound. Limited masticatory function resulting from hypoplasia of the TMJ may itself be the cause of the exaggerating deformity as growth proceeds.

the same as that of facial microsomia, hypoplasia of the TMJ, mandibular ramus, and ear being common features. However, additional malformations comprising facial skin tags, epibulbar dermoids, and vertebral anomalies distinguish Goldenhar's syndrome (Fig. 12–7). Many authors have suggested that these two conditions represent varying expressions of the same pathological entity, with between 10 and 15 per cent of cases falling within the Goldenhar group (Rollnick, 1987; Ross, 1975). Defects in other organ systems (notably cardiovascular and genitourinary) are seen in about 50 per cent, and cleft palate in about seven to 15 per cent of patients.

Nager-Reynier Syndrome (Acrofacial Dysostosis)

The abnormalities of the TMJ observed in the Nager-Reynier syndrome closely resemble those found in facial microsomia, but maldevelopment is limited to the TMJ (which may be hypoplastic or absent) and the mandibular ramus. There is usually bilateral abnormality without symmetry. The characteristic that distinguishes this condition from facial microsomia is the absence of auricular or temporal bone maldevelopment. Acrofacial dysostosis is unlikely to constitute an independent malformation syndrome, as the anomalies observed are similar to those of facial microsomia where the

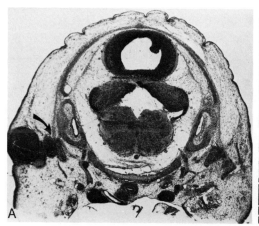
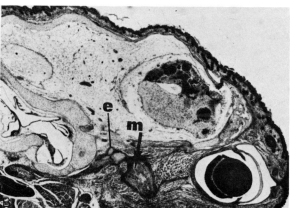

FIGURE 12–6. *A*, Localized hematoma in frontal section of tissues of right otomandibular region at day 14 of embryonic development. Note extrusion of blood clot medially to involve developing mandibular condyle (arrows). *B*, Hypoplastic changes in condyle and coronoid process (m) and fused middle ear ossicles (e) following damage by local hematoma.

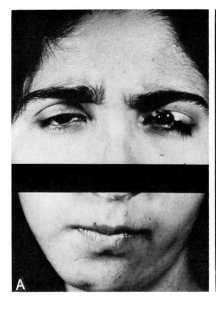
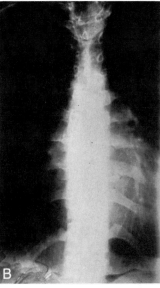

FIGURE 12–7. A, Mandibular underdevelopment and upper eyelid coloboma and B, rib and cervical spine anomalies, all features of Goldenhar's syndrome.

condyle alone, rather than the whole otomandibular apparatus, has been affected by focal hematoma formation.

Treacher Collins Syndrome (Mandibulofacial Dysostosis)

The Treacher Collins syndrome presents a characteristically symmetrical bilateral facial deformity recognized by the antimongoloid slope of the palpebral fissures, a hypoplastic mandible, deficient malar bones, and low-set, deformed ears (Fig. 12–8A and B). About 50 per cent of cases are inherited as an autosomal trait with complete penetrance; the remaining cases occur as spontaneous mutations. While the penetrance of the gene is 100 per cent, the degree of severity varies widely, even within the same family.

The TMJs exhibit hypoplasia that is usually symmetrical. It affects all elements of the joints without limiting their function. The condyle shows changes varying between near normality and complete agenesis, but is often small with a short or nonexistent neck. Its articulation with the glenoid fossa may be medially positioned and the articular eminence flattened. Although classically described as symmetrical, the skeletal changes in some patients with Treacher Collins syndrome have been shown on computed tomography scans to vary between left and right sides (Marsh, 1986). In these unusual asymmetrical forms it may be difficult to distinguish between mandibulofacial dysostosis and bilateral facial microsomia. The diagnostic distinction lies entirely in the characteristic changes observed in the middle ear in these two different conditions (Phelps, 1981) (Fig.

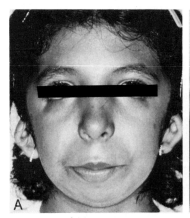
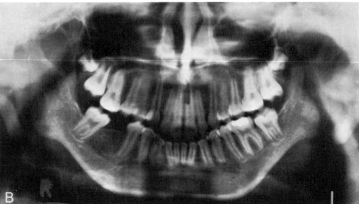

FIGURE 12–8. A, Facial characteristics and B, radiographic features of Treacher Collins syndrome.

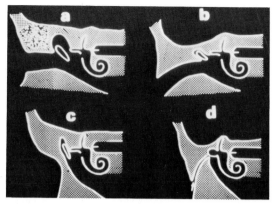

FIGURE 12–9. Four characteristic examples of anomalous development of the middle ear in Treacher Collins syndrome; note minimal descent of the tegmen tympani.

12–9). The ramus and body of the mandible are small, producing retrogenia that is further exaggerated by a high gonial angle and downward bowing of the lower border. The mandibular notch is shallow and the coronoid process frequently abnormal.

An animal model of the Treacher Collins syndrome has been described by Poswillo (1975b). The administration of 100,000 I.U. of water soluble vitamin A to pregnant Wistar rats on day 8.5 of development leads to a 100 per cent incidence in the offspring of otomandibular defects characteristic of the human Treacher Collins syndrome (Fig. 12–10). A reduction in the dosage of the teratogen has recently been found by the same author to produce bilateral asymmetry in the model of mandibulofacial dysostosis.

Observations on the serial stages of embryological development in the experimental animals indicated that the mechanism of malformation was early destruction of the neural crest cells of the facial and auditory primordia before their migration to the first and second branchial arches. Sulik (1987) using the vitamin A-like compound 13-*cis*-retinoic acid as a teratogen in mice, also found abnormalities in the region of the first and second branchial arches and the first branchial cleft, concluding that excessive cell death in these regions following migration from the neural crest was the causative mechanism (Fig. 12–11).

This cellular deficiency in the neighborhood of the optic cup enables surrounding tissues to flow toward the damaged region, resulting in a relocation of the otic pit from its position adjacent to the second branchial arch into first arch territory. Thus the future ear is over the angle of the mandible rather than further back on the head. The loss of ectomesenchymal neural crest cells from the developing face leads to hypoplasia of both skeletal and soft tissue elements of the face, jaw, and ear. That these structures are not totally absent is probably due to the survival of some of the neural crest cells and also to the contribution made by the lateral plate mesoderm.

Hallermann-Streiff Syndrome (Oculomandibulodyscephaly)

Facial deformity resembling Treacher Collins syndrome, as well as skull vault abnormalities (scaphocephaly), eye defects (congenital cataract), and proportionate dwarfism, characterize this rare syndrome in which virtually all cases occur sporadically. The face appears small in relation to the skull, the mandible is narrow,

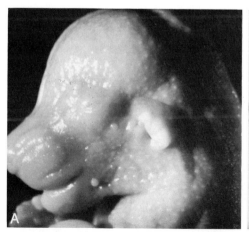

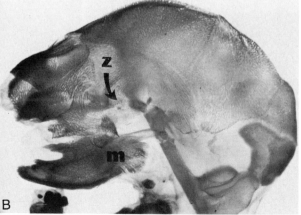

FIGURE 12–10. *A*, Abnormality of low-set ear and symmetrical maxillary and mandibular hypoplasia in rat model of Treacher Collins syndrome (day 20 of development). *B*, Alizarin-stained skull of rat head shown in A; note abnormalities in ramus of mandible (m) and deficient zygomatic arch (z).

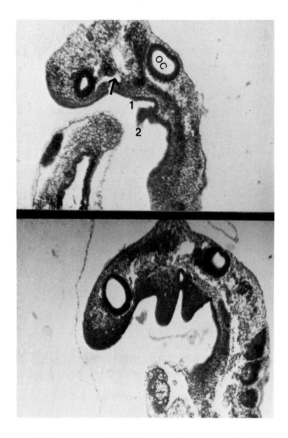

FIGURE 12–11. Normal embryo (bottom) and "Treacher Collins" rat embryo (top) showing severe loss of neural crest cells in mesencephalon (arrow), reduced branchial arch development (1,2), and upward drift of otocyst (oc) in the phenocopy of the syndrome.

and the nose is beaked, resulting in a bird-like facies (Fig. 12–12). Both bony elements of the TMJ may be hypoplastic, the condyle often being absent, and the whole joint is displaced anteriorly. In contradistinction to Treacher Collins syndrome, where the hypoplastic condyles have a normal antero-posterior relationship to the fossa, in Hallermann-Streiff syndrome the hypoplastic condyles articulate with the articular eminence (Friede, 1985). Despite this malposition of the TMJ, the underdevelopment of the mandibular ramus and body results in a class II incisor relationship, often with an anterior open bite.

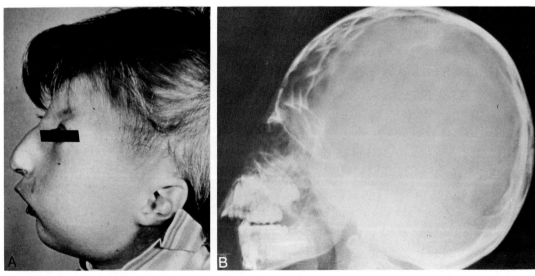

FIGURE 12–12. *A*, Photograph and *B*, radiograph of the Hallermann-Streiff facies. Note underdevelopment of mandible and anterior displacement of condyles.

Although the pathogenesis of this condition is not yet described, it seems likely that mechanisms similar to those thought to cause destruction to neural crest tissue in Treacher Collins syndrome may be at work.

Thalidomide Otomandibular Dysostosis

The combination of aural atresia and partial agenesis of the mandibular condyle and fossa was induced by the sedative thalidomide in about 30 per cent of all children with the characteristic thalidomide limb embryopathy (Kleinsasser, 1964). The variety of defects in the outer and middle ears and TMJ was similar to that found in the less severe cases of facial microsomia (Fig. 12–13). Rarely was the condyle absent, although the finding of condylar hypoplasia was common. The truncated condyle is posteriorly placed in the fossa in the position usually occupied by the endaural cartilage, which is absent. There are frequent bony defects between the middle ear and the glenoid fossa, and there may be facial palsy or paresis, although the course of the facial nerve is not grossly aberrant (Livingstone, 1965; Phelps, 1974).

Fetal Alcohol Syndrome

Children with this anomaly are the offspring of severely and chronically alcoholic women. The principal defects are CNS dysfunction, growth deficiency, and craniofacial anomalies.

The mandible is generally small at birth, and ear anomalies also occur in conjunction with some hypoplasia of the mandibular condyles. Posterior rotation of the helix is common and alteration in conchal shape occurs occasionally. In some cases, catch-up growth of the jaws is greater than that of the severely hypoplastic midfacial structures, so that an apparent prognathism may be observed at adolescence. It is unlikely that the condition would be confused with any other syndromic pattern of ear and jaw because of the characteristic facies found, especially the diminished or absent philtrum of the lip.

Deformations

Pierre Robin Anomaly and Pierre Robin Sequence

These conditions are characterized by a primary retrognathism that, in association with isolated cleft palate and glossoptosis, create severe management problems in the neonatal period. The principal distinction between the anomaly and the sequence is the association in the sequence of multiple congenital anomalies that comprise a recognized syndrome.

The causal mechanism for the anomaly is explained on the basis of animal experiments (Poswillo, 1966) in which the loss of amniotic fluid causes the lower border of the mandible to be compressed against the sternum, molding the anterior mandible and, by a domino effect,

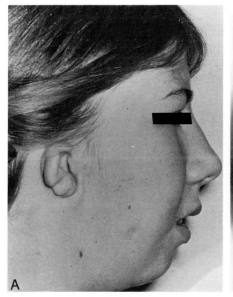 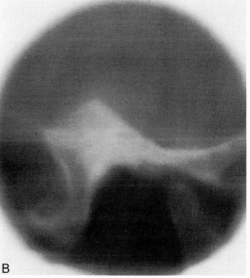

A   B

FIGURE 12–13. *A*, Photograph and *B*, radiograph of temporomandibular region in thalidomide otomandibular dysostosis. Note in A the similarity to facial microsomia, and in B the bony changes in the fossa.

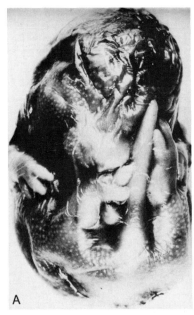
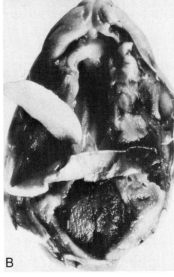

FIGURE 12–14. *A*, Postural deformation of mandible against the sternum and *B*, tongue impaction in palatal U-cleft in Pierre Robin anomaly phenocopy.

FIGURE 12–15. (*A*) Normal ovoid developing condyle and (*B*) compressed spherical condyle in phenocopy of Pierre Robin anomaly at 20 days (rat).

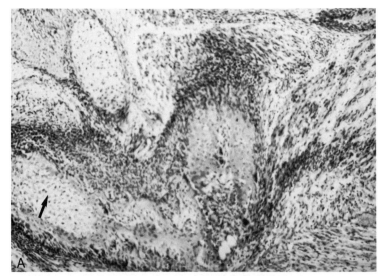
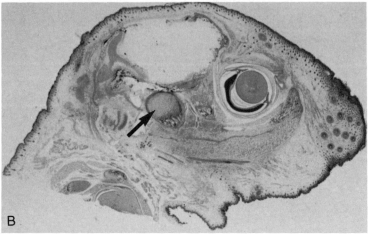

the ramus and condyle into variations from normal. The tongue frequently becomes trapped between the palatal shelves leading to a molding deformity in the midline of the palate or a complete U-shaped cleft (Fig. 12–14).

While animal experiments did not show significant change in the histological development of the condyle, growth studies (Beers, 1955; Pruzansky, 1954) have suggested that a primary delay in the development of the whole mandible may eventually be overcome, to a greater or lesser degree, by catch-up growth. The precise role of the condyle in growth of the mandible has not yet been quantified, but it seems illogical to suggest that, in a severe deformation such as the Pierre Robin anomaly, there is no change in this aspect of development (Fig. 12–15).

The etiopathogenesis of the Pierre Robin syndrome sequence is less clear. It is a regular feature of Stickler syndrome and may represent malformation rather than deformation; there is a degree of support for the proposition that those with the isolated Pierre Robin anomaly have the potential for normal growth of the mandible if airway and feeding problems are prevented, from birth, by postural nursing. However, infants with the syndrome sequence have a poorer prognosis in terms of growth and development in spite of early intervention and provision for catch-up growth of the jaws (Pashayan, 1984). This may be the significant difference between deformation and malformation of the mandible and particularly the growth element in the condyle.

Potter Syndrome and Whistling Face Syndrome

The Potter syndrome is only of academic interest in that the renal agenesis, which leads to the problem of oligohydramnios, and the underdevelopment of the chin (as occurs in the Pierre Robin anomaly), is incompatible with life. There is, therefore, no documented evidence of the effect of condylar deformation on postnatal growth (Potter, 1946).

Whistling face syndrome, or craniocarpotarsal dystrophy, is an autosomal dominant condition in which there is a microstomia and underdevelopment of the mandible in addition to many other abnormalities. It is likely that the orofacial defects may be the result of deformation, because there is some evidence based on clinical observations to suggest that arthrogryposis may play a part in the overall pattern of maldevelopment. Despite a variety of patterns of anom-

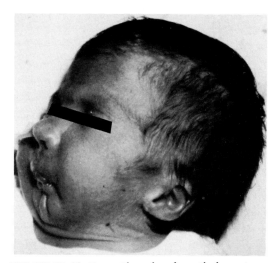

FIGURE 12–16. Face with puckered mouth, low-set ears, and underdeveloped mandible in whistling face syndrome.

alous development, general health is not affected. Because the growth disturbance has been suggested as intrinsic to bone, including the mandible, Weinstein (1969) suggested that this condition may be better described as a dysplasia. The true cause of the mandibular condition remains obscure and growth is severely retarded (Fig. 12–16).

Arthrogryposis Multiplex Congenita Syndrome

This is a rare condition in which patients present with rigid joints of the extremities, joint dislocation, absence or atrophy of muscle groups, and severe contractures. The condition may occur as a single entity or in conjunction with a number of other neurological syndromes. The etiology is unknown and may be linked to a primary lesion in the anterior horn cells, producing restricted movement. Another possible cause is oligohydramnios and subsequent limitation of movement as in the Pierre Robin and Potter syndromes.

There are few instances of TMJ involvement in arthrogryposis, if scarcity of reports in the literature is a guide to incidence (Heffez, 1985; Hodgson, 1988). In arthrogryposis of the TMJ, the articular surfaces, capsule, and disc fail to develop normally because of restrictive joint mobility. There is limitation of jaw movement, micrognathia, and lack of translation of the mandibular condyles. Micrognathia is usually the predominant feature, but Hodgson (1988) described a case in which the alteration was a severe mandibular prognathism. In general, however, muscular contracture retards mandibular growth, induces micrognathia, and accentuates antegonial notching. There is little information in the literature on methods of correcting the mandibular disability.

Disruptions
Bifid Condyle

The bifid mandibular condyle is a rare abnormality thought to be the result of trauma to the developing condyle. Two cases have been reported (Thomason, 1986) in which there was complete duplication of the condyle following fracture and dislocation, a new condyle having developed alongside the displaced original. Limitation and deviation on opening were reported in these patients, both young children. Stadnicki (1971) reported a bifid condyle in a child injured by obstetric forceps during delivery. The existence of double condyles has also been noted on dried skulls (Moffett, 1966).

Less notable duplication of the condyle is manifested as grooving or clefting of the articular surface, with reciprocal changes seen in the glenoid cavity. During prenatal life, the developing condylar cartilage is usually divided by septa from the overlying articular tissue. It is possible that the bifid condyle results from the retention of one of these bands.

Poswillo (1972) has shown that a bifid condyle can occur following condylectomy in the monkey (Fig. 12–17), and Wilkinson (personal communication) has described the persistence of the articular portion of Meckel's cartilage adjacent to the condyle formed in membrane bone in a case of Treacher Collins syndrome. Thus bifid condyle can arise from both embryological causes and trauma in early childhood.

Partial and Complete Congenital Ankylosis

Cases of authentic congenital ankylosis of the TMJ appear only rarely in the literature (see Chapter 10). Topazian (1964) stated that most so-called congenital ankyloses were secondary to trauma or infection either at, or soon after, birth. Often the limited movement resulting from a partial ankylosis is not noticed until the infant is weaned, and in many cases is not recognized until still later in childhood or adolescence.

Those ankyloses present at birth generally result from fusion between various parts of the mandible, from the alveolus to the coronoid process, and the nearby portions of the maxilla or zygoma. Rarely is the TMJ itself directly implicated. Blocks of bone forming abnormal connections between the jaws have been described by Converse (1979) and Nwoku (1986). These sites of bony fusion occurred on the medial aspect of the ramus and coronoid region, and extended across to the pterygoid plates in one instance and up to the base of the skull in the other. The mechanism of this congenital abnormality is not known. Possible causes that have been cited are necrosis resulting from some vascular event localized to the region of the developing jaws or trauma to this region during late fetal life as a result of malposition within the uterus.

Dysplasias
Aplasia of the Mandible

The most severe of the so-called first and second branchial arch anomalies is the condition of aplasia of the mandible. In this rare, lethal condition there are often multiple defects of the

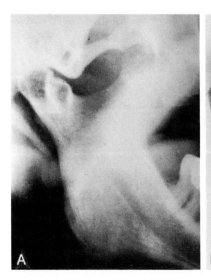
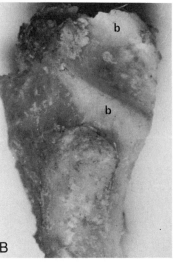

FIGURE 12–17. *A*, Human and *B*, monkey bifid condyles. The condition in B resulted from condylar regeneration after condylectomy; b,b indicates bifid articular surface.

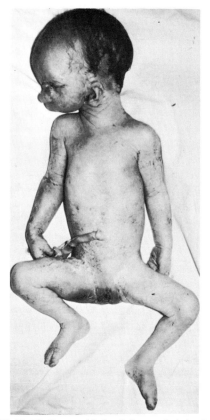

FIGURE 12–18. Otomandibular defects in lethal aplasia of the mandible.

orbit and maxilla, microstomia, low-set ears, and a partial or complete absence of the mandible and hyoid bone (Fig. 12–18). This malformation is of academic interest, but has no clinical significance. Those so affected do not survive the neonatal period. This form of aplasia presents an embryological enigma, particularly when the mandible and hyoid bone are absent and the pinnae of the ears are present and well developed, and the chain of auditory ossicles are well differentiated and intact. One possible explanation for the pathogenesis of this deformity is complete ischemic necrosis of both the mandible and the hyoid bone after separation of the mandible from the developing middle ear. Subsequent catch-up repair of the enveloping soft tissues could account for the microstomia and symmetrical low-set ears, constant findings in mandibular aplasia.

Agenesis of the Condyles

This is an exceedingly rare condition in which the condyles are symmetrically absent from birth. Radiologic examination reveals an abrupt conclusion of the mandible at the presumed developmental junction of the condylar neck and mandibular ramus (Fig. 12–19). The only likely explanation of this anomaly is a local disturbance in mesenchyme from which the cartilaginous blastema of the condyle arises relatively late in embryonic morphogenesis. It may represent either a failure of migration of specific neuroectodermal cells to the site or a breakdown in inductive or other cell-mediated processes that should establish the concentration of chondroblasts that form the condyles. There is severe and progressive underdevelopment of the height of the lower third of the face. Surgical correction is by costochondral grafts to replace the absent condyle and reconstruct the posterior mandibular height.

Hypoplasia

IDIOPATHIC

Hypoplasia of the condyle has already been referred to in specific syndromic patterns of anomalous development (see Chapter 10).

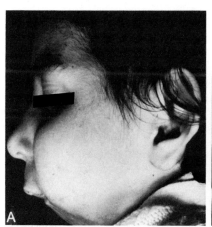

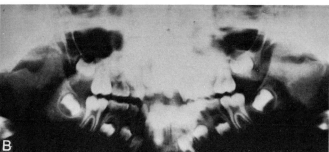

FIGURE 12–19. *A*, Facial and *B*, radiographic appearance of bilateral agenesis of the condyles at 8 years of age.

There are, however, examples of hypoplastic condyles that do not fit in any of the specified categories and can, at best, be described as idiopathic conditions because of their unknown cause. Occasionally these are small symmetrical changes that fall below the threshold of normal variation, yet are not severe enough to fit the category of agenesis. It is difficult to envisage a mode of etiopathogenesis except to speculate that these conditions are microforms of agenesis and that the same postulated mechanisms of malformation have operated, but to a lesser degree.

ATROPHIC

This condition is more readily identified and is grouped into two categories—condylysis and hemifacial atrophy.

Condylysis. Rabey (1978) called attention to eight cases of disappearing condyles none of whom had a significant family history of anomalies (see Chapter 13). This condition is not associated with oral or facial anomalies, and it has been suggested that a local lytic mechanism, perinatally or postnatally, causes lysis of the developed condyle. There is associated underdevelopment of the mandible and the stump of the condylar neck articulates with the eminence. Although most cases are bilateral, unilateral condylysis also occurs, and is most likely precipitated by trauma or infection.

While it is difficult to distinguish between condylar aplasia and some of the cases of condylysis reported by Rabey (1978), in two patients there was a postnatal history suggestive of infective lysis of the condyle, an acquired rather than a congenital anomaly.

Another patient exhibited juvenile scleroderma. It therefore seems likely that condylysis is an acquired phenomenon with a variable age of onset and that the condition is multifactorial.

Hemifacial Atrophy. Hemifacial atrophy, known also as Romberg's disease, is a progressive condition in which one half of the face, particularly the maxilla and preauricular region, slowly becomes atrophied (Figs. 12–20 and 24–10). Atrophy may spread from the dermis to the facial and masticatory muscles, cartilage, and underlying bone. The mandible may be involved up to and including the condyle (Vickery, 1972). The etiology of this disease is obscure. In about 30 per cent of cases there is a history of previous trauma, but this may be coincidental. The sympathetic trophic theory has some support. However, the link between the disease and scleroderma is still debated.

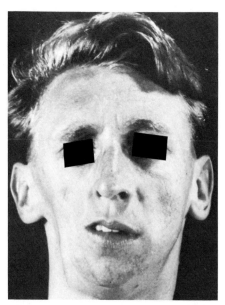

FIGURE 12–20. Severe Romberg's disease affecting right mandibular angle, ramus, and condyle (see also Fig. 24–10).

While the condition is unlikely to be congenital, it is developmental to the extent that onset may be as early as two years of age. The disease process often burns out spontaneously after a few years, but the defects left pose very considerable problems for the reconstructive surgeon who must consider tissue augmentation by vascularized free composite grafts (see Chapter 24).

Hypertrophy and Hyperplasia

Based on recent work there would appear to be four disparate entities of dysplastic overgrowth of the condyles: congenital hemifacial hypertrophy, condylar hyperplasia, hemimandibular hyperplasia, and hemimandibular elongation (see Chapter 10).

CONGENITAL HEMIFACIAL HYPERTROPHY

In congenital hemifacial hypertrophy there is gross unilateral enlargement of the glenoid fossa, and the mandibular condyle, ramus, and body. It may involve the right or left side with equal frequency. The teeth on the affected side are enlarged and this finding contributes to the differential diagnosis. Usually only the second molars are affected in the primary dentition but all teeth on the affected side may be involved in the permanent dentition (Figs. 12–21 and 24–11). Function is not significantly affected.

The clinical management of the condition is hampered by a continuation of abnormal growth

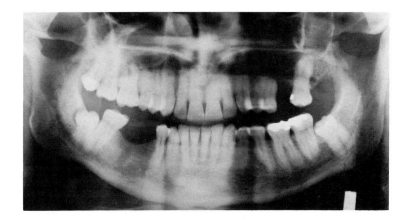

FIGURE 12–21. Radiographic appearance of patient with left congenital hemifacial hypertrophy. Note enlargement of left molars (see also Fig. 24–11).

often until late adolescence, especially in males. A limited cosmetic procedure such as reduction of the lower border of the mandible with preservation of the inferior dental nerve is the most successful method of producing facial symmetry. It is important in all cases of congenital hemihypertrophy to recognize the association of Wilms' tumor and carcinoma of the adrenal cortex with this condition. The possibility of the occurrence of these tumors on the affected side should be recognized by all clinicians who observe such cases of congenital hemifacial hypertrophy (see Chapter 24).

HYPERPLASIA

Condylar. This term refers to an isolated enlargement of the condyle (Fig. 12–22) and not to the two other and disparate hemimandibular anomalies known as hemimandibular hy-

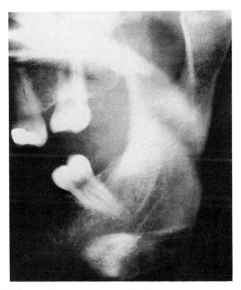

FIGURE 12–22. Radiograph of unilateral condylar hyperplasia.

perplasia and hemimandibular elongation. Obwegeser (1986) suggested that there are mixed forms of all these growth anomalies but did not identify the hemimandibular hypertrophy that is observed at birth and is accentuated at puberty. Nevertheless, for the first time, those dysplastic variations of condylar growth which have, for some time, been lumped together as variations in the extent and severity of the same condition have been classified in Obwegeser's study.

Previously all of these abnormalities of condylar and ramal growth have been accounted for by speculative mechanisms such as disturbances in lymphatic or vascular function (Egyedi, 1969), exophytic cartilage formation (Rushton, 1946), or arthrosis (Reichenbach, 1948). However, in all the histologically observed and documented cases, only actively growing normal cartilage was observed (Obwegeser, 1986). These authors make pertinent comments on the role of the condyle in normal growth, agreeing with Enlow's (1982) hypothesis that ". . . the condyle is a major field of growth . . . serving as a master center." They conclude that the genetically determined form of the normal hemimandible can only occur if a state of equilibrium exists between the growth regulators that govern the condyle, ramus, and body of the mandible on both sides, and the growth regulators of the body as a whole. In short, they ascribe abnormalities in condylar growth to imbalance in growth factors as yet unidentified.

Hemimandibular. This is a three-dimensional enlargement of the condyloid process, ramus, and body of the mandible. The anomaly commences before puberty and results in an asymmetric increase in height of the face (Fig. 12–23). Radiographs illustrate the striking unilateral enlargement of the mandible in all dimensions together with the associated downgrowth

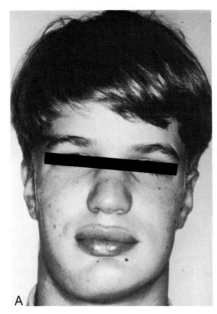
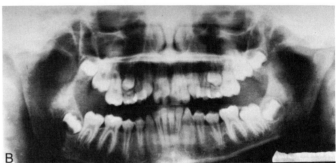

FIGURE 12–23. *A*, Facial and *B*, radiographical features of right hemimandibular hyperplasia. Note coarse trabeculation on affected side.

of the maxilla and the antrum. The mandibular canal is displaced to the lower border of the jaw. The bone on the affected side is characterized by coarse trabeculation. The condyle is large and irregularly deformed. The hyperactivity in the condyle can be clearly identified by scintigraphy (Fig. 12–24). Histological examination of the resected condyle during growth reveals broad, deep layers of fibrous tissue covering cartilage with exaggeration of the proliferative zone. Active remodeling resorption is seen in the presence of many multinucleated giant cells. Surgical correction can best be achieved after the completion of growth, as measured by serial cephalometric radiographs

or scintigraphy, by the procedure described for congenital hemifacial hyperplasia, which most closely resembles hemimandibular hyperplasia.

Hemimandibular Elongation. This condition involves an elongation of the condyloid process with normal proportions of the condyle, ramus, and body. The teeth are displaced away from the affected side, as laterognathia, with or without an open bite. There is no change in the trabecular structure of the affected side. Elongation of the neck of the condyloid process, with pronounced displacement of the chin prominence to the unaffected side (Fig. 12–25) and convex bowing of the ramus in anteroposterior view, characterizes this condition. His-

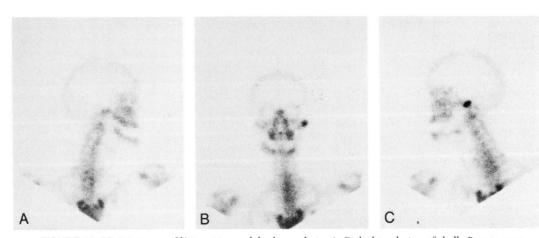

FIGURE 12–24. Scintigram of hot spot in condylar hyperplasia. *A*, Right lateral view of skull, *B*, anteroposterior view of skull, and *C*, left lateral view of skull.

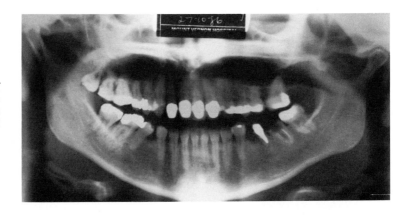

FIGURE 12–25. Radiograph of hemimandibular elongation showing overgrowth of condylar neck and deviation of chin to unaffected side.

tologically, a central core of hyperactive cartilage, with little change in shape or size of the condyle, is occasionally seen. In distinction to the other forms of dysplastic overgrowth, hemimandibular elongation may be intercepted by surgical removal of the condyloid process, at the neck, during the prepubertal growth spurt when the condition is first observed. The mandible then swings back to the affected side, the cross bite or open bite corrects spontaneously, and within a year the condyle regenerates to almost normal size and shape. The bowing of the ramus on the affected side does not disappear and remains into adult life as a marker of the onset of this growth dysplasia.

While Enlow (1982) believes that the condyle is a major field of growth, and the presence of normal condylar cartilage undoubtedly contributes to the regular growth of the ramus, there is currently insufficient information on the other regulators of growth to support the existence of a determining role for the cartilage growth center in overall growth of the mandible. Sprinz (1979), in studies with rodents, has proposed that the condylar cartilage contributes about 15 per cent of the growth of the jaw but the great variability of the ramal and condylar morphology among mammals (see Chapters 1 and 2), including the human primate, suggests that the role of the fibrocartilage cap is two-fold. First, it acts as an effective articular cover with a unique capacity to repair the ravages of masticatory overloading and second, it adds to the functional flexibility of the ramus by acting as an adjustable link between the tooth-bearing jaw and the skull.

SPECIFIC IMPLICATIONS FOR GROWTH AND INDICATIONS FOR SURGICAL INTERVENTION

The mandibular condyle combines two principal functions, namely articulation and growth,

within the covering fibrocartilage. The intimate association of these two roles makes the effect of pathological processes on the TMJ more complex and the features of the resultant deformity harder to interpret than would be the case if these functions were anatomically and physiologically distinct. There is now overwhelming evidence that the patterns of movement and function of the TMJs have a powerful influence on growth of the mandible (McNamara, 1975; Moss, 1968; Petrovic, 1975). Therefore, limitation of jaw movement, for whatever reason, may result in deficient mandibular growth, although the growth mechanisms per se are preserved intact but not fully exploited. Conversely, malformation of, or damage to, the condyle may cause deformity of the mandible by direct impairment of the mechanism for compensatory growth and adjustment between the tooth-bearing jaw and the skull. As function of the TMJ is likely to be affected by such structural alterations of mandibular form, it can be appreciated that the relationship of cause and effect remains the subject of conjecture.

Nature's own experiments, the congenital malformations, can be considered excellent sources of information on the effects of abnormalities of condylar growth on facial development. These facial deformities may have a profound effect on the appearance, function, and subsequent behavior of patients, thereby influencing the timing of treatment. It is appropriate at this stage, however, to consider the relationship of the pathogenesis of these congenital deformities to subsequent growth and rehabilitation. An appreciation of the nature and sequence of pathogenic changes leading to specific patterns of facial deformity can provide both the surgeon and the orthodontist with a biological basis on which to plan the timing and technique of surgical procedures.

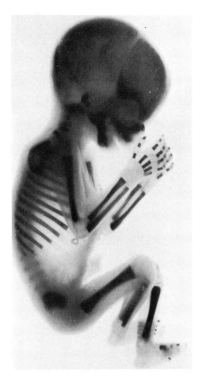

FIGURE 12–26. Symmetrical anomalous development of mandible and TMJ in 16-week human Treacher Collins fetus (alizarin-stained).

Malformations

Nonprogressive

Treacher Collins and Hallermann-Streiff syndromes are examples of malformations where the structural defects arise from a primary deficiency of ectomesenchymal tissue in the region of the developing face. The resulting dysplastic changes to skeletal elements of the face, including the condyle, are largely symmetrical (Fig. 12–26). Growth is uniform and progressive, within the limits of the dysplastic functional matrix; thus the deformity tends toward improvement as development proceeds to adulthood (Fig. 12–27).

Surgical rehabilitation in patients with this type of primary malformation depends more on augmentation of the missing contours of the face, that is the malar region, and alteration of mandibular position by orthognathic procedures, than on techniques designed to modify the form or function of the TMJs. The timing of these procedures is not governed by discrepancies in the growth rate of individual sides of the face. Symmetrical growth is maintained at any age, provided that the existing functional matrix is not seriously disturbed. Thus surgery may be done at a convenient time free of the restrictions imposed by persisting growth limitations or progressive asymmetry.

Asymmetrical and Progressive

In facial microsomia and Goldenhar's syndrome the damage to the developing derivatives of the first and second branchial arches is usually unilateral and always asymmetrical. The extent of the disruption varies from minor skeletal anomalies (often in association with microtia) to widespread deficiencies of both hard and soft tissues of the face. A useful classification based on the severity of the deformity has been proposed by Lauritzen (1985).

Where asymmetrical defects exist in the condyle, ramus, or glenoid fossa, these deficiencies in themselves may provide for differences between the two sides in the response to normal developmental stimuli. When, in addition to skeletal differences, there are asymmetrical deficiencies in the muscles and other soft tissues, there may be considerable discrepancies in subsequent growth of the left and right sides of the face. The prognosis for such cases of facial

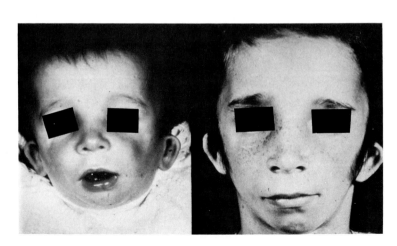

FIGURE 12–27. Human infant and adolescent facies in Treacher Collins syndrome.

microsomia is of worsening asymmetry until growth ceases.

The ideal aim of treatment should be to restore function at the earliest practical stage, if this is possible, to minimize secondary deformities. However, in the most severe cases, there may be only rudimentary muscles attached to a diminutive mandibular body with no ramus or TMJ. The functional matrix here does not exist so that tissue grafted into this environment will not have the stimulus for growth, and indeed bone grafts in this situation have been noted to resorb. Surgical rehabilitation in such severe cases is therefore dependent on passive reconstruction of facial contour by suitable hard and soft tissue grafts either at the completion of growth or as staged procedures during development.

In lesser degrees of deformity, when the muscles and other soft tissue elements of the functional matrix are spared, defects of the mandibular ramus and condyle may be effectively repaired by placement of a costochondral graft. If function of the grafted tissue within its new environment can be preserved, the costal cartilage has the potential to adapt and remodel with the growing demands of the face in the same manner as a normal functional condyle (Poswillo, 1974). Surgical intervention of this nature should aim to exploit the periods of acceleration of normal growth associated with the eruption of the permanent dentition and puberty. Orthodontic functional appliance therapy has been advocated in these patients to maximize the stimulus to growth of the affected tissues.

Deformations and Disruptions

Those conditions where normal development is physically restricted demonstrate that if the constraining influence is removed, catch-up growth is possible. Perhaps the best natural example of this phenomenon is the Pierre Robin anomaly. Restricted space in utero caused by oligohydramnios results in extreme neck flexion and hypoplasia of the mandible as the chin is pressed and molded into the chest. At birth this physical restraint is released and, provided the neonate can be nursed through the associated airway difficulties, the jaw proceeds to normal development through the childhood years.

The restriction to TMJ movement seen in congenital ankylosis requires surgical intervention to restore function, and abnormal sites of fusion between the jaws may need to be released in infancy to allow mouth opening. For-

mal reconstruction of the TMJ with a costochondral graft should ideally be undertaken at about five or six years of age before the eruption of the secondary dentition.

Dysplasias

Those dysplastic conditions where hypoplasia results in a progressive asymmetry of the face are subject to similar principles of surgical and orthodontic management as facial microsomia. The intriguing phenomenon of excessive unilateral facial growth resulting from condylar hyperplasia or hemifacial hypertrophy also presents the clinical problem of a worsening asymmetry. In this case the surgeon's task is to reduce the excessive bulk of tissue on the affected side after cessation of growth, or to limit the developing deformity by intervention. Condylar hyperplasia and its variant hemimandibular hypertrophy are associated with increased growth activity of the condyle that often continues beyond the normal growth period. Such persisting enlargement of the mandible can be detected by measurement of serial radiographs or may be predicted by bone scintiscanning. Increased uptake of bone seeking technetium 99 in one condyle indicates raised metabolic activity and possible potential for further growth (Pogrel, 1985; Robinson, 1990). Removal of the whole condyle or a high condylectomy in such cases may curtail further growth and minimize the deformity.

Deviations from the norm, particularly in dysplastic overgrowth, are excellent sources of information on the effects of aberrant growth in the region of the condyle on the shape of the face. As further information is gathered on the action of specific growth factors on condylar cartilage, the surgeon and the orthodontist will broaden the biological base from which the timing and technique of intervention will be planned. It is the ultimate hope that reconstruction will be based on a knowledge of the etiology and pathogenesis of the dysplasia, rather than on empirical surgical techniques that have been modified to suit the occasion.

FUTURE STUDIES ON CONDYLAR GROWTH AND FORM

The ultimate goal of understanding and thereby influencing the mechanisms of craniofacial development at the subcellular level remains, for the present time, the dream of developmental biologists. Progress toward this target is made with the isolation of each new gene that determines an inherited abnormality, and the identification of each previously undiscovered teratogenic agent. However, a major problem in the conversion of these basic facts concerning the causation of abnormal development into a fuller understanding of the respective resulting deformity is that even the mechanisms and controlling influences of normal mandibular development are poorly understood (Hall, 1982). In addition, most of the malformations of the TMJ are known to have a multifactorial etiology, including both inherited and environmental influences. Thus the interplay of different factors during embryogenesis poses difficulties in interpreting their relative importance. The answers to these questions and others must come from the study of cell behavior in tissue and organ culture as well as from further work on suitable animal models of TMJ deformity (Poswillo, 1976).

Advances in the clinical management of facial deformity are to be anticipated in three principal areas; namely the prevention of developmental anomalies, minimizing the effects of progressive deformity, and reconstruction of the established problem. A fertile area for effective prevention lies in the isolation of teratogens. While some teratogenic agents such as phenytoin and 13-*cis*-retinoic acid are well recognized so that their damaging effects on the fetus are theoretically preventable, other harmful environmental agents remain undiscovered, and still more await invention with the advent of new chemicals and drugs. Despite this multiplicity of teratogenic agents, their pathogenic mechanisms are probably few in number. Therefore, the identification of causal mechanisms leading to specific patterns of malformation affecting the TMJ may greatly reduce the complexities of the search for teratogenic agents. Teratogens of similar molecular configuration or biological activity may travel the same ultimate physiological pathway. By searching from the lesser to the greater, the process of inquiry may become faster and more logical.

Prevention of inherited deformity relies at present on the identification of families at risk and appropriate genetic counseling. Prenatal diagnosis of some conditions is also possible using various methods including amniocentesis, high resolution fetal ultrasonography, chorionic villous sampling, and fetoscopy. These diagnostic procedures are likely to assume an increasingly important role as techniques become safer and their results more accurate. In the future, if specific gene defects can be pinpointed, advancing techniques of genetic engineering may have the capability of correcting the affected genome in the offspring of affected patients. This possibility, however, presupposes quantum leaps in craniofacial genetic studies as well as in public opinion.

The role of specific growth factors in influencing retarded or accelerated condylar growth is as yet completely unknown, but unlikely to remain in oblivion for very much longer considering the pace of biological advances.

Minimizing the deformity and functional handicap in cases where the abnormality is progressive also is a realistic hope for the near future. Early identification of the problem will become simpler as more markers of abnormality (whether anatomic, biochemical, or genetic) are identified and the diagnostic tools for their recognition are refined. In addition, ever-improving imaging techniques, notably magnetic resonance imaging, will permit closer study of growth and development of the evolving deformity. This accumulating data base should be the foundation for a better understanding of a wide range of developmental anomalies involving the TMJ, and also provide specific direction to the treatment of the individual case.

Management of the established deformity by reconstructive surgery may also be on the brink of a new era. It is no longer adequate to plan the reconstitution of an anatomic defect without due consideration of the functional aspects of the repair. The functional unit of mastication is the TMJ and the muscles that move it; therefore, TMJ reconstruction must mean functional reconstruction of the whole masticatory apparatus. Muscle grafts to the face as a part of composite free flaps with reanastomosed vascular supply are fast becoming routine procedures, and there has been some success with free neurotized muscle transfer (Harrison, 1985). The prospect of a graft that moves itself offers exciting possibilities for the rehabilitation of patients with TMJ deformity.

It is the fruitful combination of science and surgery in the analysis of facial deformity, the understanding of factors responsible for acceleration or retardation of growth, and the development of new techniques for reconstruction that present the future biological basis for management of abnormalities of the TMJ.

CLINICAL CONSIDERATIONS

The importance of recognizing the range of severity in known or suspected cases of TMJ dysmorphogenesis cannot be overstressed. The surgeon who bases his or her plan for reconstruction on a fundamental strategy of delineating defects within a given anatomic or functional field, whether the defects are isolated or syndromic, is well equipped to assess the reconstructive procedures which may, at appropriate stages, best be utilized to remedy the defects. This knowledge, combined with an understanding of mandibular growth as thoroughly reviewed by Sarnat (1986), provides optimum opportunities for successful reconstruction and rehabilitation. John Hunter, the father of scientific surgery, encapsulated this principle in an annotation to his anatomic studies. "Not only is it important that the surgeon recognize the features of malformation but so also should he recognize those factors which lead to their occurrence; for only in this way can he give full consideration to those features in their correction which may be compromised by the phenomena which cause them."

Rare as they may be, congenital and developmental malformations of the TMJ present the clinician and the academician with some of the most perplexing problems encountered in the practice of maxillofacial surgery and orthodontics. In the forme fruste or microform of a condition, the surgical recommendations tend to be more conservative and fewer surgical risks are taken. Conversely, in the case of the worst of these deformities, where agenesis or hyperplasia of the condyle is bilateral and severe, the surgical decisions are relatively straightforward and compromised treatments have little place. These deformities have a significant and detrimental effect on facial growth, function, and appearance, and where severe asymmetry exists, these usually worsen with age. Continuing investigation of birth defects by increasingly more sophisticated cell and gene mapping will reveal more causal mechanisms in the next few years. There is the eventual hope that the primary aim of the dysmorphologist, total prevention, may be realized, but that day seems far away on the basis of present knowledge.

Advanced techniques of surgical reconstruction now permit increasingly earlier surgical intervention without compromising growth; the close collaboration of the craniofacial biologist, maxillofacial surgeon, and orthodontist now permit increasingly more accurate reconstructions of the facial skeleton and dentition where form and function have been disorganized by developmental anomalies. The most compelling pressure on the surgeon contemplating early surgical rehabilitation of these anomalies is the psychosocial attitude of the patient, the family, and society. For the benefit of all concerned, it is crucial to produce the best possible facial appearance before the child enters school. The major goal of the maxillofacial surgeon is to restore to the child the confidence and self-esteem that are essential to full participation in society at large. The problem of understanding the role of normal or abnormal growth in patients with condylar dysmorphology and the degree to which facial morphogenesis and dysmorphogenesis can be influenced by surgical and orthodontic treatment will provide clinicians and research scientists with an inexhaustible supply of questions in forthcoming years.

SUMMARY

Congenital and developmental anomalies of the condyle may result from disordered embryonic development induced by many factors, some of which may ultimately follow a common mechanistic path but lead to wide variations in ultimate pathology. The experimental teratologist has been able to add to our knowledge of the causal mechanisms of malformation and thus contribute a better understanding of the spectrum of defects that will be addressed by the attending clinicians. All of these deviations from the path of normal development of the condyle produce variation in growth and development of the mandible and often the maxilla as well. Recognition and treatment of these conditions in an ever more demanding patient population will require close collaboration among the dysmorphologist, the orthodontist, and the surgical specialist. A knowledge of craniofacial biology will continue to play a significant role in planning the timing and extent of surgical reconstruction.

As noted so appropriately by Paget in 1882, "We ought not to set them aside with idle thoughts or idle words about 'curiosities' or 'chances.' Not one of them is without meaning; not one that might not become the beginning of excellent knowledge, if only we could answer the question: why is it rare?"

REFERENCES

Beers, M. D., and Pruzansky, S.: The growth of the head of an infant with mandibular micrognathia, glossoptosis and cleft palate following the Beverly Douglas operation. Plast. Reconstr. Surg. 16:189–193, 1955.

Burck, U.: Genetic aspects of hemifacial microsomia. Hum. Genet. 64:291–296, 1983.

Converse, J. M. (with discussion by Poswillo, D. E., and Dingman, R. O.): Surgical release of bilateral, intractable temporomandibular joint ankylosis. Plast. Reconstr. Surg. 64:404–410, 1979.

Egyedi, P.: Aetiology of condylar hyperplasia. Aust. Dent. J. 14:12–17, 1969.

Enlow, D. M.: Facial Growth, 3rd ed. Philadelphia, W. B. Saunders, 1990.

Friede, H., Lopata, L., Fisher, E., and Rosenthal, I. M.:

Cardiorespiratory disease associated with Hallermann-Streiff syndrome: Analysis of craniofacial morphology by cephalometric roentgenograms. J. Craniofac. Genet. Dev. Biol. *1* (Suppl.):189–198, 1985.

Gasson, N., and Lavergne, J.: The maxillary rotation; its relation to the cranial base and the mandibular corpus. An implant study. Acta Odontol. Scand. *35*:89–94, 1977.

Hall, B. K.: How is mandibular growth controlled during development and evolution? J. Craniofac. Genet. Dev. Biol. *2*:45–49, 1982.

Harrison, D. H.: The pectoralis minor vascularized muscle graft for the treatment of unilateral facial palsy. Plast. Reconstr. Surg. *75*:206–216, 1985.

Heffez, H., Doku, H. C., and O'Donnell, J. P.: Arthrogryposis multiplex complex involving the temporomandibular joint. J. Oral Maxillofac. Surg. *45*:539–542, 1985.

Herman, G. E., Greenberg, F., and Ledbetter, D. H.: Multiple congenital anomaly/mental retardation (MCA/MR) syndrome with Goldenhar complex due to terminal deletion of (22 g). Am. J. Med. Genet. *29*:909–915, 1988.

Hodgson, P., Weinberg, S., and Consky, C: Arthrogryposis multiplex congenita of the temporomandibular joint. Oral Surg. *65*:289–291, 1988.

Houston, W. J. B.: Mandibular growth rotations—Their mechanisms and importance. Eur. J. Orthod. *10*:369–373, 1988.

Kleinsasser, O., and Schlothane, R.: Ear deformities among thalidomide embryopathies. Z. Laryngol. Rhino. Otol. *43*:344–367, 1964.

Lauritzen, C., Munro, I. R., and Ross, R. B.: Classification and treatment of hemifacial microsomia. Scand. J. Plast. Reconstr. Surg. *19*:33–39, 1985.

Livingstone, G.: Congenital ear abnormalities due to thalidomide. Proc. R. Soc. Med. *58*:493–497, 1965.

Macgregor, F. C.: Social and psychological implications of dentofacial disfigurement. Angle Orthod. *40*:231–236, 1970.

Marsh, J. L.: The skeletal anatomy of mandibulofacial dysostosis (Treacher Collins Syndrome). Plast. Reconstr. Surg. *78*:460–470, 1986.

McNamara, J. A., Connelly, T. J., and McBride, M. C.: Histological studies of temporomandibular joint adaptions. *In* McNamara, J. A. (Ed.): Determinants of Mandibular Form and Growth. Ann Arbor, University of Michigan Press, 1975.

Moffett, B. C.: The morphogenesis of the temporomandibular joint. Am. J. Orthod. *52*:401, 1966.

Moss, M. L.: The primacy of functional matrices in orofacial growth. Dent. Practit. *19*:65–73, 1968.

Nwoku, A. L.: Congenital ankylosis of the mandible. J. Maxillofac. Surg. *14*:150–152, 1986.

Obwegeser, H. L., and Makek, M. S.: Hemimandibular hyperplasia—Hemimandibular elongation. J. Maxillofac. Surg. *14*:183–208, 1986.

Paget, J.: Some Rare and New Diseases. Bradshaw Lecture. Royal College of Surgeons, London, 1882.

Pashayan, H. M., and Lewis, M. B.: Clinical experience with the Robin sequence. Cleft Palate J. *21*:270–276, 1984.

Petrovic, A. G., Stutzmann, J. J., and Oudet, C. L.: Control processes in the postnatal growth of the condylar cartilage of the mandible. *In* McNamara J. A. (Ed.): Determinants of Mandibular Form and Growth. Ann Arbor, University of Michigan Press, 1975.

Phelps, P. D.: Congenital lesions of the inner ear demonstrated by tomography. Arch. Otolaryngol. *100*:11–18, 1974.

Phelps, P. D., Poswillo, D. E., and Lloyd, G. A. S.: The ear deformities in mandibulofacial dysostosis (Treacher Collins Syndrome). Clin. Otolaryngol. *6*:15–28, 1981.

Phelps, P. D., Glyn, A. S., and Poswillo, D. E.: The ear deformities in craniofacial microsomia and oculo-auriculo-vertebral dysplasia. J. Laryngol. Otol. *96*:995–1005, 1983.

Pogrel, M. A.: Quantitative assessment of isotope activity in the temporomandibular joint regions as a means of assessing unilateral condylar hypertrophy. Oral Surg. Oral Med. Oral Pathol. *60*:15–17, 1985.

Poswillo, D. E.: Foetal posture and causal mechanisms of deformity of the palate, jaws and limbs. J. Dent. Res. *45*:584–596, 1966.

Poswillo, D. E.: The late effects of mandibular condylectomy. Oral Surg. *33*:500–512, 1972.

Poswillo, D. E.: The pathogenesis of the first and second arch syndrome. Oral Surg. *35*:302–328, 1973.

Poswillo, D. E.: Experimental reconstruction of the mandibular joint. Int. J. Oral Surg. *3*:400–411, 1974.

Poswillo, D. E.: Hemorrhage in development of the face. Birth Defects *11*:61–81, 1975a.

Poswillo, D. E.: The pathogenesis of the Treacher Collins syndrome. Br. J. Oral Surg. *13*:1–26, 1975b.

Poswillo, D. E.: Mechanisms and pathogenesis of malformation. Br. Med. Bull. *32*:59–64, 1976.

Potter, E. L.: Facial characteristics of infants with bilateral renal agenesis. Am. J. Obstet. Gynecol. *51*:885–888, 1946.

Pruzansky, S., and Richmond, J. B.: Growth of the mandible in infants with micrognathia. Am. J. Dis. Child *88*:29–42, 1954.

Rabey, G. P.: Bilateral mandibular condylysis—A morphoanalytic diagnosis. Br. J. Oral Surg. *15*:121–134, 1978.

Reichenbach, E., and Seidler, H.: Uber die sogenannte hypertrophie des kieferkopfchens. Dtsch. Zahnarztl. Z. *3*:806–810, 1948.

Robinson, P. D., Harris, K., Coughlan, K., and Altman, K.: Bone scans and the timing of surgery in condylar hyperplasia. Int. J. Oral Maxillofac. Surg. *19*:243–246, 1990.

Rollnick, B. R., Kaye, C. I., Nagatoshi, K., et al.: Oculo-auriculovertebral dysplasia and variants: Phenotypic characteristics of 294 patients. Am. J. Med. Genet. *26*:361–375, 1987.

Ross, R. B.: Lateral facial dysplasia (first and second branchial arch syndrome, hemifacial microsomia). Birth Defects *11*:51–59, 1975.

Rushton, M. A.: Unilateral hyperplasia of the mandibular condyle. Proc. R. Soc. Med. *39*:431–438, 1946.

Sarnat, B. G.: Growth pattern of the mandible: Some reflections. Am. J. Orthod. Dentofacial Orthop. *90*:221–233, 1986.

Sprinz, R.: Mandibular growth following meniscectomy in young rats. J. Dent. Res. Special Issue C *58*:1230, 1979.

Stadnicki, G.: Congenital double condyle of the mandible causing temporomandibular joint ankylosis: Report of a case. J. Oral Surg. *29*:208–211, 1971.

Sulik, V. K., Johnston, M. C., Smiley, S. J., et al.: Mandibular Dysostosis (Treacher Collins Syndrome): A new proposal for its pathogenesis. Am. J. Med. Genet. *27*:359–379, 1987.

Thomason, J. M., and Yusuf, H.: Traumatically induced bifid mandibular condyle: A report of two cases. Br. Dent. J. *161*:291–293, 1986.

Topazian, R. G.: Etiology of ankylosis of temporomandibular joint: Analysis of 44 cases. J. Oral Surg. *22*:227, 1964.

Vickery, I. M.: Hemifacial atrophy. Br. J. Oral Surg. *9*:102–109, 1972.

Weinstein, S., and Gorlin, R. J.: Craniocarpotarsal dysplasia or the whistling face syndrome. 1. Clinical consideration. Am. J. Dis. Child *117*:427–433, 1969.

Wilkinson, W. M., and Poswillo, D. E.: Asymmetry in mandibulofacial dysostosis. J. Craniofac. Genet. Dev. Biol. (*in press*).

13

EXPERIMENTAL STUDIES*

WILLIAM H. WARE, D.D.S., M.S.
and JEFFREY T. FUJIMOTO, D.D.S., M.A.

INTRODUCTION

Disorders of the temporomandibular joint (TMJ) that have received the most attention experimentally include (1) discrepancies in growth and development, (2) arthritides, (3) disc derangements, (4) traumatic injuries, (5) ankylosis, and (6) functional adaptations. Effects of other factors are less understood. This chapter discusses those experimental studies that have had an impact on current therapy.

GROWTH DISCREPANCIES

Most students of facial growth and development assign a major role to the mandibular condyle. Some controversy exists, however, as to whether the condyle is a primary growth site or if it responds secondarily to growth of the facial soft tissue matrix. Based on the early studies of Hunter (1778) and later of others

*See Chapters 4, 6, 10–12, 16, 22, and 24.

(Bjork, 1955; Brash, 1924; Brodie, 1941; Charles, 1925; Hulen, 1948; Humphry, 1864; Keith, 1922; Robinson, 1955; Sarnat, 1986), it has been assumed that skeletal growth of the face was dependent on intrinsic bony growth sites with the soft tissue being merely adaptive. Moss (1969; 1968; 1960), however, suggested that the opposite may be the case—that the facial skeleton, including the mandible, grows in response to growth of functional soft tissue matrices. The anatomic models most supportive of this hypothesis are the growth of the cranium in response to brain growth and the growth of the orbit in response to ocular growth (Sarnat, 1981). The postnatal functions of breathing, eating, and talking certainly require growth and development of the facial soft tissues, which in turn may be the primary stimulation for skeletal development. In this regard, an experiment was recently reported that tested the thesis of whether bone growth would occur without a functional soft tissue matrix. Rat heads were transplanted to recipient animals and bone growth was observed! (Hirabayashi, 1988).

While at first glance the two hypotheses appear opposed, present evidence suggests a mutually supportive role between the bony growth sites and the functional matrix.

Growth Changes

Studies of normal facial growth in both lower animals and humans have provided information on changes after condylectomy, but have given little insight into their cause. Because the condyle has been assumed to be the primary growth site of the mandible, it was appropriate to test this assumption by observing growth following removal of the condyle. In the young rodent (Das, 1965; Jarabak, 1952; Jolly, 1961; Pimenidis, 1972) remarkable regenerative powers apparently exist. Following extirpation of the mandibular condyle in these animals, partial or complete regeneration with little deformity was reported. Such experimental evidence lends support to the functional matrix hypothesis.

In young primates, presumably more like the human, removal of the condyle more often results in deformity (Fig. 13–1). Nevertheless, regeneration of the monkey condyle also has been reported. Choukas (1966) and later Skuble (1968) described the results of resecting the mandibular condyle in four- to six-month-old monkeys. The animals were observed up to 18 months following surgery. Minimal craniomandibular changes were described, with reformation of the condyle being observed within four months. Histologic studies of the reformed condyles showed a proliferating cartilaginous cap similar to the unoperated side. The authors concluded that condylectomy retards the normal increment of growth in the young monkey, induces minor skeletal changes in the zygomatic arch, but has minimal effect on function.

These findings differ somewhat from those of Sarnat (1951; 1957; 1971), who studied the effects of condylectomy in both young and adult monkeys. In a series of studies on young rhesus monkeys, regeneration of a condyle occurred, but growth of the mandible on the operated side was severely altered. In addition, the facial and neurocranial bone complexes were less developed than those on the unoperated side, resulting in asymmetry of the skull. Histologic studies of the operated joint region revealed no chondrogenic zone covering the resected stump.

These divergent findings may be explained in part by (1) the differences in age of the animals at the time of the operation and (2) the different lengths of time that elapsed between the operation and death. Sarnat's animals were eight months old at surgery and killed 31

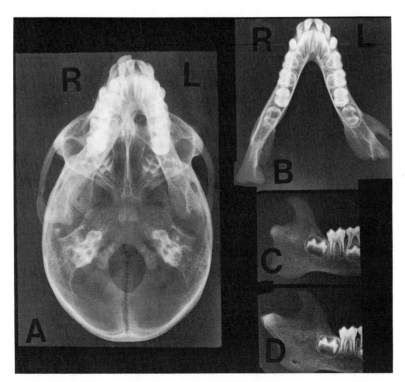

FIGURE 13–1. Effects of unilateral (left side) condylectomy on the facial skeleton of a growing monkey are demonstrated in the radiographic views of the skull one year following surgery. A, Deviation of the mandible and, to a lesser extent, the maxillary teeth to the side of condylectomy. The zygoma is shorter on the operated left side. B, Disparity in horizontal development is demonstrated in an occlusal view of the mandible. C and D, Comparison of operated side (C) with normal right side (D), illustrating the adaptive changes in the ramus following condylectomy. (From Ware, W. H., and Taylor, R. C.: Cartilaginous growth centers transplanted to replace mandibular condyles in monkeys. J. Oral Surg. 24:33–43, 1966.)

months later (Sarnat, 1951; 1957), while animals studied by Choukas (1966) and Skuble (1968) were four to six months of age at surgery and were killed two and one-half to 18 months later. Younger animals commonly exhibit greater regenerative activity within the joint. Furthermore, development of fibrocartilaginous tissue at the site of a fracture or ostectomy is a sequential part of the normal healing process. A cartilaginous covering of the condylar stump would more likely be observed within a few months following resection (Skuble, 1968). Another factor may be that in Sarnat's studies the articular disc and attachment of the lateral pterygoid muscle were also removed.

Following the studies on the growing monkeys, Sarnat (1957) concluded that the skeletal changes were the result of both growth arrest and the subsequent skeletal adaptations to altered functional stress. In later investigations where a comparable surgical procedure was performed on adult monkeys, skeletal changes similar to, but not as severe as, those occurring in the young animals were observed. Since similar skeletal changes were observed in both growing and adult animals (Sarnat, 1971; 1978), it would appear that the effects were due more to loss of articular integrity and decreased ramus height than to loss of the growth center. These findings were confirmed by Sorenson (1975), who showed that ramus shortening without removal of the condyle in growing monkeys still resulted in deformity, while alloplastic replacement in adult monkeys prevented skeletal changes. These data neither prove that the functional matrix is the primary growth organizer nor do they support the established belief that the condyle is the primary site of growth.

In a well-designed study, Bernabei (1975) has produced evidence supportive of the theory that the mandibular condyle is a primary growth site. Based on the knowledge that the adult mandible is capable of linear growth under the influence of growth hormone, Bernabei developed an experimental system to determine the general location of the growth center(s) responsible for this bodily movement. The mandible of mature rats was separated into three parts by bilateral condylotomy. Bony healing was prevented by covering the cut surfaces with acrylic. Metallic markers were placed in the skull and in mandibular fragments to be used for cephalometric measurements and evaluation of change over the experimental period. Fresh growth hormone was injected daily for 30 days. Experimental control was maintained by both sham operations and injections of sterile saline

solution in place of growth hormone. By comparisons of both experimental and control groups, it was demonstrated that (1) condyles ". . . isolated in situ responded to growth hormone in a manner consistent with a growth center while condyles without a growth promoting agent (saline) did not grow" (Bernabei, 1975), and (2) mandibular bodies isolated in situ collapsed irrespective of whether or not a growth-promoting agent was administered. The collapse was less in animals receiving growth hormone. This study supports the primacy of the condyle on linear growth of the mandible, but also demonstrates a role for the functional matrix.

Ware (1981) followed the progress of 10 growing children who received costochondral junction transplants following resection of the condyles for various problems. Transplant growth was erratic, with several patients exhibiting overgrowth of the transplant, supporting the idea of intrinsic growth potential of the transplanted costochondral growth center. Other investigators have reported similar findings (Politis, 1987).

With the development of new and improved cell culturing techniques, the phenomenon of growth has been investigated at its most basic level. Copray (1983) cultured the mandibular cartilage of 4-day-old rats in serum-free and serum-supplemented media for 28 days and compared the growth results with in vivo growth. In the serum-free and serum-supplemented cultures, proliferation, differentiation, and matrix formation continued in the condyles but differed from that observed in the functioning condyles. The stratified organization of the condyle was severely disrupted, with a reduction of the prechondroblastic and transition zones and with enlargement of the hypertrophic zone. It was concluded that the modulation mechanism in control of the rate of proliferation, differentiation, and maturation of the prechondroblasts was absent in the in vitro cultures.

Buchner (1982) found that lessening the load on the condyle in rats (by a bite-raising appliance) resulted in an increased thickness of the entire cartilaginous layer. He emphasized the importance of functional load on the regulation of condylar growth. Shimshoni (1984) cultured young rat condyle cells and discovered a significant increase in both cAMP production and [^{3}H]-thymidine incorporation when the cells were physically stimulated. It was postulated that the stimulus-receptor system for these events may lie in cellular membrane changes.

The data from cell biology research and histological studies suggest that the functional matrix may modulate intrinsic growth.

In an attempt to define extrinsic factors important in growth regulation, Duterloo (1967) transplanted condyles into the brain of rats and found chondrogenesis and growth to continue for a short time, but without mechanical influences, ossification occurred. Engelsma (1980) transplanted 4-day-old rat condyles to the site of resected 4th distal metacarpal epiphyses in 7-day-old host rats. Within one week of transplantation, there was a rapid increase in the size of the transplant until the space of the resected metacarpal epiphysis was filled. This growth spurt was interpreted to be an expression of the intrinsic growth potential of condylar cartilage in a nonfunctional position. In a position of articular function, condylar progenitor cells continued to differentiate into chondroblasts, and well-defined mandibular condyles developed without the appearance of an epiphysis. The conclusion was that articular function maintains chondrogenesis and growth, and in the absence of articular function, chondrogenesis changes to osteogenesis.

Following condylar resection in both young and adult monkeys, similar facial skeletal changes were observed, suggesting that removal of the condylar growth site was not the principal factor (Sarnat, 1978). Disruption of normal TMJ function with all of the associated ramifications was emphasized as the important determinant. Hall (1982) suggested that the basic morphogenetic properties (how many elements, what shape) are intrinsically determined by neurocrest cells or the mesenchyme that forms from them, and sympathizes with the oral surgeon ". . . whose efforts become tinkering with the accelerator and brake of the engine which is totally inaccessible to him." Epigenetic influences are obviously important in differentiation and control of growth rate, but the real question is how much of the shape of the mandible resides in the intrinsic property of the cells and how much resides in the ability of the cells to respond to environmental influences (Hall, 1982). Precious (1987) postulated that mandibular growth is a composite of the growth contributions of its various skeletal units (corpus, condyle, coronoid, angle, and dento-alveolar). The size, situation, and orientation of these units are the important factors in the ultimate expression of form and growth. It follows that soft tissue pathology may result in abnormal bone growth just as skeletal deformities may result in soft tissue imbalances. These concepts integrate elements of both the functional matrix theory and growth center theory, and may best account for the variety of altered growth patterns observed in conjunction with many clinical problems.

From a teleologic standpoint, the concept of intrinsic growth properties evolving under the influence of functional demands, as well as developing associated structures to yield a final functional unit, is most appealing. The process of natural selection would dictate such a scheme. Application of this knowledge to clinical situations, however, requires us to investigate the question of degree: the degree of intrinsic and extrinsic control of growth related to the age of development. Only with this further information can we judge when and how much to intervene in a clinical problem.

Replacement of the Condyle

Although the question of whether the mandibular condyle is a primary or secondary growth site remains unsettled, it is obvious that when it is missing in the young animal, some degree of deformity can be anticipated. The clinical problems of agenesis and ankylosis, and the need for resection of the temporomandibular joint (TMJ) in children, prompted investigators to search for means of improving both function and facial development. Replacement of the missing or defective condyle with an anatomically similar structure appeared desirable to (1) re-establish integrity of joint function, (2) establish symmetry of the mandibular rami and hence improve facial esthetics, and (3) promote harmonious facial growth.

Considerable work performed in cartilage transplantation supports the credibility of replacing the condyle with another cartilaginous growth site (Sarnat, 1954). Peer (1955) concluded not only that autogenous cartilage transplants remained viable, but also that cell division and growth continued. These observations were made on young human rib cartilage following autogenous transplantation to the abdominal wall. Lacroix (1951) had demonstrated earlier that epiphyseal cartilage removed from the distal tibia in rabbits and transplanted to the kidney continued to grow and develop, with bone replacement occurring in an organized manner.

Ring (1955) studied the regenerative properties of epiphyseal cartilage in rabbits. Excision of the cartilage columns produced no significant disturbance in growth. Excision of the reserve zone, however, caused complete arrest. Felts

(1957) excised the humeri of mice two days after birth and buried them in the abdominal wall of the mother. The bone grew to about 80 per cent of normal size if the transplantation was immediate. If the transplants were stored, growth and development were adversely affected in direct proportion to the time of storage.

Numerous studies (Campbell, 1959; Felts, 1957; Gelbke, 1951; Haas, 1958; Ring, 1955; Strobino, 1952) have shown that cartilage is extremely resistant to physical stresses. To cause growth arrest, large areas of the cells replenishing the cartilage columns have to be destroyed. In contrast to its resistance to physical trauma, epiphyseal cartilage is apparently quite responsive to biochemical change. Engfeldt (1960), using histologic, microradiographic, and autoradiographic techniques, found adverse effects in the epiphyseal regions of growing dogs within 12 hours following a single dose of aminoacetonitril (lathyrism).

Laskin (1952; 1953) and Sarnat (1954) studied the effects of transplantation on the metabolism of rabbit cartilage. Respiration and anaerobic glycolysis declined to one-half of the normal rate during the first seven days following transplantation. Both autografts and homografts were shown to behave similarly with respect to changes in these two metabolic processes. The homografts eventually were replaced with fibrous tissue, in spite of evidence of continued viability, whereas the autogenous cartilage showed no tendency to resorb. Kluzak (1960), using labeled phosphate ($^{34}PO_4$), determined that autotransplants of cartilage integrated with the metabolic processes in the host tissues within a few hours after transplantation. Schatten (1958), studying survival and growth of rib cartilage grafts in rats, concluded that autografts grew to about 70 per cent the size of in situ cartilage; homografts attained about 30 per cent of normal linear growth. Roy (1956) studied the differential growth of rabbit ribs.

Meikle (1973) determined that the proliferative zone of the condylar cartilage in young rats continues to show cell division following transplantation of the entire TMJ into the brain tissue of littermates. Meikle suggested that there was an intrinsic genetic program that accounted for the proliferative activity. While the cells continued to proliferate, they differentiated into osteoblasts rather than chondroblasts following transplantation. The multipotentiality and environmental response of these cells were demonstrated. Extrinsic mechanical stresses associated with function of the joint may be required to provide the stimulus for the cells of the proliferative zone to differentiate into chondroblasts rather than osteoblasts.

These basic studies support the concept that the growth potential of the cartilage of the mandibular condyle, rib, or epiphyseal plate is in part independent of a functional soft tissue matrix.

The discovery that autogenous cartilage grafts not only survive transplantation but also retain intrinsic growth potential stimulated clinical application. Preceding the animal studies were a number of human case reports (Dingman, 1964; Hovell, 1962; Manchester, 1965; Stuteville, 1955) in which the mandibular condyle was replaced by another cartilaginous growth center, either rib or metatarsal bone. While the reports of improved function following such operative procedures were encouraging, the question of growth and graft response were largely left unanswered. The need for further study of these processes in a more controlled manner was obvious.

The reports that followed provided additional insight not only into the biological processes associated with graft-host tissue relationship but also into the intrinsic properties of the condyle and TMJ. A review of the studies illustrates the contributions that experimental surgery had made in this particular area.

In 1965, Peskin reported on a study of autogenous condylar grafts. Thirty-one puppies were divided into three groups. In Group I (13 animals), the lateral half of the condyloid process was removed unilaterally, with a sham operation on the opposite side. In Group II (12 animals), lateral hemisections of the condylar processes were carried out bilaterally. In addition, the medial half of the condyle was removed unilaterally. The lateral halves of the condyles were then transplanted to the contralateral sides. Group III (six animals) was used as a control, with unilateral total condylectomies performed. Metallic implants were placed in a triangular pattern in the mandible for later use in direct craniometry. This experimental approach allowed comparisons of subsequent growth to be correlated with the local tissue responses occurring at the surgical sites in the several categories. Experimental variations included effects of (1) removing half a condyle, which was used as a donor, (2) utilizing half a condyle for replacement of the entire condyle, and (3) a hemicondylar transplant to replace a missing hemicondyle.

Killing of the animals at staged intervals from four to 24 weeks permitted comparisons by both direct measurement of subsequent mandibular growth and microscopic assessment of the cellular responses in the surgical region. This well-designed experiment produced several interesting results that helped to explain clinical observations and suggested further clinical applications.

Comparisons among animals with total condylectomy, hemicondylectomy, and total condylectomy with hemicondylar grafts helped to delineate the differences between functional reconstruction and regeneration of the condyle. After condylectomy, a nearly normal shape was attained with return of functional movements, but condylar cartilage did not re-form and longitudinal mandibular growth remained retarded. When only half the condyle was removed or a hemicondylar transplant was performed, complete regeneration of the condyle occurred, including the condylar cartilage, along with recovery of longitudinal growth. Functional activity was the same in all cases; the main difference was the lack of inductive stimulus where the condyle was totally removed, whereas the hemicondyle, when retained in place or transplanted, provided sufficient stimulus to induce regeneration.

In Peskin's (1965) study, reduction in the size of the condyle (hemicondylectomy) resulted in temporary reduction of longitudinal growth, suggesting that this finding might be applied to early treatment of young patients demonstrating mandibular prognathism. Theoretically, such a preventive measure has merit. If controlled regeneration of condylar growth could be achieved without significant surgical risks (which, however, are inherent in open procedures on the TMJ), then reduction of condylar size would be attractive.

Ware (1965) approached the problem of growth site transplantation by studying first the effects of replantation of the excised condyle in young monkeys. In a later study (Ware, 1966), either the distal end of the fourth metatarsal bone or the costochondral junction (CCJ) of the seventh rib was used to replace the mandibular condyle. Metallic markers were placed in the mandible and zygoma of each animal for cephalometric radiographic evaluation of growth during a three-year postsurgical period. Twenty animals were included in the studies and the manner in which they were operated on is described in Table 13–1.

The jaws of all animals were immobilized for four weeks. Cephalometric radiographs were taken at six-month intervals for periods from 24 to 36 months. Following sacrifice, the skulls

TABLE 13–1. Condylar Experiments by Ware and Taylor (1965, 1966)

NO. OF MONKEYS	EXPERIMENT
3	Controls—normal growth study only
4	Unilateral condylectomy
2	Condylectomy with immediate replantation
1	Displaced condylar fracture
4	Unilateral condylectomy with seventh rib costochondral junction transplant
6	Unilateral condylectomy with fourth metatarsal bone transplant

were prepared as dry or histologic specimens. Radioactive sulfur (^{35}S) was injected 48 hours before death in those animals slated for histological study. In addition to the routine morphologic comparisons, the chondroitin sulfate synthesis in both the operated and control condyles was assessed by standard autoradiographic techniques.

In the animals having only the unilateral condylectomies, asymmetric facial growth occurred similar to that reported in other studies (Sarnat, 1951; 1957; 1971). There was no evidence of a cartilaginous cap covering the remodeled articular surface. Those condyles that were removed and then replanted showed essentially normal growth. Based on histologic and biochemical (^{35}S uptake) comparisons, the cartilage of the replanted condyle was found to be similar to that of the unoperated side (Fig. 13–2).

The animals in which the condyle was fractured and displaced did not show the same recovery as those reported by Walker (1960). Postsurgical immobilization of the mandible may have retarded the regeneration process. The results of the transplantation of both the rib and metatarsal grafts ranged from no growth, similar to that following condylectomy, to overgrowth of the grafts (Fig. 13–3). In those animals exhibiting vigorous growth of the transplant, both the dry specimens and the histologic sections demonstrated the functional adaptations of the transplant to conform closely to the shape and size of a normal mandibular condyle. At the same time, the cartilaginous growth center retained the mosaic cellular pattern of the donor tissue. The cartilage of both the costochondral junction and the metatarsal epiphysis showed the chondrocytes to be widely separated by interposing matrix. Columns of enlarging chondrocytes extended to the underlying zone of calcification (Fig. 13–4). The chondrocytes in the cartilage of the normal

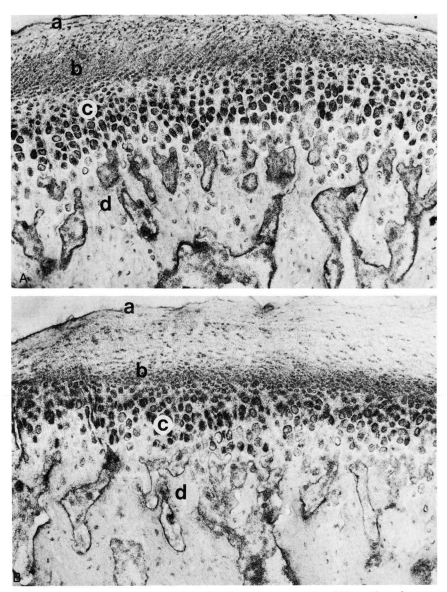

FIGURE 13–2. *A*, Autoradiograph of normal condyle demonstrating uptake of $^{35}SO_4$. The radioactive sulfate is indicated by the developed grains in the emulsion overlying the tissue. From above downward, all layers of tissue took up the ^{35}S, including the fibrous layer (a), chondroblasts (b), mature chondrocytes (c), and osseous structures (d). Heaviest labeling occurred within the mature chondrocytes (reduced 20 per cent from orginal magnification, × 150). *B*, Autoradiograph of replanted condyle exhibiting similar labeling characteristics as in *A*. A heavy band of labeling is present in the chondroblast and mature chondrocyte layers. The cartilage of the replanted condyle took up the ^{35}S to the same extent as did the normal condyle, indicating viability (reduced 20 per cent from original magnification, × 150). (From Ware, W. H., and Taylor, R. C.: Replantation of growing mandibular condyles in rhesus monkeys. Oral Surg. *19*:669–677, 1965.)

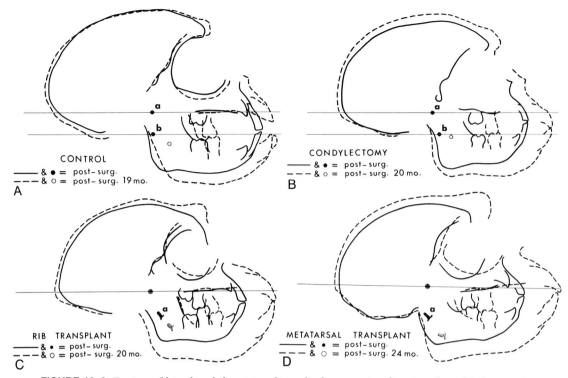

FIGURE 13–3. Tracings of lateral cephalometric radiographs demonstrating direction of mandibular growth in monkeys. *A*, Control. Tracings are oriented on zygomatic markers and the nasal floor to emphasize the effect of the mandibular growth component. *B*, Condylectomy. Direction and extent of growth differ from that observed in A. Mandibular movement carried the tantalum marker in the ramus anteriorly but only slightly inferiorly to the reference plane during the 20-month period. *C*, Rib transplant. Intraosseous wire (a) in the ramus is carried in an inferior and anterior direction similar to that observed in the control animal in A. *D*, Metatarsal transplant. Considerable vertical growth of the transplant is indicated by the position of the transosseous marker two years following surgery. (From Ware, W. H., and Taylor, R. C.: Cartilaginous growth centers transplanted to replace mandibular condyles in monkeys. J. Oral Surg. *24*:33–43, 1966.)

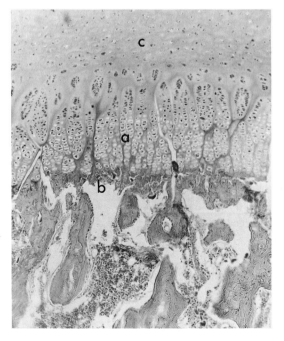

FIGURE 13–4. Section through normal costochondral junction in growing monkey demonstrating the columnation of the chondrocytes (a) near the zone of calcification (b). A similar phenomenon is observed in the cartilage of the epiphyseal plate of long bones. Note the amount of matrix surrounding the chondrocytes in the proliferative zone (c), as compared with that seen in the mandibular condyle (see Fig. 13–5). (From Ware, W. H., and Taylor, R. C.: Cartilaginous growth centers transplanted to replace mandibular condyles in monkeys. J. Oral Surg. *24*:33–43, 1966.)

mandibular condyle were more tightly but randomly arranged, with little matrix and no columnation (Fig. 13–5). The transplant, while apparently conforming to the new environment in terms of form and function, still retained the intrinsic cellular pattern characteristic of its former site (Figs. 13–6 and 13–7).

On the basis of a study in which rib cartilage was transplanted to replace missing mandibular condyles in young adult monkeys, Poswillo (1974) proposed that the mandibular condyle is not a primary growth center, but rather that it responds in a secondary and adaptive manner to growth of the soft tissue matrix. Poswillo emphasized the difference between the cartilage of a long bone epiphyseal plate and that of the mandibular condyle. The columns of cartilage cells in the epiphyseal plate predispose to

elongation of the bone in a longitudinal manner, whereas the haphazard arrangement of the condylar cartilage cells permits multidirectional growth and adaptation in response to the changing environment.

Poswillo (1974) concluded that it was irrational to use epiphyseal growth centers to replace the mandibular condyle because of anatomic and functional differences between the cartilage components. In Poswillo's study on monkeys, both sliding ramus and costochondral grafts were used, and it was felt that both procedures were acceptable for replacing a missing condyle and re-establishing ramus height. The functional condyle formed by the sliding graft, however, lacked the histological features or capacity for remodeling that both the normal condyle and the costochondral graft

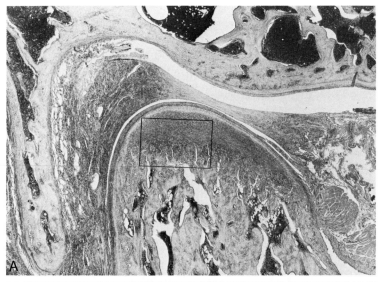
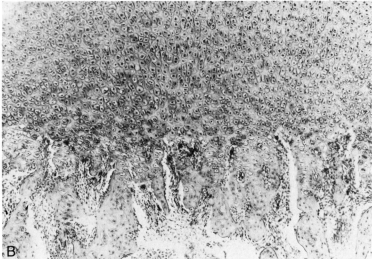

FIGURE 13–5. Normal temporomandibular joint of immature monkey. *A*, Proliferative condylar cartilage and osteogenic replacement. *B*, Higher-power view of osteogenic zone outlined in *A* demonstrating mature cartilage cells arranged in a haphazard manner (original magnification, × 150). There is little matrix between the cells. Unlike either the costochondral junction or epiphyseal plate, columnation of chondrocytes does not occur at the osteogenic interface. (From Ware, W. H., and Taylor, R. C.: Cartilaginous growth centers transplanted to replace mandibular condyles in monkeys. J. Oral Surg. *24*:33–43, 1966.)

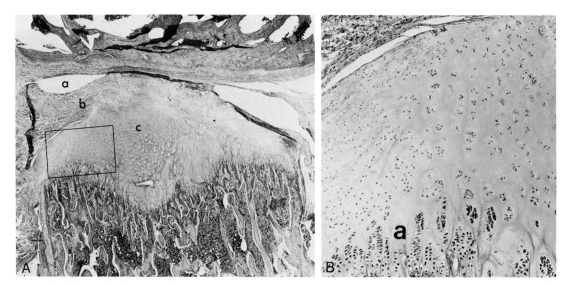

FIGURE 13–6. Rib transplant in a monkey two years following surgery. *A,* Single joint compartment (a) separates the transplant from the temporal bone. Dense fibrous tissue (b) covers the cartilage cap junction (see Fig. 13–4). *B,* Higher magnification of region marked in *A* illustrates the columnation of mature chondrocytes (a) near the zone of calcification (original magnification, × 150). The relationship of matrix to cartilage cells retains the characteristics of the costochondral junction rather than those typical of the mandibular condyle (see Fig. 13–5). (From Ware, W. H., and Taylor, R. C.: Cartilaginous growth centers transplanted to replace mandibular condyles in monkeys. J. Oral Surg. *24:*33–43, 1966.)

showed. The study suggests that the condylar cartilage and transplanted costochondral cartilage have some beneficial inductive capacity, although whether it is primary or secondary to other growth forces remains unknown. Poswillo (1979) stated, however, that the costochondral grafts are unpredictable and that further search for a more reliable graft source should continue.

On the basis of a study reported in 1969, Hunsuck suggested that the clavicle was an appropriate donor site to replace a defective mandibular condyle. The sternoclavicular joint (SCJ) and the TMJ have many similarities. The articulating surfaces of each are covered with fibrous tissue and each has a disc dividing the joint into two compartments. Also, cartilaginous zones exist in the condyles of both the mandible and the clavicle.

Hunsuck operated on eight growing monkeys, replacing the excised condyle with the sternal end of the clavicle. Following the surgical procedures, the animals' jaws were immobilized for five weeks. They were then killed in pairs at intervals up to six months. At the time of death, silicone rubber was infused into the vascular system to study more accurately the process of revascularization of the graft. The specimens were bisected, and half were used for histologic examination of the graft while the other half were processed for study of microvascular changes during healing. The grafts

healed without complications and apparently functioned extremely well as a replacement for the mandibular condyle. On the basis of the microvascular study, Hunsuck concluded that little or none of the transplanted osseous tissue survived.

In specimens obtained two weeks following surgery, there was minimal revascularization, and beginning resorption and reconstruction of the transplant were evident. By eight weeks, revascularization was complete, and the cartilaginous growth center appeared to be re-established. Hunsuck further stated that the transplanted tissue did not survive but served as a matrix and stimulus for reconstruction and regeneration. During the course of observation (six months), near-normal function returned, with no evidence of growth deficiency.

While the report is encouraging, the observation period following the surgery was too short to draw conclusions on growth of SCJ grafts to the TMJ in the rhesus monkey. Furthermore, revascularization studies, while pertinent to assessing bone vitality, are not adequate for assessing cartilage (chondrocyte) viability. Because cartilage is an avascular tissue, the metabolic exchange occurs by diffusion. The cartilaginous portion of the transplant may well retain viability even without evidence of associated bone vascularity. It is probable that the donor tissue cells, particularly the prolifer-

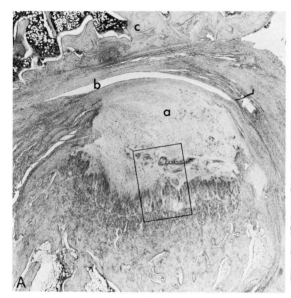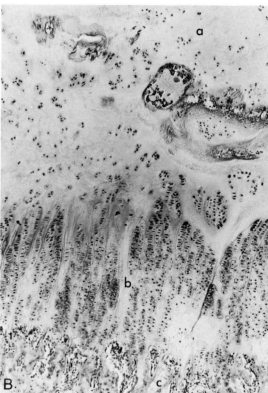

FIGURE 13–7. Metatarsal head transplant in monkey two years following surgery. *A*, Epiphyseal bone has been replaced with fibrous tissue and cartilage (a). The graft has assumed similar morphological characteristics to those observed in the rib transplant (see Fig. 13–5). A single joint compartment (b) separates the transplant from the temporal bone (c) (original magnification, × 150). *B*, Higher magnification of region outlined in *A* illustrates chondrocytes widely separated by interposing matrix material (a). Clustering of cells suggests that proliferation has been occurring. Columns of chondrocytes (b) are seen extending to the zone of calcification (c). (From Ware, W. H., and Taylor, R. C.: Cartilaginous growth centers transplanted to replace mandibular condyles in monkeys. J. Oral Surg. *24:*33–43, 1966.)

ative zone of cartilage, contributed along with the host tissue to the rebuilding and growth process.

Based on the anatomic similarity between the SCJ and the condyle, the SCJ has aroused more recent interest as a potential donor tissue (Hall, 1978). Ellis (1986) performed histomorphologic examinations of the SCJ and the costochondral junction (CCJ) during growth in the *Macaca mulatta* monkey and compared these observations with those of the normal condyle in infant, juvenile, adolescent, and adult monkeys. The TMJ and the SCJ were found to be very similar morphologically throughout growth, sharing the same stratified organization of the cartilage. The CCJ differed in organization, however, and was found to be similar to the growth plate in the long bone epiphysis. Based on these results, the authors suggested that the SCJ may be a more suitable replacement than the CCJ for the mandibular condyle.

Daniels (1987) excised the mandibular con-

dyles by performing vertical osteotomies on juvenile *Macaca mulatta* monkeys and replaced them with either CCJ grafts, SCJ grafts, or the original condyles immediately after removal. Histologic studies of the grafts were performed at five, 11, and 17 weeks. The results showed a faster incorporation of the condylar and SCJ grafts compared with the CCJ grafts. Both SCJ and condylar grafts remodeled in a similar fashion following transplantation. The CCJ graft, on the other hand, remained relatively unchanged in its organization, and a new condylar process was formed medial to the graft that had a trabecular pattern and cartilage lining similar to those of the mandibular condyle. Daniels emphasized the importance of a healthy environment and normal host structures for condylar regeneration to occur, suggesting that the SCJ may be more appropriate for condylar replacement where growth potential is desired since the SCJ graft seems to have a shorter lag period between placement and response to external stimuli. When growth is not a concern, either graft may be appropriate.

Collectively, the preceding studies by Daniels (1987), Ellis (1986), Hunsuck (1969), Peskin (1965), Poswillo (1974), and Ware (1965; 1966), have contributed significantly to the understanding of host-donor interaction in autogenous transplantation of growth centers to the TMJ. While little of a basic nature was added to the general knowledge of autogenous transplantation, specific information necessary to bridge the gap that often exists between general concepts and clinical application was accumulated. These studies provide a better basis for proceeding with clinical trials.

Substitution of the mandibular condyle with a cartilaginous growth center transplant has proved advantageous when either ankylosis or tumor requires surgical resection of the joint. The graft (1) maintains or increases ramus height following the arthroplasty, (2) forms a stable articulation, and (3) contributes to subsequent growth. Results have been less impressive, however, in instances in which growth center transplants have been attempted to treat condylar hypoplasia (or agenesis). Rather than replacing a faulty but serviceable articulation with a cartilaginous transplant, better results have been achieved by surgical elongation of the shortened hemimandible by way of a ramal osteotomy.

The interplay between the processes of experimental surgery, basic sciences, and clinical experience is especially evident in the area of growth discrepancies affecting the TMJs. Improved approaches to this most challenging problem have been developed as a result of this interplay. The process is a dynamic and evolutionary one. It is to be hoped that what is an acceptable standard at present will be replaced with significant improvements in the near future.

ARTHRITIDES

The arthritides that affect the TMJ occur with differing frequencies and with varying presentations (see Chapters 11, 16, 22, and 24). Of the various types, including rheumatoid arthritis and the seronegative spondylarthritides, osteoarthritis has received the greatest attention. Osteoarthritis refers to a degenerative joint disease characterized by degeneration `of the articular cartilage, hypertrophy of bone at the margins of the articular surfaces, and changes in the synovial membrane. This arthritic process is usually associated with advanced age; however, in the TMJ it can also be seen frequently in younger patients.

The process of osteoarthritis has been well described and well studied in its late stages, although the basic pathophysiology and initiating factors are still unclear. Autopsy studies have provided a description of the process in its later stages (DeBont, 1985). These studies, however, provide us with only a few frames of an ever-changing picture. Osteoarthritis and disc derangement may exist together (see Chapter 11) and some investigators suggest a cause and effect relationship (Anderson, 1985; Westesson, 1984). Osteoarthritis may result in disc derangement due to the roughness of the articular surfaces (DeBont, 1985) or disc derangement may precede osteoarthritis (Anderson, 1985).

Intracapsular Surgery

Removal of the articular disc for chronic TMJ pain has enjoyed popularity in the past. The procedure subsequently lost support because of the high incidence of recurrent symptoms (Poswillo, 1979). On the other hand, Eriksson (1985) found, in a long-term human study, that there was a favorable response relative to pain relief and reduction of locking following disc removal. Undoubtedly many surgical procedures have been performed on the disc while, in reality, muscular or occlusal disorders were the primary sources of the symptoms. Aside from the fact that these surgical failures prompted greater effort toward conservative care, they also stimulated efforts toward developing more acceptable surgical methods.

Another procedure recommended for chronic TMJ pain has been the intracapsular arthroplasty or high condylectomy (see Chapter 24). Murnane (1971) studied the histological sequence of healing following this procedure on adult rabbits. Initially, the cut surface was covered by fibrinoid material containing inflammatory cells. Fibroblast proliferation, with formation of collagenous fibers and ground substance, followed in the sequence characteristic of connective tissue healing. At the end of three months, a fibrocartilaginous articular surface was seen. Sprinz (1963) performed similar procedures on young rabbits. Both studies supported the thesis of condylar regeneration, with the retained disc shaping and confining the proliferative response. Poswillo's (1970) observations on repair in the adult monkey following high condylectomy differed to the extent that there was no cartilaginous regeneration noted.

The repair of the condylar stump was similar to that of a bone wound at any site. Undoubtedly rabbits and primates differ in some respects in regenerative potential and response to injury of the condyle.

The effect of functional stress on healing after arthroplasty has also been investigated (see Chapter 6). Mooney (1966) studied the influence of immobilization and motion after joint resection in rabbits. Several joints of the hindlimbs, including the metatarsophalangeal joint, were resected in a series of experiments. Following surgery, the false joints were immobilized from zero to 28 days. Animals were killed at intervals from one day to five weeks. When there was immediate mobilization of the joint, the fibrin clot was wiped away from the cut surface of the bone, delaying collagen formation. The subsequent fibrocartilage formed was thin and randomly organized. When the joint was held immobile for three weeks or more, fibrogenesis and collagen fiber orientation had progressed so that motion was unduly limited. Additional surgery was required to alter the character of the tissue and achieve normal motion. The study indicated that function and regeneration of the joint were achieved best when motion was delayed for about one week. If motion was delayed further, then restrictive scar formation was progressive. On the basis of this study, timing of mobilization following arthroplasty is quite important. Sufficient time for clot maturation should be allowed before subjecting the surgical site to the influence of motion.

Synovial Fluid Analysis

If osteoarthritis of the TMJ is the late stage of a degenerative process, then when and how should there be intervention to palliate or eliminate the disease process? Diagnostic capabilities that would indicate at what stage a patient is in the process could help in the development of a more effective array of therapies. Furthermore, more efficient diagnostic modalities could help avoid applying incorrect therapy to a given disease.

Investigators have attempted to characterize the properties of TMJ synovial fluid in animals. Hatton (1986), who attempted to identify the molecules responsible, found bovine synovial fluid to have lubrication properties similar to those of other hyaline cartilage synovial fluid. It is tempting to assume that a change in the lubricating properties of the synovial fluid may

be one of the initial changes in osteoarthritis of the TMJ.

Analysis of the synovial fluid could provide important information regarding the type and stage of the disease in the TMJ. Qualitative analysis of synovial fluid from other joints has included observation of volume, color and clarity, viscosity, and clot-forming ability (Schumacher, 1981). Quantitative analysis has consisted of cultures, light microscopic examination for cells, polarized light microscopic examination for crystals, and laboratory studies for enzymes, electrolytes, proteins, and the like (Schumacher, 1981). There have been reports, however, as to the value of synovial fluid analysis in the diagnosis of disease in other synovial joints (Francis, 1982).

Up to this point, proteolytic activity in the TMJs has received little attention. In degenerative joint disease it has been suggested that collagen is initially degraded by collagenase followed by degradation of the byproducts by gelatinase. Therefore, increased gelatinase levels may reflect the level of degenerative activity in the joint, and this could play a role in the diagnosis of degenerative joint disease. Even if the proteolytic activity is secondary to physical wear, monitoring such activity may provide a window on the entire process and allow therapeutic modalities to be more appropriately applied.

In an unpublished study we analyzed synovial fluid washings from 53 TMJs prior to open joint surgery for the treatment of TMJ dysfunction; all patients had clinical or radiologic evidence of either internal derangement or osteoarthritis. Sodium dodecyl sulfate (SDS)—polyacrylamide gel electrophoresis was used to identify gelatinolytic activity. Forty per cent of the washings examined in this manner showed such activity.

Idiopathic Condylysis

Although osteolysis has been reported in many bones of the body (Heffez, 1983), its manifestations in the maxillofacial region have been sparsely documented (see Chapter 12). Rabey (1978) may have been the first to distinguish condylar osteolysis from congenital or acquired condylar hypoplasia and condylar agenesis. In a literature review, Rabey found four cases of bilateral condylysis of unknown origin and added four new cases. The cases that Rabey reported, however, were associated with other disease processes: three with measles and prolonged purulent aural discharge and one with the later development of juvenile scleroderma. Massive osteolysis has been reported in other regions of the mandible by several authors, and associations have been made with other disease entities: progressive systemic sclerosis (PSS) (Ryatt, 1982; Seifert, 1975), Gorham's disease (Fredericksen, 1983; Heffez, 1983), and generalized osteodystrophy in chronic renal failure patients on hemodialysis (Dick, 1973).

Current data on this disease are essentially limited to case reports and literature reviews. The clinical presentation of osteolysis appears similar in most bones studied; however, the pathophysiology is incompletely understood. The disease is poorly characterized because of its rarity, and it is unclear whether the finding of bone lysis is reflective of many disease states or is a disease entity in itself.

In a well-studied case, Heffez (1983) described the clinical and histologic presentation of osteolysis involving the facial skeleton in a 22-year-old man. A proliferation of thin-walled blood and lymphatic vessels was found at the site of bony destruction. Heffez described two phases in the disease process: (1) an active phase characterized by bone destruction, mild tissue swelling and tenderness, and mild to moderate pain; and (2) an inactive, stable phase. During active bone dissolution, the process probably involves osteoclastic activity in association with the exuberant vascular channels. Initially the protective layer over the hydroxyapatite crystal may be digested by the osteocyte, thereby making the bone more accessible to the osteoclasts (Chambers, 1980).

Condylar osteolysis associated with PSS has been related to vasculitis of the small muscular perforating arteries to the condyle (Ramm, 1987). This seems reasonable because the basic pathology in PSS is thought to be a small artery vasculitis, with the collagen overproduction being a response to the inflammation and ischemia (Ramm, 1987). The basic histology, as described by light and electron microscopic studies, appears to be an exuberant proliferation of vascular and supportive elements resembling hemangiomatous tissue (Fredericksen, 1983; Heffez, 1983).

We have seen several cases of osteolysis limited to the condylar process (Fig. 13–8). Clinically, the presentation was one of a slow dissolution of the condyle, often unassociated with any signs or symptoms except a shifting occlusion. It is unclear whether these findings were related to degenerative joint disease or were a focal manifestation of condylysis. In the absence of histologic samples such a diagnostic assignment is not possible. If the dissolution was secondary to a proliferation of vascular and granulation tissue, however, it is unclear what the factors are that limit this proliferation to the condyle. Obviously, further study of this disease is needed. Such study may also add significantly to our understanding of bone metabolism.

Effects of Anti-inflammatory Agents on Joint Surfaces

Corticosteroids have been used for several decades to reverse the symptoms associated with inflammatory reactions within joints and around ligaments and tendons (see Chapters 11, 22, and 24). Horton (1953) first reported on use of intra-articular injections of hydrocortisone in treatment of painful TMJs. Numerous reports have followed on the successful reversal of symptoms using prednisone, triamcinolone, and betamethasone, as well as hydrocortisone.

While relief of pain from use of intracapsular steroids has been reported, occasional osteolytic changes observed in radiographs have stimulated interest in other than the anti-inflammatory effects on the joint surfaces. Mankin (1966) observed that cortisol caused a rapid and profound decrease in glycine utilization in articular cartilage of rabbits following intracapsular injections of hydrocortisone. Glycine utilization was equated with protein synthesis within the cartilage cells. The conclusion was that matrix synthesis was retarded in response to the cortisol.

Excessive use of corticosteroids in the TMJ has also been shown to lead to osteoarthritic changes in mice (Silbermann, 1980). The focus of corticosteroid action may be inhibition of the proliferation of chondroprogenitor cells and their differentiation into chondroblasts. Silbermann (1978) studied the condyles of immature baboons after repeated intra-articular or intramuscular steroid injections. Severe destruction of cartilage and bone was found, initially marked by fibrillation and followed by the complete disappearance of the cartilage. The subchondral bone lost its characteristic lamellar organization and took on the appearance of woven bone. This bone showed a predominance of fibrosis over ossification.

Poswillo (1970) performed six intracapsular injections of 0.1 ml (2.5 mg) of hydrocortisone acetate into the TMJs of three monkeys. Controls consisted of similar injection schedules on four animals; two received the vehicle only and the other two had only needle penetrations into the joint cavity. Histologic examination four

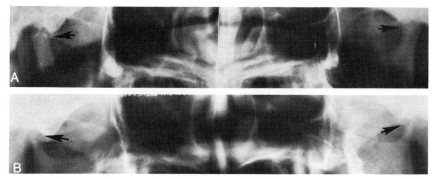

FIGURE 13–8. Idiopathic condylysis. *A,* Initial panoramic radiograph. *B,* Panoramic radiograph taken about seven years later. Note decreased dimension of the condyle in B.

months after the initial injections showed that the animals receiving the hydrocortisone had loss of the articular surface fibrous layer, erosion of the articular cartilage, and reduction of new bone formation in the subchondral layer. Poswillo postulated that the direct effect of local hydrocortisone on the cartilage was delayed turnover and repair, with consequent reduction in overall size of the condyle. Poswillo (1970) suggested that the response might be termed a pharmacological arthroplasty and explained the drug's general effectiveness in terms of circumferential reduction of the articular cap of cartilage followed by repair on a smaller scale than the original.

Controlled remodeling by pharmacological means is obviously an attractive approach to treat symptomatic degenerative and inflammatory joint disorders. The mechanism, however, needs to be better understood than it is at present. In our own unpublished experience, osteolysis with increased pain has been observed following intracapsular steroid therapy. The variable clinical responses, along with the findings from experiments such as Poswillo's (1970), indicate that intracapsular steroids, while having a place in the therapeutic regimen, are not without risk. The mechanism of action on articular tissue deserves further study.

TRAUMA

The clinical problem that has prompted the greatest controversy related to trauma of the TMJ is that of the fractured, dislocated condyloid process (see Chapter 24). The clinician called upon to treat such an injury is faced with the following questions: (1) Will adequate mandibular function and dental occlusion be achieved without anatomic reduction of the fracture? (2) If anatomic reduction appears to be indicated from a functional standpoint, is it technically feasible? e.g., is the bone comminuted? Can the condyloid process be adequately stabilized? (3) Do the risks of open reduction, primarily the potential for injury to the facial nerve, outweigh the potential benefits from anatomic realignment of the condyloid process? (4) What effect will displacement versus the surgery to reduce the fracture have on subsequent growth and development of the mandible in growing children? and (5) What effect does the condylar fracture have on the capsule and disc and how should this be managed?

The majority of surgeons treating facial trauma favor the so-called closed reduction of the displaced, fractured mandibular condyloid process. Usually, no attempt is made to reduce the fracture; treatment ordinarily consists of immobilizing the mandible in the best possible dental occlusion anywhere from two to six weeks. In fractures of other bones in the body, on the other hand, great efforts are made to achieve anatomic reduction. Why is the fractured, displaced condyloid process treated differently? Clinical results obtained with the closed method suggest that the TMJ and masticatory system have significant capacity for adaptation. Several studies have been conducted to understand further these mechanisms.

Walker in 1960 reported on two studies using young rhesus monkeys in which two methods of treatment were examined following surgical fracture and dislocation of the condyloid process. In the first study, about half of the animals had anatomic reduction of the fracture following dislocation. In the others, the condyloid process was left displaced at a right angle to its former position. The mandibles were not immobilized in either group, and the animals were killed about one and one-half years following the surgical procedures. Based on radiographic and gross examination of dried, prepared skulls, little difference in results was observed between the animals in which there had been anatomic reduction and those in which the condyloid processes were left displaced. Regeneration in the proper anatomic relationship also occurred in the latter group.

In a later study, attempts were made to follow the reformation process histologically. Animals were killed at one, two, and three months and at one year following fracture and dislocation of the condyloid process. The region in question was oriented and sectioned for microscopic study. Walker (1960) described a process of coordinated resorption, metaplasia of the cartilage, and subsequent ossification. The process resulted in reformation of a condyle similar to, if not exactly the same as, the untraumatized contralateral condyle. It was not apparent whether early mobilization of the mandible altered the process of reformation. Early movement certainly did not appear to hinder the final result.

Boyne (1967) conducted a similar study on 12 immature monkeys. Each was subjected to a bilateral subcondylar osteotomy, with displacement of the condylar fragment medially and anteriorly. Four animals were treated with open reduction and maxillomandibular fixation only, and four received no treatment. All animals healed equally well, with little deformity noted. This study again demonstrated the regenerative potential of the traumatized condyle in young monkeys. Heurlin (1961) reported on skeletal changes in the adult monkey following fracture and dislocation of the condyle. In all animals in which the procedure was unilateral, there appeared to be formation of a new false joint in an anterior position. When bilateral procedures were performed, an anterior open bite was produced. In both groups, the skeletal changes were similar to those reported in Sarnat's studies (in 1951; 1957; 1971) in which condylectomies were performed on both young and adult animals.

Results of the few experimental studies on trauma of the TMJ suggest remarkable adaptive properties of the entire masticatory system. Young animals have great potential for regeneration and reformation of the mandibular condyle. These studies support the conservative approach to clinical management of fractures of the mandibular condyloid process in children and to a lesser extent in adults. Numerous instances of regeneration of the condyle have been observed in young children following fracture and displacement. However, untoward results can occur. Significant deformity, including ankylosis, has been observed following condyloid process fractures, whether conservative treatment, open reduction, or no treatment at all was rendered. The mechanism of regeneration and remodeling needs further clarification if treatment methods are to be improved (see Chapter 6).

ANKYLOSIS: INTERPOSITIONAL ARTHROPLASTY

Autogenous Grafts

Georgiade (1957) studied the effects of interposing dermis in the ostectomy gap, first in dogs and then in monkeys (see Chapter 24). Histologic studies were performed on the animals at three-month intervals up to 18 months following surgery. Elastic fibers found in the dermis persisted, indicating the continuing viability of the tissue in its new environment. On the basis of both these studies and subsequent experiences in humans, the authors advocated that (1) the ostectomy should be through a preauricular approach and as high as possible in the mandibular neck; (2) the dermal graft should be sutured in an umbrella-like manner over the stump; and (3) early function should be instituted.

Alloplastic Materials

Cook (1972) used a polytetrafluoroethylene (Teflon) cloth to prevent bone contact following ostectomies for ankylosis. Histological studies on both rabbits and monkeys showed no inflammatory reaction around the cloth. Collagen fiber ingrowth stabilized the material in place. Silicone rubber has also been used to create pseudoarthrosis following ostectomy for ankylosis. Habbi (1970) determined that there was little or no reaction when thin sheets of silicone rubber were interposed in ostectomy sites in the mandibular necks of rabbits. The material effectively prevented bony healing for the 26 weeks of the study, and a false joint was maintained. In the control animals, complete bony union occurred at the ostectomy site within ten weeks following surgery. Tantalum foil (Goodsell, 1947), ticonium (Kent, 1972), polyethylene (Pennisi, 1965), and acrylic (Henry, 1960) have all been reported as satisfactory interpositional materials in the treatment of ankylosis. (See section on discectomy, page 223, regarding other uses of alloplastic materials in the TMJ.)

DISC DERANGEMENT

Disc Repair and Repositioning

In light of the possible relationship between disc derangement and degenerative joint disease (Westesson, 1984), disc repositioning and repair have enjoyed increasing popularity (see Chapter 24). McCarty (1979) described a technique for arthroplasty and disc repositioning that has been employed with some success in treating disc derangements. Weinberg (1984) treated patients with internal derangements with eminectomy and discorrhaphy (suturing the disc to the lateral capsule) and reported 88 per cent of the patients to be significantly improved. Hall (1984) advocated discoplasty of the superior lamina of the bilaminar zone for the treatment of anterior disc displacement and reported 65 per cent of the patients so treated to be pain-free over an average follow-up period of 18.1 months. Numerous other investigators have proposed a variety of other techniques for repositioning the displaced disc (Feinberg, 1987; Nespeca, 1987; Walker, 1987).

We have performed disc plication procedures after the methods of McCarty (1979) for the treatment of internal derangement and have enjoyed a similar success rate in the mitigation of symptoms. After a long follow-up period (greater than 18 months), we have found a number of initially supposedly cured patients who have, however, suffered a return of symptoms. It is possible that the cause of the internal derangement (biomechanical or biochemical forces) was still active, thus leading to the recurrence. Furthermore, it is plausible that there was disc deformation that precluded long-term anatomic reduction. Westesson (1985) found disc deformation to be present in 77 per cent of the autopsy specimens with complete anterior displacement. Another explanation lies in the possibility that surgery itself may lead to further degenerative changes. Wallace (1986) found that in the rabbit, incisions in the retrodiscal tissue or in the junction of the retrodiscal tissue and disc tissue healed normally, whereas incisions confined within the disc did not heal, with resultant hard and soft tissue degenerative changes. Misawa (1985) found similar results in primates.

Hall (1986) evaluated healing in five *Macaca fascicularis* monkeys after discoplasty, eminectomy, and high condylectomy. At the five-month interval, no discontinuity defects were found in the plicated discs, and all bone surfaces had new soft tissue linings but were devoid of the normal cartilage layer. The discoplasty incision was full thickness and completely within the bilaminar zone, extending into the synovium. A significant finding was the development of fibrous adhesions between the disc and either the eminectomy site or the high condylectomy site in over half of the animals.

Marciani (1987) performed bilaminar zone wedge resections or bilaminar zone freezing (cryosurgery) in 17 adult female monkeys to compare the scar-forming potential of the two procedures as a means of maintaining the repositioned disc. Marciani reported complete healing of the wedge resection with the area indistinguishable histologically from that observed in the unoperated posterior attachment tissue. Freezing of the bilaminar zone did not result in any significant scarring of the tissue, as was anticipated, and therefore it was concluded that cryosurgery may not be effective in the treatment of anteriorly displaced discs.

In the treatment of discal perforations, many investigators have attempted repair with a variety of materials. Dermal grafts have been used as a patch material in experimentally produced disc perforations in monkeys, and these grafts have been incorporated into the discal structure (Stewart, 1986). Tucker (1986) found that experimentally produced intra-articular disc perforations failed to heal in four out of five monkeys. Autogenous dermal grafts to disc perforations, however, all showed healing. One complication of dermal grafts was the development of epithelial cysts possibly related to inadequate hair follicle removal. Dermal grafts have also been used in patients with discal damage, with a resultant reduction of pain and an improvement in function (Zetz, 1984). Based on the contradictory studies, the process of repair and healing of lesions within the nonvascular portions of the disc remains controversial.

Discectomy

On occasion, repair and repositioning of the TMJ disc may be impossible because of deformation (Westesson, 1985) or degeneration of the disc. Discectomy has been the standard treatment in these cases; however, undesirable postoperative results have been encountered. Yaillen (1979) studied the effects of unilateral discectomy in four primates and compared them with one control animal. Results showed variable alterations in masticatory patterns and degenerative changes in the postsurgical joint. Furthermore, fibrous ankylosis was demonstrated in three postsurgical joints. Other investigators have found similar degenerative bony changes following discectomy in animals.

Because of the unpredictable results following discectomy, considerable attention has been directed to alloplastic replacement of the resected disc. Timmis (1986) performed discectomies on rabbit TMJs and used either reinforced silicone rubber or polytetrafluoroethylene aluminum oxide (PTFE-Al$_2$O$_3$) implants as replacements. The joints with implants were compared with sham-operated joints, with histological studies being conducted at two, four, eight, and 20 weeks after surgery. Reinforced silicone rubber implants were less stable than PTFE-Al$_2$O$_3$ implants. The foreign body reaction and articular surface destruction, however, were more intense in the PTFE-Al$_2$O$_3$–implanted joints. Other studies have reported similar histological findings in PTFE-Al$_2$O$_3$–implanted joints (Florine, 1988; Heffez, 1987) (Figs. 13–9 and 13–10) and in silicone-implanted joints (Westesson, 1987).

Bronstein (1987) compared the use of reinforced silicone rubber sheeting, HP Silastic, and Proplast II as disc replacement materials in a retrospective study in 145 patients representing 215 joints. Bronstein found that Proplast/Teflon implants produced a severe bony response characterized by flattening, sclerosis, and erosion of the fossa and the condyle. Other materials produced a less extreme radiographic response. Dolwick (1985) reported on a silicone-induced foreign body reaction with lymphadenopathy. Lagrotteria (1986) documented lymphadenopathy following the use of Proplast implant material. In 1991 the PTFE-Al$_2$O$_3$ implant was taken off the market.

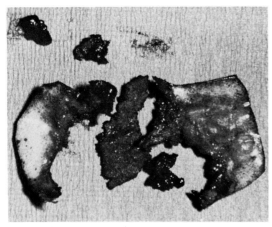

FIGURE 13–9. Polytetrafluoroethylene aluminum oxide (PTFE-Al$_2$O$_3$) implant surgically removed two years after placement in the left TMJ. Note fragmentation of the implant and the associated reactive tissue.

Clearly there exists no predictable or acceptable alloplastic replacement for the TMJ disc. Degenerative changes may be related to material failure and the subsequent foreign body reaction. The ultimate remodeling of the articular surfaces may leave the patient less symptomatic but functionally compromised.

Other materials that have been used for disc replacement include dura, fascia, dermis, and auricular cartilage. Some utility has been found in the use of a temporalis fascia and muscle flap rotated into the fossa and pedicled laterally off the periosteum of the zygomatic arch. In a few of the patients treated in this manner, return of symptoms and dysfunction has prompted reoperation. In these instances, the flap was found to be vascularized and occasionally adhesions were found on one or another of the articular surfaces. While a variety of materials have been advocated, the ideal replacement has not yet been found.

Arthroscopy

Recently, arthroscopy of the TMJ has come into vogue after the initial application by Ohnishi (1975) (see Chapter 17). Williams (1980) produced artificial lesions in the TMJs of rabbits and proceeded to examine these lesions through an arthroscope. Williams found that changes resembling some aspects of degenerative joint disease could be well visualized through the arthroscope. Furthermore, gross discal damage, condylar damage, synovial hyperplasia and acute inflammatory changes could be well visualized and diagnosed with the arthroscope. Other animal studies have documented reversible changes following arthroscopy (Hilsabeck, 1978) and have suggested that postoperative complications following human arthroscopy may be similarly reversible (Holmlund, 1986). Liedberg (1986) compared the diagnostic accuracy of TMJ arthroscopy with the findings on dissection of fresh human cadavers. Liedberg characterized arthroscopic diagnosis on the human TMJ as having high specificity but low sensitivity; pathologic entities were readily distinguishable, but may go unnoticed in certain locations.

Aside from diagnosis, arthroscopy has been used for surgical treatment of TMJ pathology. Sanders (1986) has proposed a sweeping technique with a blunt trocar in the superior joint space for lysis of adhesions and the treatment of the nonreducing anteriorly displaced disc (closed lock). In 40 arthroscopies in 25 patients, Sanders found persistent symptoms of closed lock to be eliminated in 21 joints. In a later

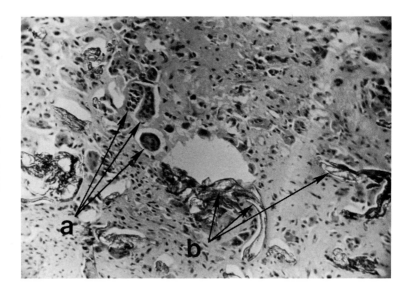

FIGURE 13–10. Photomicrograph of granulation tissue associated with PTFE-Al₂O₃ implant (see Fig. 13–9). Foreign body giant cells associated with the implant (a). Fragmented particles of PTFE-Al₂O₃ implant material (b). Clefting around particles is a preparation artifact.

study, Sanders (1987) presented results of 115 TMJ arthroscopies. Of patients with a diagnosis of internal derangement with persistent closed lock or arthrosis with capsulitis, 81.7 per cent had an excellent response as measured by a decrease in symptoms and an improvement in function. The follow-up period, however, was not specified. The authors stressed the importance of joint lavage in treatment as well as sweeping the superior joint space to lyse adhesions. Tarro (1988) described a method for triangulation of the arthroscope with a motorized cutting unit for the removal of adhesions. Of 48 surgical arthroscopies with an observation period from three weeks to 10 months, 41 surgical procedures resulted in asymptomatic joints.

The diagnostic capabilities of TMJ arthroscopy are clearly superior in certain ways to those of some of the other imaging modalities currently available. The therapeutic application of the arthroscope to intra-articular disorders, however, may become more effective with the development of more sophisticated instrumentation and a greater understanding of the pathological processes. Lysis of adhesions and joint lavage to effect a change in the immediate environment of the disc may be effective for short periods. Unless the underlying pathology is addressed, however, the benefits of all treatment directed at the manifestations of that pathology may be short-lived. Continued research is needed that will direct the timely and appropriate application of arthroscopic techniques to the treatment of TMJ derangements.

FUNCTIONAL ADAPTATIONS

The thrust for studies on the parameters of adaptability within the TMJ emanates primarily from clinicians concerned with occlusion (see Chapter 6). Orthodontists routinely are faced with occlusal disparities that could be improved through either stimulation or diminution of mandibular growth. The effects of orthopedic forces applied during growth are difficult to evaluate. The question arises whether the effect is due to the intended mechanical force or to coincidental growth. The shortcomings of such clinical studies are well recognized. Researchers have turned to animal experiments to study the relationship of altered function and joint response.

Occlusal Alterations

Many reports have described changes in the alveolar process and joint tissues as a result of dental alterations. Both cephalometric and histologic techniques have been used in these evaluations. When younger animals were used, condylar cartilage and bone exhibited significant adaptations in response to external forces (Baume, 1961; Breitner, 1933; Erlich, 1982; Hickman, 1961; Knak, 1973; Lieb, 1972; Stockli, 1971). Conversely, when older animals were used, the joint structures remained more stable or demonstrated pathologic changes in response to displacement of the mandible (Colico, 1958; Hiniker, 1966). As might be expected, the maturational level of the individual appears to be an important factor influencing the adaptive ability of the TMJ.

Perhaps the most exhaustive study performed on the adaptations of the TMJ to altered function has been by McNamara (1972) on 35 rhesus monkeys of various ages. Cephalometric, electromyographic, and histologic techniques were correlated and McNamara described the role of the masticatory muscles, particularly the lateral pterygoid, in the adaptive process. In those animals in which the mandible or maxilla was placed in a functional protrusion, the lateral pterygoid muscle appeared to assume the most active role in determination of mandibular position. A normal pattern of muscle function reappeared at 12 to 24 weeks after the functional device had been placed. In the younger animals, alterations in the amount and direction of condylar growth were evident. In the older animals, no significant condylar growth was noted. Skeletal adaptations were centered more in the alveolar processes and were achieved through tooth movement. In both young and mature animals, a correlation was evident between the appearance and disappearance of the altered neuromuscular function and the occurrence of skeletal and dentoalveolar adaptations.

Similar findings were reported in later studies. McNamara (1982) applied functional prosthetic appliances to 12 young adult female monkeys and performed histological studies on the condyle at varying periods up to 24 weeks. Changes in the TMJs were found to be qualitatively similar to changes in juvenile TMJs, but greatly reduced in magnitude. Apparently, some functional remodeling capability exists in the adult TMJ, but the potential is less with increasing age.

Studies have surveyed edentulous patients and found a significant number of them to have TMJ dysfunction (Sakurai, 1988). Axelsson (1987), in an autopsy study of 84 TMJs, also found a higher frequency of arthritic changes in edentulous specimens. A positive correlation between the severity of dental attrition or loss of teeth and degenerative joint disease is suggested by other studies (Granados, 1979). Indeed, it has been suggested that occlusal rehabilitation may influence the remodeling process and lead to a more physiological shape of the flattened (pathologic) condyle (Mongini, 1983).

Animal studies and retrospective human studies suggest a relationship between tooth loss and attrition and osteoarthrosis. The study by Christensen (1986) has shown that loss of teeth and the subsequent impaired occlusal stabilization in experimental animals results in pathologic changes in the articular cartilage, articular disc, synovium, and bony articular components. The TMJ apparatus exists as an integral functional unit with the dentition, and it is reasonable to assume that an alteration in one will result in a change in the other. Clini-

cally, most occlusal alterations may be accompanied by adaptive changes in the TMJ apparatus without pathologic changes. This may be the envelope in which we work when the occlusion is altered as part of therapy. Age may be an important factor in whether adaptation or pathology occurs. Again, reliance on adaptability is emphasized; the task is to identify the limits of adaptability (see Chapter 6).

Changes After Osteotomies

Frequently the question arises about the effect on the joint of mandibular osteotomies. The condyle may be torqued laterally or rotated anteriorly or posteriorly in conjunction with the ramal osteotomies performed to correct prognathism or retrognathism. The process of adaptation of the TMJ in response to physical stress has been well described by both Blackwood (1966) and Moffett (1964). The intermediate zone of cells within the articular surface of the TMJ evidently retains the capacity for cellular proliferation and differentiation throughout life. This zone probably is responsible primarily for the remodeling changes observed.

Boyne (1966), using tetracycline labeling, demonstrated condylar remodeling in monkeys following vertical osteotomies in the ramus with lateral displacement of the condylar fragment. The main purpose was to evaluate bony healing at the osteotomy site when the proximal fragment was left in an overlapped relation with the ramus. The study suggested that overlap of the fragments resulted in bone repair as efficient as that which occurs when decortication is performed. Callus encompassed the overlap, with bone healing progressing in the manner typical of any fracture. Examination of the TMJ showed new bone formation at the attachment of the lateral pterygoid muscle to the condyloid process within two weeks following surgery. By three weeks following surgery, evidence of remodeling of the condyle was observed. The remodeling process that occurs at a distance from the surgical site is another example of the physiological bone response to an altered function.

EFFECTS OF OTHER FACTORS

Nutrition

The circulatory pattern of the normal mandibular condyle in the guinea pig appears as a fan-like arrangement of capillaries arising from one or two small arterioles within the medullary cavity of the posterior ramus. The terminal branches that approximate and penetrate the eroded cartilage zone demonstrate a bulbar ending that conforms to the individual chondrocyte capsule. Multinucleated cells accompany the penetrating capillaries and seem to be responsible for the actual resorption of the chondrocytic capsule. The zone of calcification appears to precede the erosion front at a layer depth of three to four capsules. These findings, reported by Durkin (1969a), were similar to those observed in the articular head of the tibia, but differed from the process seen in the tibial epiphysis. While the process of erosion in the articular and mandibular condyle cartilage is dependent on chondroclastic activity, erosive activity in the tibial epiphysis is mainly by capillary penetration. Calcification of the epiphyseal cartilage proceeds along the vertical cartilaginous partitions between the columns of chondrocytes, while in both the articular and condylar cartilage calcification circumscribes the chondrocyte capsules. Since growth of the condyle is by endochondral ossification, dietary alterations that affect various cartilaginous growth centers also affect the growth and development of the mandible.

In scorbutic guinea pigs, disruption and decrease of blood supply to the condylar, articular, and epiphyseal cartilages occur. The effect of ascorbic acid deficiency on epiphyseal cartilage is apparently more pronounced than on either the articular or condylar cartilage. The epiphyseal cartilage also recovers less quickly following treatment. The capillary endothelium gives rise to those chondroclasts responsible for the normal erosive activity of the condylar cartilage in the growing animal. Ascorbic acid appears to act on the differentiation of these chondroclasts (Durkin, 1969b).

The differences between condylar and epiphyseal cartilage have been further demonstrated through studies on rachitic rats (Durkin, 1971). As with scurvy, the changes observed in the epiphysis were more rapid and more severe than those that occurred in either the articular or condylar cartilage. Increased width of the condylar cartilage, primarily of the hypertrophic type, was the most distinguishing feature. Morphologically, the cartilage took on the shape reminiscent of the carrot-shaped wedge of cartilage seen during the early development of the condyle. Vascularity and erosive activities were reduced, as was the process of calcification. The sequence of repair following administration of the vitamin D metabolite began with increased calcification. The rachitic epiphysis reverted to a more primitive arrangement similar to that seen in condylar and articular cartilage. This phenomenon suggests that epiphyseal cartilage is a more differentiated form of cartilage than the other two.

Mirsky (1984) studied the effects of an active vitamin D metabolite $(24,25\text{-}(OH)_2D_3)$ on cartilage growth in the condyle of suckling mice. The proliferative activity of the chondroprogenitor cells was found to be unaffected. The differentiation of the chondroprogenitor cells to chondroblasts, however, was inhibited, leading to an overall decrease in the number of chondroblasts and chondrocytes. Excessive vitamin D $(24,25\text{-}(OH)_2D_3)$ also resulted in metabolic and structural changes in already differentiated chondroblasts and hypertrophic chondrocytes, thereby affecting the process of endochondral bone formation. Weinreb (1986) found a significant reduction of condylar growth when either vitamin D_3 or $1,25\text{-}(OH)_2D_3$ was injected into rats. Undernourished rats showed a similar but less severe decrease in growth. Collagen synthesis in the condylar cartilage of $1,25\text{-}(OH)_2D_3$-treated suckling mice was found to be significantly inhibited (Silbermann, 1987). The inhibitory effect was the result of decreased metabolic activity of the condylar cells.

Dietary deficiency of vitamin D_3 is usually associated with undernourishment, and the effects on growth and development are well documented. Principally by examining the effects of excessive vitamin D (or metabolite) administration these studies have attempted to determine where vitamin D works. It appears that both the differentiation process of the chondroprogenitor cells and the metabolic activity of mature chondrocytes are affected. This may account for the sequence of repair seen after rachitic animals are given vitamin D.

Rachitic children exhibit clinical changes similar to those observed in rats. The reduced cartilaginous growth produces not only a shortness of the extremities but also considerable facial disharmony. In addition, delayed eruption and malpositioning of the teeth occur, since the shortened ramus does not provide adequate maxillomandibular space. Moreover, failure of the anterior border of the ramus to resorb at the time the teeth are about to erupt also contributes to the problem (Rushton, 1948).

Dietary deficiencies in pantothenic acid (Levy, 1949a), tryptophan (Bavetta, 1954), and riboflavin (Levy, 1949b) have been shown to inhibit normal growth and development of the cartilage in the mandibular condyle of mice.

Retarded condylar growth has been produced in rats by vitamin B complex deficiency (Gorlin, 1951b). Hypervitaminosis A also inhibits growth of the condylar cartilage in rats (Gorlin, 1951a). Vitamin A has also been implicated in cellular differentiation and may be involved in chondrogenesis (Kay, 1987).

Inclusions of lipid droplets within chondrocytes are apparently normal and were first reported several decades ago (Putschar, 1931). The significance of the lipid and how the fat is deposited within the cell, however, are not well known. Investigations of lipoarthrosis in rabbits have shown uptake of the lipid by the chondrocytes within four days following injections into the synovial cavity (Ghadially, 1970; Mehta, 1973). No fat droplets were demonstrated within the matrix, nor was there a diminishing concentration gradient of fat from the articular surface inward, as would be expected if the process were primarily dependent on a diffusion gradient. Degenerative changes of the articular surface and pathologic changes within the chondrocytes are thought to follow injections of lipids into the articular cavity of the TMJ (Sprinz, 1976).

While the role of the cystoplasmic lipid within chondrocytes is not well understood, apparently experimental lipoarthrosis promotes pathologic changes rather than stimulating the natural lipid metabolism. It is anticipated that, with the emerging techniques, a better understanding of the chondrocyte and its metabolism will be forthcoming. Past studies on hormonal and dietary effects were limited to relatively gross anatomic assessments because of the limited technology. With increased capabilities to study the ultrastructure, many of the earlier studies warrant repetition.

Hormones

Endocrine disturbances in animals often have a profound effect upon condylar growth (Becks, 1946; 1948; Collins, 1946; 1949). The severe and striking effects of hypothyroidism are reflected in the small stature and disproportion (Smith, 1951). Cephalometric studies of cretins revealed a generalized retardation of growth within the facial area (Engel, 1941). The head is too large for the body, and the cranial skeleton is relatively larger than the facial skeleton. The synchondroses at the cranial base and the sutures remain open. The teeth are retarded in development and eruption, but their size is not affected. Therefore, the teeth and alveolar process seem overly large for the body of the maxilla

and mandible. Retardation in anteroposterior facial growth is induced by the lag in the development of the cranial base, which normally influences the development of the upper part of the face.

A distinguishing characteristic of hyperpituitarism in the adult is overgrowth of the mandible. Evans in 1921 first induced giantism experimentally in rats with injections of pituitary extract. Since then, refined extracts have been used to produce changes resembling acromegaly in the mouse and guinea pig (Silberberg, 1943) and rat (Asling, 1965; Becks, 1946; Collins, 1949; Meyer, 1967). While the mandibular overgrowth appeared to be associated with the elevated levels of growth hormone, the studies did not determine whether the effect was directly upon the condyle or mediated through the enlarging functional matrices.

Fuller (1974), using guinea pigs, and later Bernabei (1975), using rats, attempted to answer the question by surgically isolating the condyles from the remainder of the mandible. Growth hormone injected into both growing and adult animals clearly stimulated condylar growth in the isolated condyles. At this point, the evidence supports the premise that both the condyle and soft tissue respond directly to the influence of growth hormone.

In a study of rats subjected to hypophysectomy and thyroidectomy, graded growth hormone dosages stimulated a graded response in the noncalcified region of the epiphyseal cartilage plate (Hoskins, 1977). Thyroxine augmented this response eight-fold. Hoskins found a similar response in the mandibular condyle. These findings suggest that thyroxine mediates the effect of growth hormone on condylar growth.

Irradiation

The cytotoxic effects of radiation are well established. Cell division and growth are inhibited. Progressive fibrosis of connective tissue occurs and appears to be dose-related. When joints are included in the primary beam of cancerocidal radiation, atrophy and fibrosis of pericapsular structures are commonly observed. Severe limitation of mandibular motion may occur when the TMJs receive large amounts of radiation. The specific effects of radiation on the TMJ tissues have not been widely studied. Most information has been inferred from early studies of radiation effects on epiphyseal growth (Burstone, 1950). Burstone reported pronounced retardation of condylar growth in young mice when the TMJ was subjected to a single dose of radiation varying from 1,500 to 5,000 rads. However, even in those animals receiving 5,000 rads, recovery of cellular activity was significant at six to ten weeks following irradiation.

Young rats subjected to total body irradiation of 600 rads demonstrated serious damage to the growing cartilage of the mandibular condyle. Of course, osteoblastic activity, vascularity, and hemopoietic elements were also decreased. Signs of repair were noted at seven days following irradiation and judged to be complete by four weeks (Furstman, 1970).

Sclerosing Solutions

The use of sclerosing solutions in the treatment of joint hypermobility has enjoyed some popularity in the past (see Chapter 24). The clinical practice was supported by both Schultz (1937) and Moose (1941). Schultz investigated a number of materials, finally settling on a 5 per cent solution of sodium psylliate as a nontoxic material capable of producing a controllable fibrosis of the joint capsule. In dogs, a subacute reaction occurred within 30 minutes of injection, with beginning fibrosis evident at four to six days. The injections were made into the TMJ, reportedly without any evidence of deleterious effects on the articular surfaces. Moose repeated the study on rhesus monkeys, injecting the joints weekly for several months, finding no long-term deleterious effects on the joint surfaces and only a mild thickening of the periarticular tissues.

In spite of experimental evidence supporting the benignity of the procedure, the clinical use of sclerosing solutions for treatment of the hypermobile joint has never become widespread. While restricted mandibular motion can be achieved, postinjection discomfort is frequently quite significant. Furthermore, in our own unpublished experience, occasional pronounced osteolytic changes have been observed in radiographs following the use of intracapsular injections of sclerosing solutions.

SUMMARY

Experimental studies have contributed to a better understanding of the biology of the TMJ and of possible therapeutic approaches to pathosis. Most experimentation has focused on the role of the condyle in growth and development of the face. Currently, however, there is still a question as to whether the condyle serves as a primary growth center or functions in a secondary adaptive manner. In either case, the condyle appears to play an important role.

Healing, adaptability, and regeneration of the joint tissues are better understood as a result of the surgical studies reported. Mechanisms controlling these processes, however, need to be more vigorously explored.

Inadequate development of the condyle and contiguous tissues remains a difficult management problem for the therapist. Avenues of possible exploration include (1) muscle transfer or transplantation to increase the functional matrix, (2) microvascular anastomosis to enhance transplantation of both soft and hard tissues, and (3) collaborative work on controlling immune mechanisms to permit homologous transplantation.

Further areas of research that hold promise are in the chemical analysis of the synovial fluid and soft tissues of the joint. Arthroscopic studies should continue to expand into the areas of both diagnosis and treatment of early pathosis.

Improving TMJ function in instances of debilitating arthritis or ankylosis ultimately may be approached through the implantation of an artificial joint. A usable prototype, drawing on the talents of the materials expert, mechanical engineer, and the surgeon, should not be far in the future.

REFERENCES

Anderson, Q. N., and Katzberg, R. W.: Pathologic evaluation of disc dysfunction and osseous abnormalities of the temporomandibular joint. J. Oral Maxillofac. Surg. 43:947–51, 1985.

Asling, C. W., Simpson, M. E., and Evans, H. M.: Gigantism: Its induction by growth hormone in the skeleton of intact and hypophysectomized rats, and its failure following thyroidectomy. Rev. Suisse Zool. 2:1–34, 1965.

Axelsson, S., Fitins, D., Hellsing, G., and Holmlund, A.: Arthrotic changes and deviation in the form of the temporomandibular joint—An autopsy study. Swed. Dent. J. 11:195–200, 1987.

Baume, L. J., and Derichsweiler, H.: Is the condylar growth center responsive to orthodontic therapy? An experimental study in Macaca mulatta. Oral Surg. 14:347–362, 1961.

Bavetta, L. A., Bernick, S., Geiger, E., and Bergren, W.: The effect of tryptophan deficiency on the jaws of rats. J. Dent. Res. 33:309–315, 1954.

Becks, H., Collins, D. A., Asling, C. W., et al.: The giantism produced in normal rats by injection of pituitary growth hormone. V. Skeletal changes: Skull and dentition. Growth 12:55–67, 1948.

Becks, H., Collins, D. A., Simpson, M. E., and Evans, H. M.: Growth and transformation of the mandibular joint of the rat. III. The effect of growth hormone and thyroxine injections in hypophysectomized female rats. Am. J. Orthod. Oral Surg. 32:447–451, 1946.

Bernabei, R.: A Cephalometric Investigation of the Growth, In Situ, of "Isolated" Mandibular Condyles in Adult Rats Following the Administration of Bovine Growth Hormone. Unpublished dissertation. Cleveland, Case Western Reserve University, 1975.

Björk, A.: Facial growth in man, studied with the aid of metallic implants. Acta Odontol. Scand. 13:9–34, 1955.

Blackwood, H. J. J.: Cellular remodeling in articular tissue. J. Dent. Res. 45:480–489, 1966.

Boyne, P.: Osseous healing after oblique osteotomy of the mandibular ramus. J. Oral Surg. 24:125–133, 1966.

Boyne P.: Osseous repair and mandibular growth after subcondylar fractures. J. Oral Surg. 25:300–309, 1967.

Brash, J. C.: The Growth of the Jaws, Normal and Abnormal, in Health and Disease. London, Dental Board of the United Kingdom, 1924.

Breitner, C.: Experimental change of the mesio-distal relations of the upper and lower dental arches. Angle Orthod. 3:67–76, 1933.

Brodie, A. G.: On the growth pattern of the human head from the third month to the eighth year of life. Am. J. Anat. 63:209–262, 1941.

Bronstein, S. L.: Retained alloplastic temporomandibular joint disc implants: A retrospective study. Oral Surg. 64:135–145, 1987.

Buchner, R.: Induced growth of the mandibular condyle in the rat. J. Oral Rehabil. 9:7–22, 1982.

Burstone, M. S.: The effect of x-ray irradiation on the development of the mandibular joint of the mouse. J. Dent. Res. 29:358–363, 1950.

Campbell, C. J., Grisolia, A., and Zanconato, G.: The effects produced in the cartilaginous epiphyseal plate of immature dogs by experimental surgical trauma. J. Bone Joint Surg. (Am.). 41:1221–1242, 1959.

Chambers, T. J.: Cellular basis of bone resorption. Clin. Orthod. 151:283, 1980.

Charles, S. W.: The temporomandibular joint and its influence on growth of the mandible. Br. Dent. J. 46:845–855, 1925.

Choukas, N. C., Toto, P. D., and Guccione, J. M.: Mandibular condylectomy in the rhesus monkey. J. Oral Surg. 24:422–432, 1966.

Christensen, L. V., and Ziebert, G. J.: Effects of experimental loss of teeth on the temporomandibular joint. J. Oral Rehabil. 13:587–98, 1986.

Colico, G. L.: Le modificazoni dell' A. T. M. del Macacus rhesus a sequito di apparecchi fissi. Rass. Int. Stomatol. Pra. 9(Suppl. 4):41, 1958.

Collins, D. A., Becks, H., Asling, C. W., et al.: The growth of hypophysectomized female rats following chronic treatment with pure pituitary growth hormone. V. Skeletal changes: Skull and dentition. Growth 13:207–220, 1949.

Collins, D. A., Becks, H., Simpson, M. E., and Evans, H. M.: Growth and transformation of the mandibular joint in the rat II. Hypophysectomized female rats. Am. J. Orthod. Oral Surg. 32:443–446, 1946.

Cook, H. P.: Teflon implantation in temporomandibular arthroplasty. Oral Surg. 33:706–716, 1972.

Copray, J. C. V. M., Jansen, H. W. B., and Duterloo, H. S.: Growth of the mandibular condylar cartilage of the rat in serum-free organ culture. Arch. Oral Biol. 28:967–974, 1983.

Daniels, S., Ellis, E., and Carlson, D. S.: Histologic analysis of costochondral and sternoclavicular grafts in the TMJ of the juvenile monkey. J. Oral Maxillofac. Surg. 45:675–682, 1987.

Das, A., Meyer, J., and Sicher, H.: X-ray and alizarin studies on the effect of bilateral condylectomy in the rat. Angle Orthod. 35:138–148, 1965.

DeBont, L. G. M., Boering, G., Liem, R. S. B., and Hovinga, P.: Osteoarthritis of the temporomandibular joint: A light microscopic and scanning electron microscopic study of the articular cartilage of the mandibular condyle. J. Oral Maxillofac. Surg. 43:481–488, 1985.

Dick, R., and Jones, D. M.: Temporomandibular joint changes in patients undergoing chronic hemodialysis. Clin. Radiol. 24:72–76, 1973.

Dingman, R. O., and Grabb, W. C.: Reconstruction of both mandibular condyles with metatarsal bone grafts. Plast. Reconst. Surg. 34:441–451, 1964.

Dolwick, M. F., and Aufdemorte, T. B.: Silicone-induced foreign body reaction and lymphadenopathy after temporomandibular joint arthroplasty. Oral Surg. 59:449–452, 1985.

Durkin, J. F., Heeley, J. D., and Irving, J. T.: A comparison and changes in the articular mandibular condylar and growth-plate cartilages during the onset and healing of richets in rats. Arch. Oral Biol. 16:689–699, 1971.

Durkin, J. F., Irving, J. T., and Heeley, J. D.: A comparison of the circulatory and calcification patterns in the mandibular condyle in the guinea pig with those found in the tibial epiphyseal and articular cartilages. Arch. Oral Biol. 14:1365–1371, 1969a.

Durkin, J. F., Irving, J. T., and Heeley, J. D.: A comparison of circulatory and calcification changes induced in the mandibular condyle, tibial epiphyseal and articular cartilages of the guinea pig by the onset and healing of scurvy. Arch. Oral Biol. 14:1373–1382, 1969b.

Duterloo, H. S.: In Vivo Implantation of the Mandibular Condyle in the Rat. Ph.D. Thesis, University of Nijmegen, Netherlands, 1967.

Ellis, E., and Carlson, D. S.: Histologic comparison of the costochondral, sternoclavicular and temporomandibular joints during growth in Macaca mulatta. J. Oral Maxillofac. Surg. 44:312–321, 1986.

Engel, M. B., Bronstein, I. P., Brodie, A. G., and Wesoke, P. H.: A roentgenographic cephalometric appraisal of untreated and treated hypothyroidism. Am. J. Dis. Child. 61:1193–1198, 1941.

Engelsma, S. D., Jansen, H. W. B., and Duterloo, H. S.: An in vivo transplantation study of growth of the mandibular condyle in a functional position in the rat. Arch. Oral Biol. 25:305–311, 1980.

Engfeldt, B., Tegner, B., and Berquist, E.: Early changes in the epiphyseal growth zone in experimental osteolathyrism. A histologic, microradiographic and autoradiographic study. Acta Pathol. Microbiol. Scand. (A), 49:39–54, 1960.

Eriksson, L., Westesson, P-L.: Long-term evaluation of meniscectomy of the temporomandibular joint. J. Oral Maxillofac. Surg. 43:263–269, 1985.

Erlich, J., Bol, I., Yaffe, A., and Sela, J.: Calcification patterns of rat condylar cartilage after induced unilateral malocclusion. J. Oral Pathol. 11:366–373, 1982.

Evans, H. M., and Long, J. A.: The effect of the anterior lobe administered intraperitoneally upon growth, maturity, and estrous cycles of the rat. Anat. Rec. 21:62–63, 1921.

Feinberg, S. E., and Smilack, M. S.: Technique of functional disc repositioning in internal derangements of the temporomandibular joint. J. Oral Maxillofac. Surg. 45:825–827, 1987.

Felts, W. J. L.: Tissue survival in mouse whole bone transplants. Transplantation Bull. 4:5–10, 1957.

Florine, B. L., Gatto, D. J., Wade, M. L., and Waite, D. E.: Tomographic evaluation of temporomandibular joints following discoplasty or placement of polytetrafluoroethylene implants. J. Oral Maxillofac. Surg. 48:183–188, 1988.

Francis, R. M.: Is synovial fluid analysis of diagnostic value? Br. J. Clin. Pract. 36:229–234, 1982.

Fredericksen, N. L., Wesley, R. K., Sciubba, J. L., and Helfrick, J.: Massive osteolysis of the maxillofacial skeleton: A clinical, radiographic, histologic, and ultrastructural study. Oral Surg. 55:470–480, 1983.

Fuller, D. S.: An Investigation of Growth of the Mandibular Condyle Following Condylotomy in the Guinea Pig. Unpublished dissertation. Cleveland, Case Western Reserve University, 1974.

Furstman, L.: Effect of x-irradiation on the mandibular condyle. J. Dent. Res. 49:419–427, 1970.

Gelbke, H.: The influence of pressure and tension on growing bone in experiments with animals. J. Bone Joint Surg. (Am.). 33:947–954, 1951.

Georgiade, N., Altmay, F., and Pickerell, K.: An experimental and clinical evaluation of autogenous dermal grafts used in the treatment of temporomandibular joint ankylosis. Plast. Reconstr. Surg. 19:321–336, 1957.

Ghadially, F. N., Mehta, P. N., and Kirkaldy-Willis, W. H.: Ultrastructure of articular cartilage in experimentally produced lipoarthrosis. J. Bone Joint Surg. (Am.). 52:1147–1158, 1970.

Goodsell, J. O.: Tantalum in temporomandibular joint arthroplasty: Report of case. J. Oral Surg. 5:41–45, 1947.

Gorlin, R. J., and Chaudry, A. P.: The effect of hypervitaminosis A upon the incisor and molar teeth, the alveolar bone, and temporomandibular joint of weanling rats. J. Dent. Res. 38:1008–1015, 1951a.

Gorlin, R. J., and Levy, B. M.: Changes in the mandibular joint and periodontium of vitamin B complex deficient rats and the course of repair. J. Dent. Res. 30:337–346, 1951b.

Granados, J. I.: The influence of loss of teeth and attrition on the articular eminence. J. Prosthet. Dent. 42:78–85, 1979.

Haas, S. L.: Stimulation of bone growth. Am. J. Surg. 95:125–131, 1958.

Habbi, I., Murnane, T. W., and Doku, H. C.: Silastic and supramid in arthroplasty of temporomandibular joint in the rabbit. J. Oral Surg. 28:267–272, 1970.

Hall, B. K.: Developmental and Cellular Skeletal Biology. New York, Academic Press, 1978.

Hall, B. K.: Mandibular morphogenesis and craniofacial malformations. J. Craniofac. Genet. Dev. Biol. 2:309–322, 1982.

Hall, M. B.: Meniscoplasty of the displaced temporomandibular joint meniscus without violating the inferior joint space. J. Oral Maxillofac. Surg. 42:788–792, 1984.

Hall, M. B., Baughman, R., Ruskin, J., and Thompson, D. A.: Healing following meniscoplasty, eminectomy and high condylectomy in the monkey temporomandibular joint. J. Oral Maxillofac. Surg. 44:177–182, 1986.

Hatton, M. N., and Swann, D. A.: Studies on bovine temporomandibular joint synovial fluid. J. Prosthet. Dent. 56:635–638, 1986.

Heffez, L., Doku, H. C., Carta, B. L., and Feenez, J. E.: Perspectives on massive osteolysis. Oral Surg. 55:331–343, 1983.

Heffez, L., Mafee, M. F., Rosenberg, H., and Langer, B.: CT evaluation of TMJ disc replacement with a Proplast/Teflon laminate. J. Oral Maxillofac. Surg. 45:657–665, 1987.

Henry, T. C.: Prosthetic restoration of the left temporomandibular joint in a case of partial ankylosis. Transactions of the Second Congress of the International Society of Plastic Surgeons. London, E. and S. Livingstone, 1960, pp. 159–164.

Heurlin, R. G., Gans, B. J., and Stuteville, O. H.: Skeletal changes following fracture dislocation of the mandibular condyle in the adult rhesus monkey. Oral Surg. 14:1490–1500, 1961.

Hickman, J. H., and Graziano, F. W.: The effectiveness of orthopedic forces in inhibiting mandibular growth. Am. J. Orthod. 62:634–635, 1961.

Hilsabeck, R. B., and Laskin, D. M.: Arthroscopy of the temporomandibular joint of the rabbit. J. Oral Surg. 36:938–943, 1978.

Hiniker, J. J., and Ramfjord, S. P.: Anterior displacement of the mandible in adult rhesus monkeys. J. Prosthet. Dent. 16:503–512, 1966.

Hirabayashi, S., Harii, K., Sakuri, A., et al.: An experimental study of craniofacial growth in a heterotopic rat head transplant. Plast. Reconstr. Surg. 82:236–243, 1988.

Holmlund, A., Hellsing, G., and Borg, G.: Arthroscopy of the rabbit temporomandibular joint. Int. J. Oral Maxillofac. Surg. 15:170, 1986.

Horton, C. P.: Treatment of arthritic temporomandibular joints by intra-articular injection of hydrocortisone. Oral Surg. 6:826–829, 1953.

Hoskins, W. E., and Asling, C. W.: Influence of growth hormone and thyroxine on endochondral osteogenesis in the mandibular condyle and proximal tibial epiphysis. J. Dent. Res. 56:509–517, 1977.

Hovell, J. H.: Bone grafting procedures in the mandible. Oral Surg. 15:1281–1294, 1962.

Hulen, G. H.: A Method of Roentgenographic Cephalometry as Combined with the Use of Metallic Implants in Studying the Growth of the Mandible in Experimental Animals: The Dog. Unpublished dissertation. Chicago, Northwestern University, 1948.

Humphry, G.: On the Growth of the Jaws. Cambridge, Transactions of the Philosophical Society XI, 1864.

Hunsuck, E. E.: Autogenous grafts for replacing temporomandibular joints and mandibular condyles in monkeys. J. Oral Surg. 27:167–173, 1969.

Hunter, J.: The Natural History of the Human Teeth, 2nd ed. London, J. Johnson, 1778.

Jarabak, J. R., and Vehe, K.: Condylar regeneration in the rat (abstr). J. Dent. Res. 31:510, 1952.

Jolly, M.: Condylectomy in the rat. An investigation into the ensuing repair process in the region of the temporomandibular articulation. Aust. Dent. J. 6:243–256, 1961.

Kay, E. D.: Craniofacial dysmorphogenesis following hypervitaminosis A in mice. Teratology 35:105–17, 1987.

Keith, A., and Campion, G.: A contribution to the mechanism of growth of the human face. Dent. Rec. 42:61–88, 1922.

Kent, J. N., Homsy, C. A., Gross, B. D., and Hinds, E. C.: Pilot studies of a porous implant in dentistry and oral surgery. J. Oral Surg. 30:608–615, 1972.

Kluzak, R., and Musil, J.: The use of labeled phosphorus in the study of the metabolism of cartilage grafts. Acta Chir. Plast. 2:150–159, 1960.

Knak, G., Ulrich, R., and Vierus, H.: Influence of experimentally induced alterations of the occlusion on the morphology of the temporomandibular joint in the rat. Dtsch. Stomatol. 23:422–428, 1973.

Lacroix, P.: The Organization of Bones. Translated by Gilder, S. Philadelphia, Blackstone, 1951.

Lagrotteria, L., Scapino, R., Granston, A. S., and Felgenhauer, D.: Patient with lymphadenopathy following temporomandibular joint arthroplasty with Proplast. J. Craniomandib. Pract. 4:172–178, 1986.

Laskin, D. M., and Sarnat, B. G.: The metabolism of fresh, transplanted and preserved cartilage. Surg. Gynecol. Obstet. 96:493–499, 1953.

Laskin, D. M., Sarnat, B. G., and Bain, J. A.: Respiration and anaerobic glycolysis of transplanted cartilage. Proc. Soc. Exp. Biol. Med. 79:474–476, 1952.

Levy, B. M.: Effects of pantothenic acid deficiency on the mandibular joints and periodontal structures of mice. J. Am. Dent. Assoc. 38:215–223, 1949a.

Levy, B. M.: The effect of riboflavin deficiency on the

growth of the mandibular condyle of mice. Oral Surg. 2:89–96, 1949b.

Lieb, L., and Schlagbauer, P.: Possibilities of influencing the development of the facial bones in rhesus monkeys. Fortschr. Kieferorthop. 33:113–121, 1972.

Liedberg, J., and Westesson, P-L.: Diagnostic accuracy of upper compartment arthroscopy of the temporomandibular joint: Correlation with post mortem morphology. Oral Surg. 62:618–624, 1986.

Manchester, W. M.: Immediate reconstruction of the mandible and temporomandibular joint. Br. J. Plast. Surg. 18:291–303, 1965.

Mankin, H. J., and Conger, K. A.: The acute effects of intra-articular hydrocortisone on the articular cartilage in rabbits. J. Bone Joint Surg. (Am.) 48:1383–1388, 1966.

Marciani, R. D., Traurig, H. H., White, D. K., and Roth, G. I.: Healing following conventional and cryosurgical discoplasty in the monkey temporomandibular joint. J. Oral Maxillofac. Surg. 45:1043–1050, 1987.

McCarty, W. L., and Farrar, W. E.: Surgery for internal derangement of the temporomandibular joint. J. Prosthet. Dent. 42:191–196, 1979.

McNamara, J. A., Jr.: Functional adaptations in the temporomandibular joint. Dent. Clin. North. Am. 19:457–471, 1972.

McNamara, J. A., Jr., Hinton, R. J., and Hoffman, D. L.: Histologic analysis of temporomandibular joint adaptation to protrusive function in young adult rhesus monkeys (Macaca mulatta). Am. J. Orthod. 82:288–298, 1982.

Mehta, P. N., and Ghadially, F. N.: Articular cartilage in corn oil-induced lipoarthrosis. Ann. Rheum. Dis. 32:75–82, 1973.

Meikle, M. C.: In vivo transplantation of the mandibular joint of the rat: An autoradiographic investigation into cellular changes at the condyle. Arch. Oral Biol. 8:1011–1020, 1973.

Meyer, J., Schneider, B. J., and Das, A. K.: Experimental studies on the interrelations of condylar growth and alveolar bone formation. II. Effects of growth hormone. Angle Orthod. 37:309–319, 1967.

Mirsky, N., and Silbermann, M.: Studies on hormonal regulation of the growth of the craniofacial skeleton: III. Effects of $24,25(OH)_2D_3$ on cartilage. J. Craniofac. Genet. Dev. Biol. 4:303–320, 1984.

Misawa, T., Ohnishi, M., Kino, K., and Shioda, S.: Experimental study in microtraumatic injury to the temporomandibular joint. In Hjørting-Hansen, E. (Ed.): Oral and Maxillofacial Surgery: Proceedings from the 8th International Conference on Oral and Maxillofacial Surgery. Chicago, Quintessence, 1985, pp. 187–191.

Moffett, B. C., Johnson, L. C., McCabe, J. B., and Askew, H. C.: Articular remodeling of the adult temmporomandibular joint. Am. J. Anat. 115:119–142, 1964.

Mongini, F.: Influence of function on temporomandibular joint remodeling and degenerative disease. In Symposium on Temporomandibular Joint Dysfunction and Treatment. Dent. Clin. North Am. 27:479–494, 1983.

Mooney, V., and Ferguson, A.: The influence of immobilization and motion on the formation of fibrocartilage in the repair granuloma after joint resection in the rabbit. J. Bone Joint Surg. (Am.) 48:1145–1155, 1966.

Moose, S. M.: Experimental injections of fibrosing solutions into the temporomandibular joints of monkeys. J. Am. Dent. Assoc. 28:761–765, 1941.

Moss, M., and Rankow, R.: The role of the functional matrix in mandibular growth. Angle Orthod. 38:95–103, 1968.

Moss, M. L.: Functional analysis of human mandibular growth. J. Prosthet. Dent. 10:1149–1159, 1960.

Moss, M. L., and Salentijn, L.: The primary role of functional matrices in facial growth. Am. J. Orthod. 55:566–577, 1969.

Murnane, T. W., and Doku, H. C.: Non-interpositional intracapsular arthroplasty of the rabbit temporomandibular joint. J. Oral Surg. 29:268–272, 1971.

Nespeca, J. A., and Merrill, R. G.: Sliding capsular discopexy. Oral Surg. 63:9–11, 1987.

Ohnishi, M.: Arthroscopy of the temporomandibular joint (in Japanese). J. Jpn. Stomatol. 42:251, 1975.

Peer, L. A.: Cell survival theory versus replacement theory. Plast. Reconstr. Surg. 16:161–168, 1955.

Pennisi, V. R., Shapiro, R. L., Bucher, J. H., et al.: Marlex 50 as a replacement for the mandibular condyle. Plast. Reconstr. Surg. 35:212–217, 1965.

Peskin, S., and Laskin, D. M.: Contribution of autogenous condylar grafts to mandibular growth. Oral Surg. 20:517–534, 1965.

Pimenidis, M. Z., and Gianelly, A. A.: The effect of early postnatal condylectomy on the growth of the mandible. Am. J. Orthod. 62:42–47, 1972.

Politis, C., Fossion, E., and Bossuyt, M.: The use of costochondral grafts in arthroplasty of the temporomandibular joint. J. Craniomaxillofac. Surg. 15:345–354, 1987.

Poswillo, D.: Experimental investigation of the effects of intra-articular hydrocortisone and high condylectomy on the mandibular condyle. Oral Surg. 30:161–173, 1970.

Poswillo, D.: Experimental reconstruction of the mandibular joint. Int. J. Oral Surg. 3:400–411, 1974.

Poswillo, D.: Surgery of the temporomandibular joint. In Zarb, G. A., and Carlsson, G. E. (Eds.): Temporomandibular Joint Function and Dysfunction. St. Louis, C. V. Mosby, 1979, pp. 397–432.

Precious, D., and Delaire, J.: Balanced facial growth: A schematic interpretation. Oral Surg. 63:637–644, 1987.

Putschar, W.: Uber Fett im Knorpel unter normalen und pathologischen Verhaltnissen. Beitr. Pathol. 87:526–539, 1931.

Rabey, B. P.: Bilateral mandibular condylysis—A morphoanalytic diagnosis. Br. J. Oral Surg. 15:121–134, 1978.

Ramm, Y., Sumra, H., and Oberman, M.: Mandibular condylosis and apertognathia as presenting symptoms in progressive systemic sclerosis (scleroderma). Oral Surg. 63:269–274, 1987.

Ring, P. A.: The effects of partial or complete excision of the epiphyseal cartilage of the rabbit. J. Anat. 89:79–91, 1955.

Robinson, I. B., and Sarnat, B. G.: Growth pattern of the pig mandible. A serial roentgenographic study using metallic implants. Am. J. Anat. 96:37–64, 1955.

Roy, E. W., and Sarnat, B. G.: Growth in length of rabbit ribs at the costochondral junction. Surg. Gynecol. Obstet. 102:481–486, 1956.

Rushton, M. A.: Some aspects of the anteroposterior growth of the mandible. J. Dent. Res. 68:80–87, 1948.

Ryatt, K. S., Hopper, F. E., and Colterill, J. A.: Mandibular resorption in systemic sclerosis. Br. J. Dermatol. 107:711–714, 1982.

Sakurai, K., San Giacomo, T., Arbree, N. S., and Yurkstas, A. A.: A survey of temporomandibular joint dysfunction in completely edentulous patients. J. Prosthet. Dent. 59:81–85, 1988.

Sanders, B.: Arthroscopic surgery of the temporomandibular joint: Treatment of internal derangement with persistent closed lock. Oral Surg. 62:361–372, 1986.

Sanders, B., and Buoncristiani, R.: Diagnostic and surgical arthroscopy of the temporomandibular joint: Clinical experience with 137 procedures over a 2-year period. J. Craniomandib. Disord. Fac. Oral Pain 1:203–213, 1987.

Sarnat, B. G.: Facial and neurocranial growth after removal of the mandibular condyle in the macaca rhesus monkey. Am. J. Surg. 94:19–30, 1957.

Sarnat, B. G.: Differential craniofacial skeletal changes after postnatal experimental surgery in young and adult animals. Ann. Plast. Surg. 1(2):131–145, 1978.

Sarnat, B. G.: The orbit and eye. Experiments on volume in young and adult rabbits. Acta Ophthalmol. (Suppl.) 147:1–44, 1981.

Sarnat, B. G.: Growth pattern of the mandible: some reflections. Am. J. Orthod. Dent. Orthop. 90:221–233, 1986.

Sarnat, B. G., and Engel, M. B.: A serial study of mandibular growth after removal of the condyle in the macaca rhesus monkey. Plast. Reconstr. Surg. 7:364–380, 1951.

Sarnat, B. G., and Laskin, D. M.: Cartilage and cartilage implants. Surg. Gynecol. Obstet. 99:521–541, 1954.

Sarnat, B. G., and Muchnic, H.: Facial skeletal changes after mandibular condylectomy in growing and adult monkeys. Am. J. Orthod. 60:33–45, 1971.

Schatten, W. E., Bergenstal, D. M., Kramer, W. M., et al.: Biological survival and growth of cartilage grafts. Plast. Reconstr. Surg. 22:11–28, 1958.

Schultz, L. W.: A treatment for subluxation of the temporomandibular joint. JAMA 109:1032–1035, 1937.

Schumacher, H. R.: Synovial fluid analysis. In Kelley, W. N., Harris, E. D., Ruddy, S., and Sledge, C. B. (Eds.): Textbook of Rheumatology. Philadelphia, W. B. Saunders, 1981, pp. 568–579.

Seifert, M. H., Steigerwald, J. C., and Cliff, M. M.: Bone resorption of the mandible in progressive systemic sclerosis. Arthritis Rheum. 18:507–512, 1975.

Shimshoni, Z., Binderman, I., Fine, N., and Somjen, D.: Mechanical and hormonal stimulation of cell cultures derived from young rat mandible condyles. Arch. Oral Biol. 29:827–831, 1984.

Silberberg, M., and Silberberg, R.: Influences of the endocrine glands on growth and aging of the skeleton. Arch. Pathol. 36:512, 1943.

Silbermann, M., and Finkelbrand, S.: Reversibility of systemic corticosteroid-induced mandibular osteoarthritis: An experimental study in A/J mice. J. Oral Surg. 38:660–663, 1980.

Silbermann, M., Moredohovich, D., Toister, Z., and Asaria, N.: Mechanisms involved in mandibular condylopathy secondary to intra-articular injection of glucocorticoids. J. Oral Surg. 36:112–117, 1978.

Silbermann, M., von der Mark, K., Mirsky, N., et al.: Effects of increased doses of 1,25 dihydroxy vitamin D3 on matrix and DNA synthesis in condylar cartilage of suckling mice. Calcif. Tissue Int. 41:95–104, 1987.

Skuble, D. F., Choukas, N. C., and Toto, P. D.: Craniomandibular bone changes in rhesus monkeys induced by condylectomy. J. Oral Surg. 28:273–279, 1968.

Smith, C. A., Oberhelman, H. A., Jr., Storer, E. H., et al.: Production of experimental cretinism in dogs by the administration of radioactive iodine. Arch. Surg. 63:807–821, 1951.

Sorenson, D. C., and Laskin, D. M.: Facial growth after condylectomy or ostectomy in the mandibular ramus. J. Oral Surg. 33:746–756, 1975.

Sprinz, R.: The role of the meniscus in the healing process following excision of the articular surfaces of the mandibular joint in rabbits. J. Anat. 97:345–352, 1963.

Sprinz, R., and Stockwell, R. A.: Changes in articular cartilage following intra-articular injection of tritiated glyceryl trioleate. J. Anat. 122:91–112, 1976.

Stewart, H. M., Hann, J. R., DeTomasi, D. C., et al.: Histologic fate of dermal grafts following implantation for temporomandibular joint meniscal perforation: A preliminary study. Oral Surg. 62:481–485, 1986.

Stockli, P. W., and Willert, H. G.: Tissue reactions in the temporomandibular joint resulting from anterior displacement of the mandible in the monkey. Am. J. Orthod. 60:142–155, 1971.

Strobino, L. J., French, G. O., and Colonna, P. C.: The effect of increasing tensions on the growth of the epiphyseal bone. Surg. Gynecol. Obstet. 95:694–700, 1952.

Stuteville, O., and Lanfranchi, R.: Surgical reconstruction of the temporomandibular joint. Am. J. Surg. 90:940–950, 1955.

Tarro, A. W.: Arthroscopic diagnosis and surgery of the temporomandibular joint. J. Oral Maxillofac. Surg. 46:282–289, 1988.

Timmis, D. P., Aragon, S. B., Van Sickels, J. E., and Aufdemorte, T. B.: Comparative study of alloplastic materials for temporomandibular joint disc replacement in rabbits. J. Oral Surg. 44:541–554, 1986.

Tucker, M. R., Jacoway, J. R., and White, R. P.: Autogenous dermal grafts for repair of temporomandibular joint disc perforations. J. Oral Maxillofac. Surg. 44:781–789, 1986.

Walker, R. V.: Traumatic mandibular condylar fracture dislocations. Am. J. Surg. 100:850–863, 1960.

Walker, R. V., and Kalamchi, S.: A surgical technique for management of internal derangement of the temporomandibular joint. J. Oral Maxillofac. Surg. 45:299–305, 1987.

Wallace, D. W., and Laskin, D. M.: Healing of surgical incisions in the disc and retrodiscal tissue of the rabbit temporomandibular joint. J. Oral Maxillofac. Surg. 44:965–971, 1986.

Ware, W., and Brown, S.: Growth center transplantation to replace mandibular condyles. J. Maxillofac. Surg. 9:50–58, 1981.

Ware, W. H., and Taylor, R. C.: Replantation of growing mandibular condyles in rhesus monkeys. Oral Surg. 19:669–677, 1965.

Ware, W. H., and Taylor, R. C.: Cartilaginous growth centers transplanted to replace mandibular condyles in monkeys. J. Oral Surg. 24:3–43, 1966.

Weinberg, S.: Eminectomy and meniscorrhaphy for internal derangements of the temporomandibular joint. Oral Surg. 57:241–249, 1984.

Weinreb, M., Jr., Gazit, E., and Weinreb, M. M.: Mandibular growth and histologic changes in condylar cartilage of rats intoxicated with vitamin D3 or 1,25(OH)2D3 and pair-fed (undernourished) rats. J. Dent. Res. 65(12):1449–1452, 1986.

Westesson, P-L., Eriksson, L., and Linstrom, C.: Destructive lesions of the mandibular condyle following discectomy with temporary silicone implant. Oral Surg. 63:143–150, 1987.

Westesson, P-L., and Rohlin, M.: Internal derangement related to osteoarthrosis in autopsy specimens. Oral Surg. 57:17–22, 1984.

Westesson, P-L., Bronstein, S. L., and Liedberg, J.: Internal derangement of the temporomandibular joint: Morphologic description with correlation to joint function. Oral Surg. 59:323–331, 1985.

Williams, R. A., and Laskin, D. M.: Arthroscopic examination of experimentally induced pathologic conditions of the rabbit temporomandibular joint. J. Oral Surg. 38:652–659, 1980.

Yaillen, D. M., Shapiro, P. A., Juschei, E. S., and Feldman, G. R.: Temporomandibular joint meniscectomy—Effects on joint structure and masticatory function in Macaca fascicularis. J. Maxillofac. Surg. 7:258–264, 1979.

Zetz, M. R., and Irby, W. B.: Repair of the adult temporomandibular joint meniscus with an autogenous dermal graft. J. Oral Maxillofac. Surg. 42:167–171, 1984.

PART II

Clinical Practice: Diagnosis and Treatment

14

EPIDEMIOLOGY*

ELLIOT N. GALE, Ph. D.

INTRODUCTION

Aims of Epidemiologic Studies

Epidemiology is the study of the determinants and distribution of diseases or disorders in man. The distribution of a disorder often is studied for public health reasons and to help the clinician in understanding the demographic characteristics associated with it. Once these are known, an attempt is made through epidemiological methods to explain the patterns of distribution of the disorder in relation to potential causal factors. The latter tends to be the most significant purpose of epidemiological studies.

The aims of epidemiologic studies, in addition to elucidating causal mechanisms, are to describe the natural history of a disorder and to provide guidance in the development of health care services. The temporal sequence of a disorder is also of importance. Many disorders, while unpleasant, are self-limiting. Knowledge of such factors, to be gained from epidemiologic studies, may help the clinician to determine whether to intervene when certain clusters of signs and symptoms are present. Thus, these studies help the clinician to make both diagnostic and therapeutic decisions. To understand better the value of epidemiologic

studies, certain concepts and methods used in the field need to be defined.

Definitions of Importance

There are a number of terms very specific to epidemiology that have frequently been misused in the literature on temporomandibular disorders (TMDs). Two of the most basic terms are incidence and prevalence of a disorder, sign, or symptom. *Incidence* refers to the number of cases of a disorder that come into being during a specified period of time. The *incidence rate* is the number of cases per specified unit of the population. These terms also apply to signs and symptoms. Thus, incidence is also the frequency of an event under study during a period of time or the number of new events reported during a given period. *Prevalence*, on the other hand, is a measure of all individuals exhibiting a known event (disorder) during a study period. For chronic diseases, prevalence rates would be higher than incidence rates. Thus, if the unit of time was one year and the disorder lasts for three or four years, prevalence of the disorder would be much higher than the number of new cases per year (incidence).

While it is not unusual that nonepidemiologists might confuse the concepts of incidence and prevalence, it is surprising that the re-

---

*See Chapters 8, 9, 19, 20, 25, and 26.

searchers in the field of TMD often confuse the concepts of signs and symptoms. Symptoms are defined as those factors bothering the patient and, while they may be objective, they are generally considered to be subjective. Signs, on the other hand, are generally considered to be objective and are usually elicited or noticed upon examination, manipulation, or laboratory analysis. Signs and symptoms do not always coincide; patients may not be aware of problems associated with signs but, by definition, they are aware of symptoms. Sometimes, however, the two do coincide. In TMD, for example, clicking may be both a symptom reported by the patient, and a sign heard or palpated by the examiner. The same may be true for tenderness. On the other hand, limitation of opening of the mouth may not be reported as a symptom but can be defined and considered to be the case by the examiner.

In epidemiologic studies of TMDs, many of the signs and symptoms are *elicited* by the examiner. The patient under study may not be aware of the symptom, or minimally so, until the information is elicited on examination. In most instances in which individuals seek treatment, on the other hand, the report of symptoms is usually *spontaneous* by the patient. This is a very important difference, because in most epidemiologic studies on TMDs the report of symptoms is elicited and the signs are found on examination.

One of the greatest problems in doing epidemiologic studies of TMDs is the definition of a case. There are several reasons for this. The most basic is that there is no agreement among researchers or clinicians as to what cluster of signs and symptoms is indicative of which disorder. As a result, most studies on the epidemiology of TMDs report the prevalence not of a specific disorder, but rather of the signs and symptoms associated with a group of conditions classified under the heading TMD. Without a case definition it is extremely difficult for epidemiologists to establish the incidence and prevalence of a specific disorder or to find what characteristics, whether they be anatomic, psychological, or sociodemographic, are associated with the determinants of that disorder. Epidemiologic studies are also limited by the need for relatively large populations to study. With large populations, many of the diagnostic tests, such as imaging, are too expensive to be used as an aid in the appropriate definition of a case.

Methods Used in Epidemiologic Studies

As in all scientific endeavors, the methods used in epidemiologic studies are based on the aims of the research. Different methods are used to evaluate prevalence, incidence, causation, or any combination of these factors. The most prevalent type of epidemiologic study on TMDs has been the cross-sectional study that, in essence, is a survey. A cross-sectional study evaluates factors such as signs, symptoms, or a disease in a sample and then generalizes the data from the sample to the population which it represents. In this type of study, both risk factors and disorders are assumed to be ascertained at the same time. From these types of data we can begin to understand prevalence factors and their relation to the disorder. There are several other advantages to this type of study; it provides information on the prevalence of the signs and symptoms and the prevalence of the disorder, and it is relatively inexpensive compared with other types of studies.

The second general type of epidemiologic study is the longitudinal study, which can be divided into a retrospective, prospective, and historical prospective type. With the retrospective study, individuals are diagnosed as having a disorder and compared with individuals who do not have the disorder. Those with the disorder are cases and those who do not have the disorder are controls. The purpose of a retrospective study is to determine if these two groups differ in the proportion of individuals who have a specific factor or factors that may be associated with the disorder. This is also known as the case control method. There are a number of important criteria and definitions of cases that must be maintained for the validity of retrospective studies to be high. This tends to be very difficult for TMDs.

In the retrospective study one looks for past exposure to a factor or factors in both cases and controls and attempts to determine the relationship. The major advantage of a retrospective study is that it is relatively inexpensive compared with other types of studies. The number of subjects can be much smaller than with prospective studies, even when it includes numerous controls. The results of a retrospective study can also be obtained relatively quickly and risk factors not evaluated at the initiation of the study can be evaluated at a later date.

While there are advantages to retrospective studies, there are also a number of disadvantages. First, information about past events may not be available from the record, or it may be available but inaccurately recorded. If information is sought through interview or questionnaire, the informant may have inadequate information about, or recall of, the factors in which one is interested. Information supplied by a patient or relative may be biased. When the study is being conducted, the patient has already been diagnosed as having a disorder and this may cloud the individual's perception. Patients are also attempting to give explanations for their disorder and often assign more or less significance to a sign or symptom based on their needs and desires rather than on historic facts. This is referred to as retrospective falsification.

The second type of longitudinal study, the prospective study, starts with groups of individuals all considered to be free of a given disorder. These individuals are followed over a period of time to determine differences in the rate at which the disorder develops. With TMDs, many of these individuals would already have some of the signs and symptoms associated with the disorder because many signs and symptoms, such as headaches, are so prevalent. In most prospective studies, measurements are also made on factors believed to be associated with the disorder and attempts are made to determine the association between these factors and the onset of the disorder.

One advantage of a prospective study is the total lack of bias in choosing individuals based on faulty assumptions. The prospective study also yields incidence as well as risk rates. The prospective study may also provide information about the association between etiologic factors and the disorder. When individuals are classified as having the disorder, one can also study the natural history of both treated and untreated cases (Dworkin, 1988; Von Korff, 1988). Such a study can provide information on when to and how to, or when not to treat a patient.

There are also disadvantages to this method. For a prospective study, large numbers of subjects are needed who can be followed over long periods of time. There is also the problem of attrition in this type of study. Prospective studies also assume that potential risk factors are known and that methods of measurement are adequate. The most important disadvantage of the prospective study is the high cost. The potential information to be gained from this type of study, however, is often worth the price.

The third type of longitudinal epidemiologic study, the historic prospective study, follows individuals based on a known pre-exposing factor or factors. Thus, if one expects that a factor, such as orthodontics, plays a role in the development of TMDs, patients can be selected who have had exposure to the factor and compared with controls who have not had exposure to the factor. Records are followed from the time of exposure to the present and then to the future to evaluate if those exposed to the factor develop the disorder in significantly greater numbers than those not exposed to the factor. Obviously, it is necessary to be able to establish the supposed etiologic factor before the onset of the disorder. The advantage of this type of study is that it is less costly than the prospective study, although more costly than the truly retrospective study. Unfortunately, the disadvantage is also great. Accurate records on all factors of interest must have been maintained, which is seldom the case.

RESULTS FROM EPIDEMIOLOGIC STUDIES

A number of different epidemiologic studies have been completed on temporomandibular disorders (TMDs). These include both cross-sectional and longitudinal approaches.

Cross-sectional Studies

There has been a wealth of epidemiologic studies on the signs and symptoms associated with TMDs. While some cross-sectional studies have attempted to define the disorder, most have been an evaluation of the signs and symptoms. These studies have been completed on many different types of populations, including those with variation in age, gender, socioeconomic class, and demographic characteristics. They also have been completed on urbanites, rural populations, and relatively isolated groups.

Exceedingly wide ranges have been reported for each sign and symptom. These differences may be due to the variations in sociodemographic characteristics previously mentioned. It is more likely, however, that these differences result from methodological variations in the studies. Careful attention must be given to the way a question is phrased to elicit symptoms as well as to the methods of examination used to discover signs.

Symptoms

PAIN

The most common symptom that results in the patient seeking health care is pain. It may or may not be associated with function. In the young, which includes both children and adolescents, pain unassociated with functional movements of the masticatory system has been reported in 4.6 to 16.5 per cent of the samples studied (Eskola, 1985; Moss, 1984; Solberg, 1979). Reported pain unassociated with function ranged from 5.4 to 24 per cent in broader range age groups (Abdel-Hakim, 1983; Bush, 1982; Gross, 1988b; Hansen, 1984).

Reported pain with function in an adolescent sample ranged from 3.5 to 52 per cent of the respondents (Egermark-Eriksson, 1981; Nilner, 1981a; 1981b; Solberg, 1979; Wanman, 1986). In wider-range age groups, the pain with function was reported in 3 to 6.9 per cent of the samples (Bush, 1982; Sakurai, 1988; Swanljung, 1979).

The types of questions used to elicit information about pain have varied widely and may well account for the differences in results. The following three questions serve as examples: (1) Have you ever had pain in the area in front of your ears? A 60-year-old individual who responds yes may have had pain in the area in front of the ears 40 years ago that is totally unrelated to the presence of a TMD at the present time. (2) Have you had pain in front of the ears in the last six months? This could be related to the presence of a TMD. (3) Do you have pain in the area in front of your ears? This may imply at the present time to the respondent. A negative response to this question would not rule out the presence of a TMD. This is an excellent example of the differences in, and importance of, phraseology in epidemiological research and diagnosis.

JOINT SOUNDS

Joint sounds are the most common symptom next to pain reported by patients with TMD. While there are few commonalities in the data, clicking sounds are more commonly reported than crepitation. While clicking is more common, crepitus has more clinical significance (Gale, 1985). In the younger population, joint sounds have been reported in 8.9 to 20 per cent of the samples (Egermark-Eriksson, 1981; Nilner, 1981a; 1981b; Solberg, 1979; Wanman, 1986). Joint noises were reported in 11 to 34 per cent of the sample with a broader age range (Abdel-Hakim, 1983; Bush, 1982; Gross, 1988b; Hansson, 1975; Sakurai, 1988; Swanljung, 1979; Vincent, 1988).

LIMITATION OF MOVEMENT

The definition of limitation of movement, often considered to be a cardinal symptom of a TMD, has varied from study to study. The method of questioning in this regard is also very important, but has not been given much consideration in either the clinical or epidemiological literature. Because of these variations, the reported prevalence for limitation of motion in adolescents has ranged from 1.8 to 7 per cent of the sample (Egermark-Eriksson, 1981; Nilner, 1981a; 1981b; Wanman, 1986) and from 6 to 12.6 per cent in a broader-range age population (Abdel-Hakim, 1983; Hansson, 1975; Swanljung, 1979).

While pain, joint sounds, and limited opening are the most commonly reported symptoms associated with TMD, there are a number of other symptoms that are reported and that many clinicians believe also are associated with the disorder. Of these symptoms, subluxation is the least common, with a reported prevalence of 1 to 2.5 per cent (Sakurai, 1988; Wanman, 1986). More common is the report of headache. The range reported in samples of adolescents was from 12.5 to 21.7 per cent (Nilner, 1981a; 1981b; Solberg, 1979; Wanman, 1986). With adult populations, headaches were reported in 5.5 to 18.2 per cent of the sample (Gross, 1988b; 1983; Hansen, 1984; Hansson, 1975; Nilner, 1981a).

While the percentage of the population who report one symptom associated with TMD can be fairly high, the percentage reporting two or more symptoms generally falls below 10 per cent; those who report three or more symptoms generally fall below 4 per cent (Kleinknecht, 1986; Rugh, 1985; Sakurai, 1988; Wanman, 1986).

Signs

There are as many problems with the data reported from epidemiologic studies on signs associated with TMDs as with the data reported on symptoms. One of the difficulties in comparing across studies is that the methods used to elicit the signs are not well explained and, therefore, not comparable from study to study. As with the symptom data, a wide variety of populations have been studied and there is a tremendous range of percentages associated with each sign. While some of the differences associated with the data on signs may result from variations in populations or samples, it is more likely that differences in methodology account for a greater percentage of the variance. Clinicians should take note of the relatively higher percentage of signs found than symptoms reported when interpreting a clinical examination.

PAIN

A good clinical examination of a patient complaining of a possible TMD would include palpation of both the joint and masticatory musculature. Pain elicited upon palpation of the musculature is often indicative of a TMD. A relatively high percentage of patients with no subjective complaints (symptoms) of TMD, however, also report pain upon palpation of the joint and muscles of mastication. This must be taken into consideration in evaluating such findings.

Summary data from the research on children and adolescents show a tremendous range of reported tenderness on palpation of the joint and the muscles of mastication (Egermark-Eriksson, 1981; Gazit, 1984; Kirveskari, 1986; Nilner, 1981a; 1981b; Ogura, 1985). The finding of tenderness on palpation of the masticatory muscles ranged from 7.6 to 41.8 per cent in samples of children and adolescents studied. The reported data for tenderness over palpated joints ranged from 1.7 to 30.4 per cent of the study sample. With these younger populations, the lateral pterygoid muscle seemed to be the most tender, with the reported pain response on palpation ranging from 4.5 to 30 per cent. The next two most tender muscles were the masseter (range, 17 to 26 per cent of the sample) and temporalis (range, 5 to 27 per cent of the sample). While TMDs are not usually thought of as a disorder of children or young adults, the data seem to indicate that many of these individuals show tenderness on palpation. As will be noted, these data can be very misleading.

In an older and more broad-ranged population, muscle tenderness upon palpation for all muscles ranged from 4 to 39 per cent (Abdel-Hakim, 1983; Bush, 1983; Gross, 1983; Hansson, 1975; Heft, 1984; Rao, 1981; Reik, 1981; Sakurai, 1988). Thus, about four out of every 10 patients reported pain of one or more muscles. The data for palpation of the joint are equally surprising and ranged from 2.5 to 30 per cent of the samples studied. At the high end of the range it would mean that one out of every three individuals would report tenderness on palpation of the TMJ. As was found with younger age groups, the most tender muscle reported was the lateral pterygoid (8 to 29 per cent of the sample studied) followed by the temporalis (less than 1 to 20 per cent of the sample) and the masseter (2 to 17 per cent of

the sample). As with younger age groups, interpretation of the data must be made with care.

Not all studies have reported individual muscle data and very few have reported details of the method used to palpate the areas that would enable the study to be repeated. One of the most important criteria in comparing studies would be knowledge of the amount of pressure used in the palpation procedure. While some studies do indicate moderate pressure, the amount of pressure can vary from examiner to examiner. Only a few studies gave the amount and duration of pressure used in palpation even though these are two of the most important determinants of the subject's response. Because of variations in these parameters, in studies where the percentages of positive response of specific muscles, as well as the response of any muscle, are given, those that report the highest response of any muscle also tend to report the highest rates of response for the individual muscles. These higher general and specific rates most likely come from a greater amount or longer duration of pressure being used by the investigators.

JOINT SOUNDS

The reported percentage of the adolescent population in whom joint sounds were recorded ranged from 8 to 35.8 per cent (Egermark-Eriksson, 1981; Gazit, 1984; Kirveskari, 1986; Nilner, 1981b; Ogura, 1985; Solberg, 1979). Similar data have been reported for adults, with the percentage of the population reported to have clicks ranging from 15.2 to 65 per cent (Abdel-Hakim, 1983; Bush, 1983; Gross, 1983; Hansson, 1975; Heft, 1984; Rao, 1981; Reik, 1981; Sakurai, 1988; Swanljung, 1979; Vincent, 1988).

As with pain, there are many problems in interpretation of the data reported on clicking. The method used to elicit the information is extremely important. Investigators who listened with their ears tended to report the lowest prevalence of joint sounds. Investigators who examined for palpable irregularities reported the next highest prevalence, and those who used stethoscopes tended to report the highest prevalence rates. In general, on the basis of such data, more than half the population would be expected to have joint sounds when examined using a stethoscope. If this is the case, then joint sounds would be considered normal if normality was defined as greater than 50 per cent of the population exhibiting a sign.

LIMITED OPENING OF THE MOUTH

Another problem area for both clinical and epidemiological studies lies in the definition of limited or restricted mouth opening. Based on the small number of studies reporting on restriction of opening, the percentage of young individuals with such a problem ranged from 0.3 to 3.5 per cent of the samples (Egermark-Eriksson, 1981; Gazit, 1984; Ogura, 1985; Solberg, 1979). For a broader-range age group, the reported percentage of the study samples with restricted opening ranged from 4 to 13 per cent (Abdel-Hakim, 1983; Gross, 1983; Heft, 1984; Reik, 1981; Swanljung, 1979).

The problem in both epidemiologic and clinical studies is the definition of restricted opening. In the small number of studies reported, the definition of restriction ranged from less than 35 mm to less than 40 mm of opening and either did or did not include overbite. This is a rather wide range for such a definition. It also might be argued that younger individuals, with smaller mandibles, would generally not have as large an opening as older individuals with larger mandibles.

OTHER SIGNS AND COMBINATIONS

The only other TMD sign that is commonly reported is deviation of the mandible on opening the mouth. For those samples in which this sign was evaluated, the percentage of persons who had the sign ranged from 9 to 38 per cent (Gross, 1983; Reik, 1981; Sakurai, 1988; Solberg, 1979).

While more sophisticated techniques are available for evaluating the potential for a TMD, such as the Helkimo index (Helkimo, 1974; 1976), many authors have attempted to evaluate the probability of having combinations of symptoms. The likelihood of finding a single symptom in a general population appears to be very high, ranging from a low, and very unusual, 9.8 per cent to a high of 76 per cent. The reported range for two or more symptoms was 6.4 to 37.9 per cent, and for three or more symptoms the range was 0.6 to 5.2 per cent (Gross, 1983; Nilner, 1981a; 1981b; Ogura, 1985; Solberg, 1979).

Bruxism as a Sign and Symptom

As with many of the other factors previously mentioned, bruxism (clenching or grinding of the teeth for nonfunctional use) can be a sign or a symptom. In addition, some investigators and clinicians classify bruxism as a TMD. When bruxism is considered a symptom, patients are asked if they brux. As a sign, bruxism is often defined as abnormal tooth wear. In general, the interpretation of the data reported in epidemiologic studies seems to indicate that bruxism is a fairly frequent sign and symptom. In the general population, bruxism is reported to occur in between 10 and 20 per cent of the samples studied (Nilner, 1981a; 1981b; Swanljung, 1979; Wanman, 1986).

Relationships Among Signs and Symptoms

Based on almost any conceptualization or model of TMD, one would expect that the more signs exhibited by the patient the larger the number of symptoms that would also be reported. While this has often been reported to be the case, the relationship between the number of signs and symptoms as well as between specific signs and symptoms, while significant, has often accounted for a very small percentage of the variance (Bush, 1983). There have been a number of literature reviews on the signs and symptoms of TMD (Carlsson, 1984; Clark, 1984; Given, 1986; Greene, 1982; Helkimo, 1976; Padamsee, 1985; Rieder, 1983; Rugh, 1985).

Longitudinal Studies
Case Definitions

The major problem with epidemiologic studies of TMDs has been case definition. Diagnostic skills vary and often practical means of diagnosis, such as radiography and laboratory tests, are unavailable to the epidemiologist who usually does large-scale studies. In the usual epidemiological study, signs and symptoms are recorded and the prevalence, incidence, and associated factors are determined. As Drinnan (1987) has stated, however, ". . . many diseases have overlapping symptoms, and it may need considerable diagnostic skill to differentiate one from the other." Because of this problem, although there have been occasional good retrospective studies, there have been very few good prospective studies. As more and more is known about TMD, differentiating one disorder from another may become more exacting and this will make these conditions more amenable to epidemiological studies.

Treatment and Natural History

Much of the longitudinal epidemiologic TMD research has been done on patient groups. Such studies provide insight into the natural course of the disorder. One study was completed on a population of 119 patients who were diagnosed as having TM arthropathy (Rasmussen, 1981a; 1981b). The patients were followed from one-half to five and one-half years. The author was able to divide the progress of symptoms into phases. In essence, the first phase was clicking of the joint, followed by periodic locking in the second phase. In the third and fourth phases pain was present in the joint. The last phase was an absence of major symptoms. It is difficult to tell if this was a natural course of the disorder because treatment was not described. It appears, however, that some of the patients did not receive treatment. In general, most of the patients were pain-free, restriction-free, and generally noncomplaining after four years. In patients with residual symptoms, crepitation tended to be the most frequent finding.

In a shorter-term study, patients who complained of headaches and mandibular dysfunction were fitted with new dentures (Magnusson, 1980). Of the 17 patients with recurrent headaches, 65 per cent reported less frequent headaches six months after treatment. It was also reported that signs of masticatory system dysfunction were significantly reduced.

There have been additional long-term studies on treatment effects. Usually, the findings indicate that after a period of time patients, no matter what the treatment, report significant improvement. For example, in one study, three to five years after treatment, 75 per cent reported little or no trouble, while only 7 per cent still had severe pain or mandibular dysfunction (Agerberg, 1974). In another study, 154 females were evaluated about seven years after they had treatment for TMD (Mejersjo, 1984). Poor general health was a negative influence on both the immediate response to treatment and on long-term prognosis. The authors did report, however, that there were few correlations between occlusal factors and dysfunction. The loss of molars and premolars was related to impaired function. In an additional study of 110 patients with TMD who were treated previously, interpretation of retrospective longitudinal data indicated that 85.5 per cent were not experiencing pain or were experiencing much less pain. The duration of this retrospective study was two to eight and one-half years (Okeson, 1986). All the patients in this group were administered conservative treatment.

The findings from these studies are very instructive. It is evident that in many cases patients experience relief of symptoms with conservative or no treatment. As all clinicians know, however, there are still a large number of patients who do not improve over time. Future studies must identify those characteristics that differentiate these groups. Longitudinal studies of preonset environmental and personal characteristics are best suited for this task.

Risk Factors

One of the major goals of epidemiologic research is to ascertain potential etiological factors. These can also be termed risk factors because they place the individual at risk to develop the disorder. There have been some attempts with this type of epidemiologic research to determine the potential risk factors for TMD. In a study of almost 5,000 individuals (Wigdorowicz-Makowerowa, 1979) it was concluded that functional disturbances of the masticatory system are caused by local factors. It was also concluded that ". . . psychoemotional tension" influences such functional disturbances. In addition, factors such as bruxism and malocclusion increased the frequency of TMD, and environmental factors and living conditions also exerted an influence on the potential development of these problems. Because this was a cross-sectional study, there is some question whether the conclusions can be accepted. It has served, however, as the basis for much additional research in the area.

In an attempt to evaluate genetic factors as a potential cause for myofascial pain and dysfunction, 94 sets of twins were studied (Heiberg, 1980). No differences were found in the rates of TMD between monozygous (identical) twins, and dizygous (nonidentical) twins. This led to the conclusion that it is environmental influences rather than genetic factors that give rise to a specific stress reaction pattern that leads to myofascial pain.

A number of studies have attempted to evaluate occlusion as a potential risk factor for the development of these disorders. Almost all of these studies have found some type of a relationship between occlusal factors and the development of signs and symptoms associated with TMD. The problem, as we shall see, is that there is little or no consistency among the factors found responsible for these disorders. In a study of 389 males, there were positive correlations between subjective symptoms of dysfunction and nonworking side interferences (Ingervall, 1980). Also, TMJ sounds were positively correlated with single tooth contact on the working side and muscle tenderness was found to be related to interferences in the retruded position of the mandible. In a population of 309 adolescents, those with distal occlusion were more frequently aware of symptoms of the masticatory system than those with a neutral or mesial occlusal relationship (Nilner, 1983). While not directly the opposite of the preceding study, the differences in position of the mandible related to subjective symptoms were quite different.

In another cross-sectional study (Mohlin, 1983) 272 females were examined to determine the prevalence of objective and subjective symptoms of mandibular dysfunction. The author reported a correlation between subjective symptoms and the number of tipped teeth, as well as the severity of dysfunction being related to the need for orthodontic treatment. In addition, the author reported that tenderness of the masticatory muscles upon palpation was related to the need for orthodontic or prosthetic treatment. Again, there is no concordance of findings on occlusal factors with those from the preceding two studies.

Although it was suggested that orthodontic treatment might reduce the risk for the development of TMD, some studies have questioned whether, in fact, this is the case. In one review (Kalbfleisch, 1985) it was determined that it was unlikely that orthodontic treatment resulted in the development of mandibular dysfunction or that orthodontic correction would reduce the chance of developing TMD. This implies that orthodontic treatment neither increases nor decreases the risk for the development of a TMD. It does not mean, however, that orthodontic intervention may not be an appropriate treatment for a TMD.

The best way to evaluate risk factors is through longitudinal studies. Unfortunately, there have been very few such studies related to mandibular dysfunction. In one of the better studies, longitudinal changes of signs and symptoms of mandibular dysfunction were evaluated in 240 children over a four- to five-year period (Egermark-Eriksson, 1987), and it was noted that the signs and symptoms of mandibular dysfunction increased in both frequency and severity. They were, however, mild in most cases. It was also noted that dental wear increased during the period, but there were few changes in psychological traits. Some significant correlations were reported between a number of occlusal factors and mandibular dysfunction, but probably not more than would be expected

by chance. For those that were found to be significant, the correlations were extremely low. The relationship between occlusal interferences and mandibular dysfunction did not reveal any strong correlation. The results were interpreted further as supporting a multifactorial etiology of functional disturbances of the masticatory system but the authors were unable to determine any strong risk factors.

In addition to occlusion as a potential risk factor, there have been investigations of psychosocial and demographic factors as related to risk for developing these disorders. While many studies have found various psychosocial and demographic characteristics associated with the development of TMD, as was found for occlusion, there is no consistency among them. It does not appear that these factors alone are clearly related to the risk for developing a TMD. A representative study (Kleinknecht, 1987) had a subject population of 621 and included a number of psychosocial and demographic characteristics. The factor analysis was interpreted as not indicating a single factor or group of factors that would put the individual at risk for developing a TMD. The results were interpreted as indicating that the often reported association between TMD and psychosocial factors may be associated with treatment-seeking behavior rather than risk factors.

One other area that may be considered a risk factor has unfortunately received even less research than the preceding two areas. Occupational factors could theoretically be a major area that places the individual at risk for developing these disorders. In a study of 141 female employees in a shipyard and oil refinery, 75 were classified as being at risk due to the nature of their work (Alanen, 1985). These were individuals who performed a minimum of two hours of regular typing per day. Clinical examinations and medical histories were obtained. Those subjects who were considered to be at risk had done typing for an average of 4.4 hours per day for almost 11 years. The control subjects were found not to have been exposed to the same type of physical stress. No difference was reported between the exposed and unexposed groups in the frequency of TMD, nor in the frequency of neck symptoms between the two groups. Temporomandibular dysfunction was also reported not to be associated with the length of time spent at the potential risk type occupation.

There are many potential reasons for the failure of researchers to identify risk factors associated with TMD. The methods used in many of the studies leave many areas for improvement. With very few exceptions, the sample sizes were probably not reflective of the population. In addition, there were very few longitudinal studies that evaluated risk factors. The consistent failure to find occlusal, psychosocial, demographic, and occupational factors placing the individual at risk certainly indicates the need for continued research. It also suggests that the development of the disorders may be multifactorial and indicates that there is a need to look at combinations of factors that place the individual at risk for the development of the disorders. Only long-term, large-scale epidemiologic studies, investigating many potential factors, will be able to accomplish this important goal.

CONCLUSIONS

The same problems that have plagued epidemiological research also plague clinical research. Such problems not only interfere with appropriate diagnosis, but also may result in treatment failure. It appears that those interested in epidemiologic research are now beginning to address these problems and, thus, clearer diagnostic and therapeutic approaches for the clinician may result. While some of the problems to be discussed appear to be associated only with the researcher, it is clear that they are also influential in decision-making by the health provider.

Clinical Implications

Both clinical and epidemiologic research indicate that TMDs are a diverse group of disorders (Rugh, 1985; Zarb, 1984). One of the most pressing needs for both the clinician and the epidemiologist is an adequate case definition of each of these conditions (Hansson, 1975; Rugh, 1985). Almost all of the studies reviewed have dealt with signs and symptoms of a disorder and have not combined them to give an adequate case definition. Without such a definition, how does the clinician make a correct diagnosis? It is an axiom that diseases must be understood if they are to be successfully treated. How is the disorder to be understood if there is no agreement on the definition of what constitutes a case? The number of signs and symptoms found in the general population is very high (Rugh, 1985) and, depending on the study, as much as 87.5 per cent show at least one sign or symptom. We do know, however, that the

number of signs or symptoms varies enormously from study to study (Rieder, 1983; Rugh, 1985). If we use as our definition the presence of one or more symptoms or signs as an indication of a case, the definition would result in a large portion of the population having TMD. If on the other hand, we use a strict definition of the number and intensity needed to form a case, then very few people would be defined as having the disorder and undertreatment or failure to use preventive methods could occur (Rugh, 1984).

Which signs and symptoms require treatment also needs to be determined. It has been indicated that individuals with signs and symptoms may be subclinical (Rugh, 1985). Subclinical was defined as exhibiting relatively minor signs or symptoms of dysfunction. It is extremely difficult to define which signs and symptoms would result in the need for treatment if the patient is noncomplaining. This is especially important in diagnosis of the disorder. The individual patient may report no symptoms associated with a TMD, but the examining health practitioner may be able to elicit signs that may be indicative of a disorder. Yet, if the patient does not report problems, the question remains if it is appropriate to treat. One attempt to alleviate this dilemma has been to place greater emphasis on the effect of any sign or symptom on masticatory function (Rugh, 1984). One possible solution is to question the need for treatment if there is no compromised function. While epidemiologic research has focused on signs and symptoms, very few researchers have attempted to show how elicited signs and symptoms are related to compromised function. If so-called subclinical cases do have compromised function, and if this is disturbing to the patient, there may be, in fact, a need for treatment. There is a need to do more research on compromised function.

Highly related to the preceding problem, but distinct from it, is the fact that the same disorder can be described under different names (Foreman, 1985; Laskin, 1984). Because of a lack of clear definition of a case, it is equally possible that the same name can be used for highly different disorders. Without the appropriate classification of signs and symptoms it is impossible for the epidemiologist or the diagnostician to diagnose the individual's problem appropriately. Without the knowledge of a distinct disorder, the health provider must rely on belief rather than on fact in his or her choice of treatment modalities. Such an effect is not limited to TMD but also is a problem in other masticatory disorders (Spector, 1985).

An additional factor, which is advantageous for both the researcher and clinician, is that epidemiologic research does not focus on a clinical population. Many theoretical orientations toward etiology of TMD have come from the examination of clinical populations, but many of the signs and symptoms associated with such clinical populations are also found in the general population (Kent, 1985). Such findings should indicate that treatment-seeking behavior is significantly different from the presence of signs. Thus, the clinician should be aware that even if he or she is able to elicit a sign, it is not necessarily an indication of a disorder. Signs and symptoms are evaluated by the patient; their importance is then related to the perception of the need for treatment. Epidemiologic research has certainly indicated that signs and symptoms of TMD are very common in the general population.

Although one of the major goals of epidemiologic research is to determine risk factors and perhaps reduce the risk to individuals, confusion by clinicians has resulted in less-than-adequate epidemiologic research. Without specific knowledge of the underlying pathology, the same apparent disorder may actually have vastly different etiologies and the same etiology can lead to apparently different disorders (Villarosa, 1985; Zarb, 1984). This results in confusion for both the epidemiologist and the health provider, and may lead to inappropriate treatment. As cases are better defined, the epidemiologist can focus on expected etiological factors and determine their influence on the risk of developing a disorder. As clinicians are better able to define a case, the epidemiologist can then undertake retrospective studies to build hypotheses to determine risk factors that can be investigated in prospective studies. The problem of a lack of knowledge of etiology also affects the epidemiologist and diagnostician in other areas associated with the masticatory system (Gorsky, 1987).

The variability in signs and symptoms over time, another problem that hampers the epidemiologist, should influence decision-making by the clinician. Some TMDs frequently fluctuate in their severity. If this is the case, then the ability of the clinician to make diagnostic and therapeutic decisions is based on the time he or she sees the patient. This is also true for the epidemiologist. Over a relatively short period of time, the reproducibility of a response to a questionnaire on symptoms of masticatory dysfunction can be relatively low (Kopp, 1976). Even a question on masticatory muscle pain, to

which the answer should be relatively easy to recall, showed relatively poor, but possibly acceptable, reproducibility. This could be due to at least two factors: (1) fluctuation in symptoms and (2) poor determination by patients of the masticatory pain. Not only was the reliability of some questionnaire data questionable, but also the same was true of clinical signs in patients with mandibular dysfunction (Kopp, 1977). While there was some fair agreement for palpation of the muscles and detecting TMJ sounds, it was of borderline acceptability. As with the questionnaire data, this may be due to the fluctuation of symptoms as well as to different interpretations by the examiner.

One of the greatest problems for both the epidemiologist and the clinician is the lack of consistency in examination of the samples under study (Heloe, 1984). The techniques used to examine patients as well as epidemiologic samples have varied widely and result in difficulty in defining a case. As clinicians can agree more reliably on examination techniques, better epidemiologic studies will result. There have been attempts to standardize techniques (Helkimo, 1974) but this has not been successful, nor has it been widely accepted in the field.

SUMMARY

A review of the literature in the area of epidemiology demonstrates widely varying results that should be of importance to the clinician. There is a large portion of the population that shows signs and/or symptoms of a TMD. However, signs and symptoms may be very different from having a disorder. Both the epidemiologist and clinician should be aware of the need to define a case that requires treatment and not assume that everyone with a sign or symptom is, in fact, in need of care. According to one study, if a single sign were to define a case, more than 85 per cent of the population might be in need of treatment. Epidemiologic research has shown that the epidemiologist and clinician must work more closely to obtain a better case definition as well as to define those in need of treatment.

The quality of research in epidemiology has varied widely. There is a definite need for larger, longitudinal studies to better determine risk factors associated with the development of a TMD. As this occurs, improvements in diagnosis and treatment can follow, as well as potential preventive techniques. Longitudinal epidemiologic studies can show when preventive intervention techniques are needed as well as how to determine potential etiologic factors.

REFERENCES

Abdel-Hakim, A. M.: Stomatognathic dysfunction in the western desert of Egypt: An epidemiological survey. J. Oral Rehabil. 10:461–468, 1983.

Agerberg, G., and Carlsson, G. E.: Late results of treatment of functional disorders of the masticatory system. A follow-up by questionnaire. J. Oral Rehabil. 1:309–316, 1974.

Alanen, P. J., and Kirveskari, P. K.: Occupational cervicobrachial disorder and temporomandibular joint dysfunction. J. Craniomandib. Pract. 3:70–72, 1985.

Bush, F. M., Butler, J. H., and Abbott, D. M.: The relationship of TMJ clicking to palpable facial pain. J. Craniomandib. Pract. 1:43–48, 1983.

Bush, F. M., Butler, J. H., Abbott, D. M., and Carter, W. H.: Prevalence of mandibular dysfunction: Subjective signs and symptoms. In Lundeen, H. C., and Gibbs, C. H. (Eds.): Advances in Occlusion. London, John Wright, 1982.

Carlsson, G. E.: Epidemiological studies of signs and symptoms of temporomandibular joint-pain-dysfunction. A literature review. A P S Bulletin 14:7–12, 1984.

Clark, G. T., and Mulligan, R.: A review of the prevalence of temporomandibular dysfunction. Gerodontology 3:231–236, 1984.

Drinnan, A. J.: Differential diagnosis of orofacial pain. Dent. Clin. North Am. 4:627–643, 1987.

Dworkin, S. F., LeResche, L., and Von Korff, M.: Epidemiology of TMD: Preliminary longitudinal data. Paper presented at the meeting of the International Association for Dental Research, Montreal, March, 1988.

Egermark-Eriksson, I., Carlsson, G. E., and Ingervall, B.: Prevalence of mandibular dysfunction and orofacial parafunction in 7-, 11- and 15-year-old Swedish children. Europ. J. Ortho. 3:163–172, 1981.

Egermark-Eriksson, I., Carlsson, G. E., and Magnusson, T.: A long-term epidemiologic study of the relationship between occlusal factors and mandibular dysfunction in children and adolescents. J. Dent. Res. 66:67–71, 1987.

Eskola, S., Ylipaavalniemi, P., and Turtola, L.: TMJ-dysfunction symptoms among Finnish university students. J. Am. Coll. Health 33:172–174, 1985.

Foreman, P. A.: Temporomandibular joint and myofascial pain dysfunction—Some current concepts. Part 1: Diagnosis. New Zealand Dent. J. 81:47–52, 1985.

Gale, E. N., and Gross, A.: An evaluation of temporomandibular joint sounds. J. Am. Dent. Assoc. 111:62–63, 1985.

Gazit, E., Lieberman, M., Eini, R., et al.: Prevalence of mandibular dysfunction in 10–18 year old Israeli school children. J. Oral Rehabil. 11:307–317, 1984.

Given, B. K., and Stack, B. C.: Temporomandibular joint dysfunction syndrome in children. J. Sch. Health 56:86–89, 1986.

Gorsky, M., Silverman, S., and Chinn, H.: Burning mouth syndrome: A review of 98 cases. J. Oral Med. 42:7–9, 1987.

Greene, C. S., and Marbach, J. J.: Epidemiologic studies of mandibular dysfunction: A critical review. J. Prosthet. Dent. 48:184–190, 1982.

Gross, A., and Gale, E. N.: A prevalence study of the clinical signs associated with mandibular dysfunction. J. Am. Dent. Assoc. 107:932–936, 1983.

Gross, A., Gale, E. N., and Lavoie, S. Y.: Correlation of signs and symptoms of temporomandibular disorders. Paper presented at the meetings of the International Association for Dental Research, Montreal, March, 1988a.

Gross, A. J., Rivera-Morales, W. C., and Gale, E. N.: A prevalence study of symptoms associated with temporomandibular disorders. J. Craniomandib. Disord. 2:191–195, 1988b.

Hansen, C. A., and Axinn, S.: Incidence of mandibular dysfunction symptoms in individuals who remove their complete dentures during sleep. J. Prosthet. Dent. 51:16–18, 1984.

Hansson, T., and Nilner, M.: A study of the occurrence of symptoms of diseases of the temporomandibular joint masticatory musculature and related structures. J. Oral Rehabil. 2:313–324, 1975.

Heft, M. W.: Prevalence of TMJ signs and symptoms in the elderly. Gerodontology 3:125–130, 1984.

Heiberg, A., Heloe, B., Heiberg, A. N., et al.: Myofascial pain dysfunction (MPD) syndrome in twins. Community Dent. Oral Epidemiol. 8:434–436, 1980.

Helkimo, M.: Epidemiological surveys of dysfunction of the masticatory system. Oral Sci. Rev. 7:54–69, 1976.

Helkimo, M.: Studies on function and dysfunction of the masticatory system. II. Index for anamnestic and clinical dysfunction and occlusal state. Swed. Dent. J. 67:101–121, 1974.

Heloe, B.: Epidemiological studies in the general population. Paper presented at the meeting of the National Institutes of Dental Research, Washington, D.C., October, 1984.

Ingervall, B., Mohlin, B., and Thilander, B.: Prevalence of symptoms of functional disturbances of the masticatory system in Swedish men. J. Oral Rehabil. 7:185–197, 1980.

Kalbfleisch, J. F.: Does orthodontic treatment precipitate TMJ/muscular disorders? Ontario Dent. 62:27–31, 1985.

Kent, G. G.: Prevalence vs. incidence of the mandibular pain dysfunction syndrome: Implications for epidemiological research. Community Dent. Oral Epidemiol. 13:113–116, 1985.

Kirveskari, P., Alanen, P., and Jamsa, T.: Functional state of the stomatognathic system in 5, 10 and 15 year old children in southwestern Finland. Proc. Finn. Dent. Soc. 82:3–8, 1986.

Kleinknecht, R. A., Alexander, L. D., Mahoney, E. R., and Dworkin, S. F.: Correspondence between subjective report of temporomandibular disorder symptoms and clinical findings. J. Am. Dent. Assoc. 113:257–261, 1986.

Kleinknecht, R. A., Mahoney, E. R., and Alexander, L. D.: Psychosocial and demographic correlates of temporomandibular disorders and related symptoms: An assessment of community and clinical findings. Pain 29:313–324, 1987.

Kopp, S.: Constancy of clinical signs in patients with mandibular dysfunction. Community Dent. Oral Epidemiol. 5:94–98, 1977.

Kopp, S.: Reproducibility of response to a questionnaire on symptoms of masticatory dysfunction. Community Dent. Oral Epidemiol. 4:205–209, 1976.

Laskin, D. M.: Problems of definition of TMJ disorders. Paper presented at the meeting of the National Institutes of Dental Research, Washington, D. C., October, 1984.

Magnusson, T.: Prevalence of recurrent headache and mandibular dysfunction in patients with unsatisfactory complete dentures. Community Dent. Oral Epidemiol. 8:159–164, 1980.

Mejersjo, C., and Carlsson, G. E.: Analysis of factors influencing the long-term effect of treatment of TMJ pain/dysfunction. J. Oral Rehabil. 11:289–297, 1984.

Mohlin, B.: Prevalence of mandibular dysfunction and relation between malocclusion and mandibular dysfunction in a group of women in Sweden. Europ. J. Ortho. 4:115–123, 1983.

Moss, R. A., Sult, S. C., and Garrett, J. C.: Questionnaire evaluation of craniomandibular pain factors among college students. J. Craniomandib. Pract. 2:365–368, 1984.

Nilner, M.: Prevalence of functional disturbances and diseases of the stomatognathic system in 15–18 year olds. Swed. Dent. J. 31:189–197, 1981a.

Nilner, M.: Relationships between oral parafunctions and functional disturbances in the stomatognathic system among 15- to 18-year-olds. Acta Odontol. Scand. 41:197–201, 1983.

Nilner, M., and Lassing, S. A.: Prevalence of functional disturbances and diseases of the stomatognathic system in 7–14 year olds. Swed. Dent. J. 5:173–187, 1981b.

Ogura, T., Morinushi, T., Ohno, H., et al.: An epidemiological study of TMJ dysfunction syndrome in adolescents. J. Pedod. 10:22–35, 1985.

Okeson, J. P., and Hayes, D. K.: Long-term results of treatment for temporomandibular disorders: An evaluation by patients. J. Am. Dent. Assoc. 112:473–478, 1986.

Padamsee, M., Tsamtsouris, A., Ahlin, J. H., and Ko, C. M.: Functional disorders of the stomatognathic system: Part I—A review. J. Pedod. 9:179–187, 1985.

Rao, M. B., and Rao, C. B.: Incidence of temporomandibular joint pain dysfunction syndrome in rural population. Int. J. Oral Surg. 10:261–265, 1981.

Rasmussen, O. C.: Clinical findings during the course of temporomandibular arthropathy. Scand. J. Dent. Res. 89:283–288, 1981a.

Rasmussen, O. C.: Description of population and progress of symptoms in a longitudinal study of temporomandibular arthropathy. Scand. J. Dent. Res. 89:196–203, 1981b.

Reik, L. Jr., and Hale, M.: The temporomandibular joint pain-dysfunction syndrome: A frequent cause of headache. Headache 21:151–156, 1981.

Rieder, C. E., and Martinoff, J. T.: The prevalence of mandibular dysfunction. Part II. A multiphasic dysfunction profile. J. Prosthet. Dent. 50:237–244, 1983.

Rugh, J. D.: Epidemiological measurements of mandibular function. Paper presented at the meeting of the National Institutes of Dental Research, Washington, D.C., October, 1984.

Rugh, J. D., and Solberg, W. K.: Oral health status in the United States: Temporomandibular disorders. J. Dent. Educ. 49:398–405, 1985.

Sakurai, K., San Giacomo, T., Arbree, N. S., and Yurkstas, A.A.: A survey of temporomandibular joint dysfunction in completely edentulous patients. J. Prosthet. Dent. 59:81–85, 1988.

Solberg, W. K., Woo, M. W., and Houston, J. B.: Prevalence of mandibular dysfunction in young adults. J. Am. Dent. Assoc. 98:25–34, 1979.

Spector, G. J.: "How I do it"—Head and neck and plastic surgery. A targeted problem and its solution. Classification of facial nerve disorders. Laryngoscope 95:100–103, 1985.

Swanljung, O., and Rantanen, T.: Functional disorders of the masticatory system in southwest Finland. Oral Epidemiol. 7:177–182, 1979.

Villarosa, G. A., and Moss, R. A.: Oral behavioral patterns as factors contributing to the development of head and facial pain. J. Prosthet. Dent. 54:427–430, 1985.

Vincent, S. D., and Lilly, G. E.: Incidence and characterization of temporomandibular joint sounds in adults. J. Am. Dent. Assoc. 116:203–206, 1988.

Von Korff, M., Dworkin, S. F., LeResche, L., and Kruger, A.: An epidemiologic comparison of pain complaints. Pain 32:173–183, 1988.

Wanman, A., and Agerberg, G.: Mandibular dysfunction in adolescents. I. Prevalence of symptoms. Acta Odontol. Scand. 44:47–54, 1986.

Wigdorowicz-Makowerowa, N., Grodzki, C., Panek, H., et al.: Epidemiologic studies on prevalence and etiology of functional disturbances of the masticatory system. J. Prosthet. Dent. 41:76–82, 1979.

Zarb, G. A.: Problems of definition and related aspects of TMJ disorders. Paper presented at the meeting of the National Institutes of Dental Research, Washington, D.C., October, 1984.

15

HISTORY AND PHYSICAL EXAMINATION*

DANIEL M. LASKIN, D.D.S., M.S.
and BERNARD G. SARNAT, M.D., D.D.S.

INTRODUCTION

Proper diagnosis is the key to successful therapy. The key to proper diagnosis is a thorough and accurate history and physical examination. Taking a patient's history and doing a careful physical examination is both an art and a science that merits meticulous attention in every instance. Relevant and significant facts can be overlooked, forgotten, or withheld by the patient unless drawn out by careful and systematic questioning, and pertinent physical findings can be missed unless there is a precise and orderly search. The effort devoted to these activities is well spent, for establishment of the correct diagnosis significantly reduces the time necessary to resolve the patient's problem.

All of the information gathered from the history and physical examination should be carefully recorded in a logical order. This facilitates review at subsequent visits. An outline of the information to be obtained from the history is shown in Figure 15–1. In eliciting the history, it is important to listen attentively, patiently, and understandingly, and to permit the patient sufficient time for thorough expression. This not only avoids missing significant information,

but also helps to establish the proper doctor-patient relationship necessary to treat patients with temporomandibular joint (TMJ) dysfunction successfully.

HISTORY TAKING

The history is divided into two parts—the general past history that includes medical, surgical, psychological, occupational, social, and family background; and the specific history related to the presenting complaint (onset and course). It is best to start with the specific history, because this enables better interpretation of the more general information. The questioning should begin by determining the presenting complaint and then proceeding with the gathering of information about the events that led up to the present (Fig. 15–1). The patient should be encouraged to describe these events in chronological order and to include previous treatments and their effect upon the present illness.

If not elicited from the history of the present illness reported by the patient, certain pertinent information must be obtained by secondary questioning. For example, it is important to ascertain the effect of function on the symptoms; the temporal character of the symptoms, particularly if they are worse in the morning or

---

*See Chapter 14.

249

FIGURE 15–1. Outline For Clinical History of Patient with Temporomandibular Joint Disorder

A. Personal Data
　　1. Name (complete)
　　2. Address
　　3. Telephone number
　　4. Date of birth
　　5. Age
　　6. Sex
　　7. Marital history
　　8. Occupation
　　9. Referral source

B. Present Complaint
　　List symptoms in order of importance to patient and note duration, as (1) pain in left ear for two weeks; (2) difficulty in opening mouth for five days; etc.

C. Onset and Course of Present Illness
　　Patient's story of illness, as: "Patient was entirely well until two weeks ago when she suddenly noticed. . ." (Describe symptoms in chronological order.) Include treatments for present illness and any changes in symptoms up to the current time.

D. Past History
　　1. Previous illnesses and time of occurrence: Include medications taken
　　2. Surgical procedures and anesthetics: Include method of anesthetic administration
　　3. Accidents or injuries: Type, date, complications
　　4. Habits: Clenching or grinding teeth, lip-, cheek-, or nail-biting, excessive gum chewing, biting on hard objects, tobacco, alcohol, other drugs
　　5. Allergy: Etiological agent, site(s) involved
　　6. Diet: Nutritional adequacy, consistency, recent dietary changes
　　7. Psychological background: Counseling or psychotherapy, use of tranquilizers or other psychotropic drugs, current or past stressful life situations (especially around onset of TMJ symptoms), sleep habits
　　8. Family history: Children (number and age), health status of parents, children, spouse

E. Inquiry by Systems
　　1. Eyes: Vision, pain, inflammation, tearing, diplopia
　　2. Ears: Pain, loss of hearing, noises, stuffiness, discharge
　　3. Nose: Colds, discharge, obstruction, allergy
　　4. Sinuses: Pain, swelling, nasal discharge
　　5. Salivary glands: Pain, swelling
　　6. Gastrointestinal: Appetite, pain, diarrhea, constipation, loss of weight
　　7. Nervous: Headache (time of onset, duration, periodicity, type of pain, location), dizziness, fainting, pain (other than that related to present complaint)
　　8. Musculoskeletal (other than head and neck region): Joint pain and/or stiffness, joint swelling, fractures, deformities
　　9. Oral cavity: Swelling, ulceration, dryness
　　10. Teeth: Pain, loose teeth, infections, extractions, long dental appointments, prostheses, impactions, uncomfortable bite
　　11. Temporomandibular joint: Pain, limitation or excessive movement, noise, tenderness, dislocation, locking, snapping, clicking, grating

less in the morning and increase during the day; the effect that stressful situations have on either the onset or severity of the symptoms; and what possible factors or events may have led to the problem or now cause exacerbation or remission of the symptoms. It is also of value to ask patients what they think is the cause of their problem and what condition they think they have. The answers give some insight into the patient's understanding of the illness. In some individuals, the symptoms are perpetuated by the fear of having a crippling or fatal disease, even after the initiating factors are no longer present. For such persons, reassurance that they do not have a serious condition is often therapeutic.

The information gathered from the general past history can be helpful in ruling out a systemic cause for the patient's problem, in recognizing other contributing factors, and in gaining some insight into the patient's psychological state (see Chapter 20). The information obtained by verbal questioning can be supplemented by having the patient fill out a health questionnaire (Fig. 15–2). When a questionnaire is used, it should serve merely as a guide, and additional inquiries should be made about any significant positive answers elicited.

An inquiry by systems is also a part of the history. In most instances, however, it is not necessary to include all parts of the body. The most pertinent information generally comes from questions about headache; ear problems; sinus disorders; disorders of the muscles, bones, and joints; neurological dysfunction; and particularly, conditions related to the oral cavity, teeth, and jaws. Questions about gastrointestinal disorders are also appropriate, since patients with myofascial pain dysfunction (MPD) syndrome frequently have a history of such conditions as duodenal ulcer, ileitis, or colitis.

PHYSICAL EXAMINATION

Examination of the patient should proceed in an organized, standard manner. By always following the same order, the process becomes routine, and there is less likelihood of something being overlooked. A suggested order involves starting with the general body examination, then examination of the face, followed by examination of the TMJ, the muscles of mastication and associated cervical musculature, the dentition and other oral tissues, and finally, the remaining structures of the head and neck (Fig. 15–3).

FIGURE 15–2. Temporomandibular Joint and Facial Pain Health Questionnaire

Name ....Age ....Sex ....Date ....

If you can answer YES to the question asked, put a circle around YES.
If the answer is NO to the question asked, put a circle around NO.
Answer all questions and fill in blank spaces when indicated. If you are not sure, guess.

1.	Are you being treated by a medical doctor at present?	YES	NO
	If yes, for what?		
	....		
2.	Do you suffer from any chronic (long-standing) diseases? If yes, list them.	YES	NO
	....		
	....		
3.	Do you regularly take any medication or pills? If yes, what are they?	YES	NO
	....		
4.	Do you suffer from headaches?	YES	NO
5.	Do you have any allergies?	YES	NO
6.	Do you have chronic ear pain or infections?	YES	NO
7.	Do you suffer from stomach troubles or ulcer?	YES	NO
8.	Are you suffering from rheumatism or arthritis? If yes, what kind? Rheumatoid;	YES	NO
	degenerative; traumatic; gout.		
9.	Do your muscles and joints ever feel stiff or swollen?	YES	NO
10.	Do you ever experience muscle aches or spasms? If so, where?	YES	NO
	....		
11.	Do you have frequent diarrhea?	YES	NO
12.	Have you ever had any serious accidents or injuries?	YES	NO
13.	Have you ever been hospitalized for any serious illness or surgical procedure? If	YES	NO
	so, what was the problem? When did it occur?		
	....		
	....		
14.	Do you have any oral habits such as grinding or clenching your teeth, cheek- or	YES	NO
	lip-biting, or biting on hard objects?		
15.	Have you ever has a nervous breakdown, counseling, psychotherapy,	YES	NO
	or psychoanalysis?		
16.	Do you take sedatives, tranquilizers, nerve medicine, sleeping pills, or medicine	YES	NO
	to relax?		
17.	Do you have trouble sleeping?	YES	NO
18.	Do you ever have dizzy spells?	YES	NO
19.	Do you suffer from low back pain?	YES	NO
20.	Do you have, or have you ever had, ileitis or colitis?	YES	NO
21.	Do you have any eye problems?	YES	NO
22.	Do you have any sinus problems?	YES	NO
23.	Do your saliva glands ever hurt or swell?	YES	NO
24.	Do you ever have dental pain or infection?	YES	NO
25.	Have you ever had your wisdom teeth removed?	YES	NO
26.	Do your teeth feel loose?	YES	NO
27.	Does your bite feel comfortable?	YES	NO
28.	Does your jaw ever snap or lock?	YES	NO
29.	Does your jaw crack or pop?	YES	NO
30.	Does your jaw ever feel stiff?	YES	NO
31.	Does eating make your jaw tired or hurt?	YES	NO
32.	Do you get swellings or sores in your mouth?	YES	NO
33.	Do you ever get swollen glands?	YES	NO
34.	Are you frequently confined to bed by illness?	YES	NO
35.	Are you always in poor health?	YES	NO
36.	Do you come from a sickly family?	YES	NO
37.	Has your pain made work impossible for you?	YES	NO
38.	Are you constantly made miserable by poor health?	YES	NO
39.	Do you have to lie down and rest often because of pain?	YES	NO
40.	Does your pain bother you so much you have to keep moving?	YES	NO
41.	Has your pain interfered with your sex life?	YES	NO
42.	Are you unable to do the things you want because of pain?	YES	NO
43.	Do you find that all you can think about is your pain?	YES	NO
44.	Do doctors seem to have failed you?	YES	NO
45.	Do you keep looking for a specialist to solve your case?	YES	NO
46.	Do you have trouble getting doctors to take you seriously?	YES	NO
47.	Have some doctors said your pain is imaginary?	YES	NO
48.	Do you secretly think your case may be hopeless?	YES	NO
49.	Do you have, or have you ever had, any other significant medical problems that	YES	NO
	were not mentioned above? If yes, what are they?........................		
	....		
50.	My last medical examination was on		
	My last dental examination was on		
	The name, address, and telephone number of my physician is		
	....		
	The name, address, and telephone number of my dentist is		
	....		

FIGURE 15–3. Examination of Patient with Temporomandibular Joint Disorder

A. General Body Examination (Extent determined by history)
    1. Gait ....
    2. Posture ....
    3. Joints (enlargement, tenderness, stiffness) ....
    ....
    4. Tremors ....
B. Facial Topography
    1. General expression ....
    2. Deformity ....
    3. Asymmetry ....
    4. Swellings ....
    5. Cutaneous lesions ....
    6. Scars ....
    7. Twitching or tics ....
    8. Muscle flexing ....
    9. Paralysis or paresis ....
    10. Flushing ....
    11. Sweating ....
C. Temporomandibular Joint
    1. Maximum opening of mouth (interincisal distance):
       a. Without discomfort .... mm
       b. With discomfort .... mm
    2. Movements

	Normal	Restricted	Excessive
Protrusion—			
Retrusion—			
Right lateral—			
Left lateral—			

    3. Mandibular gait
       a. Synchronous ....
       b. Asynchronous ....
    4. Mandibular deviation on opening ....
    5. Joint sounds (type and relation to function) ....
    ....
    6. Joint tenderness
       a. Intrameatal palpation ....
       b. Lateral palpation ....
    7. Swelling ....
    8. Condylar enlargement ....
    9. Condylar deficiency ....
D. Masticatory and Cervical Muscles

	Side	Sites of Tenderness	Rigidity	Masses
1. Masseter				
2. Temporalis				
3. Medial pterygoid				
4. Lateral pterygoid				
5. Sternocleidomastoid				
6. Trapezius				
7. Occipital				
8. Splenius capitis				
9. Scalenus anticus				
10. Suprahyoids				

E. Oral Tissues
    1. Mucosal lesions ....
    2. Swellings ....
    3. Periodontal disease ....
    4. Xerostomia ....
    5. Evidence of cheek- or lip-biting ....
F. Dentition
    1. Caries ....
    2. Mobile teeth ....
    3. Missing teeth ....
    4. Prosthetic replacements ....
    5. Impactions ....
    6. Supraerupted teeth ....

7. Occlusion:
   a. Normal ....
   b. Class I ....
   c. Class II ....
   d. Class III ....
   e. Open bite ....
   f. Large overjet ....
   g. Deep overbite ....
   h. Edge-to-edge ....
   i. Crossbite ....

8. Vertical dimension
   a. Increased ....
   b. Decreased ....

9. Mandibular positioning ....

10. Mandibular displacement from initial tooth contact to full closure
    a. Apparent ....
    Not apparent ....
    b. Anterior ....
    Posterior ....
    c. Right lateral ....
    Left lateral ....

11. Occlusal disharmony related to dental restorations ....

12. Attrition ....

G. Head and Neck
   1. Eyes ....
   2. Ears ....
   3. Nose ....
   4. Throat ....
   5. Sinuses ....
   6. Salivary glands ....
   7. Neck ....

H. Radiologic, MRI, Radionuclide Examination
   1. Teeth and jaws ....
   ....
   2. Temporomandibular joint ....
   ....
   3. Cervical spine ....
   ....
   4. Sinuses ....
   ....
   5. Other ....
   ....

I. Laboratory Tests (Extent determined by history and clinical findings)
   1. Complete blood cell count ....
   2. Calcium ....
   3. Phosphorus ....
   4. Alkaline phosphatase ....
   5. Uric acid ....
   6. Creatine ....
   7. Creatine phosphokinase ....
   8. Sedimentation rate ....
   9. Rheumatoid factor ....
   10. Latex fixation test ....
   11. Other ....

J. Psychological Evaluation
   ....
   ....
   ....

K. Electromyographical Examination
   ....
   ....
   ....

L. Other Examinations
   ....
   ....
   ....

M. Summary of Findings
   ....
   ....
   ....

N. Diagnosis
   ....
   ....
   ....

O. Recommended Treatment
   ....
   ....
   ....

Total Body Examination

The patient with a TMJ disorder generally does not require an extensive examination of the entire body. There are certain observations, however, that should be made that may be helpful in arriving at a definitive diagnosis (see Chapter 26). These relate mainly to diseases of the musculoskeletal system. Abnormalities in posture or gait may be indicative of bone or joint disease, muscular disorders, or diseases of the nervous system, such as Parkinson's disease or multiple sclerosis. Examination of the hands can often provide information regarding the presence of arthritis. Observation of nervous movements of the hands or feet also may offer clues regarding the individual's psychological state.

Examination of Facial Topography

Following whatever aspects of the total body examination are deemed appropriate in the particular patient, a general evaluation of the face should be done. The entire face is examined for swellings, other types of deformity, or asymmetry. The skin is examined for erythema, rash, scaling, or atrophic changes that may be indicative of a systemic connective tissue disease. The chin and submental region, especially, should be observed for scars that might be related to a past traumatic injury. The general facial appearance also should be noted, since tenseness, twitching, or flexing of the facial or masticatory muscles may be indicative of nervousness or stress. Likewise, the patient's facial expression may give some indication of the degree of pain or suffering.

Evaluation of Temporomandibular Joint Function

The TMJs are examined before the musculature and oral tissues to avoid the possibility of misdiagnosis by stimulating referred pain from the latter regions to the joint area. Function of the TMJs is evaluated both directly and indirectly. Indirect evaluation begins with measurement of the interincisal distance both at the point when discomfort is first felt, and at maximum opening, regardless of symptoms. The opening and closing movements are also evaluated for synchrony and deviation (see Chapter 24, Table 24–3). Finally, the patient is asked to perform protrusive, retrusive, and lateral movements. Variations from normal function can often be related to the observations made upon examination of the masticatory muscles.

Direct examination of the TMJ involves palpation and auscultation. Palpation of the condyle is done both in the preauricular area and via the external auditory meatus while the teeth are in occlusion and during opening and closing movements. In addition to eliciting tenderness, one may feel asynchronous movements, popping, snapping, or crepitus. It is also possible to evaluate the range of condylar movement by palpation.

Although some sounds emanating from the TMJ are clearly audible to the examiner, others reported by the patient can only be confirmed by listening to the joint with a stethoscope. The relation of the sound to the degree of opening or closing of the mouth can be of significance in determining the etiology of the problem. The character of the sound may also be significant. Crepitation is usually a sign of organic pathology in the TMJ, while clicking and popping sounds are more often indicative of functional derangements associated with masticatory muscle spasm or anatomic disc derangements due to trauma or other factors.

Examination of the Masticatory and Associated Musculature

Before palpation of the muscles for areas of tenderness, rigidity, or masses, an estimation of the patient's reaction to pain should be made by applying firm pressure bilaterally on the mastoid processes. Under normal circumstances, this should be a painless procedure. In performing this test, as with the remainder of the physical examination, one should be careful not to suggest answers by the types of information elicited. For example, rather than saying, "Does this hurt?" the patient should be asked, "What do you feel when I press here?" If the patient complains of pain in the mastoid region bilaterally and there is no indication of a reason for the pain, this should be taken into consideration in evaluating the responses to palpation during the remainder of the examination.

The major portion of the masseter and temporalis muscles can be examined extraorally. Intraoral palpation is necessary, however, to examine the anterosuperior aspect of the superficial belly of the masseter and the region of the attachment of the temporalis to the coronoid process. The muscles should be examined in both a relaxed and contracted state.

Examination of the medial pterygoid muscle is done mainly by an intraoral approach. However, the region of its attachment to the inner aspect of the angle of the mandible can be palpated best by placing one hand on the outside of the face below the lower border of the mandible. While this is being done, the submandibular gland should also be palpated, since repeating this relatively uncomfortable procedure later in the examination is then avoided.

The lateral pterygoid muscle is relatively inaccessible, and, at best, only the portion inserting on the pterygoid plate can be palpated by placing a finger behind the maxillary tuberosity. This can be an uncomfortable procedure even in an asymptomatic individual, and the response elicited is probably meaningful only if there is a difference between the two sides. This sort of judgment is also important to make when examining the medial pterygoid muscles. Another common error made when examining the lateral pterygoid is inadvertently to press the back side of the palpating finger against the attachment of the temporalis muscle on the coronoid process. Because this is a frequent site of tenderness in patients with MPD syndrome, one must be careful in determining from which site a positive response is being elicited.

The suprahyoid muscles (stylohyoid, mylohyoid, geniohyoid, and digastric), because of their role as opening muscles for the lower jaw, should also be palpated for areas of tenderness. Moreover, because pain can be referred to the orofacial region from trigger points in various muscles in the neck, particularly from the sternocleidomastoid, trapezius, occipital, splenius capitis, and scalenus anticus, these muscles should also be carefully examined.

Examination of the Dentition and Other Oral Tissues

Since various forms of oral pathology can produce both jaw dysfunction and pain resembling that associated with TMJ disorders, the hard and soft tissues of the oral cavity must be examined thoroughly. The dentition should be carefully examined for supraerupted teeth, improperly contoured restorations, prostheses that encroach excessively on the intermaxillary space, or annoying dental conditions that may predispose to clenching or grinding of the teeth. Gross malocclusions should also be noted. Conditions such as mandibular prognathism, mandibular retrognathism, or maxillary protrusion, particularly when the patient attempts to hold the mandible in a strained position to achieve a more esthetic profile or more functional bite, may lead to MPD syndrome or degenerative changes in the TMJ.

It is generally inadvisable to evaluate the occlusion for functional dental interferences in the presence of active conditions involving the muscles of mastication or the TMJ. Such disorders can produce shifts of the mandible that may be translated secondarily into an apparent disharmony between individual teeth. These interferences are difficult to distinguish from those that may have preceded the jaw dysfunction. Most of them disappear, however, when the mandible returns to its normal neuromuscularly determined position following treatment. If not, the presence of true occlusal interferences can at least be determined more accurately at that time.

Examination of the Head and Neck

Although the major portion of the physical examination focuses on the TMJ, the masticatory and cervical muscles, the dentition, and the other oral tissues, examination of the remaining structures of the head and neck for abnormalities must not be neglected, because pain from these regions can be referred to the TMJ region. This is particularly true for the ears, nose, paranasal sinuses, and the parotid gland. If all of the previous aspects of the physical examination have not revealed any significant findings, and these areas also appear normal, it is sometimes advisable for the dentist to refer the patient to an otolaryngologist to ensure that nothing has been overlooked.

Radiographic and Laboratory Examinations

Radiographic evaluation of the teeth, jaws, TMJs, and associated structures, as well as occasional radiographs of other parts of the skeleton, are essential for the establishment of a proper diagnosis. Magnetic resonance imaging and radionuclide scanning of the TMJs are also helpful procedures. These aspects of the physical examination are discussed in Chapter 16. Certain laboratory tests are also used occasionally for purposes of differential diagnosis. These include the complete blood cell count in suspected infections; serum calcium, phosphorus, and alkaline phosphatase measurement in bone diseases; serum uric acid determination in gout; serum creatinine and creatine phosphokinase as indicators of muscle disease; and sedimentation rate, rheumatoid factor, and latex fixation tests for suspected rheumatoid arthritis. Other tests may also be indicated depending upon the findings from the history and physical examination. Additionally, electromyography is a useful tool in the evaluation of muscle function.

Consultations

Based upon their interpretation of the etiology of the problem, patients may initially seek care from either the dentist or the physician. Each of these practitioners possesses certain special knowledge and skills. When the history and physical examination do not reveal any obvious basis for the patient's complaints, it is appropriate to seek consultation with those who possess this special background rather than to attempt empirical treatment or to relegate the patient to the psychoneurotic category. Thus, there may be instances when the physician may wish to have the advice of the dentist or other physicians, and where the dentist may avail himself of consultation with the internist, otolaryngologist, neurologist, psychiatrist or psychologist, or even other dentists. Such an exchange of ideas and information results in more accurate diagnosis and is consonant with the concept of providing the best in total patient care.

SUMMARY

An accurate, detailed history and physical examination are the basis for proper diagnosis. The clinician should develop an orderly, consistent approach for obtaining and recording these data so that pertinent information is neither overlooked nor forgotten. The thoroughness of the investigation in any particular patient varies with the complexity of the problem, and when clinicians reach the limits of their expertise, consultation should be sought.

The information obtained from both the history and physical examination is only useful if one is familiar with the various disorders that can affect the patient and the signs and symptoms that they can produce. This knowledge ultimately guides the extent and depth of patient evaluation.

16

IMAGING*

PER-LENNART WESTESSON, D.D.S., PH.D.

INTRODUCTION

Diagnostic imaging is used principally to document clinically suspected disorders of the temporomandibular joint (TMJ). For a long time plain film imaging was the only method used. With the development of newer modalities such as arthrography, computed tomography (CT), and, most recently, magnetic resonance imaging (MRI), the understanding of the anatomy, pathophysiology, and internal derangement of the TMJ has been greatly improved (Katzberg, 1989). Several studies have shown that it is difficult to determine accurately the intra-articular status of the joint by a clinical examination alone (Anderson, 1989; Roberts, 1985b; 1986; 1987a; 1987b; 1987c). The purpose of this chapter is to review the imaging modalities that are available for studies of the TMJ, to discuss their relative merits, and to present a strategy for the imaging of patients with symptoms related to the TMJ.

Selection of the appropriate imaging technique, and understanding and interpretation of the resulting image will require full knowledge about normal and pathologic anatomy of the joint and surrounding tissues (see Chapters 5, 9, 17, 19, and 23).

PLAIN FILM RADIOGRAPHY

Transcranial Projection

The most common and traditional radiograph of the TMJ is the transcranial projection. Ideally

---

*See Chapters 5, 6, 9–13, 17, 19, 22–24, and 26.

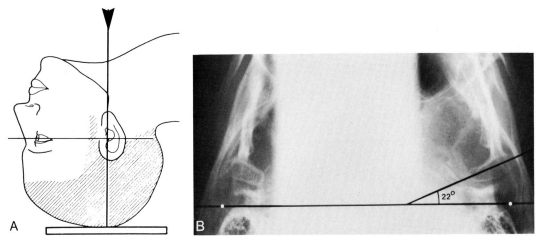

FIGURE 16–1. *A*, Schematic drawing of submentovertical projection. (From Omnell, K.-Å., and Lysell, L.: Roentgendiagnostics. *In* Krogh-Poulsen, W. (Ed.): Stomatognathic Function and Physiology, vol. 2, ed. 2. Copenhagen, Munksgaard, 1979, pp. 141–153.) *B*, Submentovertical projection of the base of the skull showing the angulation of the mandibular condyles. The horizontal line is connecting the left and right external auditory meatuses. The other line shows the angulation of the right mandibular condyle.

the x-ray beam should be parallel to the long axis of the condyle in all planes. A submentovertical projection (Fig. 16–1A) is useful to determine the horizontal angulation of the mandibular condyle (Fig. 16–1B). To avoid superimposition of the base of the skull on the joint, a vertical angulation is also needed (Fig. 16–2). Usually an angulation of 15 to 25 degrees from above is sufficient to project the joint free of the base of the skull. This angulation places the x-ray beam tangential to the lateral pole of the condyle (Fig. 16–3). Therefore, the cortical surface of the condyle seen on the transcranial radiograph represents the lateral portion of the condyle (Fig. 16–4). The central and medial parts of the joint are not clearly seen on the transcranial projection because the tangent of the x-ray beam is not parallel to this surface. This is a disadvantage of the technique. This disadvantage is compensated, however, by the fact that most early osseous changes occur laterally in the joint (Öberg, 1971).

Degenerative joint disease, limitation of condylar translation, and, very uncommonly, calcified loose bodies within the joint can be observed in transcranial radiographs. Translation of the condyle to the apex of the articular eminence or beyond is considered normal. When the condyle does not reach the apex of the eminence, however, it is considered abnormal.

Many discussions have been focused on the significance of the position of the mandibular condyle within the glenoid fossa as related to

disorders of the joint (Farrar, 1979; Katzberg, 1983). A condyle posteriorly positioned in the fossa in the closed-mouth position has been reported to be associated with an anteriorly displaced disc. This is not a reliable finding because about the same frequency of posteriorly positioned condyles has been found in patients with and without symptoms of TMJ disorders (Table 16–1) (Bean, 1987). These findings have been confirmed in a recent study in which condylar position as assessed by tomography was correlated with arthrographic diagnosis of the position of the disc (Brand, 1989). About 50 per cent of the joints with normal superior disc position demonstrated tomographic evidence of

TABLE 16–1. Condylar Position in Asymptomatic Individuals and Symptomatic Temporomandibular Joint Patients

CONDYLAR POSITION	ASYMPTOMATIC	SYMPTOMATIC
	(N = 50)	(N = 100)
Central	70 per cent	73 per cent
Anterior (narrowing of anterior joint space)	17 per cent	14 per cent
Posterior (narrowing of posterior joint space)	13 per cent	13 per cent

From Bean, L. R., and Thomas, C. A.: Significance of condylar positions in patients with temporomandibular joint disorders. J. Am. Dent. Assoc. *114*:76–77, 1987.

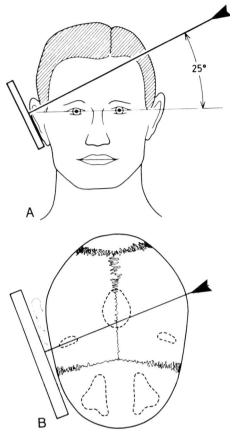

FIGURE 16–2. Schematic drawing of a transcranial projection of the right TMJ. (From Omnell, K.-Å., and Lysell, L.: Roentgendiagnostics. *In* Krogh-Poulsen, W. (Ed.): Stomatognathic Function and Physiology, vol. 2, ed. 2. Copenhagen, Munksgaard, 1979, pp. 141–153.)

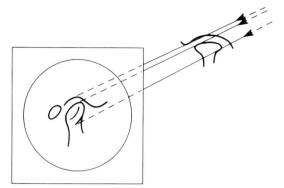

FIGURE 16–3. Schematic drawing of the transcranial projection and resulting radiograph. The condyle and temporal component of the TMJ seen in the radiograph represent the lateral part of the joint. (From Omnell, K.-Å., and Lysell, L.: Roentgendiagnostics. *In* Krogh-Poulsen, W. (Ed.): Stomatognathic Function and Physiology, vol. 2, ed. 2. Copenhagen, Munksgaard, 1979, pp. 141–153.)

Transmaxillary Projection

The transmaxillary projection (Bean, 1975; McCabe, 1959; Petersson, 1975) is made from about 10 degrees above and about 35 degrees lateral to the sagittal plane (Fig. 16–5). This projection gives an excellent image of the superior surface of the condyle and the inferior contour of the articular eminence (Fig. 16–5), provided that the patient is able to open the

a retroposition of the condyle. In the same study, about one-third of the joints with concentric or anteriorly positioned condyles had an arthrographic diagnosis of internal derangement (Brand, 1989). Based on the information in this study and others (Pullinger, 1985; 1986a; 1986b; 1987), it can be concluded that the position of the condyle in the glenoid fossa is only of limited value to determine the position of the disc.

Because the transcranial projection mainly depicts the lateral or the lateral central parts of the joint, there is a need for another projection to study the medial part of the joint. It is therefore advisable to combine the transcranial projection with another projection, such as the transmaxillary, transorbital, or anteroposterior, that depicts the central and medial parts of the joint.

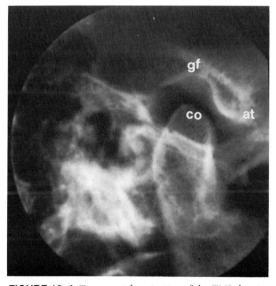

FIGURE 16–4. Transcranial projection of the TMJ showing normal osseous structures. Glenoid fossa (gf), condyle (co), and the articular eminence (tubercle) (at).

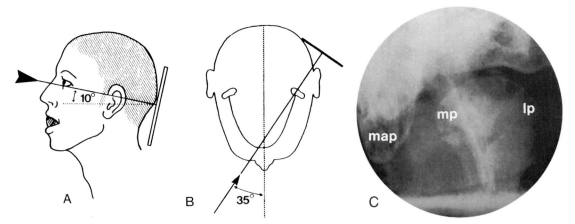

FIGURE 16–5. *A and B,* Schematic drawings of transmaxillary projection of left TMJ. (From Bean, L. R., Petersson, A., and Svensson, A.: The transmaxillary projection in temporomandibular joint radiography. Dentomaxillofac. Radiol. 4:13–18, 1975.) *C,* Transmaxillary projection showing the left mandibular condyle. There are no osseous changes. The superior part of the condyle and the inferior part of the articular eminence are clearly delineated. The mastoid process (map) and the medial (mp) and the lateral (lp) poles of the condyle are indicated on the figure.

mouth wide and translate the condyle under the articular eminence. Comparative studies have indicated that the transcranial and transmaxillary projections are complementary in the diagnosis of osseous changes of the joint (Petersson, 1975).

Transpharyngeal Projection

The transpharyngeal projection (Fig. 16–6) is another frequently used method to image the mandibular condyle (Boering, 1966; Hansson, 1978; Rasmussen, 1980; 1981; 1983; Toller, 1974b). The transpharyngeal projection is obtained with the mouth opened wide. The x-ray beam is directed through the mandibular notch on the contralateral side and the film is placed close to the skin on the side that is imaged (Fig. 16–6). Studies comparing transpharyngeal and transmaxillary projections have suggested that the transpharyngeal projection is not as effective in detecting osseous abnormalities as the transcranial projection (Hansson, 1978). Longitudinal studies with the transpharyngeal projection have indicated, however, that this radiographic technique may be valuable to follow patients with erosions of the mandibular condyle (Rasmussen, 1983; 1981; 1980).

Tomography

Tomography is a more complex radiographic method than plain film imaging and requires special equipment. Tomography involves sec-

tional imaging that is accomplished by moving the x-ray tube and the film in opposite directions during the exposure. Structures outside the tomographic plane will be blurred while structures within the tomographic plane will be reproduced clearly. The differences between the various tomographic techniques depend on the pattern of motion of the tube and film. Complex motion tomography (hypocycloidal, circular, or trispiral) provides thinner tomographic sections and superior image quality compared with linear tomography.

Tomographic sections can be obtained in any anatomic plane through the joint. In general, sagittal sections are preferred for examination of the TMJ (Fig. 16–7). The tomographic layer is usually about 3 mm thick when complex motion tomography is used (Eckerdal, 1973). Usually five 3 mm sections will cover the mediolateral dimension of the joint. The most lateral and the most medial parts of the joint are usually not possible to depict with tomography (Eckerdal, 1973), because the superior surface of the condyle is not parallel to the central x-ray beam and because the lateral and medial poles are small. Lateral tomographic sections are ideally made perpendicular to the long axis of the condyle and this specific technique is termed corrected sagittal tomography (Omnell, 1976; 1980). To determine the horizontal long axis of the condyle, a submentovertical projection can be used (Fig. 16–1).

Studies have confirmed that more information about osseous anatomy can be gained from

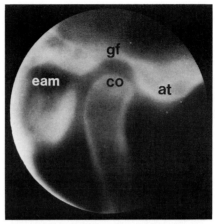

FIGURE 16–7. Corrected sagittal tomogram of right TMJ showing normal osseous structures. External auditory meatus (eam), glenoid fossa (gf), condyle (co), and articular eminence (tubercle) (at).

tomography than from a transcranial projection (Omnell, 1976). Sagittal corrected tomography probably is also one of the most reliable methods to assess the position of the condyle in the mandibular fossa at the closed-mouth position.

Tomography is sometimes also performed in the coronal plane. This plane of tomographic section can be useful to assess osseous changes of the lateral and medial poles of the condyle that are not clearly depicted on sagittal tomograms (Figs. 16–8, 16–9). Figure 16–9 shows an extensive erosive change of the lateral part of the mandibular condyle in a patient with rheumatoid arthritis. Inflammatory arthritis of the joint is usually diagnosed clinically, but radiographic examination may provide supplementary information.

Tomographic images are useful for evaluating the osseous components of the joints only and provide no information about the soft tissues.

ARTHROGRAPHY

Arthrography involves radiography of the joint after intra-articular injection of contrast medium. This technique is frequently used to examine other joints of the body. The first systematic attempt to evaluate the TMJ arthrographically was by Nørgaard (1947; 1944). The technique was adopted, however, by only a few clinicians because it was difficult to perform and painful for the patient. Additionally, and probably most importantly, the information obtained was usually of only limited value for treatment

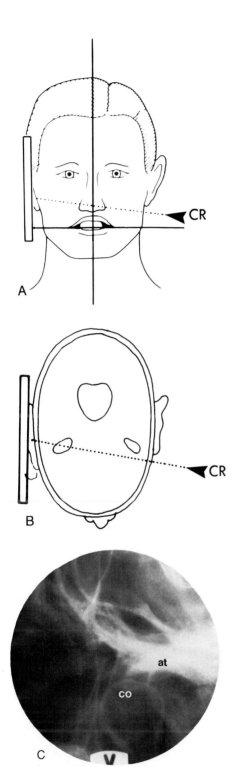

FIGURE 16–6. *A,* Schematic drawing of transpharyngeal projection in frontal view. *B,* Schematic drawing of transpharyngeal projection in axial view. (From Omnell, K.-Å.: Radiology of the TMJ. *In* Irby, W. B. (Ed.): Current Advances in Oral Surgery, vol. 3. St. Louis, C. V. Mosby, 1980, pp. 196–226.) *C,* Transpharyngeal projection. Mandibular condyle (co), articular eminence (tubercle) (at).

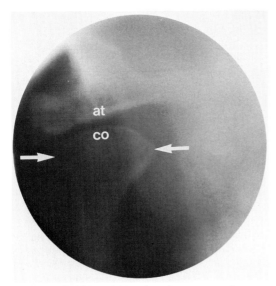

FIGURE 16–8. Coronal tomogram showing normal osseous structures. The mandibular condyle (co), articular eminence (tubercle) (at), and the lateral and medial poles (arrows) of the condyle are indicated on the figure.

planning and for evaluation of prognosis (Toller, 1974a). Only scattered descriptions of arthrography for evaluation of the TMJ appeared in the literature during the 1950s, 1960s, and 1970s (Campbell, 1965; Frenkel, 1965; Toller, 1974a). In 1978 two studies appeared that described the clinical and arthrographic characteristics of anterior displacement of the TMJ disc

(Wilkes, 1978a; 1978b). The arthrographic technique used involved injection of contrast medium into both upper and lower joint spaces and imaging the joint with tomography (Fig. 16–10). By this technique it was possible to show that the disc was anteriorly displaced in a significant proportion of patients with TMJ pain and dysfunction. These studies (Wilkes, 1978a; 1978b) substantiated speculations from several earlier studies (Annandale, 1887; Burman, 1946; Christie, 1953; Farrar 1978; 1971; Ireland, 1951; Mullen, 1937; Pringle, 1918; Silver, 1956) suggesting that displacement of the disc can occur.

Following these two studies (Wilkes, 1978a; 1978b), and another report by Farrar (1979), an explosion of literature describing the usefulness of TMJ arthrography for diagnosis of internal derangement of the TMJ occurred. The changed attitude toward TMJ arthrography can be traced back to at least three factors: (1) the use of an image intensifier to facilitate injection of the joint (Wilkes, 1978a; 1978b) and also as a method to study and document the dynamics of the joint (Bell, 1983); (2) the identification of anterior disc displacement as a common cause of TMJ pain and dysfunction (Wilkes, 1978a; 1978b); and finally, and probably most importantly, (3) the introduction of new nonsurgical (Bellavia, 1983; Dolwick, 1983; Dugal, 1982; Farrar, 1979; Lundh, 1985) and surgical (McCarty, 1979; 1982) methods to treat disc displacement that required accurate information about the status and function of the joint. The use of nonionic contrast medium, making the

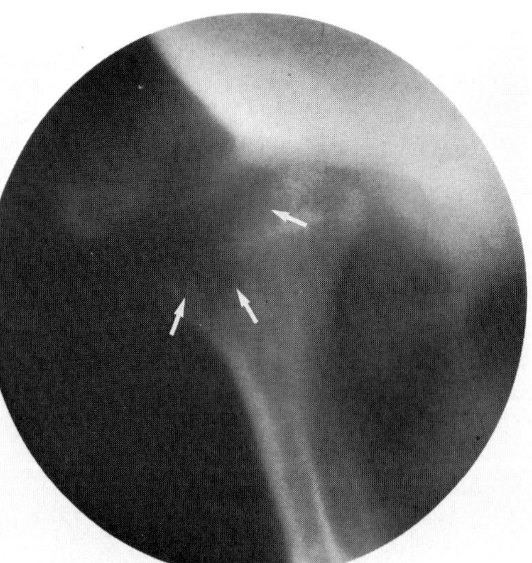

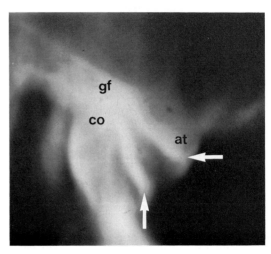

FIGURE 16–9. Coronal tomogram of right TMJ showing an extensive erosion of the lateral and central part of the mandibular condyle (arrows) in a patient with rheumatoid arthritis. (Courtesy of Dr. Arne Petersson.)

FIGURE 16–10. Dual-space arthrotomogram of right TMJ. Contrast medium was injected into the lower and upper joint spaces followed by linear tomography. Glenoid fossa (gf), condyle (co), articular eminence (tubercle) (at). The upper and lower joint spaces are indicated by arrows.

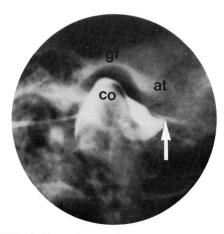

FIGURE 16–11. Single-space lower-joint compartment arthrogram showing anterior disc displacement. Glenoid fossa (gf), condyle (co), articular eminence (tubercle) (at). Contrast medium in the anterior recess of the lower joint space is indicated by an arrow.

examination less painful, probably also influenced the more frequent use of arthrography, as did the combination of arthrography and tomography (Campbell, 1965; Frenkel, 1965; Wilkes, 1978a; 1978b) that improved the quality of the radiographs. A simplification of the arthrographic technique described by Wilkes (1978a; 1978b) was made by Farrar (1979) who injected contrast medium only into the lower joint space and used a videotape recording in a transcranial projection (Fig. 16–11). Thus, the need for tomography and for injection of contrast medium into the upper joint space was

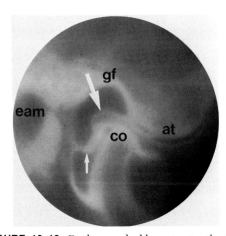

FIGURE 16–12. Dual-space double-contrast arthrotomogram. The disc is biconcave and lying superior to the condyle in this half open–mouth view. The posterior band (large arrow) is located superior and posterior to the condyle. The posterior disc attachment is redundant and hanging down (small arrow). External auditory meatus (eam), glenoid fossa (gf), condyle (co), articular eminence (tubercle) (at).

eliminated. Today the single-contrast, lower-compartment arthrographic technique (Farrar, 1979) is probably the most commonly used.

Techniques for dual-space double-contrast arthrotomography also have been described (Arnaudow, 1974; 1968; Westesson, 1984; 1983; 1982; 1980). In this technique a combination of iodine contrast medium and air is used. The dual-space double-contrast arthrotomography is superior to the single-contrast technique in its demonstration of the configuration of the disc and the posterior disc attachment (Fig. 16–12). The double-contrast technique has not gained wide acceptance, probably because it is technically more difficult to perform than single-contrast arthrography and requires specific radiography equipment such as a tomographic unit with an attached head holder for upright positioning of the patient.

Indications

The major indication for TMJ arthrography is to assess either the soft tissue component or essentially the position, function, and configuration of the disc in patients with pain and mechanical symptoms that suggest an internal derangement. Arthrography may also be indicated in patients with diffuse facial and head pain in whom differential diagnosis is essential. Frequently these patients have not responded to therapy. The arthrogram also can be used to determine a mandibular position in which the disc is in correct relation to the condyle. This position has been used for protrusive splint therapy (Manzione, 1984b; Tallents, 1985). Less frequent indications for arthrography are delineation of loose bodies within the joint spaces, evaluation of the joint after acute injury, and evaluation prior to diagnostic aspiration of joint fluid or injection of intra-articular medications such as cortisone. In these last situations, the injection of a small amount of contrast medium will help confirm the correct intra-articular position of the needle tip.

Contraindications

The main contraindication for arthrography is an infection in the preauricular region that could contaminate the joint. Previous reactions to contrast medium is a relative contraindication. Other modalities such as MRI and possibly CT scanning should be considered as an alternative for these patients. An arthrogram has been performed on such patients, however, without untoward reaction after pre-arthrography medication with an antihistamine and cortisone. Indeed, life-threatening events are rare with arthrography. Bleeding disorders and use of anticoagulation medication are other relative contraindications to arthrography. Anticoagulants can be discontinued or decreased prior to the procedure.

Radiologic Equipment

A fluoroscopy table or a C-arm with an x-ray tube and an image intensifier are useful equipment for TMJ arthrography. The patient is positioned on the side, with the head oriented so that the side under examination is located superiorly. In this way the head is slightly tilted and a transcranial projection is obtained. The best image of the joint is determined by changing the position of the head during fluoroscopy. Because of the small dimensions of the TMJ it is valuable to magnify the image up to about three times. Spot films and videotape recording are important for documentation.

Technique

The procedure is explained to the patient and all questions are answered before starting. The patient is then placed on the table and the skin is prepared with an antiseptic solution and the region is draped. Opening and closing movements are recorded fluoroscopically on a videotape. Arthrography can be performed either as a single-contrast, lower-joint space procedure or as dual-space, double-contrast arthrotomography. Because the techniques for the two examinations vary slightly they will be described separately.

Single-Contrast

The posterior superior aspect of the mandibular condyle is identified with a metal marker (Fig. 16–13). This area is then marked on the skin with a pen. A local anesthetic agent (0.5–1.0 ml of 1 to 2 per cent lidocaine) is injected into the region of joint puncture. A ¾ inch, 25-gauge scalp-vein needle and the attached tubing are filled with contrast material (Omnipaque, 300 mg iodine per ml), with care taken to eliminate air bubbles. Air bubbles injected into the joint space may simulate loose bodies. The needle is introduced in a direction perpendicular to the skin and parallel to the x-ray beam until contact with the condyle is felt. Needle position is checked fluoroscopically. The patient is then instructed to open the mouth

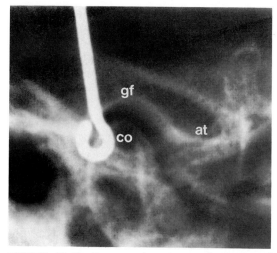

FIGURE 16–13. Transcranial projection showing metal marker indicating the position for puncture of the lower joint space. Glenoid fossa (gf), condyle (co), articular eminence (tubercle) (at).

slightly and the needle is advanced along the posterior aspect of the condyle. When correctly placed, the needle will appear to be contiguous with the posterior condylar outline. About 0.2 to 0.5 ml of contrast material is injected into the lower joint compartment under fluoroscopic observation (Fig. 16–14). The free flow of contrast medium around the condyle is an indication of correct joint puncture. If there is simultaneous filling of the upper joint compartment, this indicates perforation between the lower

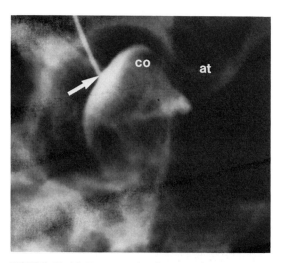

FIGURE 16–14. Transcranial arthrogram showing contrast medium being injected into the lower joint space. There is no evidence of internal derangement. The needle inserted into the lower joint space is indicated by an arrow. Condyle (co), articular eminence (tubercle) (at).

and upper joint spaces and usually requires that another 0.5 ml of contrast medium be injected for optimal visualization. The needle is withdrawn and fluoroscopic videotape images are recorded during opening and closing movements of the mouth. Spot films are then obtained at closed and maximal mouth opening, as well as at any jaw position where abnormalities are most clearly seen. An arthrotomogram can now be obtained for more complete evaluation. Complex motion tomography is optimal for this imaging.

Dual-Space Double-Contrast

The patient is positioned on the fluoroscopy table in the same way as for single-contrast arthrography. Slightly more local anesthetic is injected because catheters (Angiocath, 0.8 mm diameter and 25 mm long) are used that are thicker than the needle used for single-contrast arthrography. About 1 ml of a 2 per cent solution of a local anesthetic agent is injected in the regions of joint puncture. The lower joint space is punctured the same way as in the single-contrast technique. Thus, the catheter enters the lower joint compartment in the posterior recess along the posterior aspect of the condyle. The upper joint compartment is then cannulated in the fossa or along the posterior slope of the tubercle. The area for joint puncture is identified fluoroscopically and then the catheter is advanced until bone contact is made. When bone contact has been established, the tip of the catheter is slid along the articular surface. Correct placement of the needle tip in the joint space is indicated by the free movement of the catheter with no resistance. The inner metal needle is removed and the catheter is advanced into the joint space. An extension tube filled with contrast medium is connected to the catheter and contrast medium is injected into the lower joint space. Usually between 0.2 and 0.5 ml is adequate for visualization. Joint movements are recorded fluoroscopically. Spot films are obtained at closed and maximal mouth opening. If abnormalities are seen, these are maximized and documented on spot films. About 0.4 to 0.6 ml of contrast medium is then injected into the upper joint space. Spot films are obtained at closed and at maximal mouth opening.

The external parts of the catheters are now taped securely to the skin so that they remain in proper position in the joint spaces during the remainder of the examination. After a few opening and closing movements, as much of the contrast medium as possible is aspirated from both the upper and lower joint spaces. Only a thin layer of contrast medium should remain on the articular surfaces. The patient is moved from the fluoroscopy table to a tomography unit. A Philips Polytome with the possibility for upright positioning of the patient and a head holder, so that the patient's head can be accurately oriented and repositioned to a predetermined position, are used.

Once the patient is placed in the tomography unit, new extension tubes are connected to the catheters in the upper and lower joint spaces and two ml glass syringes filled with room air are attached to them. Glass syringes have low friction and are therefore preferred to disposable plastic syringes. About 0.5 to 1 ml of air is injected simultaneously into both upper and lower joint spaces. The correct amount of air is determined by the ease of the injections. It is essential to inject the air simultaneously into both upper and lower joint compartments so that the disc is not displaced. If too much or too little air is injected into either joint space, the disc will be insufficiently visualized. The amount of air is adjusted for each exposure. More air is usually needed for the maximal opening of the mouth than for the rest position. After air has been injected, a hemostat is placed on the extension tube to prevent back flow. Double-contrast arthrotomographic images are obtained at the rest position (Fig. 16–15A) and at maximal opening (Fig. 16–15B). Additional arthrotomograms may be obtained at positions that are necessary for documentation of abnormalities. After the examination has been completed, the air is aspirated from the joint spaces and the catheters are removed.

Book cassettes with five or seven films can be used for simultaneous tomography. In this way, multiple images can be obtained in one exposure and the position of the condyle will be the same on all cuts. Additionally, use of this cassette is not only time-saving but also reduces the radiation dosage.

Objectives

The aim of the arthrographic examination is to document intra-articular status and function. The radiographic protocol should be tailored to the clinical symptoms and the fluoroscopic findings. In patients with painful clicking of the joint and a fluoroscopic diagnosis of anterior disc displacement with reduction, a jaw position where the disc is correctly located superior to the condyle can be determined and docu-

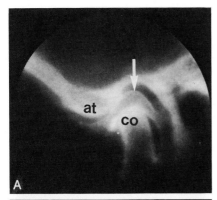

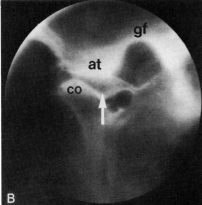

FIGURE 16–15. *A,* Dual-space double-contrast arthroto-mogram showing biconcave disc in superior position. The posterior band of the disc is indicated by an arrow. Articular eminence (tubercle) (at), condyle (co). *B,* Dual-space double-contrast arthrotomogram obtained at maximal opening. The disc is biconcave and located normally. The posterior band of the disc is indicated by an arrow. Glenoid fossa (gf), articular eminence (tubercle) (at), condyle (co).

mented by a fast-setting material injected between the teeth (Manzione, 1984b; Tallents, 1985). This jaw registration can be used by the referring clinician for the purpose of constructing a protrusive splint. In patients with disc displacement without reduction, or with disc displacement associated with perforation, the arthrotomograms provide detailed assessment of the morphology of the joint. The arthrotomogram is especially important in instances when the joint appears to be normal on fluoroscopy.

Findings

Normal

The normal TMJ is arthrographically characterized by the posterior thick part of the disc (posterior band) lying over the condyle in the closed-mouth position (Fig. 16–15A). In the single-contrast lower-space arthrogram this status is usually associated with a relatively small anterior recess (Fig. 16–16). Even in normal joints, however, substantial variation exists in the dimension of the lower joint compartment, and this recess can be relatively large even though the disc is located in the correct position (Fig. 16–17). Measurements of the size of the joint compartments in sagittal arthrotomograms also have shown great variation in normal joints (Fig. 16–18) (Westesson, 1990a). In instances where the diagnosis is not clear, contrast medium should be injected into both the upper and the lower joint space, followed by transcranial radiography or tomography.

Pathologic

The most frequent pathologic change seen during arthrography of the TMJ is displacement of the disc (Figs. 16–19, 16–20). Morphologically this is characterized by the posterior band of the disc lying anterior to the condyle in the closed-mouth position. Enlargement of the an-

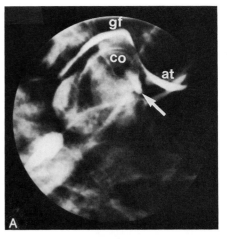

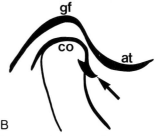

FIGURE 16–16. *A,* Single-contrast lower joint-compartment arthrogram and *B,* schematic drawing of normal joint. This arthrogram was obtained in a healthy volunteer without clinical symptoms. The anterior recess of the lower joint space (arrow) is small. Glenoid fossa (gf), condyle (co), articular eminence (tubercle) (at).

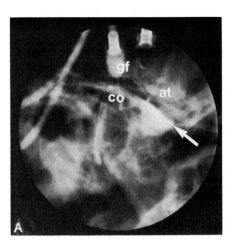

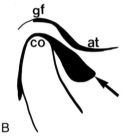

FIGURE 16–17. *A*, Transcranial arthrogram and *B*, schematic drawing of normal TMJ showing a biconcave disc located superiorly over the condyle. This arthrogram was obtained in a healthy volunteer without clinical symptoms. The anterior recess (arrow) of the lower joint space is large. Glenoid fossa (gf), condyle (co), articular eminence (tubercle) (at).

terior recess of the lower joint compartment in the single-contrast arthrography technique is a sign of this pathologic condition.

Disc displacement is functionally divided into displacements with reduction, which implies normalization of disc position during opening of the mouth (Fig. 16–19), and displacement without reduction (Fig. 16–20), which implies that the relationship between the disc and the condyle is not normal during opening (Eriksson, 1983; Katzberg, 1980; Wilkes, 1978a; 1978b).

Anterior disc displacement with reduction is usually characterized by reciprocal clicking. This means clicking during opening that is followed by clicking during closing. Disc displacement with reduction, however, may be present when only an opening click can be heard or when there is no clicking or any other acoustic phenomena (Westesson, 1985). Furthermore, arthrographic studies on patients with reciprocal clicking have demonstrated that about 15 per cent have anterior disc displacement without reduction, which means the disc is permanently anterior to the condyle in spite of reciprocal clicking (Miller, 1985). Therefore, clinically it is difficult in the individual patient to accurately diagnose disc displacement without the help of imaging.

Anterior disc displacement without reduction (Fig. 16–20) implies that the disc is lying permanently anterior to the condyle during all condylar movements. This condition is functionally different from disc displacement with reduction. Clinically, disc displacement without reduction is nearly always preceded by a history of disc displacement with reduction. Commonly the clicking is first replaced by intermittent locking and then suddenly one day the joint is completely locked. Translation and mouth opening are limited and the clicking has disappeared. Arthrographically the disc is lying anterior to the condyle and squeezed between it and the articular eminence, thereby blocking anterior translation (Fig. 16–20).

Studies have shown that the majority of pa-

FIGURE 16–18. Schematic drawing of TMJ showing mean and range of dimensions of the upper and lower joint spaces. Measurements are given in millimeters (mm). Glenoid fossa (gf), condyle (co), articular eminence (tubercle) (at). (From Westesson, P.-L., Eriksson, L., and Kurita, K.: Temporomandibular joint: Variation of normal arthrographic anatomy. Oral Surg, 69:514–519, 1990.)

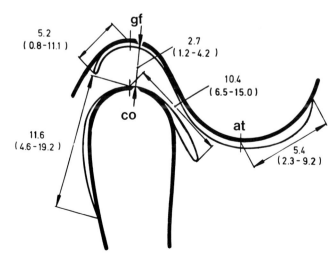

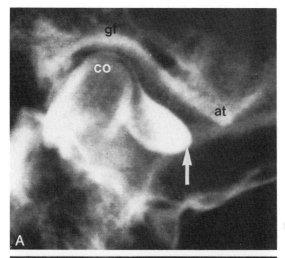

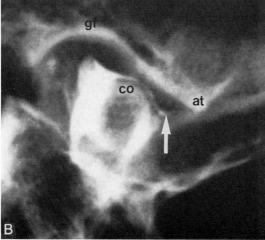

FIGURE 16–19. *A*, Lower joint-compartment arthrogram showing anterior disc displacement. The anterior recess of the lower joint space (arrow) is large, suggesting anterior disc displacement. Glenoid fossa (gf), condyle (co), articular eminence (tubercle) (at). *B*, The same joint as shown in A after reduction of the disc. The anterior recess of the lower joint compartment (arrow) is much smaller.

tients with disc displacement without reduction also have disc deformation. Prospective clinical studies (Westesson, 1989b) have suggested that patients with disc displacement with reduction and deformation of the disc have a greater likelihood of developing locking than those without disc deformation.

Until recently, not much attention was given to the possibility of medial or lateral disc displacement. This was probably caused by the difficulty in imaging such displacement using arthrography. Recent studies have indicated that the clinical presentation of patients with medial or lateral type displacements is similar to that of patients with anterior disc displacement, namely clicking, locking, pain, and irregular movements (Katzberg, 1988). The clinical significance of medial and lateral disc displacement is not known and awaits further research.

Overflow of contrast medium from the lower to the upper joint compartment suggests disc perforation. This occurs most frequently in a joint with disc displacement without reduction (Eriksson, 1983; Westesson, 1983). Only rarely are perforations seen in a joint with a reducing disc or a disc in a normal superior position. Perforations are most frequently located at the junction between the disc and its posterior attachment or in the posterior attachment. There are descriptions of false-positive arthrographic diagnoses of perforations. These might have been caused by accidentally inserting the needle through the disc. This can probably be avoided by proper cannulation technique. A false negative diagnosis of perforation is probably rare, but may occur as a result of injection of only a small amount of contrast medium in a joint with severely restricted movement. With the aid of dual-space double-contrast arthrotomography, it is sometimes possible to achieve superior delineation of a perforation (Fig. 16–21). Adhesions are another pathological entity

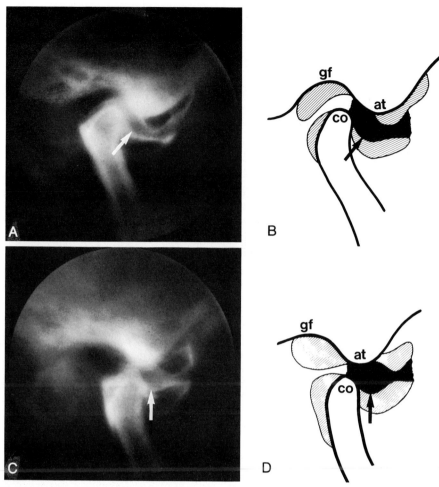

FIGURE 16–20. *A* and *C*, Dual-space double-contrast arthrotomograms and *B* and *D*, schematic drawings showing anterior disc displacement without reduction. The posterior band of the disc (arrow) is lying anterior to the condyle both at rest position *(A, B)* and at maximal mouth opening *(C, D)*. Glenoid fossa (gf), condyle (co), articular eminence (tubercle) (at).

that, in a few instances, can be diagnosed by the use of dual-space double-contrast arthrotomography (Fig. 16–22).

After Trauma

There has been no systematic arthrographic evaluation of internal derangement as related to mandibular trauma severe enough to cause fractures of either the condyle or neck of the condyloid process. Limited clinical experience with patients who have sustained mandibular fractures suggests that internal derangement does in fact occur with these injuries (Katzberg, 1989). Displacement of the condyle, however, is much more commonly found, and this makes the arthrographic diagnosis difficult. MRI is a more effective way to evaluate those patients

who have sustained acute injury to the mandible. This type of imaging will permit examination of the patient soon after the acute injury and provide a greater amount of information about the extent of soft tissue damage.

Loose Bodies

Very rarely, patients with symptoms such as clicking and locking may have loose bodies within the joint spaces (Anderson, 1984). These loose bodies may be calcified and the diagnosis already suggested on plain films. The cause of the loose bodies is unknown.

Synovial chondromatosis is a relatively rare, benign condition of the synovium characterized by metaplasia and the formation of multiple pieces of cartilage (Ballard, 1972; Blenkinsopp,

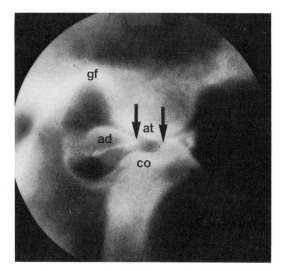

FIGURE 16–21. Dual-space double-contrast arthrotomogram obtained at maximal mouth opening. A perforation of the disc is indicated by arrows. Glenoid fossa (gf), articular disc (ad), articular eminence (tubercle) (at), condyle (co).

1978; Fechner, 1976; Jaffe, 1978; Jones, 1924; McIvor, 1962) (see page 157). The affliction is monoarticular and most commonly involves the knee. It is a rare disease in the TMJ and only about 40 cases have been reported (Arx, 1988; Eriksson, 1985). Such reports, however, have increased during the last few years (Manco, 1987; Nokes, 1987), probably as a result of improved diagnosis and increased awareness of intra-articular pathology as a source of TMJ pain and dysfunction.

In synovial chondromatosis there are multiple filling defects in combination with increased synovial thickness and irregularity seen on the arthrogram (Fig. 16–23). Synovial chondromatosis should be differentiated from loose bodies in the joint with which there are fewer filling defects. The differential diagnosis of intra-articular loose bodies, which are not attached to the bone, includes osteoarthrosis and osteochondritis dissecans (Blenkinsopp, 1978; Schellhas, 1989b; Stoneman, 1988).

Complications

Serious complications following TMJ arthrography are extremely uncommon. The joint is quite resistant to infection, and no such incident has been noted in the literature.

Transient facial nerve palsy may result from administration of the local anesthetic. This can be avoided by reducing the amount injected. Slight discomfort for one or two days after arthrography is normal. The use of nonionic contrast medium will further reduce this discomfort. If pain persists after a few days, anti-

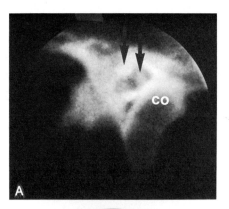

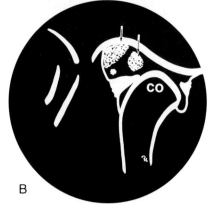

FIGURE 16–23. *A,* Dual-space double-contrast arthrotomogram and *B,* schematic drawing of patient with synovial chondromatosis of right TMJ. The disc is perforated and a few remnants remain. In the upper joint space there are loose bodies (arrows) seen. Condyle (co). (See Fig. 10–5.)

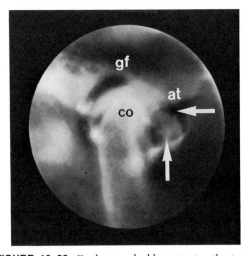

FIGURE 16–22. Dual-space double-contrast arthrotomogram showing anterior displacement and deformation of the disc. There are adhesions (arrows) between the disc and the joint capsule superiorly and inferiorly. Glenoid fossa (gf), condyle (co), articular eminence (tubercle) (at).

inflammatory agents (aspirin or acetaminophen) are given orally and warm compresses should be applied to the affected side.

COMPUTERIZED TOMOGRAPHY

Computerized tomography (CT) of the TMJ enjoyed a great deal of interest soon after the development of arthrography, partly due to its noninvasive nature (Helms, 1982; Katzberg, 1989; Manzione, 1982; Thompson, 1984). The direct-sagittal, thin-section CT of the TMJ with the mouth closed and opened, and with bone (Fig. 16–24A, 16–24B) and soft tissue settings (Fig. 16–24C, 16–24D) as well as reconstructed axial images, have been reported as useful for demonstrating internal derangement and osseous disease. The use of CT scanning for the evaluation of the TMJ has decreased dramatically, however, because MRI with surface coils is superior for soft tissue differentiation (Table 16–2). CT scanning, however, still represents the best imaging modality for detection of osseous anatomy and pathology.

CT scanning produces static images, which is a disadvantage since the dynamics of the joint are not demonstrated. Another disadvantage of the technique is the inability to detect a perforation between the upper and lower joint compartments. The application of cine-CT has been reported (Helms, 1986a). The technique has not gained wide acceptance, however, probably because of the limited availability of the scanners for cine-CT and the limitation of the spatial and contrast resolution of this technique.

Technique

Both direct-sagittal scanning and reconstruction of axial scans can be done. Direct-sagittal scanning is preferred when this is possible

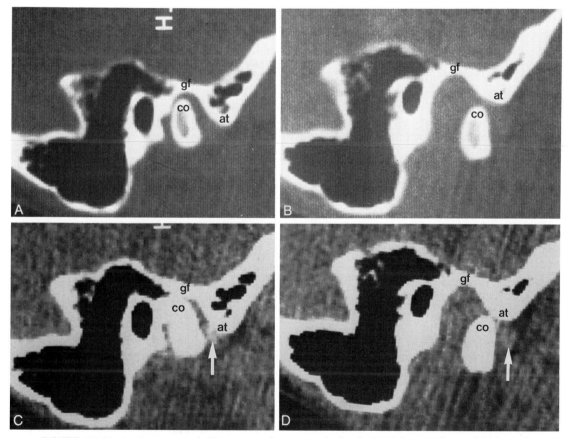

FIGURE 16–24. A, Direct sagittal–CT scanning (bone setting) of right TMJ showing the condyle located posteriorly in the fossa at the closed-mouth position. There is no evidence of osseous disease. Glenoid fossa (gf), condyle (co), articular eminence (tubercle) (at). B, Same joint with mouth open. C, Soft tissue setting for same joint showing anterior disc displacement. The radiopacity anterior to the condyle and inferior to the articular eminence represents the image of the disc (arrows). D, Same joint imaged at maximal mouth opening showing the disc (arrow) anterior to the condyle and inferior to the eminence, suggesting anterior disc displacement without reduction. (Courtesy of Dr. Richard W. Katzberg.)

TABLE 16–2. Advantages and Disadvantages of Magnetic Resonance Imaging as Compared with Computerized Tomography

ADVANTAGES
No ionizing radiation
Fewer artifacts from dense bone and metal clips
Imaging in multiple planes without moving the patient
Superior image of soft tissues
DISADVANTAGES
Slower scanning times than CT
High initial cost of the scanner
Special site planning and shielding
Danger to patients with cerebral aneurysm clips, pacemakers
Claustrophobia in MR scanner
Inferior image of hard tissues

(Manco, 1985; Manzione, 1982; 1984; Sartoris, 1984; Thompson, 1984). However, the design of many CT scanners requires an auxiliary table or adjustable stretcher to position the patient for direct-sagittal CT of the TMJ (Manzione, 1982; 1984). It is placed at about a 45-degree angle to the scanner gantry. Once the patient is correctly positioned, the TMJ is scanned from the medial to lateral poles at about 2 mm increments, depending on the type of scanner used. About six to eight scans are usually needed to cover the mediolateral dimension of the joint. A second series of scans is obtained at the maximal mouth opening. The images are filmed for optimal depiction of soft and hard tissues. In this way the use of CT scanning eliminates the need for either plain films or tomograms.

Findings

The normally positioned disc is usually not directly depicted in the CT scans. Instead, indirect signs such as the position of the lateral pterygoid fat pad and the absence of a radiopacity anterior to the condyle are used as indicators of a normal disc position. Examples of sagittal CT scans of a joint with normal superior disc position are shown in Figure 16–25. CT scans obtained with the mouth open usually provide superior detection of the disc (Fig. 16–25).

When the disc is anteriorly displaced it may appear in the CT scans as a radiopaque mass anterior to the condyle and inferior to the eminence (Fig. 16–24). The lateral pterygoid fat pad is displaced anteriorly and is helpful in determining disc position. The configuration of the disc cannot be determined from CT scans

because of inadequate resolution of the soft tissues.

If the disc reduces to a normal position on opening, it appears as a radiopacity behind the condyle in the open-mouth scans. In cases with disc displacement without reduction, the radiopaque mass will remain anterior to the condyle in the open-mouth scan. The lateral pterygoid fat pad will also be displaced anteriorly, but is sometimes compressed and therefore not clearly visible on the open-mouth scans.

The depiction of the disc by CT scanning depends on the dimensions of the disc. Thus, if the disc is thin and small, it is usually not possible to demonstrate it with CT. On the other hand, if the disc is large, it can be more easily depicted. Comparison of CT scans and corresponding cryosections are shown in Figures 16–26 and 16–27.

MAGNETIC RESONANCE IMAGING

Magnetic resonance imaging (MRI) is a recently developed modality that has been used to image the TMJ (Harms, 1985; Helms, 1986b; Katzberg, 1985; 1986; 1989; Manzione, 1986; Roberts, 1985a). The most important advantage of MRI over radiographic imaging is the absence of exposure to ionizing radiation. Unlike conventional radiography, tomography, and computerized tomography, MRI is not dependent upon differences in electron density but instead depends on the differences in proton density and tissue magnetic relaxation characteristics and blood flow.

Since the details of the physical principles of this method are not within the scope of this discussion, and have been described elsewhere (Alfidi, 1984; Bottomley, 1983; Bradley, 1983; Edelstein, 1983; Lauterbur, 1973), they will be reviewed only briefly. MRI depends on differences in hydrogen protons or water density. Hydrogen protons have a magnetic movement due to the spin of the positively charged nucleus. During normal magnetic movement, protons are randomly aligned with each other. When the patient is placed in the MRI scanner, the hydrogen protons within the body will align themselves with the external magnetic field. When a radiofrequency is supplied, the protons absorb energy and change their inner orientation from the external magnetic field. The radiofrequency is then removed and the protons realign with the external magnetic field, and in doing so they emit the energy they absorbed from the radiofrequency. This emitted energy

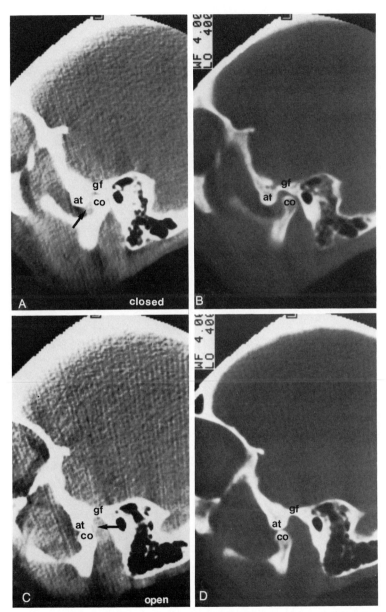

FIGURE 16–25. CT scanning of patient with normal superior disc position and no evidence of osseous disease. *A*, soft, and *B*, hard tissue settings of closed-mouth scans. *C*, soft, and *D*, hard tissue settings of open-mouth scans. The position of the disc is indicated by arrows. Glenoid fossa (gf), articular eminence (tubercle) (at), condyle (co). (Courtesy of Dr. Mario Paz.)

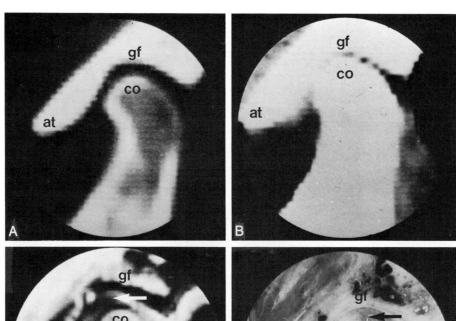

FIGURE 16–26. CT scan. *A*, soft, and *B*, hard tissue setting. *C*, MRI, and *D*, cryosection of normal TMJ. There is good correlation between the CT image of the osseous anatomy and the cryosection. The MRI *(C)* is superior in delineation of the soft tissue anatomy. The disc is indicated by arrows. Glenoid fossa (gf), condyle (co), articular eminence (tubercle) (at).

is detected by a receiver antenna (surface coil). The signals are then processed by a computer and an image is established that is dependent on differences in the emitted signal intensity within the portion of the body examined.

The objective of MRI is to detect soft tissue abnormalities in the TMJ and surrounding structures. An advantage of MRI over arthrography is the capability of also studying soft tissue structures outside the joint capsule. A comparison between arthrography and MRI of the same joint is seen in Figure 16–28.

Magnetic Field Strength and Comparison with Computerized Tomography

The strength of the magnetic field is probably the most significant characteristic of an MRI

scanner. Scanners with a magnetic field strength from 0.05 T (tesla) up to 2 T are in clinical use. A comparative study on the diagnostic accuracy and image quality of two different MRI systems with 1.5 and 0.3 T field strengths, respectively, has indicated that about a four times longer imaging time is needed with the midfield strength system (Hansson, 1989).

Some principal advantages and disadvantages of MRI compared with CT are outlined in Table 16–2. Contraindications for MR scanning are outlined in Table 16–3. MRI offers superior soft tissue resolution compared with CT, and MRI with surface coils is rapidly surpassing CT for imaging of the TMJ (Katzberg, 1989; 1986; Westesson, 1987b). Comparative studies with cryosectioned cadaver material have confirmed the superior imaging capacity of MRI over CT (Figs. 16–26, 16–27) (Westesson, 1987b) and have also illustrated the value of multiplaner imaging of the TMJ (Katzberg, 1988; Westesson, 1987).

Surface Coil and Scanning Technique

As with other imaging modalities, the standard plane of imaging is in the sagittal direction. A high-field strength system is preferred; midfield strength MR systems may require longer scanning times for a comparable image, because additional excitations are needed.

The use of a dual-surface coil technique for bilateral imaging of the TMJ has the advantage of reducing total imaging time (Hardy, 1988; Shellock, 1989). A similar pulse sequence protocol, however, can be used for imaging one side at a time. MRI is performed with the body coil as the transmitter and the two surface coils,

TABLE 16–3. Contraindications for Magnetic Resonance Imaging

ABSOLUTE
  Patients with cerebral aneurysm clips
  Patients with cardiac pacemakers
RELATIVE
  Claustrophobic or uncooperative patients
  Pregnant patients
  Metallic prosthetic heart valves
  Ferromagnetic foreign bodies in critical locations (e.g., eye)
  Implanted stimulator wires for pain control
NO CONTRAINDICATION
  Surgical clips outside the brain
  Metallic prostheses
  Orthodontic fixed appliances

6.5 cm in diameter, as receivers. The patient is placed supine in the magnet and the surface coils are located just lateral to the TMJs. Images are obtained at closed- and open-mouth posi-

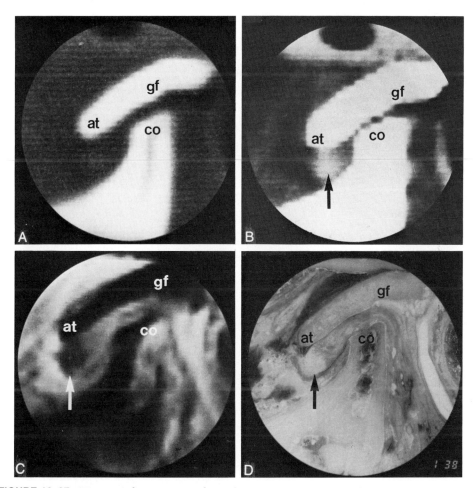

FIGURE 16–27. CT scan. *A*, bone setting and *B*, soft-tissue setting. *C*, MRI and *D*, cryosection of joint with anterior displacement and deformation of the disc (arrow). There is good correlation between the CT image of the osseous anatomy and the cryosection. The MR image (*C*) is superior for delineation of the soft tissue anatomy. Glenoid fossa (gf), articular eminence (tubercle) (at), condyle (co).

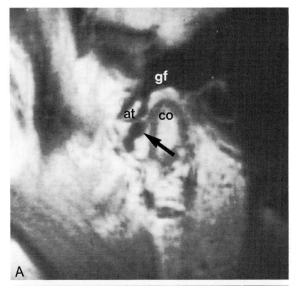

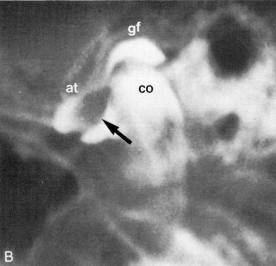

FIGURE 16–28. *A*, MRI and *B*, dual-space transcranial arthrogram of the same joint showing anterior disc displacement. In the MRI the disc is black due to its low signal intensity. In the arthrogram the disc is outlined by the radiopaque (white) contrast medium. Glenoid fossa (gf), articular eminence (tubercle) (at), condyle (co).

tions. The same scanning settings are used for both positions, with only one excitation, which reduces the imaging time by about half.

A slightly lower signal to noise ratio is usually sufficient for the open-mouth images because the disc generally is more clearly visible than in the closed-mouth position. A shorter imaging time for the open-mouth position is also helpful in reducing the risk of motion artifacts. Having the mouth open for a prolonged time is sometimes uncomfortable for the patient in the supine position because saliva collects in the back of the pharynx. Corks or plastic syringes of variable sizes are used as bite blocks during the open-mouth scanning.

The TMJ can also be imaged in the coronal plane. This is helpful in identifying medial and lateral displacements of the disc. Additionally,

the osseous anatomy of the condyle can sometimes be better evaluated with two imaging planes rather than with one.

There is no evidence that T1- or T2-weighted images provide any specific advantages for determining the position of the disc since it has a low signal intensity at all pulse sequences and the lateral pterygoid fat pad is bright on all proton-weighted sequences. The possible need to document trauma to the tissues behind the disc or fluid in the joint spaces, however, may require a T2-weighted sequence (Harms, 1985; Schellhas, 1989a; 1989b).

The use of corrected sagittal and coronal planes has recently been applied to MR imaging of the TMJ (Shellock, 1989). This implies that the plane of imaging is parallel (coronal imaging) or perpendicular (sagittal imaging) to the long axis of the condyle. The image quality can be improved with this technique compared with straight sagittal and straight coronal images.

Normal Findings

The normal TMJ, demonstrated by MRI in the sagittal and coronal planes, is illustrated in Figure 16–29. In the sagittal plane the disc has a biconcave configuration with the posterior band lying over the condyle. Due to the low signal intensity of the fibrous connective tissue of the disc, it is clearly distinguishable from the surrounding tissues that have brighter signals. The cortex of the condyle has no signal, but is well depicted because of the relatively bright signal intensity of the contiguous cartilaginous and synovial tissues superiorly, and the bright signal of the fat in the cancellous marrow of the condyle inferiorly. The posterior disc attachment has a bright signal relative to the posterior

band of the disc due to the rich network of fatty tissue in the former contrasted with the low signal intensity of the fibrous tissue in the latter. MR images are actually the only images that can distinguish the disc from its posterior attachment. In some instances there is a small region of high signal intensity in the posterior part of the posterior band of the disc. This is similar to what has been described in the meniscus of the knee and is probably a normal anatomic variation representing mucin deposits. It has no known clinical significance. The insertion of the superior belly of the lateral pterygoid muscle is sometimes demonstrated clearly on the MRI as a low-signal intensity, thread-like structure attaching on the medial aspect of the disc. In the open-mouth views the central thin part of the disc lies between the eminence and the condyle (Fig. 16–29 B). The posterior band of the disc is located behind the condyle and the anterosuperior part of the condyle articu-

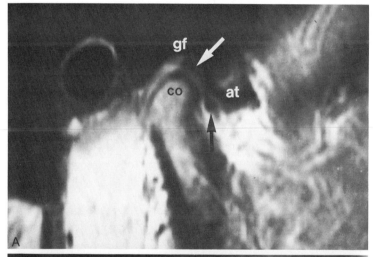

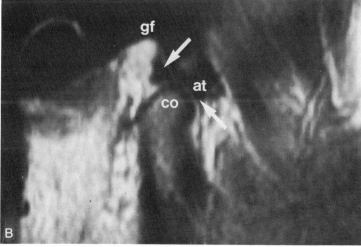

FIGURE 16–29. MRI of normal right TMJ. A, The disc (arrows) is biconcave and located superior to the condyle in the closed-mouth position. B, Open-mouth scan. The disc (arrows) is located between the condyle and articular eminence. Glenoid fossa (gf), condyle (co), articular eminence (tubercle) (at).

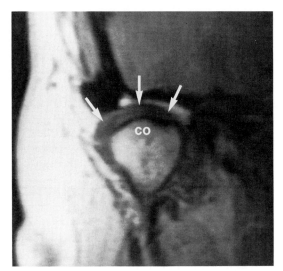

FIGURE 16–30. Coronal MR image with the mouth closed demonstrating a normal position of the arc-shaped disc (arrows). Condyle (co).

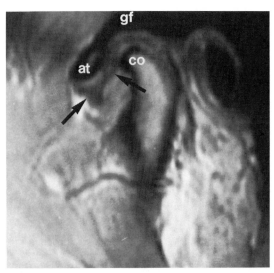

FIGURE 16–31. MR imaging of left TMJ showing anterior displacement of a biconcave disc (arrows). Glenoid fossa (gf), articular eminence (tubercle) (at), condyle (co). (Courtesy of Dr. Richard W. Katzberg.)

lates against the anterior band of the disc. In the coronal plane the disc has a crescent shape with the medial aspect attached to the capsule and medial pole of the condyle and the lateral aspect attached to the lateral pole of the condyle and the lateral capsule (Fig. 16–30).

Abnormal Findings

Anterior, anteromedial, or anterolateral displacements of the disc are the most common abnormalities. In the sagittal MR image the

displaced disc is located anterior to the condyle in the closed-mouth position (Figs. 16–31, 16–32). If there is rotational disc displacement, the coronal images show a medial (Fig. 16–33) or a lateral (Fig. 16–34) component to the displacement. When the disc is medially or laterally displaced (Liedberg, 1988), it is frequently not well visualized in the sagittal plane (Fig. 16–35). This is termed the empty fossa sign and is an indication that the disc might be displaced sideways. The open-mouth view reveals whether the disc reduces to a normal superior

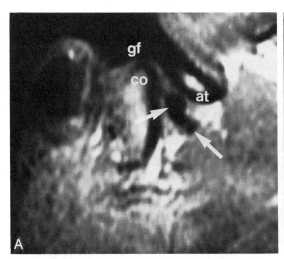

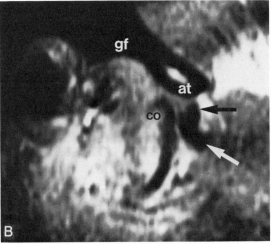

FIGURE 16–32. MR image of right TMJ in *A*, closed-mouth position and *B*, at maximal mouth opening showing anterior disc displacement without reduction. The disc (arrows) is deformed, being shorter in anteroposterior (AP) dimension, and lacking its normal biconcave appearance. Glenoid fossa, (gf), condyle (co), articular eminence (tubercle) (at).

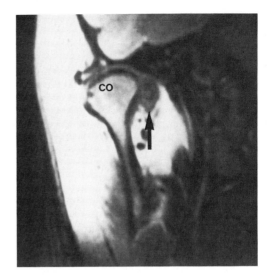

FIGURE 16–33. Corrected coronal MR image of right TMJ showing medial displacement of the disc (arrow). Condyle (co).

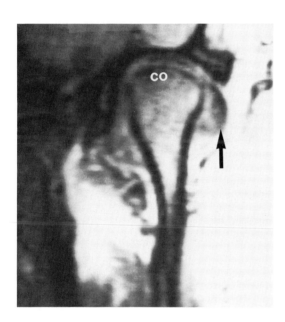

FIGURE 16–34. Coronal MR image of left TMJ showing lateral displacement of the disc (arrow). Condyle (co).

FIGURE 16–35. Sagittal MR image of the joints shown in Figure 16–31 demonstrating the empty fossa sign. When the disc is medially or laterally displaced there is frequently no image of the disc in the sagittal views. Glenoid fossa (gf), articular eminence (tubercle) (at), condyle (co).

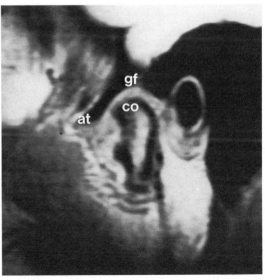

position during mouth opening (disc displacement with reduction) (Fig. 16–36) or stays anterior to the condyle (disc displacement without reduction) (Fig. 16–37). Coronal imaging obtained at the open-mouth position also may show if the medially or laterally displaced disc reduces to a normal superior position on opening.

Disc deformation and also changes in the configuration of a disc at different jaw positions are clearly visible on MR images. In disc displacement without reduction (Fig. 16–32), the disc is consistently located anterior to the condyle. Disc deformation is usually more pronounced with this condition (Eriksson, 1983). Perforations are not readily diagnosable with MR imaging. Inability to depict perforation and the limitation to static images are the disadvantages of MRI. The use of gradient recalled acquisition in the steady state (GRASS) shows some promise in depicting sequential positions of the disc (Schellhas, 1989a).

Recent literature has suggested that MRI of the TMJ has a potential also to provide information about the condition of the bone marrow of the mandibular condyle (Schellhas, 1989b). Thus, if the central area of the condyle has a low signal (decreased T1) and appears black on MRI, this has been claimed to be pathological and a sign of avascular necrosis. More research on the pathophysiology of avascular necrosis of the mandibular condyle, with histological correlation, is needed before we know what the reduced signal intensity of the bone marrow of the mandibular condyle represents. It is clear, however, that MRI represents an exciting modality to acquire an insight into the biology of the bone marrow of the mandibular condyle that is not possible with other imaging techniques.

POST-TREATMENT IMAGING

Imaging after treatment is indicated when the patient continues to have symptoms that might be related to intra-articular pathology. Arthrography has been used for this purpose, but this can be difficult to perform after surgery because of narrowing of the joint spaces or

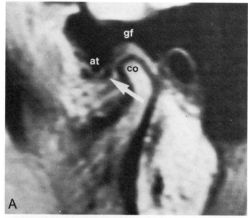

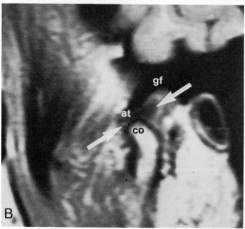

FIGURE 16–36. MR image of left TMJ showing anterior disc displacement with reduction. In *A* the disc (arrows) is anteriorly displaced in the closed-jaw position. In *B* the disc (arrows) has been recaptured to its normal superior position as demonstrated in this open-mouth view. Glenoid fossa (gf), articular eminence (tubercle) (at), condyle (co).

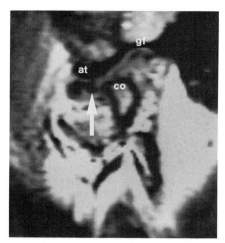

FIGURE 16–37. MR image of left TMJ showing anterior disc displacement without reduction. The disc (arrow) is lying anterior to the deformed condyle in the open-mouth view. The disc is deformed. Glenoid fossa (gf), articular eminence (tubercle) (at), condyle (co).

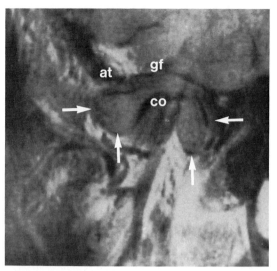

FIGURE 16–39. Postsurgical complications from teflon-proplast TMJ implant. MR image in the sagittal plane shows the implant within the fossa. There is granulation tissue (arrows) anterior and posterior to the deformed condyle. Articular eminence (tubercle) (at), glenoid fossa (gf), condyle (co). (Courtesy of Dr. Richard W. Katzberg.)

because of intra-articular adhesions. For these reasons MRI is usually preferable for examination of postoperative patients (Katzberg, 1989; Kneeland, 1987; Schellhas, 1988).

MRI may help in confirming surgical correction of disc displacement or correct placement of an implant, and also in understanding postsurgical failures. An example of a postsurgical MR image showing a teflon-proplast implant in good position is seen in Figure 16–38. A postsurgical view of a teflon-proplast implant associated with granulation tissue and condylar deformity is shown in Figure 16–39.

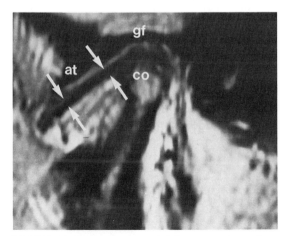

FIGURE 16–38. MR image of left TMJ with implant (arrows) in good position. There is no evidence of extensive granulation tissue around the implant. There is a thin soft tissue layer superior to the implant. Glenoid fossa (gf), articular eminence (tubercle) (at), condyle (co). (Courtesy of Dr. Richard W. Katzberg.)

CT examination represents an alternative imaging modality for the postoperative patient with a nonmetallic implant (Fig. 16–40). When erosion and osteolysis of the bone is of concern, CT might be preferred to MRI. CT provides a high degree of soft tissue differentiation and is accurate for diagnosis of osseous changes. It should be mentioned, however, that erosion and osteolysis of the bone usually are the result of inflammation in the adjacent soft tissues, changes that might be detected earlier by MRI.

Arthrography also has been used to document the intra-articular status after disc repositioning (Bronstein, 1984) and discectomy (Westesson, 1985). If the changes are in the joint capsule or outside the joint capsule, arthrography will not demonstrate these changes. MRI is then the preferred method. Arthrograms obtained after disc repositioning surgery can be difficult to interpret (Bronstein, 1984) and they have not provided a clear answer as to how often this type of surgery fails to reposition a displaced disc.

Plain film imaging (Agerberg, 1971) and tomography after discectomy (Eriksson, 1986) have demonstrated that the osseous contours of the joint will be obscure during the first year after surgery. This is interpreted as a sign of postsurgical remodeling (see Chapter 6). After about two years the sclerotic outline of the condyle is again seen (Fig. 16–41). Flattening of the condyle, progressive remodeling, and

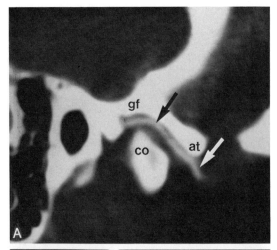

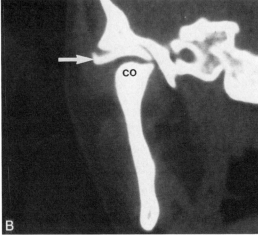

FIGURE 16–40. *A*, Direct-sagittal and *B*, coronal CT scans of a TMJ with an implant. The condyle is flattened. The implant (arrows) is located in the fossa and along the articular eminence (tubercle). Glenoid fossa (gf), condyle (co), articular eminence (tubercle) (at).

flattening of the articular tubercle are the most common findings in this stage. Arthrography before and after discectomy (Fig. 16–42) has shown that the space between the condyle and the glenoid fossa becomes filled with fibrous connective tissue (Westesson, 1985b). This means that the distance between the osseous parts of the TMJ does not decrease to the extent of the thickness of the disc that was removed.

DIAGNOSTIC ACCURACY OF ARTHROGRAPHY, COMPUTERIZED TOMOGRAPHY, AND MAGNETIC RESONANCE IMAGING

The accuracy of both single- and double-contrast arthrography, CT, and MRI have been investigated in experimental studies on fresh autopsy specimens (Westesson, 1984b; 1986; 1987a) and all techniques have demonstrated a high degree of accuracy in diagnosing the po-

sition of the disc (Table 16–4). The data were obtained with optimal imaging conditions and so it is reasonable to believe that the accuracy might have been lower in a clinical setting. The figures in Table 16–4 are relevant for comparison between the different techniques, however, because the studies were performed under similar conditions. In the clinical setting, information about the symptoms would help to improve the diagnostic accuracy. Therefore, they probably also represent a good estimate of the accuracy for the clinical use of the techniques.

RADIONUCLIDE IMAGING

Radionuclide imaging by means of conventional skeletal imaging techniques (Fig. 16–43) may be a valuable screening test for osseous diseases of the TMJ (Collier, 1983; Katzberg, 1984). The technique can be performed simply, with very minimal radiation to the patient (Katz-

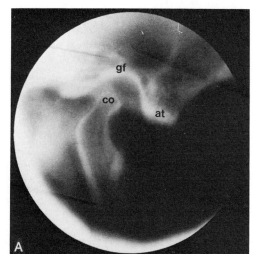

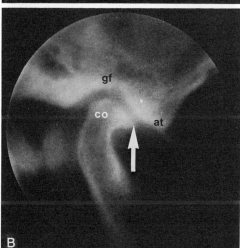

FIGURE 16–41. Corrected sagittal tomograms *A*, before and *B*, two years after discectomy. Characteristic remodeling with flattening, an anterior osteophyte (arrow) and sclerosis are seen. Glenoid fossa (gf), articular eminence (tubercle) (at), condyle (co).

TABLE 16–4. Accuracy of Different Forms of Imaging

IMAGING MODALITY	NUMBER OF JOINTS	DISC POSIT.	DISC CONFIG.	PERFORATION	ARTICULAR SURFACES
Single-space single-contrast lower-compartment videoarthrography*	58	84 per cent	N.A.	97 per cent	N.A.
Dual-space double-contrast arthrotomography†	48	92 per cent	92 per cent	100 per cent	N.A.
Computed tomography‡	15	67 per cent	N.A.	N.A.	N.A.
Magnetic resonance imaging§	15	73 per cent	60 per cent	N.A.	N.A.
Magnetic resonance imaging**	39	85 per cent	N.A.	N.A.	N.A.

N.A. = not assessed
*Westesson, 1986
†Westesson, 1984b
‡Westesson, 1987a
§Westesson, 1987b
**Hansson, 1989

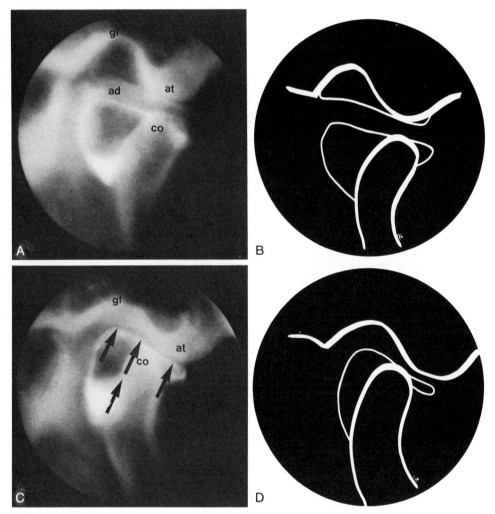

FIGURE 16–42. *A*, Arthrogram and *B*, schematic drawing before discectomy. *C* and *D* show the same joint 21 months after discectomy. The dual-space double-contrast arthrotomograms show that the soft tissue covering in the fossa (arrows in *C*) is considerably thicker after discectomy than before. Glenoid fossa (gf), articular disc (ad), articular eminence (tubercle) (at), condyle (co).

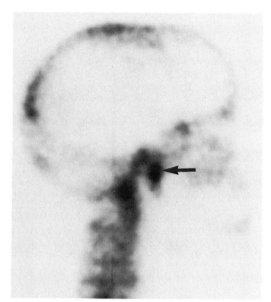

FIGURE 16–43. Radionuclide imaging of patient with suspected condylar hyperplasia. The increased activity in the area of the right TMJ (arrow) supports the clinical diagnosis. (Courtesy of Dr. Richard W. Katzberg.)

berg, 1989). Not only can disease and remodeling of the TMJ be detected, but also other pathological conditions in and around the TMJ that mimic or produce TMJ pain might be revealed.

IMAGING STRATEGY AND CLINICAL CONSIDERATIONS

The first step in the imaging of patients presenting with TMJ pain and dysfunction is the use of plain film radiography, usually in a transcranial projection. If greater detail is needed, tomography should be used. This is a screening test where a negative finding does not rule out pathologic changes in the soft tissues.

The next imaging level should be focused on the soft tissue. The choice is between MRI, arthrography, and CT. CT is no longer a competitive modality in the assessment of TMJ soft tissues, however, because MRI has been shown to have a better capability to demonstrate the soft tissues of the joint. MRI is superior to arthrography because of its lack of radiation to the patient and its capacity to demonstrate medial and lateral disc displacements as well as extracapsular changes. Therefore, MRI is the best imaging modality for most TMJ patients when a soft tissue abnormality is suspected. CT

should be considered if the status of the bone is of primary concern.

If function of the TMJ is of primary concern, arthrography is preferable. Arthrography can document a functional abnormality when combined with dynamic video fluoroscopy.

REFERENCES

Agerberg, G., and Lundberg, M.: Changes in the temporomandibular joint after surgical treatment. A radiologic follow-up study. Oral Surg. 32:865–875, 1971.
Alfidi, R. J., and Haaga, J. R.: Magnetic resonance imaging. Radiol. Clin. North Am. 22:763–969, 1984.
Anderson, G. C., Schiffman, E. L., Schellhas, K. P., and Friction, J. R.: Clinical vs. arthrographic diagnosis of TMJ internal derangement. J. Dent. Res. 68:826–829, 1989.
Anderson, Q. N., and Katzberg, R. W.: Loose bodies of the temporomandibular joint: Arthrographic diagnosis. Skeletal Radiol. 11:42–46, 1984.
Annandale, T.: Displacement of the inter-articular cartilage of the lower jaw, and its treatment by operation. Lancet 1:411, 1887.
Arnaudow M., Haage, H., and Pflaum, I.: Die Doppelkontrastarthrographie des Kiefergelenkes. Dtsch. Zahnarztl. Z. 23:390–393, 1968.
Arnaudow, M., and Pflaum, I.: Neue Erkenntnisse in der beurteilung bei der Kiefergelenktomographie. Dtsch. Zahnarztl. Z. 29:554–556, 1974.
Arx, D. P., Simpson, M. T., and Batman, P.: Synovial chondromatosis of the temporomandibular joint. Br. J. Oral Maxillofac. Surg. 26:297–305, 1988.
Ballard, R., and Weiland, L. H.: Synovial chondromatosis of the temporomandibular joint. Cancer 30:791–795, 1972.
Bean, L. R., Petersson, A., and Svensson, A.: The transmaxillary projection in temporomandibular joint radiography. Dentomaxillofac. Radiol. 4:13–18, 1975.
Bean, L. R., and Thomas, C. A.: Significance of condylar positions in patients with temporomandibular joint disorders. J. Am. Dent. Assoc. 114:76–77, 1987.
Bell, K. A., and Walters, P. J.: Videofluoroscopy during arthrography of the temporomandibular joint. Radiology 147:879, 1983.
Bellavaia, W. D.: A functional jaw device to aid in treating anterior displaced discs. J. Craniomandib. Pract. 1:53–60, 1983.
Blenkinsopp, P. T.: Loose bodies of the temporomandibular joint, synovial chondromatosis or osteoarthritis. Br. J. Oral Surg. 16:12–20, 1978.
Boering, G.: Arthrosis deformans van het kaakegewricht. Thesis. Rijksuniversiteit te Groningen, 1966.
Bottomley, P. A., Hart, H. R., Edelstein, W. A., et al.: NMR imaging/spectroscopy system to study both anatomy and metabolism. Lancet 2:273–274, 1983.
Bradley, W. C., Newton, T. H., and Crooks, L. E.: Physical principles of nuclear magnetic resonance. In Newton, T. H., and Potts, D. G. (Eds.): Advanced Imaging Techniques. San Francisco, Clavadell Press, 1983, pp. 15–61.
Brand, J. W., Whinery, J. G. Jr., Anderson, Q. N., and Keenan, K. M.: Condylar position as a predictor of temporomandibular joint internal derangement. Oral Surg. 67:469–476, 1989.
Bronstein, S. L.: Post-surgical TMJ arthrography. J. Craniomandib. Pract. 2:165–171, 1984.

Burman, M., and Sinberg, S. E.: Condylar movement in the study of internal derangement of the temporomandibular joint. J. Bone Joint Surg. 28:351–373, 1946.

Campbell, W.: Clinical radiological investigations of the mandibular joints. Br. J. Radiol. 38:401–421, 1965.

Christie, H. K.: Internal derangements of the temporomandibular joint. J. Int. Coll. Surg. 19:704–715, 1953.

Collier, D. B., Carrera, G. F., Messer, E. J., et al.: Internal derangement of the temporomandibular joint: Detection by single-photon emission computed tomography. Radiology 149:557–561, 1983.

Dolwick, M. F., and Riggs, R. R.: Diagnosis and treatment of internal derangements of the temporomandibular joint. Dent. Clin. North Am. 27:561–572, 1983.

Dugal, G. L.: Closing a minor unilateral open bite on TMJ patients. J. Craniomandib. Pract. 1:39–41, 1982–1983.

Eckerdal, O.: Tomography of the temporomandibular joint. Correlation between tomographic image and histologic sections in a three dimensional system. Acta Radiol. 329(Suppl.):103, 1973.

Edelstein, W. A., Bottomley, P. A., Art, H. R., and Smith, L. S.: Signal, noise and contrast in nuclear magnetic resonance (NMR) imaging. J. Comput. Assist. Tomogr. 7:391–401, 1983.

Eriksson, L., and Westesson, P.-L.: Clinical and radiological study of patients with anterior disc displacement of the temporomandibular joint. Swed. Dent. J. 7:55–64, 1983.

Eriksson, L., and Westesson, P.-L.: Discectomy in the treatment of anterior disc displacement of the temporomandibular joint. A clinical and radiologic one-year follow-up study. J. Prosthet. Dent. 55:106–116, 1986.

Eriksson, L., Westesson, P.-L., and Henriksson, H.: A 66-year-old male with temporomandibular joint pain, clicking and crepitation. (A case of synovial chondromatosis of the temporomandibular joint with arthrographic diagnosis.) J. Craniomandib. Pract. 3:184–187, 1985.

Farrar, W. B.: Characteristics of the condylar path in internal derangements of the TMJ. J. Prosthet. Dent. 39:319–323, 1978.

Farrar, W. B.: Diagnosis and treatment of anterior dislocation of the articular disc. NY J. Dent. 41:348–351, 1971.

Farrar, W. B., and McCarty, W. L. Jr.: Interior joint space arthrography and characteristics of condylar paths in internal derangements of the TMJ. J. Prosthet. Dent. 41:548–555, 1979.

Fechner, R. E.: Neoplasms and neoplasm-like lesions of the synovium. In Ackermann, L. V., Spjut, H. J., and Abell, M. R. (Eds.): Bones and Joints. Baltimore, Williams & Wilkins, 1976, pp. 157–186.

Frenkel, G.: Untersuchungen mit der Kombination Arthrographie and Tomographie zur darstellung des Discus articulares des Menschen. Dtsch. Zahnartzl. Z. 20:1261–1274, 1965.

Hansson, L.-G., and Petersson, A.: Radiography of the temporomandibular joint using the transpharyngeal projection. A comparison study of information obtained with different radiographic techniques. Dentomaxillofac. Radiol. 7:69–78, 1978.

Hansson, L.-G., Westesson, P.-L., Eriksson, L., et al.: Comparison of MR imaging of the temporomandibular joint: Images of autopsy specimens made at 0.3 T and 1.5 T with anatomic cryosections. AJR 152:1241–1244, 1989.

Hardy, C. J., Katzberg, R. W., Frey, R. L., et al.: Switched surface coil system for bilateral MR imaging. Radiology 167:835–838, 1988.

Harms, S. E., Wilk, R. M., Chiles, D. G., and Milam, S.

B.: The temporomandibular joint: Magnetic resonance imaging using surface coils. Radiology 157:133–136, 1985.

Helms, C. A., Gillespy, T. III, Gould, R. G., and Ware, W. H.: Cine-CT of the temporomandibular joint. J. Craniomandib. Pract. 4:246–250, 1986a.

Helms, C. A., Gillespy, T. III, Sims, R. E., and Richardson, M. L.: Magnetic resonance imaging of internal derangement of the temporomandibular joint. Radiol. Clin. North Am. 24:189–192, 1986b.

Helms, C. A., Morrish, R. B., Kircos, L. T., et al.: Computed tomography of the meniscus of the temporomandibular joint. Preliminary observations. Radiology 145:719–722, 1982.

Ireland, V. E.: The problem of "the clicking jaw." Proc. R. Soc. Med. 44:363–372, 1951.

Jaffe, H. L.: Tumors and tumorous conditions of the bones and joints. London, Klimpton, 1978, pp. 558–566.

Jones, H. T.: Loose body formation in synovial osteochondromatosis, with special reference to etiology and pathology. J. Bone Joint Surg. 6:407–458, 1924.

Katzberg, R. W.: Temporomandibular joint imaging. Radiology 170:297–307, 1989.

Katzberg, R. W., Bessette, R. W., Tallents, R. H., et al.: Normal and abnormal temporomandibular joint: MR imaging with surface coil. Radiology 158:183–189, 1986.

Katzberg, R. W., Dolwick, M. F., Helms, C. A., et al.: Arthrotomography of the temporomandibular joint. AJR 134:995–1003, 1980.

Katzberg, R. W., Keith, D. A., Ten Eick, W. R., and Guralnick, W. C.: Internal derangement of the temporomandibular joint: An assessment of condylar position in centric occlusion. J. Prosthet. Dent. 49:250–254, 1983.

Katzberg, R. W., O'Mara, R. E., Tallents, R. H., and Weber, D. A.: Radionuclide skeletal imaging and single photon emission computed tomography in suspected internal derangements of the temporomandibular joint. J. Oral Maxillofac. Surg. 42:782–787, 1984.

Katzberg, R. W., Schenck, J., Roberts, D., et al.: Magnetic resonance imaging of the temporomandibular joint meniscus. Oral Surg. 59:332–335, 1985.

Katzberg, R. W., Westesson, P.-L., Tallents, R. H., et al.: Temporomandibular joint: Magnetic resonance assessment of rotational and sideways disc displacements. Radiology 169:741–748, 1988.

Kneeland, J. D., Ryan, D. E., Carrera, G. F., et al.: Failed temporomandibular joint prosthesis: MR imaging. Radiology 165:179–181, 1987.

Lauterbur, P. C.: Image formation by induced local interactions: Examples employing nuclear magnetic resonance. Nature 242:190–191, 1973.

Liedberg, J., and Westesson, P.-L.: Sideways position of the temporomandibular joint disk: Coronal cryosectioning of fresh autopsy specimens. Oral Surg. 68:644–649, 1988.

Lundh, H., Westesson, P.-L., Kopp, S., and Tillström, B.: Anterior repositioning splint in the treatment of temporomandibular joints with reciprocal clicking. Comparison with a flat occlusal splint and an untreated control group. Oral Surg. 60:131–136, 1985.

Manco, L. G., and DeLuke, D. M.: CT diagnosis of synovial chondromatosis of the temporomandibular joint. AJR 148:574–576, 1987.

Manco, L. G., Messing, S. G., Busino, L. J., et al.: Internal derangements of the temporomandibular joint evaluated with direct sagittal CT: A prospective study. Radiology 157:407–412, 1985.

Manzione, J. V., Katzberg, R. W., Brodsky, G. L., et al.: Internal derangement of the temporomandibular joint: Diagnosis by direct sagittal computed tomography. Radiology 150:111–115, 1984a.

Manzione, J. V., Katzberg, R. W., Tallents, R. H., et al.: Magnetic resonance imaging of the temporomandibular joint. J. Am. Dent. Assoc. 113:398–402, 1986.

Manzione, J. V., Seltzer, S. E., Katzberg, R. W., et al.: Direct sagittal computed tomography of the temporomandibular joint. AJNR 3:677–679, 1982.

Manzione, J. V., Tallents, R., Katzberg, R. W., et al.: Arthrographically guided split therapy for recapturing the temporomandibular joint meniscus. Oral Surg. 57:235–240, 1984b.

McCabe, J. B., Keller, S. E., and Moffet, B. C.: A new radiographic technique for diagnosing temporomandibular joint disorders. J. Dent. Res. 38:663, 1959.

McCarty, W. L. Jr.: Surgery. In Farrar, W. B., and McCarty, W. L. Jr. (Eds.): A Clinical Outline of Temporomandibular Joint Diagnosis and Treatment, 7th ed. Montgomery, Normandie Publications, 1982, pp 155–167.

McCarty, W. L. Jr., and Farrar, W. B.: Surgery for internal derangements of the temporomandibular joint. J. Prosthet. Dent. 42:191–196, 1979.

McIvor, R. R., and King, D.: Osteochondromatosis of the hip joint. J. Bone Joint Surg. 44A:87–97, 1962.

Miller, T. L., Katzberg, R. W., Tallents, R. H., et al.: Temporomandibular joint clicking with nonreducing anterior displacement of the meniscus. Radiology 154:121–124, 1985.

Mullen, T. F.: Internal derangement of the temporomandibular joint. West. J. Surg. 45:181–187, 1937.

Nokes, S. R., King, P. S., Garcia, R. Jr., et al.: Temporomandibular joint chondromatosis with intracranial extension: MR and CT contributions. AJR 148:1173–1174, 1987.

Nørgaard, F.: Artografi av kaebeleddet. Preliminary report. Acta Radiol. 25:679–685, 1944.

Nørgaard, F.: Temporomandibular arthrography. Thesis. Copenhagen, Munksgaard, 1947.

Öberg, T., Carlsson, G. E., and Fajers, C. M.: The temporomandibular joint. A morphologic study of human autopsy material. Acta Odontol. Scand. 29:349–384, 1971.

Omnell, K.-Å.: Radiology of the TMJ. In Irby, W. B. (Ed.): Current Advances in Oral Surgery, vol. III. St. Louis, C. V. Mosby, 1980, pp. 196–226.

Omnell, K.-Å., and Lysell, L.: Roentgendiagnostics. In Krogh-Poulsen, W. (Ed.): Stomatognathic Function and Physiology, vol. 2, ed. 2. Copenhagen, Munksgaard, 1979, pp. 141–153.

Omnell, K.-Å., and Petersson, A.: Radiography of the temporomandibular joint utilizing oblique lateral transcranial projections. Comparison of information obtained with standardized technique and individualized technique. Odontol. Rev. 26:77–92, 1976.

Petersson, A., and Nathaviroj, S.: Radiography of the temporomandibular joint utilizing the transmaxillary projection. A comparison of the information obtained with the oblique lateral transcranial projection versus the transmaxillary projection. Dentomaxillofac. Radiol. 4:76–83, 1975.

Pringle, J. H.: Displacement of the mandibular meniscus and its treatment. Br. J. Surg. 6:385–389, 1918.

Pullinger, A., and Hollender, L.: Variation in condyle-fossa relationships according to different methods of evaluation in tomograms. Oral Surg. 62:719–727, 1986a.

Pullinger, A. G., Hollender, L., Solberg, W. K., and Petersson, A.: A tomographic study of mandibular condyle position in an asymptomatic population. J. Prosthet. Dent. 5:706–713, 1985.

Pullinger, A. G., Solberg, W. K., Hollender, L., and Guichet, D.: Tomographic analysis of mandibular condyle position in diagnostic subgroups of temporomandibular disorders. J. Prosthet. Dent. 55:723–729, 1986b.

Pullinger, A. G., Solberg, W. K., Hollender, L., and Petersson, A.: Relationship of mandibular condylar position to dental occlusion factors in an asymptomatic population. Am. J. Orthod. Dentofacial Orthop. 91:200–206, 1987.

Rasmussen, O. C.: Description of population and progress of symptoms in a longitudinal study of temporomandibular joint arthropathy. Scand. J. Dent. Res. 89:196–203, 1981.

Rasmussen, O. C.: Longitudinal study of transpharyngeal radiography in temporomandibular joint arthropathy. Scand. J. Dent. Res. 88:257–268, 1980.

Rasmussen, O. C.: Temporomandibular arthropathy. Clinical, radiologic, and therapeutic aspects, with emphasis on diagnosis. Int. J. Oral Surg. 12:365–397, 1983.

Roberts, D., Schenk, J., Joseph, P., et al.: Temporomandibular joint: Magnetic resonance imaging. Radiology 155:829–830, 1985a.

Roberts, C. A., Tallents, R. H., Espeland, M. A., et al.: Mandibular range of motion versus arthrographic diagnosis of the temporomandibular joint. Oral Surg. 60:244–251, 1985b.

Roberts, C. A., Tallents, R. H., Katzberg, R. W., et al.: Clinical and arthrographic evaluation of temporomandibular joint sounds. Oral Surg. 62:373–376, 1986.

Roberts, C. A., Tallents, R. H., Katzberg, R. W., et al.: Comparison of internal derangements of the TMJ to occlusal findings. Oral Surg. 63:645–650, 1987a.

Roberts, C. A., Tallents, R. H., Katzberg, R. W., et al.: Clinical and arthrographic evaluation of the location of TMJ pain. Oral Surg. 64:6–8, 1987b.

Roberts, C. A., Tallents, R. H., Katzberg, R. W., et al.: Comparison of arthrographic findings of the temporomandibular joint with palpation of the muscles of mastication. Oral Surg. 64:275–277, 1987c.

Sartoris, D. J., Neumann, C. H., and Riley, R. W.: The temporomandibular joint: True sagittal computed tomography with meniscus visualization. Radiology 150:250–254, 1984.

Schellhas, K. P., and Wilkes, C. H.: Temporomandibular joint inflammation: Comparison of MR fast scanning with T1- and T2-weighted imaging techniques. AJNR 10:589–594, 1989a.

Schellhas, K. P., Wilkes, C. H., El Deeb, M., et al.: Permanent proplast temporomandibular joint implants: MR imaging of destructive complications. AJR 151:731–735, 1988.

Schellhas, K. P., Wilkes, C. H., Fritts, H. M., et al.: MR of osteochondritis dissecans and avascular necrosis of the mandibular condyle. AJNR 10:3–12, 1989b.

Shellock, F. G., and Pressman, B. D.: Dual-surface-coil MR imaging of bilateral temporomandibular joints: Improvements in the imaging protocol. AJNR 10:595–598, 1989.

Silver, C. M., Simon, S. D., and Savastano, A. A.: Meniscus injuries of the temporomandibular joint. J. Bone Joint Surg. (Am.) 38A:541–552, 1956.

Stoneman, D. S., Speck, J. E., Weinberg, S., and Moch, D.: Chondrometaplasia involving the temporomandibular joint. Oral Surg. 49:556–559, 1980.

Tallents, R. H., Katzberg, R. W., Miller, T. L., et al.: Arthrographically assisted splint therapy. J. Prosthet. Dent. 53:235–238, 1985.

Thompson, J. R., Christiansen, E. L., Hasso, A. N., and Hinshaw, D. B.: The temporomandibular joint: High-resolution computed tomographic evaluation. Radiology 150:105–110, 1984.

Toller, P. A.: Temporomandibular arthropathy. Proc. R. Soc. Med. 67:153–159, 1974a.

Toller, P. A.: Opaque arthrography of the temporomandibular joint. Int. J. Oral Surg. 3:17–28, 1974b.

Westesson, P.-L.: Double contrast arthrography and internal derangement of the temporomandibular joint. Swed. Dent. J. (Suppl. 13) 1–57, 1982.

Westesson, P.-L.: Double contrast arthrotomography of the temporomandibular joint: Introduction of an arthrographic technique for visualization of the disc and articular surfaces. J. Oral Maxillofac. Surg. 41:163–172, 1983.

Westesson, P.-L.: Arthrography of the temporomandibular joint. J. Prosthet. Dent. 51:535–543, 1984a.

Westesson, P.-L., and Bronstein, S. L.: Temporomandibular joint: Comparison of single- and double-contrast arthrography. Radiology 164:65–70, 1987a.

Westesson, P.-L., Bronstein, S. L., and Liedberg, J.: Temporomandibular joint. Correlation between single contrast videoarthrography and postmortem morphology. Radiology 160:767–771, 1986.

Westesson, P.-L., and Eriksson, L.: Diskectomy of the temporomandibular joint: A double contrast arthrotomographic follow-up study. Oral Surg. 59:435–440, 1985.

Westesson, P.-L., Eriksson, L., and Kurita, K.: Temporomandibular joint: Variation of normal arthrographic anatomy. Oral Surg., 69:514–519, 1990.

Westesson, P.-L., Katzberg, R. W., Tallents, R. H., et al.: CT and MRI of the temporomandibular joint: Comparison with autopsy specimens. AJR 148:1165–1171, 1987b.

Westesson, P.-L., Katzberg, R. W., Tallents, R. H., et al.: Temporomandibular joint: Comparison of MR images with cryosectional anatomy. Radiology 164:59–64, 1987c.

Westesson, P.-L., and Lundh, H.: Arthrographic and clinical characteristics of patients with disc displacement who progressed to closed lock during a six months period. Oral Surg., 67:654–657, 1989.

Westesson, P.-L., Omnell, K.-A., and Rohlin, M.: Double contrast tomography of the temporomandibular joint. A new technique based on autopsy specimen examinations. Acta Radiol. (Diagn.). Stockh. 21:777–784, 1980.

Westesson, P.-L., and Rohlin, M.: Diagnostic accuracy of double contrast arthrotomography of the temporomandibular joint: Correlation with postmortem morphology. AJNR 5:463–468, 1984, and AJR 143:655–660, 1984b.

Wilkes, C. H.: Arthrography of the temporomandibular joint in patients with the TMJ pain-dysfunction syndrome. Minn. Med. 61:645–652, 1978a.

Wilkes, C. H.: Structural and functional alterations of the temporomandibular joint. Northwest Dent. 57:287–294, 1978b.

Wilkes, C. H.: Internal derangements of the temporomandibular joint. Arch. Otolaryngol. Head Neck Surg. 115:469–477, 1989.

17

ARTHROSCOPY*

ANDERS B. HOLMLUND, D.D.S., PH.D.,
and GUSTAF HELLSING, D.D.S., PH.D.

INTRODUCTION

The key to successful therapy is proper diagnosis. The temporomandibular joint (TMJ), for several reasons, offers difficulties in this respect. First, joint position under the skull base complicates clinical and radiographic examination. Second, the close relationship between the jaw muscles and joint structures complicates the distinction between signs and symptoms caused by muscular hyperactivity and those caused by organic joint disease. The use of new diagnostic and therapeutic methods, earlier developed for the knee joint, have therefore gained particular interest. The first arthroscopic examination of the TMJ was reported by Ohnishi in 1975, and during the last decade diagnostic arthroscopy has been thoroughly evaluated (Blaustein, 1988; Goss, 1986; 1987; Heffez, 1987; Holmlund, 1985; 1986; 1987; 1988a; 1988b; 1988c; Murakami, 1985; 1986a; 1986b; Ohnishi, 1975; 1980). Other reports also indicate a potential for various transarthroscopic surgical procedures (McCain, 1988; Nuelle, 1986; Ohnishi, 1986; Sanders, 1986).

DIAGNOSTIC ARTHROSCOPY

Indications

Arthroscopy provides valuable information regarding intra-articular structures that cannot

be obtained by other methods. The indications for arthroscopy are thus related to what cannot be achieved by other diagnostic methods. Although arthroscopy is well tolerated by patients, and complications are extremely rare, it is a surgical intervention and as such requires clear indications. Arthroscopy is only one of several diagnostic methods, and by no means is it a substitute for a thorough case history, clinical examination, and indirect imaging. Indications for diagnostic arthroscopy are suspected internal derangements, osteoarthrosis, diseases primarily affecting the synovium (rheumatoid arthritis, psoriatic arthritis, gout, pseudogout, synovial chondromatosis), the examination and biopsy of suspected neoplastic disease, and the investigation of post-traumatic complaints.

Internal derangements (anterior disc displacement, disc derangement) are a clear indication for arthroscopic examination. Although clicking may be difficult to reproduce during the examination due to interference from the arthroscope, other significant pathological changes can be demonstrated (Fig. 17–1A through C). Arthroscopy also provides valuable information about the degree of inflammation and cartilage and bone destruction.

Osteoarthrosis is best evaluated during arthroscopy. The different stages of the disease are accurately displayed (Fig. 17–1D through I). This is of considerable help when determining whether to use nonsurgical or surgical treat-

---

* See Chapters 5, 11, 16, and 21–24

289

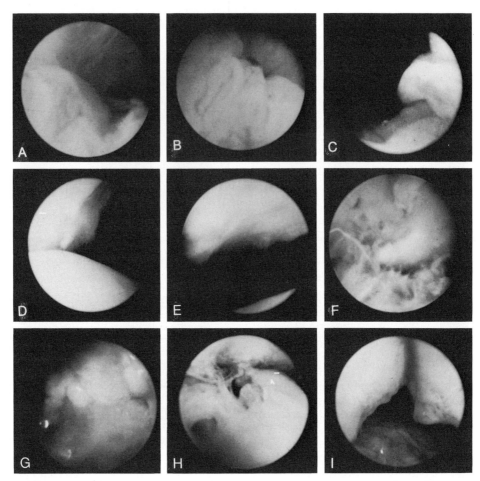

FIGURE 17–1. *A*, Right joint, superior compartment. Folding of the posterior disc attachment and increased vascularity of the synovial lining indicates disc derangement and localized synovitis. *B*, Right joint, superior compartment. Folding of the posterior disc attachment indicates disc derangement. *C*, Left joint, superior compartment. Folding of the posterior disc attachment and capillary hyperemia of the synovial lining indicates disc derangement and localized synovitis. *D*, Left joint, superior compartment. There are early signs of osteoarthrosis (fibrillation) of the fibrocartilage above. The disc surface below is unaffected. *E*, Left joint, superior compartment. Slight fibrillation of the fibrocartilage of the posterior slope of the eminence indicates early osteoarthrosis. *F*, Right joint, superior compartment. Advanced osteoarthrosis. There is pronounced fibrillation of the central part of the disc. The posterior slope of the eminence above has lesions of the fibrocartilage and bone exposure. *G*, Right joint, superior compartment. Advanced osteoarthrosis. There is pronounced change of the fibrocartilage of the posteromedial part of the glenoid fossa (irrigation fluid removed). *H*, Right joint, superior compartment. Advanced osteoarthrosis. A small perforation of the central part of the disc can be seen. The eminence above has discolored fibrocartilage. *I*, Left joint, superior compartment. Advanced osteoarthrosis. Part of a large disc perforation can be seen. Fibrocartilage lesions and bone exposure are present on the condylar surface.

ment. When rheumatoid arthritis is suspected, arthroscopy is of great importance not only because it permits thorough examination of the tissues, but also because it provides an opportunity for biopsy of the synovium. Arthroscopy is also sometimes indicated in patients with post-traumatic complaints. Contraindications for arthroscopy are infections in the joint region and extreme impairment of joint mobility.

Radiography

The prearthroscopy radiographic examination involves submentovertex and transcranial projections, and corrected sagittal tomography (see Chapter 16). The use of standardized techniques that produce images of good quality is a necessary prerequisite to provide valuable information regarding width of joint spaces, thickness and configuration of the subchondral bone, and translatory capacity of the disc-condyle complex.

Equipment

The equipment used for arthroscopy consists of a small-diameter arthroscope (needlescope), sharp and blunt trocars, arthroscopic sheath and outflow cannula, a fiber light cable, a light source, and photographic and video documentation sets (Fig. 17–2). The optics of the arthroscope are constructed from small glass rods (rod-lens system) tightly put together or from a single glass rod, with the lens treated chemically with cesium (Selfoc system). A rod-lens model is shown in Figure 17–2A. An optimal arthroscope should have a direction of view of 30 degrees for maximal field of vision.

A light source should be chosen that fits directly to the arthroscope to reduce further loss of light from intervening adapters. Photographic documentation is facilitated by the use of an articulated optical arm (Fig. 17–2B). Video documentation has improved vastly during the last few years. Video recordings produce magnified frames of the arthroscopic examination that provide a record of functional impairments and facilitate teaching (Fig. 17–2C).

Anesthesia

Although frequently done under general anesthesia, diagnostic arthroscopy may also be performed under local anesthesia on outpatients (Holmlund, 1988b; 1988c; 1986; Murakami, 1985), thus requiring fewer resources. Local anesthesia also permits the patient to cooperate,

which facilitates intra-articular access and functional observations. Effective anesthesia is achieved by blocking the auriculotemporal nerve posterior to the condylar neck and by infiltrating the lateral joint area with about 3 ml of lidocaine containing epinephrine (10 mg/ml).

Puncture Technique

The patient is placed in a supine position to reduce the risk of initiating a vasovagal reaction. Careful palpation reveals the lateral contour of both the glenoid fossa and the articular eminence. A guideline from the posterior midpoint of the tragus to the lateral canthus may be of great help to the inexperienced surgeon in determining the correct puncture site (Holmlund, 1985). This should be about 12 mm anterior to the posterior midpoint of tragus and about 2 mm below the canthal-tragal line. The selected puncture point is marked on the skin with dye. The patient is instructed to open the mouth to move the disc-condyle complex out of the glenoid fossa, thereby enlarging the posterior joint space. Distention of the joint space is obtained by injecting an isotonic saline solution using a 5 ml syringe with a 27 gauge needle. The needle is inserted in a medial and slightly anterosuperior direction until the posterior part of the articular eminence is gently contacted. To distend the inferior compartment the needle is withdrawn and redirected more perpendicular to the sagittal plane until the posterosuperior part of the condyle is gently contacted. The joint spaces are slowly distended. About 3 ml is needed for the superior compartment and 1.5 ml for the inferior compartment. Usually resistance will be noted when distention is complete, and the patient will experience a slight downward and forward displacement of the mandible. If no resistance is experienced after injecting 4 ml, the capsule may have been ruptured inadvertently and further distention should be avoided.

About a 3 mm vertical skin incision is made at the injection site and, using a sharp trocar surrounded by the arthroscopic sheath, the lateral capsule is punctured. The direction of the trocar is the same as for the distention needle. Slight resistance will usually be encountered when the trocar penetrates the capsule. In some joints the lateral capsule offers more resistance, indicating a fibrotic thickening. After penetrating the capsule, the sharp trocar is exchanged for the blunt one and the arthroscopic sheath is introduced farther into

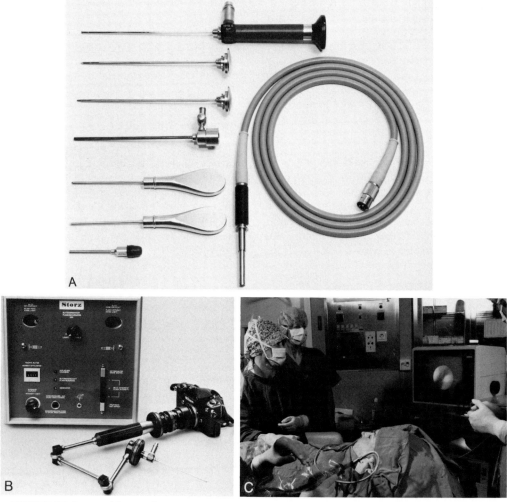

FIGURE 17–2. *A*, Rod-lens 30-degree arthroscope, trocars, arthroscopic sheath, outflow cannula with trocars, and fiber light cable. *B*, Light source and camera. An articulated optical arm is used for photographic and teaching purposes. *C*, Videoscopy. The magnified frames on the monitor facilitate visualization and teaching. Recording of functional impairment is possible.

the upper joint space. The fibrous layer of the glenoid fossa, or the posterior part of the articular eminence, is gently palpated to confirm proper placement. Mean puncture depth, i.e., the distance from the skin surface to the posterocentral part of the eminence, is about 27 mm (Holmlund, 1985). A graded trocar sleeve is useful to prevent the trocar from penetrating too deeply and to avoid accidental perforation of the medial capsule.

The blunt trocar is now exchanged for the arthroscope and proper entrance is confirmed. A second portal is then created on the canthal-tragal line about 5 mm anterior and 3 mm inferior to the arthroscopic sheath for outflow. A 2.0 mm diameter short cannula is suitable for this purpose. The joint is then continuously

irrigated during the arthroscopic procedure with either isotonic saline or lactated Ringer's solution.

The inferolateral approach (Fig. 17–3) offers good access to the superior compartment. A posterolateral approach has also been suggested for examination of the superior joint space (Murakami, 1985). This, however, offers no advantage over the inferolateral approach in terms of access, but involves an increased risk of bleeding from the temporal vessels. Different approaches have been proposed for the inferior compartment (Johnson, 1981; Murakami, 1985), but all involve a considerable risk of damage to extra-articular and intra-articular tissues. Puncture of the inferior compartment should therefore be avoided in routine examinations.

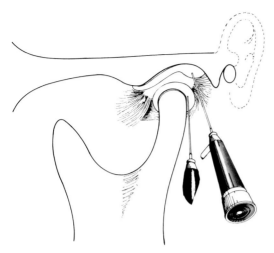

FIGURE 17–3. Diagram of inferolateral approach. Puncture directions are shown for entering the superior and inferior compartments.

Arthroscopic Anatomy

Superior Compartment

The synovial lining is well developed in the posterior part of the joint. The vascularized synovial lining clearly contrasts with the relatively avascular fibrous tissue covering of the fossa and articular eminence. The amount of vascularity seen depends on the degree of pressure from distention of the joint and the temperature of the irrigation fluid. The posterior band of the disc often appears protruded and is thus, in most cases, distinguished from the posterior disc attachment (Fig. 17–4A). The medial capsule shows a fibrous reinforcement in the posterior third (Fig. 17–4B). Anteriorly the capsule is extremely thin and the vascularity of the synovial lining is less pronounced (Fig. 17–4C). The central part of the joint is narrow. The fibrous tissue covering of the temporal bone and the superior disc surface appears smooth and glossy white (Fig. 17–4D).

Inferior Compartment

The posterior capsule attaches to the condylar neck and creates a rather deep recess. Compared with the superior compartment, vascularity of the synovial lining is less pronounced (Fig. 17–4E). Above the condyle the joint space is generally too narrow to allow passage of the arthroscope into the anterior recess (Fig. 17–4F). The anterior capsule is extremely thin and lies directly over the inferior belly of the lateral pterygoid muscle (Fig. 17–4G).

Arthroscopic Examination

The visual examination follows mainly the principles described in the orthopedic literature (Johnson, 1982; 1981). The surgeon must be

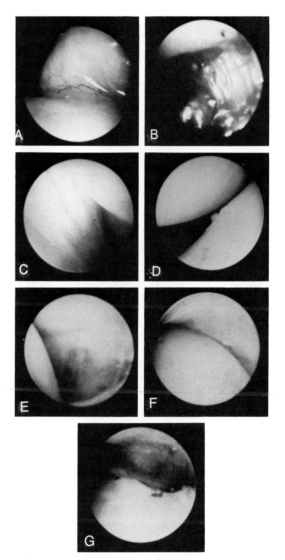

FIGURE 17–4. Arthroscopic anatomy. A, Right joint, superior compartment showing posterior disc attachment near the posterior part of the disc (irrigation fluid removed). B, Left joint, superior compartment showing posterior part of the medial capsule. The posterior part of the eminence can be seen above (irrigation fluid removed). C, Left joint, superior compartment, anterior capsule. The anterior part of the eminence can be seen above. D, Left joint, superior compartment. The posterior part of the eminence is seen above and the disc is seen below. E, Left joint, inferior compartment, posteromedial part of the disc and the posterior disc attachment. The posterosuperior part of the condyle is to the left. F, Left joint, inferior compartment, posterosuperior part of the condyle. The central part of the disc is seen above. G, Left joint, inferior compartment, anterior capsule. A small amount of remodeling can be seen on the condylar surface below.

familiar with procedures such as rotation, scanning, pistoning, and palpation (Johnson, 1981; 1982). Rotation of the telescope, often overlooked by the surgeon, increases the field of vision considerably. Pistoning means that the telescope is moved back and forth toward the object; it is helpful in estimating the correct size. A probe inserted through the outflow cannula allows for palpation of internal joint structures.

Adequate distention of the joint with saline solution seems to improve access to the different joint regions, but it is also possible to examine the joint without distention. Distention with gas instead of fluid has been proposed (Ohnishi, 1980; 1975), but should be avoided because emphysema may result. The arthroscopic landmarks have been described (Holmlund, 1988b; 1988c; Murakami, 1985), and proper knowledge of their location is of great importance so as not to lose orientation during the examination. Training on cadavers before clinical application is extremely helpful, and must be emphasized.

Examination of the superior compartment starts by identifying the posterior disc attachment (retrodiscal tissue) and the posterior synovial recess (Fig. 17–4A). The synovial lining is inspected for signs of inflammation such as increased vascularity and capillary hyperemia (Fig. 17–1A, C). Pronounced folding or hyperplasia of the posterior disc attachment may indicate disc derangement (Fig. 17–1A, B, C).

Anterior to the posterior recess, the posterior band of the disc can be visualized. In most cases the avascular posterior band is easily distinguished from the vascularized disc attachment (Fig. 17–4A). During alternate opening and closing movements of the mouth the posterior part of the disc is clearly identified and possible impairment of translation of the disc-condyle complex may be seen. The arthroscope is then moved further anteriorly to visualize the posterior part of the medial capsule. The capsule normally has a fibrous reinforcement (Fig. 17–4B). Increased vascularity of the capsule indicates synovitis.

Following examination of the posterior aspect of the joint space the arthroscope is slightly withdrawn and then directed anteromedially. The patient is instructed to close the mouth gently and the arthroscope is pushed under the articular eminence into the anterior recess. Under general anesthesia the mandible is manipulated by the assistant either by using the thumb and fingers on the anterior part of the mandible or by using a guiding clamp at the

angle of the mandible. The anterior part of the superior joint compartment (Fig. 17–4C) is examined in the same way as described for the posterior recess. Rotation of the arthroscope is important to enlarge the field of vision.

During withdrawal of the arthroscope the temporal bone and the superior disc surfaces are scanned for signs of arthrotic changes and remodeling (Fig. 17–4D). The lateral capsule is difficult to inspect with the 30-degree arthroscope. A scope with 90-degree viewing can overcome this problem. Deviation from the optical axis, however, makes orientation difficult.

The inferior joint compartment is examined in the same way as the superior compartment. The condylar surface and the inferior disc surface are identified and inspected. The joint space is too narrow to allow passage into the anterior recess without damage to the disc surface and the condylar fibrous tissue covering (Fig. 17–4E). It is, however, sometimes possible to examine the anterior recess from the superior compartment through a disc perforation (Fig. 17–4G). As mentioned earlier, puncture of the inferior compartment involves a risk of damage to internal joint structures. The limited information obtained seems, at present, not to justify routine examination of the inferior compartment.

Upon completion of the arthroscopic examination the joint cavity is thoroughly irrigated to remove debris and small blood clots. The cannulas are removed and the incisions are closed with surgical tape; there is usually no need for sutures. The patient is put on a soft, nonchewy diet for a few days. Antibiotics are not necessary (Holmlund, 1986; 1988a; 1988b; 1988c).

Postoperative Course

Perioperative and postoperative complications are rare (Goss, 1986; Holmlund, 1986; 1987; 1988a; 1988b; 1988c; Murakami, 1985). Perioperative bleeding from the temporal vessels may occur and is mainly caused by incorrect placement of the puncture point. Damage of the temporal and zygomatic branches of the facial nerve may be associated with an anterolateral approach. No such damage has been associated with an inferolateral approach. The risk of postoperative infection is low (Goss, 1986; Holmlund, 1986; 1987; 1988b; 1988c; Murakami, 1985), although single cases have been reported (Sanders, 1986). Serious complications are extremely rare. Damage to the middle ear may occur if the trocar is directed posteriorly during puncture. The trocar may perforate the anterior wall of the cartilaginous portion of the ear canal and, if further advanced, damage the middle ear. Although the glenoid fossa may be thin medially, much force must be used to perforate into the middle cranial fossa. Extreme care is recommended, however, when severe arthrosis is present. Tomograms of good quality prearthroscopically may prevent this dreaded complication. Functional impairment following arthroscopy is infrequent, minor, and transient (Goss, 1986; Holmlund, 1986; 1987; 1988a; 1988b; 1988c; Murakami, 1985).

ARTHROSCOPIC SURGERY

Several surgical procedures on the knee joint, which previously required open surgery, are now performed under arthroscopic control (Johnson, 1981; 1982; Oretorp, 1979). The postoperative period has thus been reduced. Postoperative infection, originally a dreaded complication, is today practically nonexistent. It is, therefore, not surprising to find reports advocating various transarthroscopic surgical procedures for the TMJ (McCain, 1988; Nuelle, 1986; Sanders, 1986). Arthroscopic surgery of the TMJ is more difficult to perform than knee joint surgery for many reasons. Experience with diagnostic arthroscopy and well-designed training programs are prerequisites.

Indications

At the present time, biopsy, lavage, lysis of adhesions, smoothing procedures, and restriction of disc movement can be accomplished arthroscopically.

To obtain a representative synovial specimen a biopsy is best performed with a small forceps using a second portal or a double cannula (Figs. 17–5, 17–6). The material obtained must be sufficient for histologic examination and the forceps, therefore, must not be too small.

The efficiency of lavage has been reported in both the knee joint and the TMJ (Holmlund, 1986; Sanders, 1986), and may be explained by removal of debris and other inflammatory products from the joint cavity. Isotonic saline or lactated Ringer's solutions may be used. Lavage can also be combined with other treatments such as instillation of corticosteroids or sodium hyaluronate.

Lysis has also been advocated in the treatment of disc derangement and arthritides when adhesions are present (Sanders, 1986). The procedure may be performed as a closed technique or under direct vision. With the former technique, the adhesions are released using the blunt trocar in sweeping movements (Sanders, 1986). Once the joint is freed and translation of the disc-condyle complex is achieved, physiotherapy is immediately undertaken to either maintain or increase the achieved range of motion. The lysis technique may be an important alternative to open surgery in the future.

So-called minishavers are now available that may be useful in patients with osteoarthrosis. Interfering irregularities of the fibrocartilage and disc can be smoothened and joint function improved.

Restriction of the posterior disc attachment has also been attempted in patients with repeated chronic dislocation (Ohnishi, 1986). In these instances the formation of scar tissue is induced arthroscopically using a laser technique or cautery (Ohnishi, 1986). The incision is made in the posterior disc attachment parallel to the posterior band. Studies on a larger number of patients are necessary to evaluate these techniques more accurately.

Equipment

Various instruments are available for arthroscopic surgery. One useful set of instruments is described in Figure 17–5. Knives, scissors, shavers, and other instruments must be of impeccable quality, as broken instruments inside the joint may be difficult to remove even at open surgery. To maintain sterility, the different procedures are best performed by videoscopy rather than direct vision.

Technique

A second cannula is recommended for insertion of the surgical instruments (Fig. 17–6A). The second puncture is performed about 10 mm anterior and 5 mm below the first puncture site, immediately anterior to the most inferior point of the eminence. This allows for the triangulation necessary for safe orientation of the instruments (McCain, 1988). The available space for the second puncture is, however, rather small and there is a risk of damage to the temporal branch of the facial nerve. A double-cannula technique (Fig. 17–6B) may therefore be an alternative. The fine instruments should be surrounded by a sheath. Irrigation is maintained through the arthroscopic sheath and outflow through the second cannula.

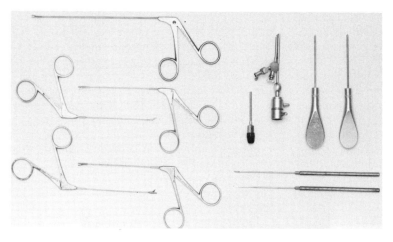

FIGURE 17–5. Instruments for arthroscopic surgery. Biopsy forceps, scissors, grasping forceps, and knives.

In some cases an outflow cannula may be placed between the working cannula and the arthroscope.

Well-designed "hands on" courses to practice triangulation, manipulation, and videoscopy with nondominant hand control are essential.

SUMMARY

TMJ arthroscopy provides valuable diagnostic data that cannot be obtained by other methods.

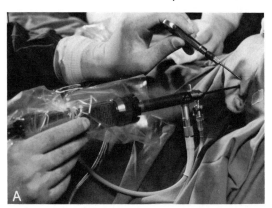

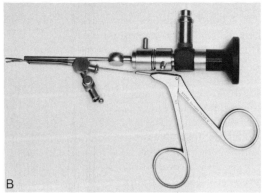

FIGURE 17–6. *A,* Clinical view of triangulation technique. A second portal is used for the surgical instruments. *B,* Double cannula. The two sheaths are connected, thereby facilitating orientation of the surgical instruments.

In agreement with earlier studies regarding the knee joint, TMJ arthroscopy has shown high diagnostic accuracy (Goss, 1987; Holmlund, 1985; 1987) and low risk of postoperative complications. Diagnostic arthroscopy can be performed on outpatients, thus requiring less resources (Holmlund, 1986; 1987; 1988a; 1988b; 1988c; Murakami, 1985).

Techniques for surgery under arthroscopic control have been developed (McCain, 1988; Nuelle, 1986; Sanders, 1986) and it is reasonable to assume that this field will grow considerably in the future. The potentials for research are substantial and well-designed correlative studies must be carried out to delineate more clearly the diagnostic and therapeutic benefits of this technique.

REFERENCES

Blaustein, D., and Heffez, L.: Diagnostic arthroscopy of the temporomandibular joint. Part II. Arthroscopic findings of arthrographically diagnosed disc displacements. Oral Surg. 65:135–141, 1988.

Goss, A. N., and Bosanquet, A. G.: Temporomandibular joint arthroscopy. J. Oral Maxillofac. Surg. 44:614–617, 1986.

Goss, A. N., Bosanquet, A. G., and Tideman, H.: The accuracy of temporomandibular joint arthroscopy. J. Craniomaxillofac. Surg. 15:99–102, 1987.

Heffez, L., and Blaustein, D.: Diagnostic arthroscopy of the temporomandibular joint. Part I. Normal arthroscopic findings. Oral Surg. 64:653–670, 1987.

Holmlund, A.: Arthroscopy of the Temporomandibular Joint. Dissertation. Karolinska Institute, Huddinge, Tiba Tryck AB, 1987.

Holmlund, A., and Hellsing, G.: Arthroscopy of the temporomandibular joint. An autopsy study. Int. J. Oral Surg. 14:169–175, 1985.

Holmlund, A., and Hellsing, G.: Arthroscopy of the temporomandibular joint. Occurrence and location of osteoarthrosis and synovitis in a patient material. Int. J. Oral Maxillofac. Surg. 17:36–40, 1988a.

Holmlund, A., Hellsing, G., and Wredmark, T.: Arthroscopy of the temporomandibular joint. A clinical study. Int. J. Oral Maxillofac. Surg. *15*:715–721, 1986.

Holmlund, A., and Nordenram, A.: Temporomandibular joint arthroscopy. *In* Parisien, J. S. (Ed.): Arthroscopic Surgery. New York, McGraw-Hill, 1988b, pp. 307–312.

Holmlund, A., and Nordenram, A.: Arthroscopy of the temporomandibular joint. *In* Keith, D. A. (Ed.): Surgery of the Temporomandibular Joint. Boston, Blackwell Scientific Publications Inc., 1988c, pp. 47–54.

Johnson, L.: Diagnostic and Surgical Arthroscopy: Knee and Other Joints. St. Louis, C. V. Mosby, 1981.

Johnson, L.: Diagnostic and surgical arthroscopy. Clinical symposia. CIBA *34*:1–32, 1982.

McCain, J.: Arthroscopy of the human temporomandibular joint. J. Oral Maxillofac. Surg. *46*:648–655, 1988.

Murakami, K.-I., and Ito, K.: Arthroscopy of the temporomandibular joint. *In* Watanabe, M. (Ed.): Arthroscopy of Small Joints. Tokyo, Igaku Shoin, 1985, pp. 128–139.

Murakami, K.-I., Matsuki, M., Iizuka, T., and Ono, T.: Diagnostic arthroscopy of the temporomandibular joint. Differential diagnosis in patients with limited jaw opening. J. Craniomandib. Pract. *4*:117–126, 1986a.

Murakami, K.-I., and Ono, T.: Temporomandibular joint arthroscopy by inferolateral approach. Int. J. Oral Maxillofac. Surg. *15*:410–417, 1986b.

Nuelle, D. G., Alpern, M. C., and Ufema, J. W.: Arthroscopic surgery of the temporomandibular joint. Angle Orthod. *56*:118–142, 1986.

Ohnishi, M.: Arthroscopy of the temporomandibular joint (in Japanese). Jpn. J. Stomatol. *42*:207–213, 1975.

Ohnishi, M.: Clinical application of arthroscopy in temporomandibular joint diseases. Bull. Tokyo Med. Dent. Univ. *27*:141–150, 1980.

Ohnishi, M.: Arthroscopic surgery of temporomandibular joint diseases. Abstract no. 173. 9th ICOMS Conference, Vancouver, Canada, 1986.

Oretorp, N., and Gillquist, J.: Transcutaneous meniscectomy under arthroscopic control. Int. Orthop. *3*:19–25, 1979.

Sanders, B.: Arthroscopic surgery of the temporomandibular joint. Treatment of internal derangement with persistent closed lock. Oral Surg. *62*:361–372, 1986.

18

TEMPOROMANDIBULAR DISORDERS: The Evolution of Concepts*

CHARLES S. GREENE, D.D.S.

* See Chapters 5–9, 14, 17, 19–21, and 23–26

CURRENT STATUS OF CONCEPTS ABOUT THE ETIOLOGY AND TREATMENT OF TEMPOROMANDIBULAR DISORDERS

Understanding the Controversies

Beginning to Resolve the Controversies: Contributions from Research

EMERGENCE OF A MEDICAL ORTHOPEDICS VIEWPOINT

Recognition That Temporomandibular Disorders Are Similar to Other Musculoskeletal Disorders

Differential Diagnosis and Classification of Temporomandibular Disorders

Recognition of the Multifactorial Etiology of Various Temporomandibular Disorders

Recognition That Psychological Factors Can Affect the Onset, Progression, and Remission of Many Temporomandibular Disorders

Utilization of General Principles of Orthopedic Medicine in Treating Temporomandibular Disorders

Judicious Use of Surgical Procedures in Appropriate Situations

CHRONIC PAIN RELATED TO TEMPOROMANDIBULAR DISORDERS

Understanding Modern Concepts of Chronic Pain

Management of Patients with Chronic Temporomandibular Disorders

SUMMARY

INTRODUCTION

In recent years significant progress has been made in many scientific and clinical areas related to temporomandibular disorders (TMDs) within and outside the dental profession. Technological developments have enabled both normal and abnormal jaw function to be studied in the laboratory in ways that were not previously possible. During this same period, several excellent clinical studies have produced important findings on the diagnosis and treatment of symptomatic patients. Epidemiologic studies have also begun to yield reliable data about the incidence and distribution of TMD in the general population. There is, however, still some disagreement about the interpretation of certain aspects of these studies. Moreover, despite these advances, diversity of opinion about nearly every major issue related to TMD still persists, and indeed several new controversies have arisen (see Chapters 14 and 19).

To understand the paradox of how a clinical discipline can have true progress occur in the midst of apparent chaos, one must study the field from a historic perspective (Greene, 1980). In doing so, it becomes clear that powerful personalities and anecdotal success stories, rather than research-based thinking, combined with a lack of systematic teaching about TMDs in the professional schools, have led to the polarization of opposing groups that characterizes so much of this field. Despite this situation, however, some basic scientists and clinical investigators have managed to apply the principles of sound research to this difficult subject, and in doing so they have produced valid information that makes real progress possible. Much of that information is presented throughout this book.

EARLY CONCEPTS OF TEMPOROMANDIBULAR DISORDERS

Overclosure of the Mandible

The earliest reports by dentists on the subject of TMDs were generally in agreement about one thing: overclosure of the mandible was responsible for their patients' problems. This viewpoint received substantial support from the writings of Costen (1934), who attributed 11 symptoms to the pressure of overclosed condyles on posterior joint structures. All of these early authors recommended essentially the same treatment approach: namely, to open the vertical dimension of the bite with dental prostheses. The apparent clinical successes that were obtained with this approach seemed to be confirmation of its validity, thereby beginning a cycle of fallacious reasoning from cure to cause that has persisted to this day.

Posterior Displacement of the Mandible

The concept of vertical overclosure of the mandible was partially replaced about 20 years later by a horizontal displacement concept. This notion was advocated primarily by orthodontists such as Thompson (1962) and Ricketts (1964), who used various radiographic techniques to determine condylar positions. These investigators correlated orthodontic malocclusions and so-called condylar displacements, with special emphasis placed on Class II, Division 2 patients, who were presumed to have incisal interferences during jaw closure that dictated a posterior shift of the mandible. As might be expected, this concept led practitioners to a treatment approach in which the mandible was protruded with various bite appliances, followed by permanent repositioning via orthodontic and/or prosthetic treatment. Once again, the apparent clinical successes that occurred were seen as a validation of the entire concept.

EARLY NEUROMUSCULAR-OCCLUSAL DISHARMONY CONCEPTS OF TEMPOROMANDIBULAR DISORDERS

Basic Neurophysiological Concepts of Muscular Dysfunction

During the first quarter-century of clinical interest in TMDs, little or no mention was made of neuromuscular factors. Instead, the focus was on mechanical displacements of the mandible, as previously described. While Seaver did report on a neuromuscular basis for TMD as early as 1937, this concept was not widely discussed until the 1950s. The basis for associating TMD pain with muscular dysfunction derives from general medical principles of muscle pathophysiology: functional fatigue, nociceptive reflexes, hyperactivity, inflammation, and so forth (see Chapter 9).

Occlusal Disharmony as a Cause of Muscular Dysfunction

The linkage between occlusal disharmonies and TMDs was proposed originally as an alternative to the mechanical displacement theories. In this concept, abnormal tooth-to-tooth relationships of various kinds are seen as a burden on masticatory muscles trying to function normally. These dental interferences are believed to elicit nociceptive reflexes that lead to continuous or intermittent increases in jaw muscle activity, which in time result in muscular pain and dysfunction (Shore, 1959). Initial support for this viewpoint came from the work of several electromyographers (Jarabak, 1956; Moyers, 1950; Perry, 1957) who reported above-normal jaw muscle activity in groups of symptomatic TMD patients.

Variations of this concept included the occlusal disharmony theories of bruxism, in which oral parafunctional habits were seen as nothing more than a reflexive response to dental interferences (Ramfjord, 1961). Because prolonged bruxism obviously can produce muscular fatigue, this became another major pathway for the dental occlusion to be responsible for TMD symptoms. In another version of the neuromuscular concept, mandibular displacement was still the major problem, but it was attributed to muscular accommodation to occlusal disharmonies rather than just mechanical displacement (Dawson, 1974). In this concept the direction of the displacement was presumed to be anterior, which was the opposite of that described by Thompson (1962).

Contradictory Evidence Against Occlusal Disharmony Concepts

It is not difficult to understand why the original occlusal disharmony concepts of neuromuscular dysfunction were appealing. In addition to their superficial logic, they seemed to have some scientific basis for being correct. Ramfjord published a classic clinical study in 1961, showing that symptomatic TMD patients had elevated electromyographic (EMG) readings. After equilibration, however, there was a reported cessation of bruxism and an improvement in symptoms as well as a decrease in EMG activity, so there seemed to be little left to doubt. Over the years, however, that study became the classic model for both inadequate research methodology and fallacious interpretations of experimental results. The failure to control for significant procedural errors in EMG utilization, combined with the failure to consider alternative reasons for the experimental outcomes, ultimately rendered this report obsolete. Rugh (personal communication) has made the interesting observation that this report was still being widely cited in the 1980s, but about two-thirds of the time it was cited either incorrectly or inappropriately.

The major arguments against the occlusal disharmony theories of muscular dysfunction arise from a combination of clinical studies (Droukas, 1984; Posselt, 1971; Solberg, 1972) and epidemiologic studies (Carlsson, 1984b; Nilner, 1981; Sadowsky, 1984) that show no consistent occlusal differences between TMD patients and normal individuals. The mere presence of some form of occlusal irregularity is so common that it makes the notion of an ideal occlusion seem to be little more than an abstraction. While some occlusionists still argue for their viewpoint by saying that TMD patients are the ones whose muscles are unable to cope with their occlusal disharmony, the more likely conclusion is that most occlusal relationships are well within the broad range of normal neuromuscular accommodation (see Chapter 9). Of course, the ultimate argument of the occlusionists that their occlusally treated patients have responded positively to therapy (Dawson, 1974; Ramfjord, 1961) can no longer be considered persuasive, especially after so many studies have demonstrated that reversible treatment approaches produce results that are equal or superior (Greene, 1983; Mjersjo, 1983). However, because some new occlusal concepts of TMD etiology have made a resurgence in recent years, this issue will be discussed further on.

PSYCHOPHYSIOLOGICAL CONCEPTS OF TEMPOROMANDIBULAR DISORDERS

Basic Concepts of Stress-Disease Relationships

The idea that emotional stress and tension could affect an individual's physical well-being has long been recognized on an empirical level. It was not until the 1930s, however, that Selye first demonstrated experimental evidence of these relationships. Selye's studies showed specific structural changes in organs, such as the adrenal glands and thymus, as well as functional changes in endocrine metabolism. These findings became the basis for a stress-disease concept of pathogenesis for certain clinical disorders (Selye, 1950; 1956).

A direct relationship between stress and muscular hyperactivity was postulated by Selye, but the original experimental evidence for this came from the work of Wolff (1948), who studied tension headache and other muscular pain syndromes. This was supported by the later work of Goldstein (1964a; 1964b) as well as by that of Malmo (1951). Their studies of response specificity showed that each individual has a tendency to respond physiologically to stress in a specific way, and for many it is by muscular hyperactivity. This was a major step forward in psychophysiological thinking, because it provided an explanation for different individuals having different stress-related disorders.

Stress as a Cause of Temporomandibular Problems

The possibility of a relationship between psychological stress and TMJ dysfunction was mentioned superficially by several investigators during the early 1950s, but the research conducted by Schwartz at Columbia University firmly established this concept (Schwartz, 1958; 1959). Schwartz proposed that so-called TMJ dysfunction symptoms were due to masticatory muscle incoordination and spasm, which could be related to increased psychological stress as well as excessive muscle function. Schwartz also stated that prolonged grinding and clenching habits (bruxism) produced chronic masticatory muscle pain, initiating a vicious cycle in which pain leads to more spasm and increased pain. Schwartz held that malocclusion, no matter what the degree of aberration, was not as important as the response of the patient's stomatognathic system to stress.

The main theoretical support for Schwartz's psychophysiological concept came from a combination of experimental and clinical findings reported by Travell (1952; 1960), Kraus (1963), and Moulton (1955; 1966). Travell (1952) earlier had established the general mechanisms for the genesis of myofascial pain, and later (1960) applied these concepts specifically to the pain of TMJ dysfunction. Kraus (1963), a student of functional muscle disorders for many years as a physiatrist, subsequently applied concepts of hyperkinetic disease to the study of the masticatory muscles and the role they play in TMJ dysfunction. Information about the role of emotional factors was obtained from the observations of Moulton (1955), a psychiatrist, who studied a number of patients with chronic facial pain. Moulton reported that psychiatric symptoms could be discerned in most of these patients and advised great caution in using treatments with irreversible effects. When the work of these researchers was combined with clinical investigations made by Schwartz, an etiological concept was formulated that differed considerably from previous concepts for the pain-dysfunction syndrome (Schwartz, 1959).

During the next few years, other researchers throughout the world began to follow similar paths of inquiry, and many reports appeared relating psychological factors, stress, muscle spasm, and bruxism to the pain-dysfunction syndrome. Franks (1964; 1965) stated that environmental stress factors predisposed certain patients to muscular hyperactivity in the form of grinding and clenching habits, and that this resulted in jaw symptoms. Molin (1966), in relating psychological stress to various neurasthenic symptoms, concluded that it was highly unlikely that psychological problems in TMJ patients were the result of occlusal disorders.

A number of researchers used electromyography to study patients with TMJ symptoms, and their findings offered further support for the psychophysiological concept of etiology. Kydd (1959) found that symptomatic TMJ patients showed generalized skeletal muscle hyperfunction, including hyperactive masticatory muscles. Perry (1960) studied a group of non-symptomatic students preparing for examinations to determine the effects of stress on the masticatory muscles. Electromyographic recordings were made before and after the examination, and the investigators concluded that situational stress could produce masticatory muscle hyperactivity in predisposed individuals.

Important contributions to this concept also have been made by Yemm (1969; 1971; 1979), who conducted a number of studies to investigate the relationships between various stressors and masticatory muscle activity. These studies not only consistently demonstrate that direct relationships between stress and masticatory muscle response do exist, but, in addition, they appear to support the viewpoint that such relationships must be of central nervous system origin. Yemm has argued convincingly that peripheral reflexive responses to noxious stimuli, such as dental interferences, could hardly account for the variety of oral motor behaviors and responses that occur in humans (see Chapter 9).

Myofascial Pain-Dysfunction Syndrome

Schwartz's psychophysiological concepts were modified about 10 years later by Laskin (1969), who proposed an entire theoretic system of etiology (see Chapter 19). In addition to the alternative theory of masticatory muscle dysfunction, Laskin also proposed a change in nomenclature to separate these muscle disorders from intracapsular TMJ problems: myofascial pain-dysfunction (MPD) syndrome. While clicking and other signs of disc derangement, if they were present, were considered at that time to be part of this syndrome, a patient with either radiographic evidence of joint pathology, primary joint symptoms, systemic articular problems, or a recent history of TMJ trauma was excluded from this diagnostic category.

Laskin's psychophysiological concepts were based on five types of supporting evidence (see Chapter 19). These included a variety of psychological studies that seemed to show personality state and trait differences between MPD patients and normal subjects (Lupton, 1966; 1969), although Rugh (1976) later concluded that no such psychological differences could be demonstrated consistently. In addition, there were stress response studies that showed a predilection for MPD patients to respond to stress with increases in masticatory muscle activity (Johnson, 1972). These responses were not only greater than other physiological responses, such as heart rate and palmar sweating, but also greater than the other skeletal muscle responses (Mercuri, 1979). This indicated a specificity of response to stress in the stomatognathic system similar to that reported in other psychophysiological disorders (Goldstein, 1964a), and it offered an explanation for MPD patients developing symptoms in the musculature of the head and face.

In a more recent publication updating the views on these matters, Greene (1982b) discussed the overall relationship of psychological factors to the onset, progression, and treatments of MPD syndrome, concluding that one could not justify a simple cause-and-effect psychological explanation for the etiology of this syndrome. However, enough experimental evidence existed to consider stress as one of the major etiologic factors in the development of muscle hyperactivity and, in some cases, muscle pain and dysfunction. In addition, psychological factors clearly have an effect on the progression of painful symptoms and on their treatment (see Chapter 20).

RESURGENCE OF THE OCCLUSAL DISHARMONY THEORIES FOR TEMPOROMANDIBULAR DISORDERS

Gnathological Viewpoints

The origins of gnathological concepts of occlusion can be traced back to the early writings of McCollum (1938), Stuart (1960), and Stallard (1963). It was not until the late 1960s, however, that these occlusal concepts became the dominant ones in American dentistry and strongly influenced clinical approaches to the diagnosis and treatment of TMDs. According to gnathological theory, the TMJs are the most important determinant of how the jaws work, and occlusal relationships must be in harmony with these determinants to ensure comfortable and healthy joints. Therefore, the diagnostic workup of symptomatic TMD patients should primarily focus on occlusal/TMJ relationships, and therapy should be directed toward improvement of these relationships. For some time this mechanistic viewpoint became the most widely accepted explanation of the etiology of TMDs. With refinements by second generation occlusionists such as Guichet (1969) and Dawson (1973), the study of TMDs became synonymous with the study of occlusion, and clinical investigations clearly reflected this influence.

Hybrid Theories (Stress and Occlusal Disharmony)

An attempt to bridge the gap between stress theories and occlusal concepts of TMD etiology occurred in the 1960s and 1970s. This viewpoint, as exemplified by Ramfjord (1966), held that a combination of adverse occlusal relationships and environmental stress could precipitate bruxism and other parafunctional oral habits, ultimately resulting in symptomatic muscle hyperactivity. On an intellectual level, this was a way of explaining why 95 per cent or more of the population could have occlusal disharmonies while only a few of them would have symptoms. On the practical level, however, the stress factors were minimized or considered untreatable, and the emphasis in therapy was placed almost entirely on occlusal corrections.

Radiographic Assessments of Condylar Positions

While several early theories of TMDs attributed symptoms to displacement of the mandible (either vertically or horizontally), one of the first to discuss them in radiographic terms was Thompson (1964). His evaluations were done on lateral cephalometric radiographs, which do not show the condyle or fossa in the closed position. Therefore, Thompson used an open-mouth film to trace the condyle and then overlaid it on the closed-mouth film. Using this approach, every symptomatic patient turned out to have a posterosuperior condylar displacement, and every treatment situation required anteroinferior repositioning of the mandible.

A more realistic approach to radiographic analysis of condylar position came from the early work of Ricketts (1964), who measured condyle-fossa relationships on TMJ tomograms and correlated them with various types of orthodontic malocclusions. Unlike Thompson, Ricketts found a variety of condyle-fossa relationships, but made the mistake of concluding that concentric positions were normal or ideal. This error was compounded by the later work of Weinberg (1972; 1979), who used the most distorted radiographic view (transcranial plain films) to determine condyle-fossa relationships. Like Ricketts, Weinberg concluded that concentric relationships were ideal, and considered the others to be abnormally displaced (Weinberg, 1977). This approach to diagnosis of TMD problems is, in effect, another variation of the occlusal disharmony concept, because it presumes that an adverse occlusal relationship forces the condyle to become malpositioned and this must be corrected to permit the condyle to return to its normal concentric position.

Treatment by Mandibular Repositioning and Occlusal Stabilization

The major difference between the early occlusal concepts of TMD etiology and the more recent theories is quite significant: the former calls for minor occlusal adjustments (equilibration) (Ramfjord, 1966; Shore, 1959), while the latter requires mandibular repositioning followed by major occlusal change to stabilize the new position (Gelb, 1975; Weinberg, 1979). In terms of invasiveness, both approaches are irreversible, but the second is obviously much more aggressive.

Over the years, the rationale for mandibular repositioning has gone considerably beyond the original mechanistic or radiographic concepts of right and wrong jaw position. Now we are told also that three-dimensional analysis of craniomandibular landmarks may indicate the need for realignment of a malaligned mandible (Gelb, 1977), or that an incorrect jaw position may cause symptoms elsewhere in the body (Goodheart, 1976a; 1976b). In addition, a new basis for mandibular repositioning has arisen from the discovery that TMJ discs can be displaced and may be recaptured by a repositioning procedure. All of these concepts will be discussed in more detail in the sections following.

EMERGENCE OF DISC DISPLACEMENT AND DYSFUNCTION IN TEMPOROMANDIBULAR DISORDERS

Documentation of Disc Displacement by Arthrography

The idea that a TMJ disc could be displaced, and that this displacement could be the basis for various symptoms, was considered as early as the 1940s. Norgaard's (1947) early study on arthrography and Ireland's (1951) study on TMJ clicking were seminal works, but they did not receive much attention since most clinicians were focused on jaw displacement, muscle dysfunction, occlusion, and stress.

The revival of interest in disc displacement came from the sophisticated arthrographic techniques devised by Wilkes (1978a), and employed later by Dolwick (1983), Katzberg (1980), and many others. Through the use of cinefluoroscopic imaging of TMJs injected with radiopaque contrast medium, it became possible to visualize both the static and dynamic aspects of disc displacement. Tomographic films taken in closed-, half-open–, and open-mouth positions confirmed that a displaced disc was reduced or recaptured when an opening click occurred, and became displaced again when the mouth was closed.

Confirmation of Disc Displacements by Direct Observation

Cadaver Studies

Reports of displaced discs in cadavers appeared as early as 1933, when Steinhardt presented histologic pictures showing this phenomenon. Many other reports mentioned this finding, but it was the work of investigators such as Hansson (1977) and Isberg-Holm (1980) that finally brought it to the attention of the dental and medical community. Hansson (1980) showed not only that these disc displacements occurred in both young and older populations, but also that various deviations in form occurred in the discs as well as in other joint structures. Isberg-Holm (1980) correlated gross anatomic findings with histologic findings, sound recordings, and movies of functional disc reductions. Combined with the work of many other investigators, these findings made it clear that discs were capable of assuming abnormal anatomic positions and causing various dysfunctions (clicking, sticking, locking) (Wilkes, 1978b). Less clear, however, was the role that displaced discs might play in causing pain in the TMJ region or in causing eventual degeneration of joint structures.

Surgical Reports

Further confirmation of disc displacement came from open surgical procedures performed on human TMJs to correct clinical problems (Dolwick, 1985; Walker, 1987). During these

procedures, one could demonstrate the clicking caused by a displaced disc by manipulating the mandible while the TMJ was surgically exposed. The direct observations also revealed a significant medial component to many of the anterior displacements noted on lateral arthrotomographic films, as well as a variety of three-dimensional alterations of disc morphology that were not visualized on such films. Postsurgical histological studies of excised discs and/or condylar tissue showed significant changes, similar to those reported in cadavers by Hansson (1977). Later, Scapino (1983) published a landmark study detailing these changes.

Change of Focus from Myofascial Pain-Dysfunction Syndrome to Intracapsular Derangements

The net result of all the discoveries described in the preceding section was a sudden and massive shift in approaches to clinical management of TMD patients. As noted in a previous publication (Greene, 1988a): "The discovery of internal derangements (has) led to the greatest rash of revisionist thinking in the history of the dental profession. Practically overnight, MPD was proclaimed dead and the age of disc derangements was begun; muscles were out and discs were in; (and) arthritis became the new bogeyman to threaten every patient with a clicking jaw. . . ." This change of focus led to significant changes in many clinicians' attitudes about TMD patients, especially if they had clicking, popping, or grating sounds in the TMJ. Even otherwise asymptomatic individuals who were discovered to have such sounds during routine checkups or epidemiological examinations were considered to have a premorbid condition, and they were urged to seek early treatment to prevent subsequent damage. Many of these patients also were subjected to painful diagnostic arthrograms to document the displacement of their discs.

Empirical Development of Treatments for Disc Displacements

Prosthetic Recapturing of Displaced Discs

The earliest concepts about TMJ clicking included ideas about how to return the displaced disc to a normal position. In 1954 a study was published on the posterosuperior displacement of the condyle, which according to Thompson (1954) could cause the condyle to slip off the back end of the biconcave disc.

Thompson was among the first to advocate a forward positioning of the mandible to recapture the disc. Although current evidence shows clearly that discs slip forward and medially rather than that condyles slip backward, an aggressive concept of recapturing the disc has become more widespread in the past 20 years.

Despite the lack of either basic or clinical research to support these procedures, clinicians began to devise remarkable intraoral appliances that could bring the mandible forward and (hopefully) into the center of the displaced disc. The foremost proponent of this approach in the 1970s was Farrar (1971), who designed anterior repositioning appliances and recommended procedures for eventually "walking the disc" back to create a more normal alignment of condyle, disc, and fossa. It was not long, however, before Farrar and others realized that a complete return of the condyle and disc to a normal centric TMJ relationship generally could not be accomplished in this manner (Clark, 1984; Moloney, 1986), and this led to the conclusion that both the condyle and disc would have to be maintained forever in a protruded position by means of major dental procedures (orthodontics, orthognathic surgery, and prosthetic rehabilitation) if clicking was to be eliminated permanently.

Surgical Correction or Removal of Displaced Discs

Soon most dentists discovered that a large number of displaced discs could not be recaptured by prosthetic or manipulative procedures. Some could be recaptured temporarily, but would slip out again during function, while others simply were displaced too far anteriorly to be repositioned by these mechanical methods. Farrar and McCarty (1982) were among the first to recognize this phenomenon and reported on surgical approaches to these problems. Using surgical procedures developed initially by orthopedic surgeons, oral surgeons began either to reposition displaced discs over condyles, or to remove them and insert alloplastic materials to substitute for the natural disc. The current status of these surgical concepts is described in more detail in Chapter 24.

Arthroscopy

With the development of miniaturized arthroscopes, it has become possible to use these instruments inside the TMJ (Neulle, 1986). The indications for, and outcomes of, arthroscopic procedures on TMJ patients are still not clear, but some early clinical reports are favorable. However, a recent study by Gabler (1989), using pre- and postoperative magnetic resonance imaging (MRI) of arthroscopically treated patients, showed that both condyles and discs moved farther anteriorly in successfully treated patients, but that the discs did not become recaptured by this procedure. On a clinical basis, 11 of 12 patients reported great improvement in opening the mouth and relief from pain. Further discussion of this modality can be found in Chapters 17 and 24.

DECLINE OF IMPORTANCE OF DISPLACED DISCS IN THE FIELD OF TEMPOROMANDIBULAR DISORDERS

Early Concepts of Progression and Morbidity

There is still considerable controversy about the clinical significance of internal derangements of the TMJ. The concept that disc displacements always represent a serious biological problem in the human TMJ appears to have followed directly from the technological studies that demonstrated their existence. It almost seemed as if one day they were discovered, the next day they were described as pathological or premorbid, and the following day clinical treatments were proposed. In retrospect, it seems that the conceptual basis for predicting negative sequelae in patients with clicking was derived from three assumptions (Farrar, 1971; 1982; Neulle, 1986): a properly positioned disc is essential for normal TMJ comfort and function; displacement of a disc will result in pain as the condyle then articulates on sensitive retrodiscal tissues. Finally, the joint tissues will become more vulnerable to arthritic degeneration if the disc is not properly interposed between the condyle and eminence, especially if the retrodiscal tissue becomes perforated. Most of these assumptions, however, have proved to be partially or totally incorrect. Normal position of the disc has not been found to be absolutely essential for normal function, whereas discs in abnormal position have turned out to be something to which many TMJs can accommodate.

The acceptance of such assumptions, however, has led many practitioners to further assumptions about how to deal clinically with patients who have clicking (Eriksson, 1986; Farrar, 1971). These include the belief that displaced discs must be repositioned between the condyle and eminence by some form of dental or surgical treatment; that early intervention to correct disc displacement is desirable to avoid irreversible deformity of the disc; that repositioning (recapturing) a disc is so important that it is acceptable to reposition the mandible permanently in an anterior location with appliances and to keep it there with major dental procedures (stabilization); and finally, that if the disc cannot be prosthetically repositioned within a reasonable time, it may be necessary to perform surgery to either reposition or replace it. The results of numerous epidemiological studies, however, fail to support these concepts (see Chapter 14).

Epidemiologic Studies

General Population Studies

The initial epidemiologic studies to determine the incidence and prevalence of TMDs were reported from the Scandinavian countries (Helkimo, 1974; Molin, 1976), but later studies came from other countries as well (Solberg, 1979). While there were some serious criticisms about the methodology of some of these studies (Greene, 1982a), the objective reports of TMJ sounds could not be disputed. These sounds were by far the most ubiquitous finding in every study, being present in one-third to two-thirds of every population surveyed. The most important aspect of this finding, however, was the lack of clinical symptoms of pain or dysfunction in the vast majority of individuals with TMJ clicking, not only at the time of the study but also during preceding years. These cross-sectional studies later were supplemented by longitudinal surveys of child, adolescent, and adult populations (Magnusson, 1986; Wanman, 1986). They showed that joint sounds either fluctuated or remained consistent over time, but only rarely became worse.

Cadaver Studies

Autopsies conducted on a large number of cadaver specimens showed a surprisingly high incidence of intracapsular derangements and deformities in the TMJs of nearly every age group (Hansson, 1980; Westesson, 1984). At this histological level, there usually was evidence of regressive remodeling in the affected joints. At first, these findings were presented as evidence for the pathologic potential of disc derangements, but in time they came to be recognized as adaptive compensatory changes

that enabled joints to function adequately despite having displaced tissues (Solberg, 1985). One of the most important observations, later confirmed in surgical specimens, was that retrodiscal tissues could undergo a metaplastic conversion to dense fibrous tissue that functioned as a pseudodisc for many patients (Blaustein, 1986).

Geriatric Population Studies

Surveys of elderly populations by Heft (1984) and Clark (1984b) showed that the prevalence of TMD signs and symptoms in these groups was as low as or lower than in younger populations. Instead of popping or clicking sounds, one was more likely to find grating or crepitant sounds in their TMJs, but the myofascial complaints that are typical of younger individuals were less common in these patients. These findings argued against the popular notion that untreated disc displacement would inevitably lead to progressive joint degeneration and increasing signs and symptoms of dysfunction.

Taken together, the three types of epidemiologic studies previously described indicate that the concerns of early investigators about the pathological potential of disc displacements were largely unfounded. While there may have been some theoretic basis for their concern (Katzberg, 1983), the evidence is becoming increasingly clear that most individuals with such displacements live asymptomatically and adapt anatomically, histologically, and physiologically to their condition (see Chapter 6).

Failure of Prosthetic Recapturing Techniques

The early enthusiasm about recapturing displaced discs with intraoral appliances began to fade as certain facts began to emerge. For one thing, Tallents (1985) showed that most repositioning appliances actually failed to place the condyle and disc in normal alignment. Using a cinefluoroscopic technique, Tallents showed that it was possible to align these structures in some instances, but in general it required even more mandibular protrusion than had previously been thought necessary. Around the same time, other investigators also began to report both short-term and long-term failure of attempts to recapture discs and stabilize them permanently in their new positions (Clark, 1984a; Moloney, 1986). One study of over 300 patients reported a 90 per cent success rate after six months of anterior repositioning appliance therapy, only to have many of them end up with a superior repositioning splint that put their condyles back into a centric relation position (Williamson, 1985). If it is true that most displaced discs cannot be prosthetically maintained in a normal centric position, and all available evidence seems to indicate that this is so, then these patients' discs merely took a round trip journey while symptoms diminished during the treatment period.

Longitudinal Studies of Symptomatic Patients

Only three studies have looked specifically at the outcome of patients with anterior disc displacement who were treated conservatively in a TMJ clinic. One (Helkimo, 1987) showed no significant difference between these patients and nonclicking TMJ patients after one year, while the second (Lundh, 1987) reported that only six of 70 patients with clicking progressed to locking after three years. In 1988, Greene and Laskin published a study of a large clinical population of conservatively treated patients who were followed over longer periods of time (up to 15 years in some cases) (Greene, 1988b). These patients included 132 University TMJ Clinic subjects and 58 from private practice, all of whom had symptomatic TMD problems that included clicking sounds when they came for initial treatment. At the time of follow-up, about one-third of these patients no longer had clicking, one-third had reduced clicking, and one-third were essentially unchanged. Only three of the 190 subjects reported progression to worse clicking or disc dysfunction (sticking, locking, and so on).

While disc derangement remains an important feature of many TMDs, it is becoming increasingly clear that most individuals who have clicking of the TMJ can be left alone if they are otherwise asymptomatic, and they can be treated later if they become symptomatic. The goal of such treatment generally is simply to reduce symptoms while allowing the body time to adapt to the internal derangement (see Chapter 23 for more specific information on the nonsurgical management of patients with symptomatic internal derangements). Only if there is persistent pain or if significant locking develops should surgery be considered.

EMERGENCE OF TECHNOLOGICAL METHODS FOR EVALUATING AND TREATING TEMPOROMANDIBULAR DISORDERS

Technological Methods for Diagnosis

The traditional approach to differential diagnosis of craniofacial pain has been the classical history and physical examination, with an emphasis on the timing and quality of pain episodes (see Chapter 25). With the development of various technological methods to study the anatomy and function of the TMJ, there have been some attempts to apply these methods to clinical diagnosis. For example, electromyography (EMG) has been used to study the activity of various jaw muscles in both normal and symptomatic subjects, and several interesting differences between these groups have been observed (Hannam, 1977). However, when an attempt is made to use EMG as a clinical diagnostic procedure, the findings in an individual patient are generally not clear enough to establish a clinical diagnosis. This is due to such confounding factors as the high variability of normal EMG readings, inconsistent electrode placement, recording problems, and a frequent lack of clear-cut positive findings that would indicate muscle dysfunction (Lavigne, 1983; Lund, 1989).

A similar analysis can be made in regard to jaw tracking machines, joint sound recording machines, and thermography, where the correlations between symptoms and positive findings are variable enough to make accurate differential diagnosis impossible. In the case of conventional radiographs, although they are helpful when gross changes are present, the controversy has been compounded by the attempts of some clinicians to use these distorted images to determine the correctness of condyle-fossa spatial relationships (Thompson, 1964; Weinberg, 1979). After many years of studies and arguments, it has become quite clear not only that such relationships cannot be reliably determined from plain radiographs, but also that the great variability of "normal" positions makes any conclusions about pathology based on spatial TMJ relationships highly suspect (Blaschke, 1981; Pullinger, 1985). Currently, the only valid diagnostic interpretations of TMJ images are those made from arthrotomograms or magnetic resonance imaging (MRI) regarding disc displacement, or those made from tomograms, CT scans, or plain films regarding gross bony changes in the joint structures.

Clinical diagnosis of TMJ problems still must be made primarily by direct examination rather than by diagnostic machines or devices. While this may be disappointing to some, it should be remembered that the nature and location of TMDs at least makes them accessible to direct examination—unlike such disorders as cardiovascular disease or liver dysfunction, which absolutely require some form of technological testing to be discovered and analyzed accurately. Differential diagnosis of craniofacial pain remains a difficult challenge for the clinician, but the required skills can be learned by those who care to do so (see Chapters 8 and 25).

Technological Methods for Treatment

Most of the traditional treatments for TMDs have been nontechnological, but some recent therapeutic developments in physical medicine also have been applied to TMD patients. While the definitive clinical studies needed to confirm their effectiveness generally are lacking, clinical experience suggests that some traditional physical therapy methods can be helpful (Abramovitch, 1988). Diathermy, ultrasound, and electrogalvanic stimulation, along with certain manipulative techniques, seem to be useful adjuncts to other treatments for relief of pain and restoration of normal TMJ function. Biofeedback also has been shown to be useful in teaching patients to reduce muscle tension and control pain (Gale, 1983).

HOLISTIC CONCEPTS OF TEMPOROMANDIBULAR DISORDERS

The original development of holistic thinking about the TMJ came from a chiropractic concept known as applied kinesiology (Goodheart, 1976a; 1976b), a concept that has nothing in common with the medical discipline of kinesiology, i.e. the study of body movements. This concept was based on alleged whole body relationships between various structures. As described by Goodheart (1976a; 1976b), Eversaul (1977), and others (Diamond, 1979), every organ dysfunction has an associated weak muscle. Thus, virtually any disease state of the body will have a structural manifestation—a specific muscle weakness pattern that can be used for making the diagnosis. This diagnosis can be established by a method known as therapy localization, in which the patient places his own hand on the area that is bothering him, and the corresponding indicator muscle is tested for strength or weakness. Goodheart (1976a) states that ". . . therapy localization is capable of identifying virtually all faults and dysfunctions which have an effect on the nervous system."

The dental version of this concept involves testing arm muscle strength while various interocclusal wafers are used to alter vertical dimension (Eversaul, 1977; Goodheart, 1976b). When the correct vertical position is obtained, it is claimed that the arm strength will be maximal. Also, therapy localization is used by having the patient place his hand over the sore TMJ area, and appropriate indicator muscles are tested. Athletes are believed to become stronger and faster with proper biteplates placed in their mouths.

According to this "neurophysiological concept," it is presumed that dysfunctioning muscles or organs send some kind of message to the central nervous system and that a return message is transmitted peripherally to an otherwise innocent and healthy indicator muscle. Learning to read this peculiar version of body language is supposed to provide diagnostic information. This type of testing currently is going on in many dental offices throughout the world, despite the fact that there is practically no independent scientific evidence to support either the validity of this concept or the efficacy of treatment based on these findings (Greene, 1984).

Another major avant-garde concept in the TMD field is that of "dental stress" (Fonder, 1977; Gelb, 1977). This idea differs from the kinesiology theory in that it places the craniomandibular articulation in the primary position. In this concept, an improperly aligned mandible produces dental stress and becomes the basis for widespread body symptoms and dysfunctions. The neurophysiological basis for this phenomenon is described as dysponetic reflexes, which are presumed to go to the brain and then out to the rest of the body (Whatmore, 1974). A more chiropractic version of this idea states that the malaligned mandible affects the spine and thereby produces effects on other structures throughout the body.

Thus, the mere existence of the improper mandibular relationship is in itself the stressor, and the conditions produced are attributed to dental stress. This type of thinking comes from individuals within our profession (Fonder, 1977; Gelb, 1977) beginning as long as 30 years ago, and the modern versions are growing in popularity. The advocates of this peculiar stress concept often invoke Selye's general adaptation syndrome (Selye, 1950; 1956) in an attempt to legitimize their position.

CURRENT STATUS OF CONCEPTS ABOUT THE ETIOLOGY AND TREATMENT OF TEMPOROMANDIBULAR DISORDERS

Understanding the Controversies

Rarely in the history of medicine and dentistry in the twentieth century have so many researchers labored so hard and for so long, only to end up with the kind of controversial status that the subject of TMDs has reached today. By using a historic perspective, we can try to understand why this is so: (1) The disorders themselves are complex and often difficult to distinguish from other craniofacial problems; (2) The methods of diagnosis have necessarily been limited to direct examination and history taking procedures; (3) Theories of etiology have been spun from the minds of clinicians rather than developed through scientific research; and perhaps most important, (4) Various treatment approaches have been used and they seem to have produced, in general, largely favorable outcomes. The combination of these factors has led to understandable differences among clinicians and even among researchers. To express this another way, the clinical successes obtained under so many different theoretic frameworks have reinforced the convictions of those who subscribe to each theory.

Beginning to Resolve the Controversies: Contributions from Research

While the controversial situation previously described is a long way from being totally resolved, some important research findings over the past 20 years have begun to make an impact on this field. The etiologic assumptions of many clinicians have been challenged by a combination of correlational and clinical outcome studies and many theories have been found to be either incorrect or lacking validation. For example, the idea that various occlusal factors (vertical dimension, malocclusion, occlusal interferences, missing teeth, and so forth) are a prime

cause of TMDs has not been supported by either epidemiological (Carlsson, 1984a; Greene, 1982a) or correlational (Droukas, 1985; Zarb, 1988) data.

These kinds of occlusal factors appear to be fairly ubiquitous, and they do not occur more often in patients with symptoms than they do in age- and sex-matched random populations. Likewise, psychological states and traits that once were thought to be more prevalent in patients than in normal individuals have not been found to be so in large population studies (Malow, 1981; Rugh, 1983). It would be fair to conclude at this time that no single etiologic factor, or any known combination of factors, can totally explain why most people get various TMDs. The only exceptions are the obvious ones attributable to extrinsic or intrinsic trauma to temporomandibular structures: auto accidents, fists hitting chins, biting on hard objects, subluxations when yawning, and so forth.

The second group of studies that have influenced contemporary viewpoints about TMDs are those that have evaluated short-term and long-term clinical responses to various treatment approaches. At first, each study of this type was nothing more than an attempt to measure the efficacy of a particular treatment approach. With the introduction of placebo control groups, however, it became increasingly clear that TMD patients could be very responsive to *any* treatment—even a fake or placebo treatment (Goodman, 1976; Greene, 1971; Laskin, 1972). Comparative studies generally showed that one treatment approach was not significantly better than another, but that both helped a large percentage of symptomatic patients (Greene, 1983). Long-term studies conducted years after treatment confirmed this observation. They also showed that successfully treated patients, regardless of *how* they were treated, tended to stay well years after their initial recovery (Greene, 1974; Mjersjo, 1983). Most important, these long-term studies showed that irreversible treatments that had been presumed to be necessary or definitive (e.g., occlusal equilibration, bite-opening, orthodontics, surgical procedures) produced no better results than programs using entirely reversible treatments (Greene, 1983). As Moulton (1966) pointed out, however, the worst outcome cases were those involving patients who became entrapped in the search for a definitive treatment after failing to respond initially to some type of irreversible therapy.

EMERGENCE OF A MEDICAL ORTHOPEDICS VIEWPOINT

Recognition That Temporomandibular Disorders Are Similar to Other Musculoskeletal Disorders

The early concepts of TMDs were influenced in a major way by dental-oriented thinking. Problems affecting this region were described in terms of occlusal relationships, condylar positions, or skeletal asymmetries, while focusing on the unique characteristics of the human TMJ. Recently, however, it has become increasingly apparent that disorders of this joint are nearly identical to those affecting all synovial joints and their associated structures: anatomic derangements, intracapsular inflammation and degeneration, local myofascial disorders, systemic connective tissue diseases, congenital and developmental anomalies. This change in perspective has made it possible to discuss diagnosis, etiology, and treatment of TMDs in a more rational framework of medical orthopedics (Greene, 1984).

Differential Diagnosis and Classification of Temporomandibular Disorders

The first problem in differential diagnosis of craniofacial pain is to identify the general source of the problem (see Chapter 25 for detailed discussion). If the source appears to be the TMJ structures, then a differentiation between extracapsular or intracapsular problems is necessary. As in other areas of orthopedic medicine, this kind of diagnostic subclassification requires a thorough understanding of various signs and symptoms that are characteristic for each disorder. In the final analysis, orthopedic diagnosis is nothing more than determining what is happening, and in which tissue(s). One should not minimize the difficulty of accomplishing this goal. Working within this orthopedic framework, we should utilize the language of medical pathology and dysfunction, while avoiding the use of special labels such as condylar malposition, mandibular malalignment, and TMJ syndrome.

Recognition of the Multifactorial Etiology of Various Temporomandibular Disorders

While some patients with TMDs report specific events that initiated their problems, most of them do not. In the past, it was common to blame some observed structural fault for causing the TMD to occur. The etiology of musculoskeletal pain and dysfunction can be quite complex. In a general sense, three types of factors are likely to be involved in the onset of such disorders: (1) predisposing factors, (2) precipitating factors, and (3) perpetuating factors. For example, a patient may be predisposed to develop a TMD by virtue of congenital or acquired anatomic factors that make him or her susceptible to an anatomic displacement or a functional overload, and this condition may be perpetuated by life stress factors or systemic illness.

Although this is a useful theoretic framework for understanding the development of clinical orthopedic problems, in practice it has limited applications. Specific identification of etiologic factors is possible at times, but most often it cannot be done scientifically because of the confusing overlap of normal variations in form and function. This situation holds true for the etiology of TMDs just as it does for other orthopedic problems, and in the end we have only reasonable assumptions to work with clinically.

Recognition That Psychological Factors Can Affect the Onset, Progression, and Remission of Many Temporomandibular Disorders

Psychological factors have long been recognized as playing an important role in the course of various physical disorders (see Chapter 20). When asked to classify all human disorders on a scale from one to six, with one being purely physical and six being purely psychological, it was suggested that the first step was to eliminate one and six from the scale.

In the case of TMDs, psychological factors went from being totally unrecognized to being named as the major cause of certain disorders. Various personality states or traits were described as etiologic factors, and environmental stress was blamed for the development of bruxism as well as for development of clinical symptoms. Over time, these etiologic assumptions failed to stand up to careful scrutiny (Rugh, 1976; 1983) and for some people this signaled the end of psychological factors as meaningful variables in TMDs. A more reasonable conclusion, however, was suggested by Greene (1982b). Psychological factors can precipitate the onset of an acute myofascial pain episode or cause chronic muscle tension, and they also can perpetuate the symptoms in a chronic pain condition. In addition, psychological factors may play a definite role in the response of patients to various physical and pharmacological therapies, and some psychological treatment approaches can provide significant relief for certain patient subgroups (Marbach, 1975; Pomp, 1974).

Utilization of General Principles of Orthopedic Medicine in Treating Temporomandibular Disorders

In the final analysis, the significance of the medical orthopedic point of view in the field of TMDs lies in its treatment ramifications. The traditional dental-structural viewpoint invariably led to treatments that were intended to correct mechanical and morphofunctional problems, and as a result it was expected that pain would disappear and normal function would return. By utilizing a medical orthopedic framework, however, the goals as well as the methods of treatment change considerably. Reduction of pain and inflammation in tissues becomes the primary goal, with reduction of muscle hyperactivity being an important secondary objective (see Chapter 9). After tissues have been allowed to heal, resumption of normal function is accomplished by using various rehabilitative techniques such as physical therapy and exercise.

Research has shown that this therapeutic approach to TMDs works very well for most patients, even when joint tissues are compromised by anatomic derangements or deformities. Unfortunately, many clinicians who still subscribe to dental-structural theories use a medical orthopedic approach for initial treatment (Phase I), but then go on to perform irreversible dental treatments after the symptoms have resolved (Phase II), despite the lack of convincing evidence that Phase II therapy is really necessary in most cases (see Chapter 21).

Judicious Use of Surgical Procedures in Appropriate Situations

According to the medical orthopedic point of view, some patients with musculoskeletal disorders will require surgical treatment to get relief from their problems. The classic argument in that field, however, is over which patients really need such treatment. Failure to respond to nonsurgical therapy is not sufficient grounds for proceeding with surgery. Rather, the patient must have an anatomic or pathologic condition

that correlates closely with the clinical symptoms of pain and dysfunction; the condition must be operable in a predictable manner; the use of appropriate nonsurgical therapy should have been tried long enough to be sure it is not successful; and finally, the patient must have the final decision about whether his or her quality of life is bad enough to justify attempting a surgical procedure (Greene, 1988a) (see Chapter 24).

CHRONIC PAIN RELATED TO TEMPOROMANDIBULAR DISORDERS

Understanding Modern Concepts of Chronic Pain

Physicians traditionally have been concerned about, and responsible for, managing a broad spectrum of acute and chronic pain problems. Dentists have mainly been concerned with acute orofacial pain problems arising from specific dental pathology. Chronic pain problems can arise in the orofacial region just as they do elsewhere in the body (Bonica, 1980). Phenomena such as idiopathic facial pain, atypical odontalgia, lower-half headache, and chronic myofascial pain have been described. Therefore, those clinicians who are responsible for treating head and neck pain have had to change their thinking about what pain really means so that they could become better pain therapists (see Chapter 25).

Most dentists currently practicing were trained according to the concept of pain being a signal that travels along simple electrical wiring that serves as a danger alert system for the body. This has led many a dentist on a merry diagnostic chase to find out exactly what and where the source of the pain may be. Furthermore, the traditional notion of pain always being a symptom of specific pathology has led to many treatments that were intended definitively to remove the cause of the pain. In terms of the traditional dentist-patient relationship, those unfortunate pain patients who failed to respond to our best treatment efforts often were placed in perjorative categories such as crock, neurotic, complainer, psychogenic, and so forth.

A large body of research conducted during the past 30 years has expanded our understanding of pain phenomenology. Beginning with the placebo studies of Beecher (1955), and supported by the gate-control theories of Melzack (1965), it has become obvious that pain does not always have a direct correlation with tissue injury or pathology. These findings, along with extensive clinical observations, led Crue (1975) to define chronic pain patients as ". . . those who complain chiefly of pain, but whose suffering is due either to unknown etiology and mechanism, or to trauma or disease that is considered too minor, or to have occurred so long ago, that it no longer can be regarded as a valid explanation for their symptoms." Instead, behavioral theorists such as Sternbach (1974) and Fordyce (1976) have postulated that chronic pain is another form of learned (conditioned) behavior, in which positive reinforcers from the patient's environment serve to perpetuate the painful state. Further discussion of these issues can be found in a review study by Greene (1981).

Management of Patients with Chronic Temporomandibular Disorders

Every dentist can expect that some of the TMD patients whom he or she treats will fail to respond to therapy, while also encountering some colleagues' failures. The first problem when this occurs is to deal with one's own feelings and attitudes about such patients. In the past, it was common for dentists either to escalate the intensity of therapy for nonresponding patients (for example, by performing a surgical procedure), or to regard these patients as having psychological problems. An awareness of some of the factors discussed earlier should lead to more enlightened attitudes about such matters. As a result, these unfortunate patients may be able to receive more modern methods of treatment for chronic pain.

Studies have been reported in which nonresponding TMD patients were treated successfully in various ways. The most promising results have been obtained with either individual (Pomp, 1974) or group (Marbach, 1975) psychotherapy. Good results also have been reported with various relaxation training methods such as biofeedback, guided imagery, and progressive relaxation (Dohrmann, 1978; Gale, 1983; Malow, 1981). The inpatient type of behavior modification program described by Fordyce (1976) has not been reported yet for MPD patients, but many patients with chronic headache problems have been successfully treated in this manner.

In addition, Clark (1987) described a limited function protocol for TMD patients who do not respond favorably to treatment. By staying within prescribed limits, many of these patients can manage their own problems and live an adequate life, thereby avoiding the risks or trauma of additional therapy. Over a long period of time, some of these patients will gradually experience relief (Greene, 1974).

SUMMARY

Dentistry is at a crossroads regarding the development of professional attitudes toward TMDs as well as toward chronic pain. When the dominating influence of the technically oriented clinician is finally replaced by a broader perspective and a more scientific approach to the study of stomatognathic system anatomy and physiology, we will achieve a more comprehensive understanding of how this vital complex functions and dysfunctions. If the next generation of dentists can be encouraged to study craniofacial pain and dysfunction with the same enthusiasm that they have applied to caries and periodontal disease, we may make some real progress toward a more rational system of diagnosis and treatment for TMDs that closely parallels the medical orthopedic and chronic pain models.

REFERENCES

Abramovitch, K., Langlais, R. P., and Bradley, G. R.: Physical therapy. In Mohl, N. D., Zarb, G. A., Carlsson, G. E., and Rugh, J. D. (Eds.): A Textbook of Occlusion. Chicago, Quintessence, 1988, pp. 333–350.

Beecher, H. K.: The powerful placebo. JAMA 159:1602–1605, 1955.

Blaschke, D. D., and Blaschke, T. J.: Normal TMJ bone relationships in centric occlusion. J. Dent. Res. 60:98–104, 1981.

Blaustein, D. I., and Scapino, R. P.: Remodelling of the temporomandibular joint disc and posterior attachment in disc displacement specimens in relation to glycosaminoglycan content. Plast. Reconstr. Surg. 78:756–764, 1986.

Bonica, J. J. (Ed.): Pain. New York, Raven Press, 1980.

Carlsson, G. E.: Epidemiologic studies of signs and symptoms of temporomandibular joint pain-dysfunction. A literature review. Australian Soc. Prosthod. Bull. 14:7–12, 1984a.

Carlsson, G. E., and Droukas, B.: Dental occlusion and the health of the masticatory system—A literature review. J. Craniomandib. Pract. 2:142–147, 1984b.

Clark, G. T.: Treatment of jaw clicking with temporomandibular repositioning: Analysis of 25 cases. J. Craniomandib. Pract. 2:263–270, 1984a.

Clark, G. T., and Mulligan, R.: A review of the prevalence of temporomandibular dysfunction. Gerodontology 3:231–236, 1984b.

Clark, G. T.: Diagnosis and treatment of painful temporomandibular disorders. Dent. Clin. North Am. 31:645–673, 1987.

Costen, J. B.: A syndrome of ear and sinus symptoms dependent upon disturbed function of the temporomandibular joint. Ann. Otol. Rhinol. Laryngol. 43:1–15, 1934.

Crue, B. L.: The present status of therapy for chronic pain states. In Crue, B. L. (Ed.): Pain: Research and Treatment. New York, Academic Press, 1975.

Dawson, P. E.: Temporomandibular joint pain-dysfunction problems can be solved. J. Prosthet. Dent. 29:100–112, 1973.

Dawson, P. E.: Evaluation, Diagnosis, and Treatment of Occlusal Problems. St. Louis, C. V. Mosby, 1974.

Diamond, J. D.: Behavioral Kinesiology. New York, Harper & Row, 1979.

Dohrmann, R. J., and Laskin, D. M.: An evaluation of electromyographic biofeedback in the treatment of myofascial pain-dysfunction syndrome. J. Am. Dent. Assoc. 96:656–662, 1978.

Dolwick, M. F., Katzberg, R. W., and Helms, C. A.: Internal derangements of the temporomandibular joint: Fact or fiction? J. Prosthet. Dent. 49:415–418, 1983.

Dolwick, M. F., and Sanders, B.: TMJ Internal Derangements and Arthrosis. St. Louis, C. V. Mosby, 1985.

Droukas, B., Lindee, C., and Carlsson, G. E.: Relationship between occlusal factors and signs and symptoms of mandibular dysfunction. A clinical study of 48 dental students. Acta Odontol. Scand. 42:277–283, 1984.

Droukas, B., Lindee, C., and Carlsson, G. E.: Occlusion and mandibular dysfunction: A clinical study of patients referred for functional disturbances of the masticatory system. J. Prosthet. Dent. 53:402–406, 1985.

Eriksson, L., and Westesson, P-L.: Diskectomy in the treatment of anterior disc displacement of the temporomandibular joint. A clinical and radiologic one-year follow-up study. J. Prosthet. Dent. 55:106–116, 1986.

Eversaul, G.: Dental Kinesiology. Las Vegas, NV, George Eversaul, 1977.

Farrar, W. B.: Diagnosis and treatment of anterior dislocation of the articular disc. NY J. Dent. 41:348–351, 1971.

Farrar, W. B., and McCarty, W. L. Jr.: A Clinical Outline of Temporomandibular Diagnosis and Treatment. Montgomery, AL, Normandie Publications, 1982.

Fonder, A. C.: Dental Physician. Blacksburg, VA, University Publications, 1977.

Fordyce, W. E.: Behavioral Methods for Chronic Pain and Illness. St. Louis, C. V. Mosby, 1976.

Franks, A. S. T.: The social character of temporomandibular joint dysfunction. Dent. Pract. 15:94–100, 1964.

Franks, A. S. T.: Masticatory muscle hyperactivity and temporomandibular joint dysfunctions. J. Prosthet. Dent. 15:1122–1131, 1965.

Gabler, M., Greene, C. S., Palacios, E., et al.: Effect of arthroscopic TMJ surgery on articular disc position. J. Craniomandib. Disord. Facial Oral Pain, 3:191–202, 1989.

Gale, E. N.: Behavioral management of MPD. In Laskin, D. M., Greenfield, W., Gale, E., et al. (Eds.): The President's Conference on the Examination, Diagnosis, and Management of Temporomandibular Disorders. Chicago, Am. Dent. Assoc., 1983, pp. 161–166.

Gelb, H.: Evaluation of static centric relation in the temporomandibular joint dysfunction syndrome. Dent. Clin. North Am. 19:519–530, 1975.

Gelb, H. (Ed.): Clinical Management of Head, Neck, and TMJ Pain and Dysfunction. Philadelphia, W. B. Saunders, 1977.

Goldstein, I. B.: Role of muscle tension in personality theory. Psychol. Bull. 61:413–425, 1964a.

Goldstein, I. B., Grinker, R. R., Heath, H. P., et al.:

Study in psychophysiology of muscle tension: I. Response specificity. Arch. Gen. Psychiatry. 11:322–330, 1964b.

Goodheart, G. J.: Applied Kinesiology, ed. 12. Workshop Procedure Manual, Detroit, George Goodheart, 1976a.

Goodheart, G. J.: Kinesiology and dentistry. J. Am. Soc. Prev. Dent. 6:16–18, 1976b.

Goodman, P., Greene, C. S., and Laskin, D. M.: Response of patients with myofascial pain-dysfunction syndrome to mock equilibration. J. Am. Dent. Assoc. 92:755–758, 1976.

Greene, C. S.: Myofascial pain-dysfunction syndrome: The evolution of concepts. In Sarnat, B. G., and Laskin, D. M. (Eds.): The Temporomandibular Joint: A Biological Basis for Clinical Practice, 3rd ed. Springfield, IL, Charles C Thomas, 1980, pp. 277–288.

Greene, C. S.: A critique of nonconventional treatment concepts and procedures for TMJ disorders. Compendium of Continuing Dental Education 5:848–852, 1984. (Originally presented at ADA President's Conference on Temporomandibular Disorders, 1982.)

Greene, C. S.: The application of modern pain management concepts to the myofascial pain-dysfunction (MPD) syndrome. In Kawamura, Y., and Dubner, R. (Eds.): Oral-Facial Sensory and Motor Functions. Chicago, Quintessence, 1981, pp. 283–291.

Greene, C. S.: Temporomandibular disorders. In Clark, J. W. (Ed.): Clinical Dentistry. Philadelphia, Harper & Row, 1984, Chapter 37.

Greene, C. S.: The relationship between pain, pathology, and surgery in the treatment of temporomandibular disorders. In Keith, D. A. (Ed.): Surgery of the Temporomandibular Joint. Boston, Blackwell Scientific, 1988a.

Greene, C. S., and Laskin, D. M.: Meprobamate therapy for the myofascial pain-dysfunction (MPD) syndrome: A double-blind evaluation. J. Am. Dent. Assoc. 85:587–590, 1971.

Greene, C. S., and Laskin, D. M.: Long-term evaluation of conservative treatment for myofascial pain-dysfunction syndrome. J. Am. Dent. Assoc. 89:1365–1368, 1974.

Greene, C. S., and Laskin, D. M.: Long-term evaluation of treatment for myofascial pain-dysfunction syndrome: A comparative analysis. J. Am. Dent. Assoc. 107:235–238, 1983.

Greene, C. S., and Laskin, D. M.: Long-term status of clicking in patients with myofascial pain and dysfunction. J. Am. Dent. Assoc. 117:461–465, 1988b.

Greene, C. S., and Marbach, J. J.: Epidemiologic studies of mandibular dysfunction: A critical review. J. Prosthet. Dent. 48:184–190, 1982a.

Greene, C. S., Olson, R. E., and Laskin, D. M.: Psychological factors in the etiology, progression, and treatment of MPD syndrome. J. Am. Dent. Assoc. 105:443–448, 1982b.

Guichet, N. F.: Applied gnathology: Why and how. Dent. Clin. North Am. 16:687–700, 1969.

Hannam, A. G., DeCou, R. E., Scott, J. D., et al.: The relationship between dental occlusion, muscle activity, and associated jaw movement in man. Arch. Oral Biol. 22:25–32, 1977.

Hansson, T.: Temporomandibular joint changes related to dental occlusion. In Solberg, W. K., and Clark, G. T. (Eds.): Temporomandibular Joint Problems: Biologic Diagnosis and Treatment. Chicago, Quintessence, 1980, p. 129.

Hansson, T., and Nordstrom, B.: Thickness of soft tissue layers and articular disc in temporomandibular joints with deviations in form. Acta Odontol. Scand. 35:281–288, 1977.

Heft, M. W.: Prevalence of TMJ signs and symptoms in the elderly. Gerodontology 3:125–130, 1984.

Helkimo, E.: Studies on the function and dysfunction of the masticatory system. III. Analyses of anamnestic and clinical recordings of dysfunction with the aid of indices. Swedish Dent. J. 67:165–181, 1974.

Helkimo, E., and Westling, L.: History, clinical findings, and outcome of treatment of patients with anterior disc displacement. J. Craniomandib. Pract. 5:269–276, 1987.

Ireland, V. E.: The problem of "the clicking jaw." Proc. R. Soc. Med. 44:363–372, 1951.

Isberg-Holm, A.: Temporomandibular Joint Clicking. Dissertation. Karolinska Institute, Stockholm, 1980.

Jarabak, J. R.: An electromyographic analysis of muscular and temporomandibular joint disturbances due to imbalances in occlusion. Angle Orthod. 26:170–190, 1956.

Johnson, D. L., Shipman, W. G., and Laskin, D. M.: Physiologic responses to stressful stimuli in patients with myofascial pain-dysfunction (MPD) syndrome. IADR Program and Abstracts of Papers, Chicago, IADR, 1972, p. 96.

Katzberg, R. W., Dolwick, M. F., Helms, C. A., et al.: Arthrotomography of the temporomandibular joint. Am. J. Roentgenol. 134:995–1003, 1980.

Katzberg, R. W., Keith, P. A., Guralnick, W. C., et al.: Internal derangements and arthritis of the temporomandibular joint. Radiology 146:107–112, 1983.

Kraus, H. T.: Muscle function and the temporomandibular joint. J. Prosthet. Dent. 13:950–955, 1963.

Kydd, W. L.: Psychosomatic aspects of temporomandibular joint dysfunction. J. Am. Dent. Assoc. 59:31–45, 1959.

Laskin, D. M.: Etiology of the pain-dysfunction syndrome. J. Am. Dent. Assoc. 79:147–153, 1969.

Laskin, D. M., and Greene, C. S.: Influence of the doctor-patient relationship on placebo therapy for patients with myofascial pain-dysfunction (MPD) syndrome. J. Am. Dent. Assoc. 85:892–894, 1972.

Lavigne, G., Frysinger, R., and Lund, J. P.: Human factors in the measurement of the masseteric silent period. J. Dent. Res. 62:985–988, 1983.

Lund, J. P., and Widmer, C. G.: An evaluation of the use of surface electromyography in the diagnosis, documentation, and treatment of dental patients. J. Craniomandib. Disord. Facial Oral Pain 3:125–137, 1989.

Lundh, H., Westesson, P.-L., and Kopp, S.: A three-year followup of patients with reciprocal temporomandibular joint clicking. Oral Surg. 63:530–533, 1987.

Lupton, D. E.: A preliminary investigation of the personality of female TMJ patients. Psychother. Psychosom. 14:199–216, 1966.

Lupton, D. E.: Psychological aspects of temporomandibular joint dysfunction. J. Am. Dent. Assoc. 79:131–136, 1969.

Magnusson, T., Egermark-Eriksson, I., and Carlsson, G. E.: Five-year longitudinal study of signs and symptoms of mandibular dysfunction in 119 young adults. J. Craniomandib. Pract. 4:338–344, 1986.

Malmo, R. B., Shagass, C., and Davis, J. F.: Electromyographic studies of muscular tension in psychiatric patients under stress. J. Clin. Exp. Psychopathol. 12:45–66, 1951.

Malow, R. M., Olson, R. E., and Greene, C. S.: Myofascial pain-dysfunction syndrome: A psychophysiologic disorder. In Golden, C., Alcaparras, S., Strider, F., and Graber, B. (Eds.): Applied Techniques in Behavioral Medicine. New York, Grune & Stratton, 1981, pp. 101–133.

Marbach, J. J., and Dworkin, S. F.: Chronic MPD, group therapy, and psychodynamics. J. Am. Dent. Assoc. 90:827–833, 1975.

McCollum, B. B.: Considering the mouth as a functioning unit as the basis of a dental diagnosis. J. South Calif. Dent. Assoc. 5:268–276, 1938.

Melzack, R., and Wall, P. D.: Pain mechanisms: A new theory. Science 150:971–979, 1965.

Mercuri, L. G., Olson, R. E., and Laskin, D. M.: The specificity of response to experimental stress in patients with myofascial pain-dysfunction syndrome. J. Dent. Res. 58:1866–1871, 1979.

Mjersjo, C., and Carlsson, G. E.: Long-term results of treatment for temporomandibular joint pain-dysfunction. J. Prosthet. Dent. 49:809–815, 1983.

Molin, C., Carlsson, G. E., Friling, B., et al.: Frequency of symptoms of mandibular dysfunction in young Swedish men. J. Oral Rehabil. 3:9–18, 1976.

Molin, C., and Levi, L.: Psycho-odontologic investigations of patients with bruxism. Acta Odontol. Scand. 24:373–391, 1966.

Moloney, F., and Howard, J. A.: Internal derangements of the temporomandibular joint. III. Anterior repositioning splint therapy. Aust. Dent. J. 31:30–39, 1986.

Moulton, R. E.: Emotional factors in non-organic temporomandibular joint pain. Dent. Clin. North Am. 13:609–620, 1966.

Moulton, R. E.: Psychiatric considerations in maxillofacial pain. J. Am. Dent. Assoc. 51:408–414, 1955.

Moyers, R. E.: An electromyographic analysis of certain muscles involved in temporomandibular movement. Am. J. Orthod. 36:481–515, 1950.

Neulle, D. G., Alpern, M. C., and Ufema, J. W.: Arthroscopic surgery of the temporomandibular joint. Angle Orthod. 56:118–142, 1986.

Nilner, M., and Lassing, S. A.: Prevalence of functional disturbances and diseases of the stomatognathic system in 7 to 14 year olds. Swed. Dent. J. 5:173–187, 1981.

Norgaard, F.: Temporomandibular Arthrography. Copenhagen, Munksgaard, 1947.

Perry, II. T.: Muscular changes associated with temporomandibular joint dysfunction. J. Am. Dent. Assoc. 54:644–653, 1957.

Perry, H. T., Lammie, G. A., Main, J., et al.: Occlusion in a stress situation. J. Am. Dent. Assoc. 60:626–633, 1960.

Pomp, A. M.: Psychotherapy for the myofascial pain-dysfunction (MPD) syndrome: A study of factors coinciding with symptom remission. J. Am. Dent. Assoc. 89:629–632, 1974.

Posselt, U.: The temporomandibular joint syndrome and occlusion. J. Prosthet. Dent. 25:432–438, 1971.

Pullinger, A. G., Hollender, L., Solberg, W. K., et al.: A tomographic study of mandibular condyle position in an asymptomatic population. J. Prosthet. Dent. 53:706–713, 1985.

Ramfjord, S. P.: Dysfunctional temporomandibular joint and muscle pain. J. Prosthet. Dent. 11:353–374, 1961.

Ramfjord, S. P., and Ash, M. M.: Occlusion. Philadelphia, W. B. Saunders, 1966.

Ricketts, R. M.: Roentgenography of the temporomandibular joint. In Sarnat, B. G. (Ed.): The Temporomandibular Joint, 2nd ed. Springfield, IL, Charles C Thomas, 1964, pp. 102–132.

Rugh, J. D.: Personal communication.

Rugh, J. D.: Psychological factors in the etiology of masticatory pain and dysfunction. In Laskin, D. M., Greenfield, W., Gale, E., et al. (Eds.): The President's Conference on the Examination, Diagnosis, and Management of Temporomandibular Disorders. Chicago, Am. Dent. Assoc. 1983, pp. 85–94.

Rugh, J. D., and Solberg, W. K.: Psychological implications in temporomandibular pain and dysfunction. Oral Sci. Rev. 7:3–30, 1976.

Sadowsky, C., and Polson, A. M.: Temporomandibular disorders and functional occlusion after orthodontic treatment. Am. J. Orthod. 86:386–390, 1984.

Scapino, R. P.: Histopathology associated with malposition

of the human temporomandibular joint disc. Oral Surg. 55:382–397, 1983.

Schwartz, L.: Conclusions of the temporomandibular joint clinic at Columbia. J. Periodontol. 29:210–212, 1958.

Schwartz, L.: Disorders of the Temporomandibular Joint. Philadelphia, W. B. Saunders, 1959.

Seaver, E. P.: Temporomandibular joint malocclusion and the inner ear: A neuromuscular explanation. Ann. Otol. Rhinol. Laryngol. 46:140–149, 1937.

Selye, H.: The Physiology and Pathology of Exposure to Stress. Montreal, Medical Publications, 1950.

Selye, H.: The Stress of Life. New York, McGraw-Hill, 1956.

Shore, N. A.: Occlusal Equilibration and Temporomandibular Joint Dysfunction. Philadelphia, J. B. Lippincott, 1959.

Solberg, W. K., Flint, R. T., and Brantner, J. P.: Temporomandibular joint pain and dysfunction: A clinical study of emotional and occlusal components. J. Prosthet. Dent. 28:412–422, 1972.

Solberg, W. K., Hansson, T., and Nordstrom, B.: The temporomandibular joint in young adults at autopsy: A morphologic classification and evaluation. J. Oral Rehabil. 12:303–321, 1985.

Solberg, W. K., Woo, M. W., and Houston, J. B.: Prevalence of mandibular dysfunction in young adults. J. Am. Dent. Assoc. 98:25–34, 1979.

Stallard, H., and Stuart, C. E.: What kind of occlusion should recusped teeth be given? Dent. Clin. North Am. 10:591–606, 1963.

Steinhardt, G.: Zur Pathologie und Therapie des Kiefergelenk-knackens. Dtsch. Z. Chir. 241:531–552, 1933.

Sternbach, R. A.: Pain Patients: Traits and Treatments. New York, Academic Press, 1974.

Stuart, C. E., and Stallard, H.: Principles involved in restoring occlusion to natural teeth. J. Prosth. Dent. 10:304–313, 1960.

Tallents, R. H., Katzberg, R. W., Miller, T. L., et al.: Evaluation of arthrographically assisted splint therapy in the treatment of TMJ disc displacement. J. Prosthet. Dent. 53:836–838, 1985.

Thompson, J. R.: Concepts regarding function of the stomatognathic system. J. Am. Dent. Assoc. 48:626–637, 1954.

Thompson, J. R.: Abnormal function of the stomatognathic system and its orthodontic implications. Am. J. Orthod. 48:758–765, 1962.

Thompson, J. R.: Temporomandibular disorders: Diagnosis and treatment. In Sarnat, B. G. (Ed.): The Temporomandibular Joint, 2nd ed. Springfield, IL, Charles C Thomas, 1964, pp. 146–184.

Travell, J.: Temporomandibular joint pain referred from muscles of the head and neck. J. Prosthet. Dent. 10:745–763, 1960.

Travell, J., and Rinzler, S. H.: Scientific exhibit: The myofascial genesis of pain. Postgrad. Med. 11:425–433, 1952.

Walker, R. V., and Kalmachi, S.: A surgical technique for management of internal derangement of the temporomandibular joint. J. Oral Maxillofac. Surg. 45:299–305, 1987.

Wanman, A., and Agerberg, G.: Two-year longitudinal study of signs of mandibular dysfunction in adolescents. Acta Odontol. Scand. 44:333–342, 1986.

Weinberg, L. A.: Correlation of temporomandibular dysfunction with radiographic findings. J. Prosthet. Dent. 28:519–539, 1972.

Weinberg, L. A.: Posterior unilateral condylar displacement: Its diagnosis and treatment. J. Prosthet. Dent. 37:559–569, 1977.

Weinberg, L. A.: Role of condylar position in TMJ dysfunction-pain syndrome. J. Prosthet. Dent. 41:636–643, 1979.

Westesson, P-L., and Rohlin, M.: Internal derangement related to osteoarthrosis in temporomandibular joint autopsy specimens. Oral Surg. 57:17–22, 1984.

Whatmore, G., and Kohli, D.: The Physiopathology and Treatment of Functional Disorders. New York, Grune & Stratton, 1974.

Wilkes, C. H.: Arthrography of the temporomandibular joint in patients with the TMJ pain-dysfunction syndrome. Minn. Med. 61:645–652, 1978a.

Wilkes, C. H.: Structural and functional alterations of the temporomandibular joint. Northwest Dent. 57:287–294, 1978b.

Williamson, E. H., and Sheffield, J. W.: The non-surgical treatment of internal derangement of the temporomandibular joint: A survey of 300 cases. Facial Orthopedics and Temporomandibular Arthrology 2:18–21, 1985.

Wolff, H. G.: Headache and Other Head Pain. New York, Oxford University Press, 1948.

Yemm, R.: Temporomandibular dysfunction and masseter muscle response to experimental stress. Br. Dent. J. 127:508–510, 1967.

Yemm, R.: A comparison of the electrical activity of masseter and temporalis muscles of human subjects during experimental stress. Arch. Oral Biol. 16:269–273, 1971.

Yemm, R.: Neurophysiologic studies of temporomandibular joint dysfunction. In Zarb, G. A., and Carlsson, G. E. (Eds.): Temporomandibular Joint: Function and Dysfunction. Copenhagen, Munksgaard, 1979, pp. 215–237.

Zarb, G. A., and Mohl, N. D.: Occlusion and temporomandibular disorders: A prologue. In Mohl, N. D., Zarb, G. A., Carlsson, G. E., and Rugh, J. D. (Eds.): A Textbook of Occlusion. Chicago, Quintessence, 1988, pp. 377–383.

19

TEMPOROMANDIBULAR DISORDERS: Diagnosis and Etiology*

DANIEL M. LASKIN, D.D.S., M.S.

INTRODUCTION

The disorders that involve the temporomandibular joint (TMJ) are no different from those that involve other joints in the body. Thus, one can encounter patients with congenital and developmental anomalies (see Chapter 12), traumatic injuries and ankylosis (see Chapter 24), neoplastic diseases (see Chapter 10), various forms of arthritis (see Chapter 11), and internal derangements (see Chapters 17 and 23). In addition, there is an even larger group of patients with primarily a masticatory muscle disorder (myofascial pain-dysfunction [MPD] syndrome, primary masticatory myalgia) that is often confused with some forms of TMJ pathology because it produces rather similar signs and symptoms. These two groups of patients comprise the spectrum of what has been referred to as temporomandibular disorders (TMDs) (Bell, 1983).

Many of the pathologic conditions involving the TMJ, such as the congenital and developmental anomalies or the neoplastic diseases, are nonpainful and have specific diagnostic criteria. Others, such as the traumatic injuries, have an acute onset of pain that is associated with a specific cause and easily recognized clinical and radiographic findings. The diagnostic difficulties that arise are most often related to the similarity in signs and symptoms produced by MPD syndrome, degenerative joint disease, and internal derangements of the TMJ. The emphasis in this chapter, therefore, will be placed on the differential diagnosis and etiology of these conditions as a basis for establishing rational therapy. For information on the diagnosis and etiology of the congenital and developmental anomalies, traumatic injuries and ankylosis, neoplastic diseases, and the other forms of arthritis, see Chapters 10, 11, 12, and 24.

---

*See Chapters 9–12, 16–18, and 20–26.

316

DIAGNOSIS OF THE MYOFASCIAL PAIN-DYSFUNCTION SYNDROME (PRIMARY MASTICATORY MYALGIA)

Because of the confusing terminology used to describe MPD syndrome in the past, and the differences of opinion regarding the principal signs and symptoms, it is important before discussing etiology to consider the essential findings that place a patient in the category of MPD syndrome. Pain of unilateral origin is the most common symptom (Greene, 1969). This pain usually is described by the patient as a dull ache in the ear or preauricular region that frequently radiates to the temporal region, the frontal region, deep to the eye, the angle of the mandible, or the lateral cervical or occipital regions. It may also be described as a jawache, earache, or headache. The pain can be relatively constant, but more often is worse upon arising in the morning, or is relatively mild or absent in the morning but gradually worsens as the day progresses. The pain is frequently exacerbated by use of the mandible.

Masticatory muscle tenderness is the next most common finding (Greene, 1969). Although usually not reported by the patient, this symptom can be elicited easily by the examiner. The most frequent areas of tenderness are found over the neck of the condyloid process, in the area distal and superior to the maxillary tuberosity, in the anterior temporal region, and over the mandibular angle and temporal crest. These sites of tenderness are presumed to be regions of spasm in the masticatory muscles.

Limitation of mandibular movement is the third cardinal symptom of the MPD syndrome. It may manifest itself either by inability to open the mouth as wide as usual, deviation of the mandible on opening, or both.

A clicking or popping sound in the TMJ is another common finding associated with MPD syndrome. Although there are other causes of such joint noise (see section on the etiology of internal derangements), both the lateral pterygoid muscle spasm and the chronic clenching noted in many patients with MPD syndrome can also be etiologic factors. Thus, although clicking or popping sounds are not an initial cardinal symptom, they can be a secondary phenomenon in some MPD patients. The occurrence of such joint sounds alone, however, is not sufficient to make a diagnosis of MPD syndrome; they must be accompanied by symptoms of myofascial pain and tenderness unrelated to muscle splinting.

Along with having one or more of the three cardinal symptoms of pain, muscle tenderness, and limitation of mouth opening, patients with MPD syndrome usually have an absence of clinical, radiographic, or biochemical evidence of organic changes in the TMJ. These negative characteristics are significant in establishing the diagnosis, since they indicate that the primary site of the problem is not in the articular structures. This distinction forms the essential basis for understanding the pathogenesis of the MPD syndrome.

Although MPD syndrome generally begins as a functional, muscular disorder, it ultimately can lead to degenerative arthritis as well as internal derangements in the TMJ. The past history of the disorder is often helpful in determining whether these changes are primary or secondary.

There are a number of conditions other than MPD syndrome that can produce similar symptoms of facial pain and jaw dysfunction. Some are nonarticular problems that merely mimic MPD syndrome; others are true pathologic conditions of the TMJ. All of these must be considered and eliminated before a final diagnosis of MPD syndrome is made (see Chapters 25 and 26).

ETIOLOGY OF THE MYOFASCIAL PAIN-DYSFUNCTION SYNDROME: PSYCHOPHYSIOLOGIC THEORY

In 1955, Schwartz reported that he was able to delineate from the large group of patients with supposed "temporomandibular joint (TMJ) syndrome" a more definitive group of individuals with painful, limited mandibular movement due to spasm in the muscles of mastication. He termed this condition TMJ pain-dysfunction syndrome. The subsequent studies of Schwartz (1959) emphasized the psychological characteristics of the patients and represented the first major shift away from the narrow mechanical concept of an occlusal etiology. These studies had a profound influence on the thinking of many investigators interested in TMJ problems and led to new areas of basic and clinical research. As a result of such investigations, the psychophysiologic theory for explaining the etiology of MPD syndrome was introduced by the author (Laskin, 1969). While differing somewhat from the concept proposed by Schwartz (1959), the two theories are not mutually exclusive.

As suggested by Schwartz (1959), masticatory

muscle spasm is considered the primary factor responsible for the signs and symptoms of MPD syndrome (Fig. 19–1). This muscle spasm can be initiated in any of four ways: trauma, muscular overextension, muscular overcontraction, or muscular fatigue. Since spasm of traumatic origin is not difficult to diagnose and is usually a self-limiting episode of short duration, it is not considered in this discussion. Examples of some of the conditions that can cause overextension and spasm of the various masticatory muscles are overly contoured dental restorations or fixed and removable prostheses that excessively encroach upon the intermaxillary space. Overcontraction, on the other hand, can result from bilateral loss of posterior teeth or from the "settling" of partial dentures replacing them. Similarly, it can occur from excessive alveolar bone resorption in patients wearing complete dentures.

Although these kinds of adverse mechanical factors can cause MPD syndrome, most patients do not acquire the problem in this way. Rather, in the majority of cases the cause appears to be muscular fatigue produced by muscle hyperactivity (Fig. 19–1). This hyperactivity usually takes the form of chronic parafunctional habits, such as clenching or grinding the teeth. These habits sometimes can be initiated by a dental irritation, such as an improperly occluding restoration, an overhanging margin, or a tooth with periodontitis. Generally, however, they are an involuntary tension-relieving mechanism in response to psychological stress.

Stress can also generate masticatory muscle hyperactivity directly without the clinical manifestations of clenching or grinding (Copland, 1954; Franks, 1965; Kydd, 1959; Newton, 1969). In these instances, such actions as excessive gum chewing, prolonged opening of the mouth, or chewing hard foods can add to the pre-existing muscle hyperactivity and fatigue and thereby trigger the syndrome. This accounts for most of the patients who deny pernicious oral habits and relate the onset of their problem to a specific episode.

Once spasm develops in the muscles of mastication, regardless of whether it was caused by fatigue, overcontraction, or overextension, the patient has pain and limitation of mandibular movement, i.e., MPD syndrome. At this stage, it is still a functional disorder. However, if the condition persists, it can ultimately lead to organic changes in the dentition, muscles, and TMJ (Fig. 19–1).

Unilateral spasm of one or more of the muscles of mastication, particularly the lateral pterygoid, can produce a slight shift in jaw position so that the teeth do not occlude properly. This has been referred to as an acute malocclusion (Bell, 1990). If the abnormal jaw relationship persists for several days or longer, the teeth may gradually shift and accommodate to the new position. In such cases, the discrepancy is not seen when the patient is asked to occlude the teeth. However, when the spasm is relieved and the rebalanced musculature returns the jaws to their original relationship, the patient exhibits occlusal disharmony.

The shift in jaw position accompanying persistent myospasm also can produce anatomic derangement of the joint structures as well as

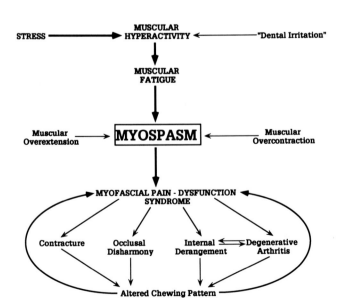

FIGURE 19–1. Etiology of the myofascial pain-dysfunction (MPD) syndrome. Although the diagram shows three means of entry into the syndrome, the *broader arrows* indicate the most common path. The mechanism whereby stress leads to myospasm is termed the *psychophysiologic theory* of MPD syndrome. (Modified from Laskin, D. M.: Etiology of the pain-dysfunction syndrome. J. Am. Dent. Assoc. 79:147–153, 1969.)

ultimately lead to degenerative arthritis in the TMJ as a result of continued function with the condyle in an abnormal position. Constant loading and unloading of the joint by clenching or grinding the teeth can add to the rapid progress of the degenerative changes and severity of the symptoms, as well as cause disc displacement by altering the frictional properties of the joint (Fig. 19–1). Since the TMJs are functionally one unit, the changes can ultimately involve both sides (see Chapters 10, 11, and 24).

Muscle contracture is the least common of the organic changes that may follow the onset of MPD syndrome. It is a slowly developing condition that ultimately leads to painless shortening of the muscles with resultant limitation of opening of the mouth.

Although MPD syndrome originates as a functional disorder, if it persists long enough, the development of secondary organic changes in the dentition, masticatory muscles, and TMJ tend to complicate the problem (Naeije, 1986; Westesson, 1985). The condition then becomes self-perpetuating, because these changes result in an altered chewing pattern with attendant reinforcement of the initial spasm and pain (Michler, 1988; Mongini, 1984) (Fig. 19–1).

The psychophysiological theory for explaining the pathogenesis of the MPD syndrome has a number of advantages over the previous occlusal theories (see Chapter 18). Not only does it adequately explain the origin of the various signs and symptoms, but also it shows how occlusal disharmonies can arise in a functioning dentition as a result rather than as a cause of the problem. This is a concept diametrically opposed to that suggested by most of the previous investigators. Furthermore, since there are three paths of entry into the syndrome (Fig. 19–1), the suggested scheme also explains how diverse etiologic factors can produce like symptoms. On a similar basis, it offers a logical explanation of how different forms of therapy sometimes may be successful in what symptomatically appears to be the same condition.

EXPERIMENTAL EVIDENCE FOR THE PSYCHOPHYSIOLOGIC THEORY

A great deal of experimental evidence has been developed that supports the psychophysiological theory of etiology for the MPD syndrome and indicates that it is primarily a muscular disorder. This evidence can be divided into five main categories: epidemiologic, radio-graphic, psychological, biochemical, and physiological.

Epidemiologic Studies

A number of epidemiologic studies have contributed to current understanding of the MPD syndrome. For example, analysis of the data on a series of 277 consecutive patients with supposed TMJ problems revealed over 80 per cent with masticatory muscle tenderness (Greene, 1969). The data on another series of patients showed that about 80 per cent presently or previously had other psychophysiologic diseases such as peptic (gastric or duodenal) ulcer, ulcerative colitis, migraine headache, asthma, or dermatitis (Lupton, 1966). Seventy-seven per cent also reported having chronic oral habits such as clenching or grinding the teeth, excessive gum chewing, or biting on hard objects. A high incidence of stress-related illnesses and oral habits in patients with MPD syndrome has also been found by other investigators (Agerberg, 1973; Berry, 1969; Gold, 1975).

While not directly supporting the psychophysiologic theory, there are a number of epidemiologic studies that support it indirectly by refuting the idea of occlusal disharmony being the causative factor (Bush, 1983). For example, the same types of occlusal disharmonies repeatedly are found equally distributed in patients with MPD syndrome and in randomly selected normal individuals (Posselt, 1971; Solberg, 1972; Thomson, 1971). Moreover, in numerous studies, at least four out of every five patients with MPD syndrome are female (Carraro, 1969; Helkimo, 1976; Schwartz, 1957), yet consistent differences in occlusion between the sexes have not been demonstrated. These findings tend to undermine the assumption that occlusal disharmonies are the most important factor in the origin of MPD problems.

Radiologic Studies

Transcranial view radiographs of the TMJs, cephalometric headplates, panoramic radiographs, and even standard tomographic techniques induce distortions that can easily be misinterpreted as evidence of pathologic changes (see Chapter 16). Moreover, many clinicians, when interpreting radiographs, fail to consider the normal variations in condylar morphology (Yale, 1966), as well as the fact that the fibrous tissue and cartilage covering the condyle can compensate in vivo for radiographically demonstrable bony defects. These factors account for the apparently high incidence of pathologic change or alteration in the spatial relationships of the joint components that have been reported by numerous investigators. When the technique of corrected tomography (Rosenberg, 1967) is used, less than nine per cent of all patients with TMJ problems have radiographic evidence of pathologic involvement of the joint structures (Markovic, 1976). This lack of significant radiographic change in the TMJs supports the contention that the joint itself is not the primary site of involvement in patients with MPD syndrome.

Psychologic Studies

Numerous studies indicate that patients with MPD syndrome are in a state of greater anxiety than normal individuals (Kydd, 1959; McCall, 1961; Molin, 1973; Solberg, 1972). It has also been clearly established that such an altered emotional state can elicit muscle hyperactivity (Dahlstrom, 1989; Goldstein, 1964a; Lundeen, 1987; Malmo, 1951; Thomas, 1973; Yemm, 1969a; 1969b; 1976). Since the psychophysiological theory implicates stress-related muscular hyperactivity as the primary cause of most cases of MPD syndrome, these findings are among the most important data supporting this concept.

While it has not been possible to distinguish a specific personality type associated with MPD syndrome, most of the patients have behavioral characteristics that make it more likely for them to become involved in psychologically stressful situations, to have greater than normal difficulty in dealing with psychologic stress, and to somatize rather than exteriorize when attempting to cope with such situations. The reason that all individuals with such characteristics do not develop MPD syndrome relates to their response specificity (Goldstein, 1964; Johnson, 1972; Mercuri, 1979) as well as to their individual ability to cope with tension-producing problems. Because of response specificity, individuals with similar personality characteristics may develop different psychophysiological disorders, such as low back pain (Sternbach, 1973), chronic obesity, duodenal ulcer, and hypertension, when stressed (Lupton, 1966).

The ability to treat patients with MPD syndrome effectively using psychologic methods is further supportive evidence for the psychophysiological theory. A program of dental therapy combined with psychological counseling provides better therapeutic results than dental therapy alone (Lupton, 1969). Moreover, psychological counseling alone, or in combination with psychotropic drugs, has proved to be an effective means of alleviating symptoms in many patients (Gessel, 1975; Marbach, 1975; Pomp, 1974). The high degree of responsiveness to placebo drugs (Greene, 1971; Laskin, 1972), placebo bite plates (Greene, 1972), and mock equilibration (Goodman, 1976) is a further indication of the role of psychological factors in the etiology of MPD syndrome. It also offers an additional explanation of why so many diverse modalities can be used to treat this condition successfully.

Biochemical Studies

There is biochemical as well as psychological evidence that individuals with MPD syndrome are under a greater than normal amount of stress. When urinary concentrations of catecholamines and 17-hydroxysteroids were compared in MPD patients and a control group, the former had significantly higher levels of both substances (Evaskus, 1972). Although muscular activity can also increase the concentration of catecholamines (Euler, 1952) this observation is still compatible with the psychophysiologic concept.

Biochemically, the state of the masticatory muscles is altered in MPD syndrome (Evaskus, 1977). Since the serum levels of lactic dehydrogenase (LDH), LDH isoenzymes, and creatine phosphokinase (CPK) are an accurate indicator of changes in the intracellular metabolism of skeletal muscle, it was hypothesized that patients with MPD syndrome would show changes in the serum levels of these substances if their masticatory muscles were in spasm. Such changes were found when a group of 16 patients with MPD syndrome and 24 normal subjects, carefully screened to eliminate those with coexisting disorders known to alter these enzyme patterns, were compared. Patients in remission and those with chronic MPD syndrome had enzyme and isoenzyme levels similar to those of the control group. However, the patients with acute MPD syndrome had reduced serum LDH and CPK levels. These decreases were interpreted as being a result of the increased utilization of the enzymes, a finding that is compatible with persistent muscle spasm.

Physiological Studies

Physiological studies indicate that the jaw muscles of patients with MPD syndrome are hyperactive (Griffin, 1971; Perry, 1957; Reuben, 1977). There are also studies supporting the concept that stress can induce such masticatory muscle hyperactivity (Dahlstrom, 1989; Haber, 1983; Lundeen, 1987; Thomas, 1973; Yemm, 1985). Perry (1960) observed such changes electromyographically in the masseter and temporalis muscles of dental students when they were subjected to a stressful interview and anticipated examinations. Yemm (1971; 1969b) confirmed these observations in normal subjects under stress from a challenging manual task. Similar increases in masticatory muscle activity have also been reported with other experimentally induced stress situations of both a physical (Drinkwater, 1968) and a psychological nature (Chaney, 1972). Johnson (1972) and Mercuri (1979) found even greater masseter responses in patients with MPD syndrome than in normal individuals, particularly when they were subjected to psychologic stress. The results reported by Yemm (1969a) using a stressful task agree with this finding.

There is also extensive evidence from studies of both masticatory and other body muscles that hyperactivity can produce symptoms of pain and dysfunction (Christensen, 1970; DeVries, 1966; Direnfeld, 1967). When a group of normal subjects was asked to grind their teeth for 30 minutes, Vestergaard Christensen (1970) found that pain having a similar location and character as that noted with MPD syndrome developed in almost all instances. Direnfeld (1967), using a muscle endurance test to fatigue the masticatory muscles, reported similar findings. Furthermore, Direnfeld showed evidence of concomitant limitation of opening of the mouth in a number of the subjects.

In addition to those physiological studies directly supporting the psychophysiological concept that stress produces muscle hyperactivity, which in turn leads to pain and dysfunction, there are several other studies that provide indirect evidence of the involvement of the masticatory muscles in MPD syndrome. Bessette (1971) showed that about half the patients with MPD syndrome have a prolonged masseteric silent period. Moreover, when the other three muscles of mastication also were studied, Skiba (1976) found that every patient had at least one or more extended silent periods. The temporalis muscle was affected in 91 per cent of the cases, the masseter in 55 per cent, the lateral pterygoid in 24 per cent, and the medial pterygoid in 18 per cent. With successful treatment the prolonged silent periods returned to normal limits (Krell, 1977).

Study of the consistency of tooth contact associated with normal jaw closing using the Occlusograph also indicated indirectly that patients with MPD syndrome have masticatory muscle dysfunction (Edmiston, 1978). When patients were symptomatic, their patterns of contact on repeated closure were erratic (Fig. 19–2). However, following treatment, which generally consisted of diazepam and sodium salicylate, but never involved alteration of the occlusal surfaces of the teeth, resolution of symptoms was accompanied by improved consistency on the Occlusograph.

An explanation of why only certain individuals develop MPD syndrome can be found in the studies comparing the response specificity of MPD patients with that of a normal control group (Johnson, 1972; Mercuri, 1979). Electromyographic activity in the masseter, frontalis, and gastrocnemius muscles; galvanic skin response; and heart rate were monitored simultaneously while the subjects were stressed psychologically as well as by induced pain and startling noise. The results showed that individuals with a history of MPD syndrome tended to respond to stress with greater masticatory and facial muscle activity than normal subjects whose major response within the parameters measured was an increase in autonomic nervous system activity. These findings suggest that patients who are prone to develop psychophysiologic disorders will develop symptoms in their target area of response to stress. Patients with fibrositis (Traut, 1968) and low back pain (Sternbach, 1973) are examples of muscle responders with different areas of expression.

IMPLICATIONS OF THE PSYCHOPHYSIOLOGICAL THEORY

Although there are still some gaps in our total understanding of the etiology of MPD syndrome, integration of the findings from the various epidemiologic, radiographic, psychological, biochemical, and physiological studies forms a solid basis for the validity of the psychophysiological theory. This position is strengthened further when one includes the data derived from animal and human studies related to the concept of occlusal disharmony as the primary etiological factor in MPD syndrome. As Yemm (1976) has pointed out, there is presently no experimental proof that premature contact between opposing teeth can initiate or maintain prolonged hyperactivity of the jaw-closing muscles or forceful clenching or grind-

Pre-treatment

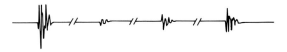

Post-treatment

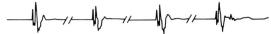

FIGURE 19–2. Occlusogram, from patient with MPD syndrome. *Upper Recording,* Inconsistent pattern of tooth contact before treatment. *Lower Recording,* Consistent pattern following treatment with diazepam and sodium salicylate. (From Edmiston, G. F., and Laskin, D. M.: Changes in consistency of occlusal contact in myofascial pain-dysfunction [MPD] syndrome. J. Dent. Res. 57:27–30, 1978.)

ing. In fact, most experiments have shown that mechanical stimulation of the teeth reduces or inhibits activity of the jaw-closing muscles (Anderson, 1958; Christensen, 1970; Hannam, 1969; Kidokoro, 1968). The theory of occlusal disharmony as the etiologic factor seems to have gained its greatest support from the clinical observation that some patients with MPD syndrome are relieved of their symptoms by grinding the teeth (Dawson, 1974; McHorris, 1985; Ramfjord, 1983; Shore, 1976). However, this concept is challenged by the finding that 64 per cent of a series of patients treated by mock equilibration also showed total or near total improvement in symptoms after only two such treatments (Goodman, 1976).

Based on the psychophysiologic concept of etiology of MPD syndrome, one can derive certain general conclusions regarding the management of this condition. First, because the initiating factors for the syndrome are generally emotional rather than physical, treatment must be directed toward this aspect of the problem, as well as toward the management of the physical symptoms and the organic sequelae (McNeill, 1990) (see Chapter 21). Disregard for this principle probably is responsible for most of the therapeutic failures encountered. Second, in the functional stage of the syndrome, when primarily the masticatory muscles are involved, there are obviously no indications for such drastic forms of therapy as joint surgery, intra-articular drug injections, or extensive forms of occlusal equilibration or reconstruction. It is even questionable whether these procedures generally are indicated in the later stages because the muscles of mastication are still the major site of involvement. Third, it must be realized that correction of the underlying emo-

tional conflicts leading to production of the syndrome may not always be possible, even when the patient receives psychotherapy.

It is not mere rationalization, therefore, to assume that a small number of patients will never be completely cured. However, one should not use this as a license to relegate any difficult problem to the incurable category before all logical forms of treatment have been tried. On the other hand, excessively radical therapeutic measures should not be attempted in desperation, because these may only induce iatrogenic problems that further complicate the situation.

DIAGNOSIS AND ETIOLOGY OF TEMPOROMANDIBULAR JOINT DISORDERS

Degenerative Joint Disease (Osteoarthritis)

Diagnosis

The distinction between MPD syndrome and degenerative joint disease (DJD) in the TMJ can be confusing because they both produce pain and jaw dysfunction. However, the muscle pain associated with MPD syndrome is diffuse and radiating, while that resulting from DJD is more localized. Thus, the patient with the former condition usually will relate the pain to an area rather than a specific site, while the patient with the latter condition will generally point directly to the TMJ when asked where it hurts.

Both patients with MPD syndrome and those with DJD will have limited jaw movement, the latter due to protective joint splinting as well as the primary disease, but the amount of limitation is usually greater in those patients with MPD syndrome. The extent and degree of masticatory muscle tenderness is also greater in the latter group. They generally also complain of pain and tenderness in the cervical and shoulder muscles because myofascial pain tends to be a regional phenomenon.

Although both patients with MPD syndrome and those with DJD can have clicking or popping sounds in the TMJ, crepitant sounds are associated with degenerative joint disease. The presence of radiographic changes in the TMJ of patients with DJD can also be a distinguishing characteristic (see Chapter 16). However, because chronic MPD syndrome can lead to DJD in some patients (see Fig. 19–1) one needs to rely more on the history and the differences in the other clinical findings to make the differential diagnosis.

Etiology

The etiology of DJD is unknown. It appears to be the result of a complex interaction of adverse mechanical, biochemical, and enzymatic events (Mankin, 1989a; 1989b). Prolonged overuse and acute or chronic trauma are common initiating factors. The earliest finding is a decrease in the concentration of the proteoglycans in the region of the chondrocytes. This is followed by an increased formation of bone in the subchondral region, which results in the cancellous tissue becoming stiffer and subject to microfractures. The callus formation that accompanies these fractures causes more stiffness, additional microfractures, and the initiation of a vicious cycle. These changes in the physical properties of the subchondral bone are associated with a fibrillation, roughening, and then a loss of the articular surface; exposure of the underlying bone; and subsequent erosion, osteophyte formation, or eburnation.

Internal Derangement

Diagnosis

There are basically three types of disc derangement that can occur, either initially or as a progressive series of events: an incoordination phase, anterior disc displacement with reduction (clicking); and anterior disc displacement without reduction (locking) (Fig. 19–3). The incoordination phase is characterized by a loss of the smooth movement that normally occurs when the mouth is opened and closed and its replacement by a painless and noiseless sensa-

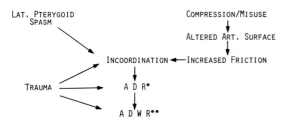

ETIOLOGY OF INTERNAL DERANGEMENTS
OF THE TEMPOROMANDIBULAR JOINT

FIGURE 19–3. Diagram showing the three types of internal derangement of the temporomandibular joint and their causes.

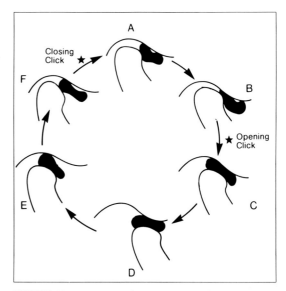

FIGURE 19–4. Diagram showing anterior displacement of the intra-articular disc with reduction on opening the mouth. A clicking or popping sound occurs as the disc returns to its normal position in relation to the condyle. During closure the disc again becomes anteriorly displaced, sometimes accompanied by a second sound (reciprocal click). (Modified from McCarty, W.: Diagnosis and treatment of internal derangements of the articular disc and mandibular condyle. *In* Solberg, W. K., and Clark, G. T. [Eds.]: Temporomandibular Joint Problems: Biologic Diagnosis and Treatment. Chicago, Quintessence, 1980, p. 155.)

tion of hesitation or catching. This sensation is caused by a change in the frictional properties of the joint resulting from alterations in the articulating surfaces of the condyle, disc, and articular eminence.

Anterior disc displacement with reduction (ADR) is characterized by an initial catching or locking sensation as the mouth is opened, followed by a popping or clicking sound. It results from looseness of the capsule and ligaments that normally maintain the disc-condyle relationship, allowing the disc to assume a more anterior position (Fig. 19–4). As the mouth is opened, the condyle presses against the posterior band of the disc, pushing the disc forward until the retrodiscal ligament becomes sufficiently taut to permit the condyle to slip over the posterior band into its normal relation with the disc. Once the normal condyle-disc relationship has been reestablished, further mouth opening is unimpeded. As the mouth is closed, however, the loose retrodiscal ligament fails to counterbalance the pull of the superior head of the lateral pterygoid muscle and the disc slips forward into an anteriorly displaced position, again predisposing to clicking or popping when the mouth is opened. When this terminal disc displacement results in a sound, it is referred to as a reciprocal click. Although this sound is not always heard, because it can be extremely faint, the sensation produced by the disc slipping forward can be felt either over the joint or by placing a finger over the angle of the mandible.

ADR is frequently associated with pain because the condyle functions partially against the highly innervated retrodiscal tissue when the disc is in an anterior position. Painless clicking or popping can occur, however, even when the disc is anteriorly displaced, if the displacement develops gradually and the retrodiscal tissue has an opportunity to undergo adaptive fibrotic changes (Scapino, 1983).

Anterior disc displacement without reduction (ADWR) is characterized by an inability to open the mouth more than 20 to 30 mm, and is due to the disc being displaced completely anterior to the condyle and acting as a mechanical barrier (Fig. 19–5). Because the retrodiscal ligament is very stretched and loose, it never becomes taut enough when the mouth is opened to hold the disc firmly and allow the condyle to slip over the posterior edge into a reduced position as happens when clicking or popping occurs. Anterior displacement without reduction is frequently associated with pain

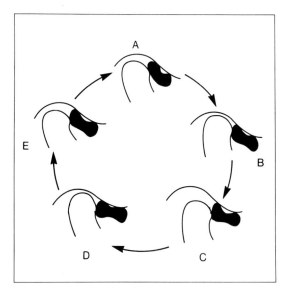

FIGURE 19–5. Diagram showing anterior displacement of the intra-articular disc without reduction on attempted mouth opening. The displaced disc acts as a barrier and prevents full translation of the condyle. (Modified from McCarty, W.: Diagnosis and treatment of internal derangements of the articular disc and mandibular condyle. *In* Solberg, W. K., and Clark, G. T. [Eds.]: Temporomandibular Joint Problems: Biologic Diagnosis and Treatment. Chicago, Quintessence, 1980, p. 151.)

because the condyle functions entirely against the innervated retrodiscal tissue. Although there are many other causes for limitation of mandibular movement (see Chapter 24, Table 24–4), the history provided by the patient usually helps to establish the diagnosis of a nonreducing disc. When the locking is of discal origin, patients will generally indicate that before the onset of limitation they clicked almost constantly when opening their mouths or that the problem began soon after they were involved in a traumatic accident.

There are some patients who vacillate between clicking and locking phases. These patients usually have initial difficulty in opening the mouth and either manually or functionally manipulate the mandible until a disc-condyle relationship is established that permits clicking, disc reduction, and mouth opening to occur. If untreated, such patients eventually end up with a totally nonreducing disc and locking.

There is also a group of patients who have pain and limitation of mouth opening in whom imaging does not show significant disc displacement (see Chapter 16). These individuals have adhesions between the disc and the articular eminence that prevent condylar translation and therefore limit mouth opening mainly to a hinge movement.

In addition to disc derangements, it is also possible for perforations in the disc to occur. Such perforations can result from the osteophytes that accompany degenerative joint disease wearing a hole in the disc. More frequently, however, a perforation will occur at the junction of the disc and the retrodiscal ligament in patients with anterior disc displacement due to constant pressure against this area during function. Perforations are usually associated with crepitant sounds during jaw movement and can be recognized arthrographically by both joint spaces filling simultaneously when the first one is injected with the contrast medium.

Because incoordination of the articular disc is silent and nonpainful, patients with this condition seldom complain about it. The diagnosis is therefore dependent on a careful history being taken of all patients in which they are asked if their jaw joint moves smoothly or if they feel any sensation of catching or hesitation. Patients should also be asked if they hear any sounds in the TMJ. Such sounds may sometimes be audible to the naked ear of the clinician, but other times they are heard only by the patient and require a stethoscope to be heard by the examiner. Lateral or intrameatal palpation of the TMJ may also elicit an altered tactile sensation when clicking or popping is occurring.

Crepitant sounds are generally indicative of bone-to-bone contact, and involve either perforation of the disc by an osteophyte accompanying degenerative joint disease or a separation or tearing of the retrodiscal ligament from the disc when there is anterior disc displacement. Although neither of these conditions is actually included in the definition of internal derangements, the latter is a sequela of such derangements.

Arthrography (Dolwick, 1979), a CT scan (Helms, 1984), or magnetic resonance imaging (MRI) (Vogler, 1987) can be used to confirm the diagnosis of anterior disc displacement. However, only arthrofluoroscopy provides a truly dynamic evaluation of the disc-condyle relationships during function, and only arthrography can be used to diagnose a perforation. The main disadvantage of the arthrographic techniques is the fact that they are invasive, while CT and MRI are not.

Although arthrography, arthrofluoroscopy, CT, and MRI are very helpful diagnostic tools, their routine use is probably not indicated. Since the mechanisms of clicking and locking are now understood, there is no reason to subject every patient with such problems to one of these procedures merely to confirm what can be determined clinically. Rather, they should be reserved for those patients in whom the clinical diagnosis is unclear. In most instances these will be individuals with limited opening and without a specific history of antecedent clicking or popping in the TMJ.

Etiology

There are three mechanisms that can lead to derangements of the intra-articular disc: lateral pterygoid muscle spasm, trauma, and chronic parafunctional compression (clenching) (see Fig. 19–3). Of the three, only trauma can directly lead to either incoordination, clicking, or locking. Lateral pterygoid spasm and chronic clenching first cause incoordination, which can then progress sequentially to clicking and locking.

Lateral pterygoid spasm, part of MPD syndrome, can cause anterior disc displacement in some patients because the superior head of the muscle fails to relax during the opening movement and the disc is pulled downward and forward with the condyle rather than being allowed to rotate posteriorly. This can initially produce a slight hesitation or a catching sensa-

tion due to the improper disc-condyle relationship. It also produces an abnormal stretching of the retrodiscal ligament that, if it continues, allows the disc to move slightly anterior to the condyle during the closing movement and causes clicking on opening.

Trauma is the most common cause of disc derangements. Mild trauma may merely cause some damage to the articular surfaces and produce increased friction during mandibular function (incoordination phase). If severe enough, however, such frictional change can limit the ability of the disc to pivot posteriorly during the opening movement and subsequently lead to stretching of the retrodiscal ligament, anterior disc displacement, and clicking. If the condition is left untreated, the constant impingement of the condyle against the posterior band of the disc can ultimately cause sufficient looseness of the retrodiscal ligament to result in permanent anterior disc displacement and locking.

More severe trauma can result directly in stretching of the retrodiscal ligament, with anterior disc displacement and clicking. This situation sometimes can be encountered in patients whose mouth opened abruptly and widely during a whiplash injury (Pullinger, 1988; Weinberg, 1987). The condition can remain static or it can eventually lead to locking, as previously described. It is also possible for trauma to be sufficiently great to cause anterior disc displacement and locking initially.

Patients with MPD syndrome who are prone to chronic clenching are also candidates to develop disc derangements. Such parafunctional activity has two effects on the articulating surfaces. First, the constant isometric loading and unloading of the joint can lead to degenerative changes. Second, it squeezes the synovial fluid out of the articulating surfaces and reduces the effectiveness of weeping lubrication, a mechanism that normally provides the most effective reduction in friction by releasing synovial fluid at the various points of maximum compression during mandibular movement. Through these two adverse effects, friction in the joint is increased and, instead of a smooth movement occurring between the condyle and disc, there is a catching sensation. Each time the mouth is opened the disc is prevented from pivoting posteriorly without friction and instead it is first pushed slightly forward by the condyle. Ultimately, this continuous forward movement results in stretching of the retrodiscal ligament and the sequelae of clicking and locking.

SUMMARY

There are two factors involved in the successful management of any disease process—an accurate diagnosis and an understanding of etiology. Unless these conditions are fulfilled, it is not possible to develop a rational treatment plan. Because the specific etiologies of most of the temporomandibular disorders are unknown, treatment often has to be empirical, involving the management of symptoms rather than cause. Under such circumstances, establishing an accurate diagnosis assumes even greater significance. For this reason, the emphasis in this chapter has been on those conditions in which similarity in signs and symptoms causes diagnostic difficulties, in an attempt to define the distinguishing characteristics more clearly. Theories and concepts of etiology have also been discussed to show directions of thinking and to provide guidelines for attempts by clinicians to establish rational approaches to therapy. This information also indicates the various areas of controversy and deficiency, and thus provides the basis for future basic and clinical research that will help to resolve these issues.

REFERENCES

Agerberg, C., and Carlsson, G.: Functional disorders of the masticatory system. II. Indices for symptoms in relation to impaired mobility of the mandible as judged from investigation by questionnaire. Acta Odontol. Scand. 31:335–347, 1973.

Anderson, D. J., and Picton, D. C.: Masticatory stresses in normal and modified occlusion. J. Dent. Res. 37:312–317, 1958.

Bell, W. E.: Classification of TM disorders. In Laskin, D. M., Greenfield, W., Gale, E., et al. (Eds.): The President's Conference on the Examination, Diagnosis and Management of Temporomandibular Disorders. Chicago, Am. Dent. Assoc., 1983, pp. 24–29.

Bell, W. E.: Temporomandibular Disorders. Classification, Diagnosis, Management, 3rd ed. Chicago, Year Book Medical, 1990.

Berry, D.: Mandibular dysfunction, pain, and chronic minor illness. Br. Dent. J. 127:170–175, 1969.

Bessette, R., Bishop, B., and Mohl, N.: Duration of masseteric silent period in patients with TMJ syndrome. J. Appl. Physiol. 30:864–869, 1971.

Bush, F.: Occlusal etiology of myofascial pain-dysfunction syndrome. In Laskin, D. M., Greenfield, W., Gale, E., et al. (Eds.): The President's Conference on the Examination, Diagnosis, and Management of Temporomandibular Disorders. Chicago, Am. Dent. Assoc., 1983, pp. 95–203.

Carraro, J. J., Caffesse, R. G., and Albano, E. A.: Temporomandibular joint syndrome. Oral Surg. 28:54–62, 1969.

Chaney, D. S., and Andreason, L.: Relaxation and neuromuscular tension control and changes in mental performance under induced tension. Percept. Mot. Skills 34:677–678, 1972.

Christensen, J.: Effect of occlusion-raising procedures on the chewing system. Dent. Pract. Dent. Rec. 20:233–238, 1970.

Copland, J.: Abnormal muscle tension and the mandibular joint. Dent. Rec. 74:331–338, 1954.

Dahlstrom, L.: Electromyographic studies of craniomandibular disorders: A review of the literature. J. Oral Rehabil. 16:1–20, 1989.

Dawson, P. R.: Evaluation, Diagnosis and Treatment of Occlusal Problems. St. Louis, C. V. Mosby, 1974.

DeVries, H. A.: Quantitative electromyographic investigation of the spasm theory of muscle pain. Am. J. Phys. Med. 45:119–124, 1966.

Direnfeld, V. N., and Laskin, D. M.: A muscle endurance test in patients with temporomandibular joint dysfunction. IADR Program and Abstracts of Papers. Chicago, IADR, 1967, p. 56.

Dolwick, M. F., Katzberg, R. W., Helms, C. A., and Bales, D. J.: Arthrotomographic evaluation of the temporomandibular joint. J. Oral Surg. 37:793–799, 1979.

Drinkwater, B. L., Flint, M. M., and Cleland, T. S.: Somatic responses and performance levels during anticipatory physical-threat stress. Percept. Mot. Skills 27:539–552, 1968.

Edmiston, G. F., and Laskin, D. M.: Changes in consistency of occlusal contact in myofascial pain-dysfunction (MPD) syndrome. J. Dent. Res. 57:27–30, 1978.

Euler, U. S., von, and Hellner, S.: Excretion of noradrenaline and adrenaline in muscular work. Acta. Physiol. Scand. 26:183–191, 1952.

Evaskus, D. S., and Laskin, D. M.: A biochemical measure of stress in patients with myofascial pain-dysfunction (MPD) syndrome. J. Dent. Res. 51:1464–1466, 1972.

Evaskus, D. S., Schriar, R., and Laskin, D. M.: Serum enzymes and isoenzymes in myofascial pain-dysfunction syndrome. J. Dent. Res. 56B:140, 1977.

Franks, A. S. T.: Masticatory muscle hyperactivity and temporomandibular joint dysfunction. J. Prosthet. Dent. 15:1122–1131, 1965.

Gessel, A. H.: Electromyographic biofeedback and tricyclic antidepressants in myofascial pain-dysfunction syndrome: Psychological predictors of outcome. J. Am. Dent. Assoc. 91:1048–1052, 1975.

Gold, S., Lipton, J., Marbach, J., and Gurion, B.: Sites of psychophysiological complaints in MPD patients: II. Areas remote from the orofacial region. J. Dent. Res. 54A:165, 1975.

Goldstein, I. B.: Physiological responses in anxious women patients. Arch. Gen. Psychiatry 10:382–388, 1964a.

Goldstein, I. B., Grinker, R. R., Heath, H. A., et al.: Study in psychophysiology of muscle tension: Response specificity. Arch. Gen. Psychiatry 11:312–330, 1964b.

Goodman, P., Greene, C. S., and Laskin, D. M.: Response of patients with myofascial pain-dysfunction syndrome to mock equilibration. J. Am. Dent. Assoc. 92:755–758, 1976.

Greene, C. S., and Laskin, D. M.: Meprobamate therapy for the myofascial pain-dysfunction (MPD) syndrome: A double blind evaluation. J. Am. Dent. Assoc. 82:587–590, 1971.

Greene, C. S., and Laskin, D. M.: Splint therapy for the myofascial pain-dysfunction syndrome: A comparative study. J. Am. Dent. Assoc. 84:624–628, 1972.

Greene, C. S., Lerman, M. D., Sutcher, H. D., and Laskin, D. M.: The TMJ pain-dysfunction syndrome: Heterogeneity of the patient population. J. Am. Dent. Assoc. 70:1168–1172, 1969.

Griffin, C. J., and Munro, R. R.: Electromyography of the masseter and anterior temporalis muscles in patients with temporomandibular dysfunction. Arch. Oral Biol. 16:929–949, 1971.

Haber, J. D., Moss, R. A., Kuczmiercrzk, A. R., and Garrett, J. C.: Assessment and treatment of stress in myofascial pain-dysfunction syndrome. A model for analysis. J. Oral Rehabil. *10*:187–196, 1983.

Hannam, A. G., and Matthews, B.: Reflex jaw opening in response to stimulation of periodontal mechanoreceptors in the cat. Arch. Oral Biol. *14*:415–419, 1969.

Helkimo, M.: Epidemiological surveys of dysfunction of the masticatory system. Oral Sci. Rev. 7:54–66, 1976.

Helms, C. A., Vogler, J. B., and Morrish, R. B.: Temporomandibular joint internal derangements: CT diagnosis. Radiology *152*:459–465, 1984.

Johnson, D. L., Shipman, W. G., and Laskin, D. M.: Physiological responses to stressful stimuli in patients with myofascial pain-dysfunction (MPD) syndrome. IADR Program and Abstracts of Papers. Chicago, IADR, 1972, p. 96.

Kidokoro, Y., Kubota, K., Shuto, S., and Sumino, R.: Reflex organization of masticatory muscles in the cat. J. Neurophysiol. *31*:695–708, 1968.

Krell, M., and Laskin, D. M.: Measurement of masseteric silent period for diagnosis and treatment evaluation in MPD syndrome. J. Dent. Res. *56B*:61, 1977.

Kydd, W. L.: Psychosomatic aspects of temporomandibular joint dysfunction. J. Am. Dent. Assoc. 59:31–44, 1959.

Laskin, D. M.: Etiology of the pain-dysfunction syndrome. J. Am. Dent. Assoc. 79:147–153, 1969.

Laskin, D. M., and Greene, C. S.: Influence of the doctor-patient relationship on placebo therapy for patients with myofascial pain-dysfunction (MPD) syndrome. J. Am. Dent. Assoc. 85:892–894, 1972.

Lundeen, T. F., Sturdevant, J. R., and George, J. M.: Stress as a factor in muscle and temporomandibular joint pain. J. Oral Rehabil. *14*:447–456, 1987.

Lupton, D. E.: A preliminary investigation of the personality of female temporomandibular joint dysfunction patients. Psychother. Psychosom. *14*:199–216, 1966.

Lupton, D. E.: Psychological aspects of temporomandibular joint dysfunction. J. Am. Dent. Assoc. 79:131–136, 1969.

Malmo, R. B., Shagass, C., and Davis, J. K.: Electromyographic studies of muscular tension in psychiatric patients under stress. J. Clin. Exp. Psychopathol. *12*:45–66, 1951.

Mankin, H. J.: Clinical features of osteoarthritis. *In* Kelly, W. N., Harris, E. D. Jr., Ruddy, S., and Sledge, C. B. (Eds.): Textbook of Rheumatology, 3rd ed. Philadelphia, W. B. Saunders, 1989a, pp. 1480–1500.

Mankin, H. J., and Brandt, K. D.: Pathogenesis of osteoarthritis. *In* Kelly, W. N., Harris, E. D. Jr., Ruddy, S., and Sledge, C. B. (Eds.): Textbook of Rheumatology, 3rd ed. Philadelphia, W. B. Saunders, 1989b, pp. 1469–1479.

Marbach, J. J., and Dworkin, S. F.: Chronic MPD, group therapy and psychodynamics. J. Am. Dent. Assoc. 90:827–833, 1975.

Markovic, M. A., and Rosenberg, H. M.: Tomographic evaluation of 100 patients with temporomandibular joint symptoms. Oral Surg. *42*:838–846, 1976.

McCall, C. M., Szmyd, L., and Ritter, R. M.: Personality characteristics in patients with temporomandibular joint symptoms. J. Am. Dent. Assoc. 62:694–698, 1961.

McHorris, W. H.: Occlusal adjustment via selective cutting of natural teeth. Part I. Int. J. Periodont. Rest. Dent. 5:8–25, 1985.

McNeill, C., Mohl, N. D., Rugh, J. D., and Tanaka, T. T.: Temporomandibular disorders: Diagnosis, management, education, and research. J. Am. Dent. Assoc. *120*:253–263, 1990.

Mercuri, L. G., Olson, R. E., and Laskin, D. M.: The specificity of response to experimental stress in patients with myofascial pain-dysfunction syndrome. J. Dent. Res. 58:1866–1871, 1979.

Michler, L., Moller, E., Bakke, M., et al.: On-line analysis of natural activity in muscles of mastication. J. Craniomandib. Pract. 2:65–82, 1988.

Molin, C., Edman, G., and Schalling, D.: Psychological studies of patients with mandibular pain-dysfunction syndrome (MDS). II. Tolerance for experimentally induced pain. Swed. Dent. J. 66:15–23, 1973.

Mongini, F., and Tempia-Valenta, G.: A graphic and statistical analysis of the chewing movements in function and dysfunction. J. Prosthet. Dent. 22:647–651, 1984.

Naeije, M., and Hansson, T. L.: Electromyographic screening of myogenous and arthrogenous TMJ dysfunction patients. J. Oral Rehabil. *13*:433–441, 1986.

Newton, A. V.: Predisposing causes for temporomandibular joint dysfunction. J. Prosthet. Dent. 22:647–651, 1969.

Perry, H. T.: Muscular changes associated with temporomandibular joint dysfunction. J. Am. Dent. Assoc. 54:644–653, 1957.

Perry, H. T., Lammie, G. A., Main, J., and Teuscher, G. W.: Occlusion in stress situations. J. Am. Dent. Assoc. 60:626–633, 1960.

Pomp, A. M.: Psychotherapy for the myofascial pain-dysfunction (MPD) syndrome: A study of factors coinciding with symptom remission. J. Am. Dent. Assoc. 89:629–632, 1974.

Posselt, V.: The temporomandibular joint syndrome and occlusion. J. Prosthet. Dent. 25:432–438, 1971.

Pullinger, A. G., and Monteilo, A. A.: Historical factors associated with temporomandibular disorders. J. Oral Rehabil. *14*:117–124, 1988.

Ramfjord, S. P., and Ash, M. M.: Occlusion, 3rd ed. Philadelphia, W. B. Saunders, 1983.

Reuben, B., and Laskin, D. M.: Electromyographic analysis of masticatory muscle activity in myofascial pain-dysfunction syndrome. J. Dent. Res. *56B*:232, 1977.

Rosenberg, H. M.: Laminagraphy: Methods and application in oral diagnosis. J. Am. Dent. Assoc. 74:88–96, 1967.

Scapino, R. P.: Histopathology associated with malposition of the human temporomandibular joint disc. Oral Surg. 55:382–397, 1983.

Schwartz, L. L.: Disorders of the Temporomandibular Joint. Philadelphia, W. B. Saunders, 1959.

Schwartz, L. L.: Pain associated with the temporomandibular joint. J. Am. Dent. Assoc. 51:394–397, 1955.

Schwartz, L., and Cobin, H. P.: Symptoms associated with the temporomandibular joint. Oral Surg. 10:339–344, 1957.

Shore, N. A.: Temporomandibular Joint Dysfunction and Occlusal Equilibration, 2nd ed. Philadelphia, J. B. Lippincott, 1976.

Skiba, T. J., and Laskin, D. M.: Masticatory muscle silent periods in patients with MPD syndrome. J. Dent. Res. *55B*:249, 1976.

Solberg, W. K., Flint, R. T., and Brantner, J. P.: Temporomandibular joint pain and dysfunction: A clinical study of emotional and occlusal components. J. Prosthet. Dent. 28:412–422, 1972.

Sternbach, R. A., Wolf, S. R., Murphy, R. W., and Akeson, W. H.: Aspects of chronic low back pain. Psychosomatics *14*:52–56, 1973.

Thomas, L. J., Tiber, N., and Schireson, S.: The effects of anxiety and frustration on muscular tension related to the temporomandibular joint syndrome. Oral Surg. 36:763–768, 1973.

Thomson, H.: Mandibular dysfunction syndrome. Br. Dent. J. *130*:187–193, 1971.

Traut, E. J.: Fibrositis. J. Am. Geriatr. Soc. *13*:531–538, 1968.

Vestergaard Christensen, L.: Facial pain and internal pressure of masseter muscle in experimental bruxism in man. Arch. Oral Biol. 16:1021–1031, 1971.

Vestergaard Christensen, L.: Jaw muscle fatigue and pains induced by experimental tooth clenching: A review. J. Oral Rehabil. 8:27–36, 1981.

Vogler, J. B., Dolan, E., Martinez, S., and Spritzer, C.: Internal derangements of the temporomandibular joint: Diagnosis by magnetic resonance imaging. J. Craniomandib. Disord. 1:157–162, 1987.

Weinberg, S., and Lapointe, H.: Cervical extension-flexion injury (whiplash) and internal derangement of the TMJ. J. Oral Maxillofac. Surg. 45:653–656, 1987.

Westesson, P.-L.: Structural hard tissue changes in temporomandibular joints with internal derangements. Oral Surg. 59:220–224, 1985.

Yale, S. H., Allison, B. D., and Hauptfuehrer, J. D.: An epidemiological assessment of mandibular condyle morphology. Oral Surg. 21:169–177, 1966.

Yemm, R.: A comparison of the electrical activity of masseter and temporal muscles of human subjects during experimental stress. Arch. Oral Biol. 16:269–273, 1971.

Yemm, R.: A neurophysiological approach to the pathology and etiology of temporomandibular disorders. J. Oral Rehabil. 12:343–353, 1985.

Yemm, R.: Neurophysiological studies of temporomandibular joint dysfunction. Oral Sci. Rev. 7:31–53, 1976.

Yemm, R.: Temporomandibular dysfunction and masseter muscle response to experimental stress. Br. Dent. J. 127:508–510, 1969a.

Yemm, R.: Variations in the electrical activity of the human masseter muscle occurring in association with emotional stress. Arch. Oral Biol. 14:873–878, 1969b.

20

TEMPOROMANDIBULAR DISORDERS: Psychological and Behavioral Aspects*

JOHN D. RUGH, PH.D., and SUZANNE E. DAVIS, M.M.S.

INTRODUCTION

The clinical management of patients with temporomandibular disorders (TMDs) is often difficult and perplexing. Procedures have been developed to identify and correct structural problems of the joint and teeth. Clinicians have found, however, that accomplishing these procedures does not consistently result in pain-free, appreciative patients. Fifteen to 35 per

*See Chapters 7–9, 18, 19, 21, 25, and 26.

cent of patients do not show the expected therapeutic results of decreased pain and increased function (Cohen, 1978; Eriksson, 1986; Greene, 1983; Heloe, 1980a; Marciani, 1987; Mejersjo, 1983; Okeson, 1986; Pedersen, 1987; Zarb, 1970). These patients continue to have symptoms, are at risk of becoming patients with chronic pain, and are increasingly likely to file malpractice suits. Such treatment failures may result from a host of problems, including misdiagnosis, inappropriate treatment, and/or failure to control the original etiologic factors. This chapter focuses on the behavioral and psychological factors that are crucial in the diagnosis and management of patients with TMDs.

Although substantive knowledge regarding psychological factors in TMDs is rapidly accumulating, this knowledge remains inadequate to understand these patients fully (Greene, 1982; Marbach, 1987; Melamed, 1981; Moss, 1984a; Rugh, 1983; Scott, 1981; Speculand, 1985). Thus, much of the material presented in this chapter is based on patients with other illnesses or is derived from clinical experience rather than well-controlled experimental research. Throughout the chapter, we have attempted to indicate the basis of the information. References are provided to original research and review papers in specific areas.

PSYCHOLOGICAL FACTORS MODULATING ILLNESS BEHAVIOR

Patient Pain Presentations

Reporting pain, eating soft food, taking medications, staying home from work, and seeking care are referred to as illness behaviors. The significance of psychological factors in modifying illness behaviors is often apparent at the initial office visit when the patient describes the chief complaint and how the pain affects his or her life. One patient may appear emotionally distraught and report being physically disabled and socially crippled by what is identified as only a periodic mild muscular tenderness. This patient may demand aggressive treatment for what he or she perceives as a condition that is ruining his or her life. In contrast, another patient with a similar condition may show no signs of distress and report being only slightly bothered by the pain. This patient's life has not been disrupted, the pain is not disabling, and the patient may be reluctant to accept treatment.

These two contrasting patients exemplify the important principle that there is not a simple relationship between the gravity of the pathology and the patient's illness behavior. Patients with identical illnesses in terms of tissue damage and pathology may present with dramatically contrasting verbal reports and perceptions of pain. In fact, illness behavior can occur without illness or nociception. The key point is that illness behavior and pathology are two separate issues. Although the two phenomena are often related, each may exist independently, with or without the presence of the other.

Understanding this concept is perhaps the most important message in this chapter. Since the patient's verbal reports (illness behaviors) are a key feature in diagnosis and decisions regarding treatment, it is crucial to understand the many psychological factors that may influence the patient's report of pain independent of the pathology.

Patients' illness behaviors may be influenced by any or all of a variety of factors. These include depression, anxiety, secondary gain, beliefs, focused attention, and pathology. Each of these is briefly discussed in the following sections. Several authors have provided in-depth reviews of these factors (Craig, 1986; Fordyce, 1986; Liebeskind, 1977; Marbach, 1987; Payne, 1986; Rugh, 1987a; Skevington, 1986; Turk, 1986).

Secondary Gain

In the past two decades, doctors have become increasingly aware of how reinforcement contingencies in the patient's natural environment encourage a patient to exaggerate pain reports and other illness behaviors (Marciani, 1987). This concept is referred to as secondary gain (Fordyce, 1976). Desired conditions such as sympathy, attention, and escape from work are often contingent upon illness behaviors. Being sick allows one to relinquish responsibilities of school, work, and parenting. Reade (1985) described a patient with a temporomandibular joint (TMJ) disorder whose marriage was characterized by frequent arguments over finances and child rearing. She felt powerless in these conflicts. Her continuing pain condition legitimized her dependent role with her family and provided a means to handle marital strife. The principle is that being sick has some obvious advantages at certain times and such behavior can be used to deal with the environment (Fordyce, 1976).

Pending litigation often provides an economic incentive for continued illness behaviors. Brooke (1978) suggested that pending litigation is a factor in treatment failures of patients with myofascial pain-dysfunction (MPD) syndrome. Litigation is such a powerful reinforcement for illness behavior that some clinicians prefer not to attempt to treat a patient until the litigation is settled (Sternbach, 1978).

A relatively common clinical problem following TMJ surgery is continued reports of pain related to secondary gain. Pain and limited function may be minimal. The patient, however, may overdramatize relatively minor symptoms to maintain advantageous reinforcement patterns established before surgery. Clinical observations suggest that the probability of postsurgery secondary gain is higher in patients who have had long periods (more than six months) of pain before surgery and whose lifestyles have been significantly altered by the pain. During a prolonged period of illness, permanent behavioral patterns may be established.

In general, secondary gain often emerges near the end of the healing period. In early stages of an illness, the patient's behavior is more likely related to actual tissue damage, such as might occur with inflammation or trauma. After healing, however, illness behaviors may continue due to the advantages that they provide.

Secondary gain is also recognized to be a factor in under-reporting pain in some circumstances, such as when reporting an illness may be disadvantageous to the patient. This is particularly obvious for the child who, if sick, must stay home from the movies, go to the doctor, and, worst of all, possibly receive an injection. It is not surprising that children often under-report or minimize illness (Kononen, 1987). Males in western cultures have also been noted to under-report symptoms of illness (Theorell, 1987). This sociocultural pattern may partially explain the relatively low percentage of males who seek care for TM pain conditions.

Identifying Secondary Gain

Few clinicians question the concept of secondary gain; however, it is not easy to identify. The clinician must determine which aspects of a patient's illness report are related to secondary gain and which are related to pathology. Direct questions regarding secondary gain are often threatening to the patient and should be pursued carefully. Insight may be gained by asking the patient what the pain prevents him or her from doing. Inconsistencies, such as an inability to care for children, yet no difficulties with pleasant activities such as shopping, water skiing, or tennis, should raise suspicion. Patterns of exacerbations of the pain sometimes also provide insight. The fact that flareups precede potentially undesirable life events provides a lead for discussion. Charting illness behavior in a pain diary over a 30-day period is often useful to help identify reinforcement contingencies (Andrasik, 1981). Family members are sometimes able to provide insight and, in fact, are often unknowingly a source of re-

inforcement that may maintain illness behaviors (Fordyce, 1976).

A positive response to a placebo does not provide either a definitive insight into the role of secondary gain or other psychological factors (Greene, 1982). Patients with identifiable pathology also respond to placebos. Thus, a positive response to a placebo neither points to a psychological problem nor does it rule out organic disease.

In summary, it is reasonable that sick people should be helped and be relieved of certain responsibilities. A serious problem develops, however, when illness behaviors outlast the normal healing time or when the patient begins using pain behaviors to manage his or her life or to manipulate the lives of others. It is the responsibility of the clinician to be aware of and watchful for illness behaviors that outlast the normal healing time.

Search for the Definitive Treatment

In addition to secondary gain, there are several other reasons why patients may overemphasize their pain conditions. Many chronic TMD patients have sought help from several different doctors. Appropriate palliative therapy for a recurrent stress-related problem may have been provided by each therapist. Some patients, however, consider this therapy insufficient and desire a definitive cure. To resolve this problem, some patients overstate the level of pain and disability under the assumption that it is only with extreme levels of pain and disability that a definitive treatment will be provided. This puts the patient at risk for inappropriate, irreversible therapy.

This situation results in part because clinicians have failed to explain adequately to the patient the nature of the TM pain condition. The patient must understand that TM pains are not signs of a life threatening illness, that these conditions, when chronic, are rarely completely cured, and that there are no definitive treatments for all human pain. These important concepts must be explained to the patient to reduce the probability of doctor shopping and inappropriate overtreatment.

Learned Helplessness

Another important concept in understanding illness behaviors is that of learned helplessness (Seligman, 1975). After experiencing months or years of failure to find relief from pain, some patients understandably give up trying. They perceive that their own actions are futile in terms of resolving their problems. This attitude may generalize to other aspects of their daily lives. These patients often become resistant to self-care programs, become noncompliant, and are at high risk for depression and chronic pain.

Learned helplessness can usually be identified during the history. When asked what he or she can do to relieve or prevent the pain, the patient reports, "Nothing." These patients paint a picture of being brought to their knees by a pain over which they have no control. The pain has overpowered them.

Psychological consultation may be necessary to develop a program to reverse learned helplessness. Tolerance of pain can be improved when patients perceive that they have some degree of control over their pain condition (Langer, 1983).

Apprehensive Disuse Atrophy

Patient beliefs about the meaning of pain following TMJ surgery or injury can result in pain behaviors that disrupt healing and delay the return of normal function. Some patients continue a limited function protocol long after the normal healing time because they believe they will reinjure the joint. Significant disuse atrophy may develop so that fatigue and pain result even with such function. The patient interprets this pain as an indication of more damage to the joint. Use of the mandible is further curtailed, resulting in additional atrophy. This condition must be identified and reversed by changing the patient's belief about the meaning of the pain and by beginning a regimen of supervised physical exercise to reverse the muscle atrophy. Discussions with the patient should emphasize an image of a healing and functioning joint.

Sociocultural Factors

Illness behaviors appear highly dependent upon sociocultural influences. Cultural expectations often prescribe how one responds to pain, how much pain should be tolerated, and when one should seek treatment. Individuals of Italian or Jewish descent, for example, are believed to be more likely to express pain and suffering and are contrasted with the stoic response to pain of the Irish. Caucasians are better able to tolerate pain than Asian-Americans and some report that men reliably show more tolerance to painful stimuli than women (Melzack, 1982). Biological mechanisms have

not been found to account for these differences, and it is postulated that the differences are due to learned sex roles and cultural expectations (Otto, 1985). An awareness of these cultural differences allows the clinician better to interpret the significance of pain reports.

PSYCHOLOGIC FACTORS MODULATING THE EXPERIENCE OF PAIN (see pages 455–458)

Pain is a complex multifaceted personal experience involving sensory, cognitive, and emotional aspects. The perception of pain, tolerance of pain, and behavioral response to pain are modified by numerous psychosocial factors, which include anxiety, depression, beliefs about the origin of the pain, attention, personality, and cultural factors. There is ample evidence that a relatively large subgroup of TMD patients have emotional, behavioral, or personality characteristics that may modify their experience of pain (Eversole, 1985; Fricton, 1985; Greene, 1982; Gregg, 1978; Heloe, 1980b; Malow, 1981b; Melamed, 1981; Moss, 1984a; Rugh, 1979; 1984b; 1987a; Schumann, 1988; van der Laan, 1988).

Anxiety

In general, anxiety appears to make pain conditions worse. Pain thresholds are lowered, and patients are less willing to tolerate pain when anxious (Melzack, 1984; 1986). Patients with TMD as a group are more anxious than normal individuals, and subgroups of TMD patients experience significant anxiety as either a result (Gale, 1978) or a cause of their condition (Rugh, 1979). Fricton (1985) found 26 per cent of 164 MPD patients to be clinically anxious. As many as 17 per cent may suffer from severe anxiety (Gerschman, 1987), which may lower pain thresholds and significantly complicate the management of these patients.

Patients with chronic MPD syndrome have a generalized change in pain perception. Molin (1973) reported that MPD patients had lower pain thresholds than controls. More recently, Malow (1980) demonstrated that MPD patients had both lower pain thresholds and a greater tendency to report experimental pain than non-MPD patients. In a follow-up study, Malow (1981a) found that successfully treated patients had an increase in pain threshold and a decreased tendency to report experimental pain applied to the finger, thus strengthening the hypothesis that lower pain thresholds may contribute to the patient's pain condition.

In addition to lowering the pain threshold, anxiety reduces the patient's willingness to tolerate even minor pain or dysfunction and may thus be a factor in the patient's decision to seek care. Marbach (1978) found that 62 per cent of a patient population had major life events preceding the decision to seek treatment, a result compatible with this concept. Anxiety related to these events may modify both the patients' experiences of pain and their willingness to tolerate a longstanding, but relatively minor, pain condition.

Anxiety also plays a role in a patient's experience of pain following surgery. Of particular relevance to the surgeon is the finding that levels of postoperative pain and analgesic requirements have been related to a patient's trait anxiety rather than acute or situational anxiety about the surgery (Taenzer, 1986). Trait anxiety refers to a patient's general or typical emotional reactions. Thus, in trying to predict which patients may have difficulty with postsurgical pain, the surgeon should be more concerned with evaluating patients' general emotional responses than their anxieties over the particular surgical procedure in question.

Beliefs About Cause of Pain

The level of anxiety accompanying pain is often related to the beliefs the patient has regarding the origin of the pain. Believing that pain signifies a life-threatening condition can result in significant emotional distress. This distress is sometimes worse than the original pain condition and may result in a series of problems. It is essential that the clinician alleviate the patient's misconceptions and concerns about a life-threatening disease by providing an explanation of the origin and significance of the pain. Clarifying patients' beliefs regarding their pain conditions is perhaps one of the most important aspects of therapy. It is particularly crucial today with the fear of cancer so prevalent in our society. The basic principle is that pain hurts more, causes more anxiety, and is less tolerable when its origin is unknown or misinterpreted (Ciccone, 1984; Lowery, 1983; Turk, 1986).

Perceived Control

Pain is also more bothersome when the patient believes he or she has no control over it (Bowers, 1968; Gatchel, 1980). For this reason,

it is important to assist the patient in identifying specific behaviors that are related to symptom onset and that the patient can control. In addition, it is important to provide specific self-care routines that the patient can apply when the pain appears. Depending on the specific condition, self-care programs may include use of soft diet, jaw exercises, self-relaxation, meditation, moist heat, and perhaps the direct application of transcutaneous electrical nerve stimulation. Patients are better able to cope with pain when they have knowledge of how to control its onset and/or modify its intensity or duration. This is particularly important for the recurrent TM conditions that require long-term management.

Attention Patterns

The perception and tolerance of pain can be dramatically modified by focusing attention away from the pain (McCaul, 1984). Most clinicians have experienced the frustration of dealing with a patient who spends 95 per cent of his or her waking hours focusing on what appears to be a minor pain condition. One pictures these patients sitting by the bed periodically probing the site, waiting for the pain to strike. With this intense degree of vigilance, low levels of nociception are identified that may not be perceived by another individual who, because of social and economic responsibilities, is less vigilant. Postsurgical patients often focus a great deal of attention on the surgical site and concern themselves with low levels of nociception. Clinical observations suggest that surgical patients who involve themselves in an active pace of life shortly after surgery generally have fewer problems with postsurgical pain.

Depression

Marciani (1983) described a surgical patient in whom good objective improvements were observed after discoplasty (improved opening and no further occasions of jaw locking). The patient reported, however, that the operation did not produce any relief. This patient had a longstanding diagnosis of depression. A good objective but poor subjective outcome is common among patients with depression. Depression is believed to lower the threshold for pain and decrease the patient's willingness to tolerate the pain.

Studies assessing depression in facial pain and TMD patients vary with respect to the prevalence of depression. Gerschman (1987)

TABLE 20–1. Characteristics Suggestive of Depression

Difficulty staying asleep
Fatigue and no energy
Loss of appetite
Change in appearance
Loss of sexual desires
Irritability
Poor compliance
Numerous and vague somatic
   complaints

found 52 per cent of 368 chronic facial pain patients to be moderately depressed using the Hamilton Depression Scale. Eighteen per cent were severely depressed. Fricton (1985) reported depression in 23 per cent of 164 patients. Marbach (1981), on the other hand, found that as a group, facial pain patients were not more depressed than a control group. Although group differences may not be found, it is reasonable to expect that a number of patients with TMD will have depression as a result of their pain condition or as a factor maintaining the condition.

Characteristics of depression are listed in Table 20–1. Patients exhibiting three or more of these characteristics should be questioned further and possibly referred for psychological evaluation. It is also important to recognize that depression is often masked and not readily apparent. A careful workup by either a psychologist or psychiatrist is usually necessary to identify patients with masked depression.

A significant improvement in patients' ability to tolerate pain is frequently reported with a regimen of antidepressants (Feinmann, 1984; Gessel, 1975; Lascelles, 1966; Lindsey, 1981). Often these patients have failed to respond to varied dental treatment. Hersh (1987) reviewed the clinical management of chronic orofacial pain patients using tricyclic antidepressants. The mechanism of action of antidepressants is unclear. It is hypothesized that they may modify the receptor and pain perceptual systems through the gate control mechanism (Melzack, 1984). Sharav (1987) provided evidence that amitriptyline affected levels of pain independent of its effect on mood. Regardless of the mechanism, the clinical outcome studies mentioned previously document the efficacy of antidepressants for a subgroup of TMD patients. It is likely that the use of this treatment will increase as the limitations of structural treatments are further delineated.

Summary

In the first two sections, we have discussed how patients' perception of pain, tolerance of pain, and behavioral and emotional response to pain are modified by psychological factors. These modifying factors include emotional conditions such as anxiety and depression; cognitive factors such as beliefs about the origin, meaning, and control of the pain; and attentional factors such as focusing on relatively minor conditions. In addition, we discussed the important distinction between illness behaviors and illness. As depicted in Figure 20–1, pain behaviors such as reporting pain, staying in bed, seeking care, and requesting surgery can all occur independently of pathology or nociception.

The clinician faces a difficult problem. Seventy to 80 per cent of the population has one or more signs or symptoms of TMD yet it is estimated that only five per cent of this group is in need of aggressive treatment (Rugh, 1985). The decision to treat is predominantly based on the medical history and patient reports of pain and disability, yet psychosocial factors cause some patients to overdramatize symptoms and demand unneeded, irreversible treatment. These patients have a poor prognosis because the original psychosocial problem has not been addressed. It is important that the clinician carefully analyze verbal reports and the pain behaviors of patients to determine how they have been modified by the various psychological factors discussed in these two sections.

PSYCHOLOGICAL FACTORS IN THE ETIOLOGY OF TEMPOROMANDIBULAR DISORDERS

Thus far, discussion has been limited to how psychological factors can modify the perception, tolerance, and response to a painful condition. Psychological variables, however, can also serve as primary etiologic factors. This section discusses a subgroup of TMD patients whose condition results from, or is aggravated, by stress-related muscle hyperactivity.

Oral Habits and Muscle Hyperactivity

Oral habits have long been implicated as factors in the development and perpetuation of TMDs (Laskin, 1969; Moulton, 1966), and there is now reasonably strong evidence supporting the etiological role of oral habits in these disorders (Moss, 1984b; Rugh, 1984a). Brooke (1977), for instance, noted that 80 per cent of

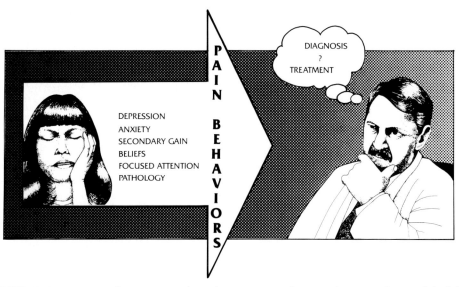

FIGURE 20–1. Diagnosis and treatment are dependent, in part, on the patient's reports of pain and disability. It is crucial to recognize that these pain behaviors are influenced by many cognitive, emotional, learning, and sociocultural factors. Pathology is only one of several conditions that may elicit or maintain pain behaviors, making diagnosis and management very difficult.

194 MPD patients reported destructive oral habits such as clenching or grinding of the teeth.

There are many causes of destructive oral habits. Some may be related to occupational jaw posturing. Muscle and joint problems have been reported in violinists and scuba divers (Pinto, 1966; Rieder, 1976). Other oral habits may be learned. Subtle peer pressure may encourage patients with a retrognathic mandible to adopt a chronic forward posturing of the mandible to minimize their weak-chinned appearance (Rugh, 1984a). The habit of unilateral chewing resulting from a toothache or missing teeth may persist long after the dental problem has been successfully resolved. These are examples of oral habits that evolve as learned avoidance responses.

Other oral habits and behaviors include stress-induced masticatory muscle hyperactivity. The relationships between muscle hyperactivity and stress, and between muscle hyperactivity and TMDs, have been established through studies in both experimental and natural environments.

Experimentally Induced Myofascial Pain

Several studies have described specific patterns of muscle contraction that have produced facial pain symptoms in normal subjects similar to those symptoms reported by TMD-MPD patients (Bowley, 1987; Christensen, 1971;

1978; 1979; 1985; Doerfler, 1984; Scott, 1980; Villarosa, 1985). In these studies, the pain symptoms were elicited through prolonged rhythmic or sustained clenching, chewing, or jaw thrusting patterns involving the masseter, temporalis, and medial and lateral pterygoid muscles (Fig. 20–2). The results of these studies support the theory that oral habits and masticatory hyperactivity may result in myofascial pain symptoms. These results are consistent with the literature regarding other muscle contraction disorders (Bakal, 1975; Haynes, 1981; Martin, 1972; Wolff, 1963).

Stress-Induced Muscle Hyperactivity and Pain

Emotional states such as anxiety may elicit a variety of oral habits. Lip-biting or cheek-biting, tooth clenching or grinding, nail-biting, and general masticatory muscle tension are believed to be manifestations of anger, anxiety, frustration, boredom, or fear. Although each of these behaviors may seem innocuous and transient, prolonged or frequent occurrences of specific oral habits may initiate and/or exacerbate TM pain and dysfunction, especially when superposed on existing TM derangements (Carlsson, 1976; Laskin, 1969; Moss, 1984b; Moulton, 1966; Villarosa, 1985; Westling, 1988).

The results of several studies show that certain individuals tend to respond to stress with

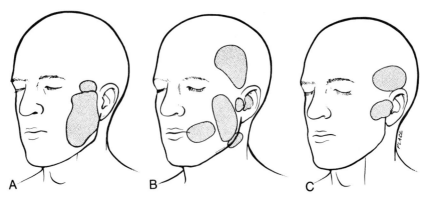

FIGURE 20–2. Jaw and facial pain have been experimentally produced in healthy subjects through oral behaviors, including tooth grinding *(A)*, forward thrusting of the mandible *(B)*, and voluntary retrusive positioning of the mandible *(C)*. (Data from Christensen, L. V.: Facial pain and internal pressure of masseter muscle in experimental bruxism in man. Arch. Oral Biol. *16*:1021, 1971; Doerfler, L. F., and Rugh, J. D.: Voluntary mandibular retrusion exercises and facial pain. J. Dent. Res. *63*:288, Abstract 1059, 1984; Scott, D. S., and Lundeen, T. F.: Myofascial pain involving the masticatory muscles: An experimental model. Pain *8*:207–215, 1980.)

significant and/or prolonged masticatory muscle activity (Dordick, 1978; Johnson, 1972; Mercuri, 1979; Perry, 1960; Rao, 1979; Rugh, 1987; Thomas, 1973; Yemm, 1971; 1976). In these studies, stress was induced through a variety of stimuli and/or manual tasks under various experimental conditions using both control and patient populations. Studies using portable EMG monitoring equipment in patients' natural environments have also found muscle hyperactivity and pain related to emotional stress (Finlayson, 1982; Funch, 1980; Rugh, 1975; 1983).

Controversy remains as to whether patients respond to stress specifically in the masticatory system or through a generalized somatic response (Gold, 1975; Heiberg, 1978; Lundeen, 1987; Mercuri, 1979; Rugh, 1987). Masticatory muscle hyperactivity has been a fairly consistent finding, however, in studies with TMD patient groups.

Stress and Temporomandibular Disorders

It is a common clinical experience to find high correlations between muscular pain symptoms and stressful life events (Brooke, 1977; Duinkerke, 1985; Lundeen, 1987; Lupton, 1969; Rugh, 1983). Patients with TMDs were found by Speculand (1984) to experience more than twice as many stressful life events as a control population. Conversely, symptoms have been reduced following a variety of behavioral or psychological treatment programs designed to reduce stress and muscular tension (Crockett, 1986; Dahlstrom, 1984; Dohrmann, 1978; Graff-Radford, 1987; Miller, 1987; Olson, 1986; Sol-

berg, 1972; Stam, 1984). Treatment effects may depend upon an increase in the patient's perceived control (Hijzen, 1986).

In summary, diurnal muscle hyperactivity related to stressful life events and emotional tension appears to be an important etiologic factor in a subgroup of patients. Clinicians must be alert to the likelihood of stress and masticatory muscle hyperactivity in TMD patients. The American Association of Oral and Maxillofacial Surgeons Criteria for TMJ Meniscus Surgery (1984) emphasize the need to identify and manage muscular components before surgery to avoid failures. Treatment of physical signs and symptoms without routine screening for stress or psychological factors may result in poor treatment outcomes.

Identification of Oral Habits and Muscle Hyperactivity

Destructive oral habits may be identified with the aid of thorough patient interviews, questionnaires, and daily pain charting.

Patient Interviews

Patients are sometimes aware of oral habits and are able to report specific maladaptive behaviors. The clinician should also observe and identify oral habits performed by the patient during the interview process. Often, firsthand observation will identify behaviors of which the patient is unaware.

Questionnaires

The use of questionnaires is an efficient and organized method to gather information to be used to supplement the oral history or interview. Questions should be in lay language and move from queries regarding general oral symptoms and associated medical conditions to questions about lifestyle and family, economic, and associated medical problems. The interview and questionnaire must be cautiously interpreted, as many patients are unaware of oral habits.

Pain and Activity Charting

Having the patient self-chart symptoms and activities every four hours over a two- or four-week period gives the clinician valuable insights regarding cyclical trends and emotion-symptom interactions. The written pain diary also often serves to educate patients in the relationship between their habits and painful symptoms, and involves the patients in their own treatment planning program (Rugh, 1982).

Electromyographic Recordings

Most oral habits are correlated with an increase in masticatory muscle activity, which may be detected electromyographically. To aid in the identification of oral habits, Rugh (1984a) suggested electromyographic recordings of facial and jaw muscles in the patient's natural environment. Solberg (1972) reported that patients were surprised at the frequency of their EMG-identified diurnal oral habits and that this new awareness was a significant factor in the ensuing reduction of the destructive behaviors. The development of portable EMG instruments (Burgar, 1983) has allowed the recording of jaw muscle activity during the patient's normal waking and sleeping hours, which provides the clinician with information about oral muscle hyperactivity in the patient's natural environment (Rugh, 1978). EMG evaluations of resting muscle activity in the clinic have not been shown to be of diagnostic value.

Management of Oral Habits and Diurnal Muscle Hyperactivity

The most significant factor in the management of oral habits is the identification of the destructive habit by both the clinician and the patient. Patients are often able to modify their behavior once it is identified and the adverse effects are discussed. Other options include counseling to deal with emotional difficulties, relaxation and biofeedback training, behavior modification techniques, and stress management (Cannistraci, 1987; Dahlstrom, 1984;

Dohrman, 1978; Gale, 1986; Lupton, 1969; Miller, 1987; Olson, 1986; Solberg, 1972; Wilkinson, 1987). Behaviorally oriented psychologists and physical therapists are usually skilled with these techniques. Short-term administration of antianxiety medication and analgesics may also be necessary. The prognosis for improvement in symptoms is dependent upon the motivation of the patient and a well-structured team approach to the multifactorial nature of these cases.

For many patients, pain and dysfunction are self-limiting because they are related to a temporary stressful life event. Feinmann (1984) found that patients who had the best prognosis were those whose pain conditions were associated with specific adverse life situations. For other patients, however, TM conditions are only one manifestation of a more chronic emotional condition or stressful lifestyle. Lupton (1969) reported that 80 per cent of the female TMJ patients he examined had a history of other stress-related disorders. It is common to find that TM patients have frequent tension headaches and neckaches. Comprehensive stress control and a relaxation program are often helpful (Gale, 1986; Mealiea, 1987).

Nocturnal Bruxism

Nocturnal bruxism is the grinding or clenching of teeth during sleep. Bruxism may involve rhythmic, chewing-like patterns and/or sustained contractions in an eccentric or intercuspal position (Rugh, 1988). Nocturnal bruxism has been implicated as an important etiologic factor in temporomandibular and myofascial pain disorders (Clark, 1981; Glaros, 1977; Hijzen et al., 1986; McGlynn, 1985; Wannam, 1986). Chronic nocturnal bruxism may result in masticatory muscle tenderness, facial pain and/or headache, limited jaw movements, joint noise, and locking of the jaw (Berlin, 1954; Clark, 1981; Magnusson, 1979). Other conditions seen in severe bruxists include subluxation and remodeling of the condyles of the mandible (Molin, 1966; Mongini, 1975).

The etiology of nocturnal bruxism is not fully understood, but it commonly occurs during stressful life situations and decreases or disappears when the life crises resolve (Carlsson, 1976; Funch, 1980; Rugh, 1975; 1988). Clark (1980) found that increased levels of urinary catecholamines correlated with high levels of nocturnal masseter activity.

Ware (1988) recently identified a group of severe bruxists whose grinding occurred primarily during rapid eye movement (REM) sleep and was related to depression rather than anxiety. In contrast to the stress-related bruxist population, these patients clenched at high levels each night without the usual fluctuation over time. They were more likely to do severe damage to the TMJ. Experimental treatment with REM-suppressing antidepressants has shown some promise in managing these patients.

Identification of Nocturnal Bruxism

Two factors complicate the identification of nocturnal bruxism in patients with TMDs. First, self-report is largely unreliable, as most are unaware of their bruxist behavior unless a roommate or sleeping partner tells them (Reding, 1966). Secondly, nocturnal bruxism levels are highly variable over time, which may necessitate several visits or prolonged screening periods. The following signs and symptoms are suggestive of nocturnal bruxism:

1. Excessive tooth wear, mobility, and/or fractured cusps.
2. Wear on an occlusal appliance.
3. Nocturnal grinding noises.
4. Facial muscle or TMJ pain, stiffness, or fatigue upon awakening.
5. Masseter muscle hypertrophy.
6. Temporal headache.

The use of a portable EMG unit to record nocturnal masseter activity over a ten-day period may prove to be a useful diagnostic aid. Rugh (1988) also suggests the administration of 5 mg of diazepam at bedtime for seven days after baseline pain measurements. As diazepam tends to decrease bruxism (Fig. 20–3), a reduction in reported symptoms during the trial period would provide further evidence of nocturnal bruxist behavior.

Management of Nocturnal Bruxism

The management of nocturnal bruxism includes both symptomatic treatment and patient education regarding stress management and lifestyle changes appropriate to each individual case. Symptoms that wax and wane according to daily stress levels imply that although short-term treatments may relieve symptoms temporarily, lifestyle changes may be required to prevent recurrence of bruxism and its clinical sequelae.

Symptomatic treatment may include physical therapy, pharmacological agents such as diaze-pam to chemically reduce bruxism levels, EMG nocturnal biofeedback, and the use of an intraoral occlusal appliance during sleep.

EMG nocturnal biofeedback uses an alarm device to awaken the patient when each bruxing episode begins. Although it has not been shown to provide any long-term benefits (Funch, 1980; Kardachi, 1977; 1978; Johnson, 1981; Pierce, 1988; Rugh, 1975; 1981), nocturnal biofeedback trials may be useful to alleviate temporarily severe and disabling bruxist behavior (see reviews by Cassisi, 1987 and McGlynn, 1985).

The occlusal bite appliance is at present the most common device used to reduce the symptoms of nocturnal bruxism because of its effectiveness, patient acceptance, convenience, low cost, and minimal side effects (Clark, 1984; Fuchs, 1975; Mejias, 1982; Sheikholesham, 1986). Although the majority of patients experience reduction of symptoms, the actual level of grinding does not always decrease (Clark, 1979). Therefore, a redistribution of the excessive masticatory forces of bruxism is suggested as the mechanism of the appliance's effectiveness. Use of the occlusal appliance will also protect the teeth from further trauma or wear even if the bruxism continues.

As with the treatment of other stress-related disorders, stress management programs and significant changes in lifestyle are the preferred methods to manage stress-related nocturnal bruxism. Casas (1982) showed that stress reduction skills learned while awake can reduce nocturnal bruxism. Although patient motivation and education are key factors in treatment success, these factors are often inadequately emphasized by the clinician. The patient must be informed of the importance of compliance and involvement in a behavioral change program. Good doctor-patient rapport is required to help these individuals recognize the role of stress in the development and perpetuation of their symptoms.

Summary

Diurnal oral habits and nocturnal bruxism are highly correlated with TMD. In some patients, these are primary etiologic factors. In others, these behaviors aggravate the condition. Oral habits and bruxism that continue after surgery or dental reconstructive work may destroy the surgical or prosthodontic repair. Management of these patients must include identification of oral habits and bruxism. Patient awareness of oral habits and involvement in the treatment process are often essential to successful treat-

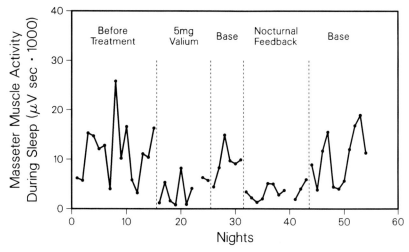

FIGURE 20–3. Nocturnal bruxism may often be temporarily reduced in patients with administration of 5 mg of diazepam, given 30 minutes before bedtime, or by nocturnal EMG feedback. The patient's responses may assist with diagnosis and be useful in cases with acute symptoms related to a short-term emotional crisis. Long-term management may require occlusal appliance therapy and/or changes in lifestyle.

ment outcome. Education of patients must emphasize that emotional or stress-related interactions do not discredit or trivialize reported symptoms. Rather, these factors necessitate a multidisciplinary approach to achieve successful management of TMD-MPD.

CHRONIC PAIN

The cumulative effects of prolonged pain, anxiety, depression, focused attention, negative beliefs, and disability sometimes result in a chronic pain condition. The patient now has an additional condition that may have a life of its own independent of the original acute problem. The chronic pain condition has been characterized as a syndrome of persistent pain lasting longer than the normal healing time. It includes learned pain behaviors, reduced social and physical activities, depression, drug dependency and excessive use of health care professionals (Fordyce, 1986; Osterweis, 1987; Sanders, 1985). Chronic pain patients often have a history of being unresponsive to conventional treatment and may have made relatively permanent changes in lifestyle such as quitting a job. They are often physically and socially inactive. The normal healing time has passed, and the pain or disability has become the central focus of their lives. Secondary gain and learned helplessness are common in these patients.

The International Association for the Study of Pain has published a classification of chronic pain conditions (IASP, 1986). Turk (1987) assessed the reliability of this classification

scheme, and Dworkin (1987) compared it with the revised DSM-III-R classification. Reviews of recent conceptualizations of chronic pain also have been published by Keefe (1985), Sanders (1985), and Turk (1987). These are useful for the dentist who attempts to manage TMD patients with chronic pain.

Assessment

A careful review of the patient's history and lifestyle usually provides the best assessment of a chronic pain condition. In addition, several inventories may assist in the assessment. These inventories include the West Haven-Yale Multidimensional Pain Inventory (Kerns, 1985), the Beck Depression Inventory (Beck, 1961), the McGill Pain Questionnaire (Melzack, 1975), and the Millon Behavioral Health Inventory (Millon, 1982). Speculand (1983), in a study of 100 TMD patients, found that the Illness Behavior Questionnaire (IBQ) could be used to screen patients for abnormal illness behavior. The MMPI has not been found practical for such screening (Millstein-Prentky, 1979). However, Eversole (1985) found significant differences in certain MMPI scales between MPD and TMJ internal derangement patients. As with most psychological assessment instruments, interpretation of these inventories requires appropriate training.

Recently, there have been two scales developed specifically for use by dentists on patients with TMD. These assessment tools are the TMJ Scale (Lundeen, 1986) and the IMPATH (Fricton, 1987). The IMPATH is administered to patients via an IBM-compatible personal computer. It requires about 60 minutes for patients to complete and provides a very comprehensive assessment of factors that cause or maintain TM pain conditions. There is evidence that patients do not mind using the computer for health questionnaires (Moore, 1984). The TMJ Scale is a paper and pencil questionnaire requiring about 15 minutes to administer and is computer-scored. Both provide a computer printout and aid in the identification of chronic pain conditions in addition to other aspects of the patient's condition. Favorable data on the validity and reliability of the IMPATH (Fricton, 1987) and the TMJ Scale (Levitt, 1988) have been published.

Management

TMD patients often have a musculoskeletal condition that cannot be totally resolved with the treatments currently available. The dentist should continue to manage the remaining pain as necessary. However, the main focus of therapy at this point should not be on the pain, but rather on the patient's lifestyle and emotional response to the pain. Techniques should be taught to help the patient cope with the pain and live an active, productive life in spite of the disability.

The management approach for each patient will be different, but may involve (1) antidepressants, (2) behavior modification, (3) counseling regarding motivation and attitude, (4) substance abuse counseling, (5) increasing social and physical activities, (6) stress management, (7) self-control procedures such as biofeedback and systematic relaxation, (8) assertiveness training, and (9) vocational rehabilitation. Appropriate management often involves family members who may be asked to change the reinforcement contingencies for illness behaviors; that is, to stop reinforcing the illness behavior. A subgroup of TMD patients has poor capacity for contact with other people or lacks long-lasting interpersonal relationships (Heloe, 1980). These patients may require long-term counseling.

The overall thrust of the chronic pain program is basically to return the patient to an active, functional life in spite of lingering pain and/or partial disability. Referral to a chronic pain clinic, psychologist, or psychiatrist who specializes in chronic pain is often a useful approach (Aronoff, 1983; Follick, 1985). Keefe (1982; 1985) has provided reviews of research studies. Fordyce (1976), Sternbach (1978), and

Brena (1985) have provided reviews of the clinical procedures. Finally, the National Institutes of Health (NIH, 1986) has published a consensus conference report outlining current concepts of assessment and management of chronic pain. This document emphasizes the need for a multidisciplinary approach.

Although chronic pain is most likely to follow a prolonged condition, it has also been found following trauma or surgery. Patient evaluation and management are similar and have been reviewed by Kelley (1986).

DOCTOR-PATIENT RELATIONSHIPS

Establishing a positive doctor-patient relationship is particularly important with TMD patients (Laskin, 1972). This involves projecting a caring and understanding attitude and demonstrating an interest in the patient and his or her problem. It requires careful listening to the patient and providing sufficient time for the patient to present his or her concerns. It is also critical to enlist patients' participation in management of their problems. A clear explanation so that a patient understands the problem helps establish this self-care orientation.

These doctor-patient skills are developed over time and are not easily fabricated. Clinicians should recognize their limitations in this area and consider a referral when faced with a patient with whom they are having difficulty communicating or establishing an appropriate relationship.

SUMMARY

The diagnosis and management of TMDs have been problematic because of the many pathologic conditions that may affect the soft and hard tissues of the masticatory system and the varied etiologic factors that are just now beginning to be identified. The situation is further complicated by psychosocial factors that sometimes precipitate or cause the condition, sometimes result from the condition, and sometimes simply blur the picture of the pathology. These issues have been discussed in this chapter and are summarized in Table 20–2. Patients may have psychological conditions that are unrelated to their TM disorders but that still make both diagnosis and treatment difficult.

Evidence regarding the heterogeneity of the conditions affecting TMD patients and their causes is abundant (Greene, 1969; Rugh, 1979; Zarb, 1979). Because of this heterogeneity, in-

TABLE 20–2. Checklist of Psychological and Behavioral Factors

1. History of stress-related disorders
2. Major changes in lifestyle preceding the condition
3. Inconsistencies and/or vague reports of pain
4. Pain duration of more than 6 months
5. Symptoms that vary with life events
6. Overdramatization of symptoms
7. Evidence of anxiety or depression
8. Evidence of secondary gain and disruption of life activities
9. Pending litigation or compensation
10. Evidence of nocturnal bruxism or destructive oral habits
11. Repeated failures with conventional therapies
12. Inconsistency in response to drugs or evidence of drug abuse

vestigators have been unable to identify factors that reliably predict treatment outcome (Okeson, 1986; Wedel, 1985) or to identify one treatment modality that works much better than another (Magnusson, 1980). Seventy to 85 per cent of patients seem to show improvement in symptoms with any one of several treatments (Greene, 1983; Kopp, 1979; Wedel, 1985). About the same number seem to show improvements with placebo treatment or no treatment. These observations, coupled with the risks of irreversible therapies, encourage a conservative approach to the management of most patients with TMD. Psychological and behavioral factors play a key role in these therapies.

There are specific conditions for which nonreversible procedures are indicated. These are described elsewhere in this book. The important point of this chapter is that both reversible and irreversible treatments for TMD are likely to be more successful when the clinician attends to the behavioral and emotional aspects of the patient as well as to his or her pain condition.

REFERENCES

AAOMS: Criteria for TMJ Meniscus Surgery. Chicago, AAOMS, 1984, p. 33.
Andrasik, F., Blanchard, E. B., Ahles, T., et al.: Assessing the reactive as well as the sensory component of headache pain. Headache 21:218–221, 1981.
Aronoff, G. M., Evans, W. C., and Enders, P. L.: A review of follow-up studies of multidisciplinary pain units. Pain 16:1–11, 1983.
Bakal, D.: Headache: A biopsychological perspective. Psychol. Bull. 82:369–382, 1975.
Beck, A. T., Ward, C. H., Mendelson, M., et al.: An inventory for measuring depression. Arch. Gen. Psychiatry 4:561–571, 1961.
Berlin, R., Dessner, L., and Aberg, S.: Diagnosis of headache and its relation to the temporomandibular joint syndrome. Svens. Laekartidn. 51:11, 1954.
Bowers, K.: Pain, anxiety and perceived control. J. Consult. Clin. Psychol. 32:596–603, 1968.
Bowley, J. F., and Gale, E. N.: Experimental masticatory muscle pain. J. Dent. Res. 66:1765–1769, 1987.
Brena, S. F., and Chapman, S. L. (Eds.): Clinics in Anesthesiology: Chronic Pain-Management Principles. London, W. B. Saunders, 1985.
Brooke, R. I., and Stenn, P. G.: Postinjury myofascial pain-dysfunction syndrome: Its etiology and prognosis. Oral Surg. 45:846–850, 1978.
Brooke, R. I., Stenn, P. G., and Mothersill, K. J.: The diagnosis and conservative treatment of myofascial pain dysfunction syndrome. Oral Surg. 44:844–852, 1977.
Burgar, C. G., and Rugh, J. D.: An EMG integrator for muscle activity studies in ambulatory subjects. IEEE Trans. Biomed. Eng. 3:66–69, 1983.
Cannistraci, A. J., and Friedrich, J. A.: A multidimensional approach to bruxism and TMD. NY State Dent. J. 53:31–34, 1987.
Carlsson, G. E., Ingervall, B., Lewin, T., and Molin, C.: Relation between functional disturbances of the masticatory system and some anthropometric, physiological and psychological variables in young Swedish men. J. Oral Rehabil. 3:305–310, 1976.
Casas, J. M., Beemsterboer, P., and Clark, G. T.: A comparison of stress-reduction behavioral counseling and contingent nocturnal EMG feedback for the treatment of bruxism. Behav. Res. Ther. 20:9–15, 1982.
Cassisi, J. E., McGlynn, F. D., and Belles, D. R.: EMG-activated feedback alarms for the treatment of nocturnal bruxism: Current status and future directions. Biofeedback Self Regul. 12:13–30, 1987.
Christensen, L. V.: Facial pain and internal pressure of masseter muscle in experimental bruxism in man. Arch. Oral Biol. 16:1021–1031, 1971.
Christensen, L. V.: Integrated electromyography of experimental tooth clenching in man. J. S. Afr. Dent. Assoc. 33:477, 1978.
Christensen, L. V.: Some subjective-experimental parameters in experimental tooth clenching in man. J. Oral Rehabil. 6:119, 1979.
Christensen, L. V., and Radue, J. T.: Lateral preference in mastication: An electromyographic study. J. Oral Rehabil. 12:429–434, 1985.
Ciccone, D. S., and Grzesiak, R. C.: Cognitive dimensions of chronic pain. Soc. Sci. Med. 19:1339–1345, 1984.
Clark, G. T.: A critical evaluation of orthopaedic interocclusal appliance therapy: II. Specific symptom effectiveness. J. Am. Dent. Assoc. 108:364–368, 1984.
Clark, G. T., Beemsterboer, P. L., and Rugh, J. D.: Nocturnal masseter muscle activity and the symptoms of masticatory dysfunction. J. Oral Rehabil. 8:279–287, 1981.
Clark, G. T., Beemsterboer, P. L., Solberg, W. K., and Rugh, J. D.: Nocturnal electromyographic evaluation of myofascial pain dysfunction in patients undergoing occlusal splint therapy. J. Am. Dent. Assoc. 99:607–611, 1979.
Clark, G. T., Rugh, J. D., and Handelman, S. L.: Nocturnal masseter muscle activity and urinary catecholamine levels in bruxers. J. Dent. Res. 59:1571–1576, 1980.
Cohen, S. R.: Follow-up evaluation of 105 patients with myofascial pain-dysfunction syndrome. J. Am. Dent. Assoc. 95:825–828, 1978.
Craig, K. D.: Social modeling influences: Pain in context. In Sternbach, R. A. (Ed.): The Psychology of Pain, Ed 2. New York, Raven Press, 1986, pp. 67–95.
Crockett, D. J., Foreman, M. E., Alden, L., and Blasberg, B.: A comparison of treatment modes in the management

of myofascial pain dysfunction syndrome. Biofeedback Self Regul. 11:279–291, 1986.

Dahlstrom, L., and Carlsson, S. G.: Treatment of mandibular dysfunction: The clinical usefulness of biofeedback in relation to splint therapy. J. Oral Rehabil. 11:277–284, 1984.

Doerfler, L. F., and Rugh, J. D.: Voluntary mandibular retrusion exercises and facial pain. J. Dent. Res. 63:288, Abstract 1059, 1984.

Dohrmann, R. J., and Laskin, D. M.: An evaluation of electromyographic biofeedback in the treatment of myofascial pain-dysfunction syndrome. J. Am. Dent. Assoc. 96:656–662, 1978.

Dordick, B., and Gallon, R.: Development of a model to study bruxism in the laboratory. J. Dent. Res. 57(Special Issue A):366, Abstract 1165, 1978.

Duinkerke, A. S., Luteijn, F., Bouman, T. K., and de Jong, H. P.: Relations between TMJ pain dysfunction syndrome (PDS) and some psychologic and biographic variables. Community Dent. Oral Epidemiol. 13:185–189, 1985.

Dworkin, S. F., and Burgess, J. A.: Orofacial pain of psychogenic origin: Current concepts and classification. J. Am. Dent. Assoc. 115:565–571, 1987.

Eriksson, L., and Westesson, P-L.: Diskectomy in the treatment of anterior disk displacement of the temporomandibular joint: A clinical and radiologic one-year follow-up study. J. Prosthet. Dent. 55:106–116, 1986.

Eversole, L. R., Stone, C. E., Matheson, D., and Kaplan H.: Psychometric profiles and facial pain. Oral Surg. 60:269–274, 1985.

Feinmann, C., Harris, M., and Cawley, R.: Psychogenic facial pain: Presentation and treatment. Br. Med. J. 288:436–438, 1984.

Finlayson, R. S., Rugh, J. D., and Dolwick, M. F.: Electromyography of myofascial pain patients and controls in the natural environment. J. Dent. Res. 61:277, Abstract 887, 1982.

Follick, M. J., Ahern, D. K., Altanasio, V., and Riley, J. F.: Chronic pain programs: Current aims, strategies, and needs. Ann. Behav. Med. 17:17–20, 1985.

Fordyce, W. E.: Behavioral Methods for Chronic Pain and Illness. St. Louis, C. V. Mosby, 1976.

Fordyce, W. E.: Learning processes in pain. In Sternbach, R. A. (Ed.): The Psychology of Pain, Ed 2. New York, Raven Press, 1986, pp. 49–65.

Fricton, J., Kroening, R., Haley, D., and Siegert, R.: Myofascial pain syndrome of the head and neck: A review of clinical characteristics of 164 patients. Oral Surg. 60:615–627, 1985.

Fricton, J. R., Nelson, A., and Monsein, M.: IMPATH: Microcomputer assessment of behavioral and psychological factors in craniomandibular disorders. J. Craniomandib. Pract. 5:372–381, 1987.

Fuchs, P.: The muscular activity of the chewing apparatus during night sleep. J. Oral Rehabil. 2:35–48, 1975.

Funch, D. P., and Gale, E. N.: Factors associated with nocturnal bruxism and its treatment. J. Behav. Med. 3:385–397, 1980.

Gale, E. N.: Psychological characteristics of long-term female temporomandibular joint pain patients. J. Dent. Res. 57:481–483, 1978.

Gale, E. N.: Behavioral approaches to temporomandibular disorders. Ann. Behav. Med. 8:11–16, 1986.

Gatchel, R. J.: Perceived control: A review and evaluation of therapeutic implications. In Baum, A., and Singer, J. E. (Eds.): Advances in Environmental Psychology, Ed. 2. Hillsdale, NJ, Lawrence Erlbaum Associates, 1980, pp. 1–22.

Gerschman, J. A., Wright, J. L., Hall, W. D., et al.: Comparisons of psychological and social factors in patients with chronic oro-facial pain and dental phobic disorders. Aust. Dent. J. 32:331–335, 1987.

Gessel, A. H.: Electromyographic biofeedback and tricyclic antidepressants in myofascial pain-dysfunction syndrome: Psychological predictors of outcome. J. Am. Dent. Assoc. 91:1048–1052, 1975.

Glaros, A. G., and Rao, S. M.: Bruxism: A critical review. Psychol. Bull. 84:767–781, 1977.

Gold, S., Lipton, J., Marbach, J., and Gurion, B.: Sites of psychophysiological complaints in MPD patients: II. Areas remote from the orofacial region. J. Dent. Res. 54(Special Issue A):165, Abstract 480, 1975.

Graff-Radford, S. B., Reeves, J. L., and Jaeger, B.: Management of chronic head and neck pain: Effectiveness of altering factors perpetuating myofascial pain. Headache 27:186–190, 1987.

Greene, C. S., and Laskin, D. M.: Long-term evaluation of treatment for myofascial pain-dysfunction syndrome: A comparative analysis. J. Am. Dent. Assoc. 107:235–238, 1983.

Greene, C. S., Lerman, M. D., Sutcher, H. D., and Laskin, D. M.: The TMJ pain-dysfunction syndrome: Heterogeneity of the patient population. J. Am. Dent. Assoc. 79:1168–1172, 1969.

Greene, C. S., Olson, R. E., and Laskin, D. M.: Psychological factors in the etiology, progression and treatment of MPD syndrome. J. Am. Dent. Assoc. 105:443–448, 1982.

Gregg, J. M.: Central nervous system factors in the myofascial pain dysfunction syndrome. J. Ala. Dent. Assoc. 62:22–26, 1978.

Haynes, S. N.: Muscle contraction headache: A psychophysical perspective of etiology and treatment. In Haynes, S. N., and Gannon, L. R. (Eds.): Psychosomatic Disorders: A Psychophysiological Approach to Etiology and Treatment. New York, Praeger Press, 1981.

Heiberg, A. N., Heloe, B., and Krogstad, B. S.: The myofascial pain dysfunction syndrome: Dental symptoms and psychological and muscular function: An overview. Psychother. Psychosom. 30:81–97, 1978.

Heloe, B., and Heiberg, A. N.: A follow-up study of a group of female patients with myofascial pain-dysfunction syndrome. Acta Odontol. Scand. 38:129–134, 1980a.

Heloe, B., Heiberg, A. N., and Krogstad, B. S.: A multiprofessional study of patients with myofascial pain-dysfunction syndrome (I). Acta Odontol. Scand. 38:109–117, 1980b.

Hersh, E. V.: Tricyclic antidepressant drugs: Pharmacologic implications in the treatment of chronic orofacial pain. Compend. Contin. Educ. Dent. 8:688–694, 1987.

Hijzen, T. H., Slangen, J. L., and Van Houweligen, H. C.: Subjective, clinical and EMG effects of biofeedback and splint treatment. J. Oral Rehabil. 13:529–539, 1986.

IASP: Subcommittee on taxonomy, classification of chronic pain: Descriptions of chronic pain syndromes and definitions of pain terms. Pain (Suppl. 3):S1–S225, 1986.

Johnson, D. L., Shipman, W. G., and Laskin, D. M.: Physiologic responses to stressful stimuli in patients with myofascial pain-dysfunction (MPD) syndrome. J. Dent. Res. 51:15, Abstract 191, 1972.

Kardachi, B. J., and Clarke, N. G.: The use of biofeedback to control bruxism. J. Periodontol. 48:639–642, 1977.

Kardachi, B. J. R., Bailey, J. O. Jr., and Ash, M. M. Jr.: A comparison of biofeedback and occlusal adjustment on bruxism. J. Periodontol. 49:367–372, 1978.

Keefe, F. J.: Behavioral assessment and treatment of chronic pain: Current status and future directions. J. Consult. Clin. Psychol. 50:896–911, 1982.

Keefe, F. J., and Gil, K. M.: Recent advances in the

behavioral assessment and treatment of chronic pain. Ann. Behav. Med. 17:11–16, 1985.

Kelley, J. T.: Chronic pain and trauma. Adv. Psychosom. Med. 16:141–152, 1986.

Kerns, R. D., Turk, D. C., and Rudy, T. E.: The West Haven-Yale Multidimensional Pain Inventory (WHYMPI). Pain 23:345–356, 1985.

Kononen, M., Nystrom, M., Kleemola-Kujala, E., et al.: Signs and symptoms of craniomandibular disorders in a series of Finnish children. Acta Odontol. Scand. 45:109–114, 1987.

Kopp, S.: Short-term evaluation of counseling and occlusal adjustment in mandibular dysfunction patients. J. Oral Rehabil. 6:101–109, 1979.

Langer, E.: The Psychology of Control. London, Sage, 1983.

Lascelles, R. G.: A typical facial pain and depression. Br. J. Psychol. 112:651–659, 1966.

Laskin, D. M.: Etiology of the pain-dysfunction syndrome. J. Am. Dent. Assoc. 79:147–153, 1969.

Laskin, D., and Greene, C. S.: Influence of the doctor-patient relationship on placebo therapy for patients with myofascial pain-dysfunction (MPD) syndrome. J. Am. Dent. Assoc. 85:892–894, 1972.

Levitt, S. R., McKinney, M. W., and Lundeen, T. F.: The TMJ Scale: Cross-validation and reliability studies. J. Craniomandib. Pract. 6:18–25, 1988.

Liebeskind, J. C., and Paul, L. A.: Psychological and physiological mechanisms of pain. Ann. Rev. Psychol. 28:41–60, 1977.

Lindsey, P. G., and Wycoff, M.: The depression-pain syndrome and its response to antidepressants. Psychosomatics 22:571–577, 1981.

Lowery, B. J., Jacobsen, B. S., and Murphy, B. B.: An exploratory investigation of causal thinking of arthritics. Nurs. Res. 39:157–162, 1983.

Lundeen, T. F., Levitt, S. R., and McKinney, M. W.: Discrimination ability of the TMJ Scale: Age and gender differences. J. Prosthet. Dent. 56:84–92, 1986.

Lundeen, T. F., Sturdevant, J. R., and George, S. M.: Stress as a factor in muscle and temporomandibular joint pain. J. Oral Rehabil. 14:447–456, 1987.

Lupton, D. E.: Psychological aspects of temporomandibular joint dysfunction. J. Am. Dent. Assoc. 79:131–136, 1969.

Magnusson, T., and Carlsson, G. E.: Headache and mandibular dysfunction in two groups of dental patients. J. Dent. Res. 58:2296, Abstract 29, 1979.

Magnusson, T., and Carlsson, G. E.: Treatment of patients with functional disturbances in the masticatory system. A survey of 80 consecutive patients. Swed. Dent. J. 4:145–153, 1980.

Malow, R. M., and Olson, R. E.: Changes in pain perception after treatment for chronic pain. Pain 11:65–72, 1981a.

Malow, R. M., Grimm, L., and Olson, R. E.: Differences in pain perception between myofascial pain dysfunction patients and normal subjects: A signal detection analysis. J. Psychosom. Res. 24:303–309, 1980.

Malow, R. M., Olson, R. E., and Greene, C. S.: Myofascial pain dysfunction syndrome: A psychophysiological disorder. In Golden, C., Alcaparras, S., Strider, F., and Graber, B. (Eds.): Applied Techniques in Behavioral Medicine and Medical Psychology. New York, Grune & Stratton, 1981b, pp. 101–133.

Marbach, J. J., and Lipton, J. A.: Aspects of illness behavior in patients with facial pain. J. Am. Dent. Assoc. 96:630–638, 1978.

Marbach, J. J., and Lipton, J. A.: Biopsychosocial factors of the temporomandibular pain dysfunction syndrome: Relevance to restorative dentistry. Dent. Clin. North Am. 31:473–486, 1987.

Marbach, J. J., and Lund, P.: Depression, anhedonia and anxiety in temporomandibular joint and other facial pain syndromes. Pain 11:73–84, 1981.

Marciani, R. D., and Ziegler, R. C.: Temporomandibular joint surgery: A review of fifty-one operations. Oral Surg. 56:472–476, 1983.

Marciani, R. D., Haley, J. V., Moody, P. M., and Roth, G. I.: Identification of patients at risk for unnecessary or excessive TMJ surgery. Oral Surg. 64:533–535, 1987.

Martin, M. J.: Muscle-contraction headache. Psychosom. 13:16–19, 1972.

McCaul, K. D., and Malott, J. M.: Distraction and coping with pain. Psychol. Bull. 95:516–533, 1984.

McGlynn, F. D., Cassisi, J. E., and Diamond, E. L.: Bruxism: A behavioral dentistry perspective. In Daitzman, R. J. (Ed.): Diagnosis and Intervention in Behavior Therapy and Behavioral Medicine, vol. 2. New York, Springer, 1985, pp. 28–87.

Mealiea, W. L. Jr., and McGlynn, D.: Temporomandibular disorders and bruxism. In Hatch, J. P., Fisher, J. G., and Rugh, J. D. (Eds.): Biofeedback: Studies in Clinical Efficacy. New York, Plenum Press, 1987, pp. 123–151.

Mejersjo, C., and Carlsson, G. E.: Long-term results of treatment for temporomandibular joint pain-dysfunction. J. Prosthet. Dent. 49:809–815, 1983.

Mejias, J. E., and Mehta, N. R.: Subjective and objective evaluation of bruxing patients undergoing short-term splint therapy. J. Oral Rehabil. 9:279–289, 1982.

Melamed, R. G., and Mealiea, W. L. Jr.: Behavioral intervention in pain-related problems in dentistry. In Ferguson, J. M., and Taylor, C. B. (Eds.): The Comprehensive Handbook of Behavioral Medicine, vol. 2, New York, Spectrum Inc., 1981, pp. 241–259.

Melzack, R.: The McGill Pain Questionnaire: Major properties and scoring methods. Pain 1:277–299, 1975.

Melzack, R.: Neuropsychological basis of pain measurement. In Kruger, L., and Liebeskind, J. C. (Eds.): Advances in Pain Research and Therapy. New York, Raven Press, 1984, pp. 323–339.

Melzack, R.: Neurophysiological foundations of pain. In Sternbach, R. A. (Ed.): The Psychology of Pain, Ed 2. New York, Raven Press, 1986, pp. 1–25.

Melzack, R., and Wall, P. D.: The Challenge of Pain. Hamondsworth, UK, Penguin, 1982.

Mercuri, L. G., Olson, R. E., and Laskin, D. M.: The specificity of response to experimental stress in patients with myofascial pain dysfunction syndrome. J. Dent. Res. 58:1866–1871, 1979.

Miller, C. S., Thrash, W. J., Glass, B. J., et al.: Progressive deep muscle relaxation for the treatment of myofascial pain dysfunction. J. Oral Med. 42:216–220, 1987.

Millon, T., Green, C., and Meagher, R.: Millon Behavioral Health Inventory Manual. Minneapolis, National Computer Systems, 1982.

Millstein-Prentky, S., and Olson, R. E.: Predictability of treatment outcome in patients with myofascial pain-dysfunction (MPD) syndrome. J. Dent. Res. 58:1341–1346, 1979.

Molin, C., Edman, G., and Schalling, D.: Psychological studies of patients with mandibular pain dysfunction syndrome. Swed. Dent. J. 66:15–23, 1973.

Molin, C., and Levi, L.: A psycho-odontological investigation of patients with bruxism. Acta Odontol. Scand. 24:373–391, 1966.

Mongini, F.: Dental abrasion as a factor in remodeling of the mandibular condyle. Acta Anat. 92:292–300, 1975.

Moore, N. C., Summer, K. R., and Bloor, R. N.: Do patients like psychometric testing by computer? J. Clin. Psychol. 40:875–877, 1984.

Moss, R. A., and Garrett, J. C.: Temporomandibular joint

dysfunction syndrome and myofascial pain dysfunction syndrome: A critical review. J. Oral Rehabil. *11*:3–28, 1984a.

Moss, R. A., Ruff, M. H., and Sturgis, E. T.: Oral behavioral patterns in facial pain, headache and non-headache populations. Behav. Res. Ther. *22*:683–687, 1984b.

Moulton, R. D.: Emotional factors in non-organic temporomandibular joint pain. Dent. Clin. North Am. 609–620, 1966.

National Institutes of Health: The integrated approach to the management of pain. Consensus Development Conference Statement. US Government Printing Office, No. 491-292-41148, *6*, 1986.

Okeson, J. P., and Hayes, D. K.: Long-term results of treatment for temporomandibular disorders: An evaluation by patients. J. Am. Dent. Assoc. *112*:473–478, 1986.

Olson, R. E., and Malow, R. M.: The effects of relaxation training on myofascial pain dysfunction syndrome patients. Clin. J. Pain *1*:217–220, 1986.

Osterweis, M., Kleinman, A., and Mechanic, D. (Eds.): Pain and Disability: Clinical and Public Policy Perspectives. Washington, DC, National Academy Press, 1987.

Otto, M. W., and Dougher, M. J.: Sex differences and personality factors in responsivity to pain. Percept. Motor Skills *61*:383–390, 1985.

Payne, B., and Norfleet, M. A.: Chronic pain and the family: A review. Pain *26*:1–22, 1986.

Pedersen, A., and Hansen, H. J.: Long-term evaluation of 211 patients with internal derangement of the temporomandibular joint. Community Dent. Oral Epidemiol. *15*:344–347, 1987.

Perry, H. T., Lammie, G. A., Main, J., and Teuscher, G. W.: Occlusion in a stress situation. J. Am. Dent. Assoc. *60*:626–633, 1960.

Pierce, C. J., and Gale, E. N.: A comparison of different treatments for nocturnal bruxism. J. Dent. Res. *67*:597–601, 1988.

Pinto, O. F. P.: Temporomandibular joint problems in underwater activities. J. Prosthet. Dent. *16*:772–781, 1966.

Rao, S. M., and Glaros, A. G.: Electromyographic correlates of experimentally induced stress in diurnal bruxists and normals. J. Dent. Res. *58*:1872–1878, 1979.

Reade, P. C., Wardrop, R. W., Holwill, B. J., et al.: Management of patients with acute temporomandibular joint disorders. J. Prosthet. Dent. *54*:110–113, 1985.

Reding, G. R., Rubright, W. C., and Zimmerman, S. O.: Incidence of bruxism. J. Dent. Res. *45*:1198–1204, 1966.

Rieder, C. E.: Possible premature degenerative temporomandibular joint disease in violinists. J. Prosthet. Dent. *35*:662–664, 1976.

Rugh, J. D.: Electromyographic analysis of bruxism in the natural environment. *In* Weinstein, P. (Ed.): Advances in Behavioral Research in Dentistry. Seattle, WA, University of Washington Press, 1978, pp. 68–83.

Rugh, J. D.: Psychological factors in the etiology of masticatory pain and dysfunction. *In* Laskin, D. M., Greenfield, W., Gale, E., et al. (Eds.): The President's Conference on the Examination, Diagnosis and Management of Temporomandibular Disorders. Chicago, Am. Dent. Assoc. 1983, pp. 85–94.

Rugh, J. D.: Psychological components of pain. Dent. Clin. North Am. *31*:579–594, 1987a.

Rugh, J. D., and Harlan, J.: Nocturnal bruxism and temporomandibular disorders. Adv. Neurol. *49*:329–341, 1988.

Rugh, J. D., and Johnson, R. W.: Temporal analysis of nocturnal bruxism during EMG feedback. J. Periodontol. *52*:263–265, 1981.

Rugh, J. D., and Lemke, R. R.: Oral habits. *In* Matarazzo, J. D. (Ed.): Behavioral Health: A Handbook of Health Enhancement and Disease Prevention. New York, John Wiley & Sons, 1984a, pp. 947–966.

Rugh, J. D., and Montgomery, G. T.: Physiologic reactions of patients with TM disorders vs. symptom-free controls on a physical stress task. J. Craniomandib. Disord. *1*:243–250, 1987b.

Rugh, J. D., and Robbins, J. W.: Oral habit disorders. *In* Ingersoll, B. (Ed.): Behavioral Aspects in Dentistry. New York, Appleton-Century-Crofts, 1982, pp. 179–202.

Rugh, J. D., and Solberg, W. K.: Electromyographic studies of bruxist behavior before and during treatment. J. Calif. Dent. Assoc. *3*:56–59, 1975.

Rugh, J. D., and Solberg, W. K.: Psychological implications in temporomandibular pain and dysfunction. *In* Zarb, G. A., and Carlsson, G. E. (Eds.): Temporomandibular Joint Function and Dysfunction. Copenhagen, Munksgaard, 1979, pp. 239–268.

Rugh, J. D., and Solberg, W. K.: Oral health status in the United States: Temporomandibular disorders. J. Dent. Educ. *49*:398–405, 1985.

Rugh, J. D., Jacobs, D. T., Taverna, R. D., and Johnson, R. W.: Psychophysiological changes and oral conditions. *In* Cohen, L. K., and Bryant, P. S. (Eds.): Social Sciences and Dentistry: A Critical Bibliography, vol. II. London, Quintessence, 1984b, pp. 19–83.

Sanders, S. H.: Chronic pain: Conceptualization and epidemiology. Ann. Behav. Med. *7*:3–5, 1985.

Schumann, N. P., Zwiener, U., and Nebrich, A.: Personality and quantified neuromuscular activity of the masticatory system in patients with temporomandibular joint dysfunction. J. Oral Rehabil. *15*:35–47, 1988.

Scott, D. S.: Myofascial pain-dysfunction syndrome: A psychobiological perspective. J. Behav. Med. *4*:451–465, 1981.

Scott, D. S., and Lundeen, T. F.: Myofascial pain involving the masticatory muscles: An experimental model. Pain *8*:207–215, 1980.

Seligman, E. P.: Helplessness: On Depression, Development and Death. San Francisco, W. H. Freeman, 1975.

Sharav, Y., Singer, E., Schmidt, E., et al.: The analgesic effect of amitriptyline on chronic facial pain. Pain *31*:199–209, 1987.

Sheikholesham, A., Holmgreen, K., and Riise, C.: A clinical and electromyographic study of the long-term effects of an occlusal splint on the temporal and masseter muscles in patients with functional disorders and nocturnal bruxism. J. Oral Rehabil. *13*:137–145, 1986.

Skevington, S. M.: Psychological aspects of pain in rheumatoid arthritis: A review. Soc. Sci. Med. *23*:567–575, 1986.

Solberg, W. K., and Rugh, J. D.: The use of biofeedback devices in the treatment of bruxism. J. Calif. Dent. Assoc. *40*:852, 1972.

Speculand, B., and Goss, A. N.: Psychological factors in temporomandibular joint dysfunction pain: A review. Int. J. Oral Surg. *14*:131–137, 1985.

Speculand, B., Goss, A. N., Hughes, A., et al.: Temporomandibular joint dysfunction: Pain and illness behavior. Pain *17*:139–150, 1983.

Speculand, B., Hughes, A. O., and Goss, A. N.: The role of recent stressful life events experience in the onset of TMJ dysfunction pain. Community Dent. Oral Epidemiol. *12*:197–202, 1984.

Stam, H. S., McGrath, P. A., and Brooke, R. I.: The effects of a cognitive-behavioral treatment program on temporo-mandibular pain and dysfunction syndrome. Psychosom. Med. *46*:534–545, 1984.

Sternbach, R. A.: Treatment of the chronic pain patient. J. Human Stress *4*:11–15, 1978.

Taenzer, P., Melzack, R., and Jeans, M. E.: Influence of psychological factors on post-operative pain, mood and analgesic requirements. Pain 24:331–342, 1986.

Theorell, T.: Stress syndrome. Ann. Clin. Res. 19:53–61, 1987.

Thomas, L. J., Tiber, N., and Schireson, S.: The effects of anxiety and frustration on muscular tension related to the temporomandibular joint syndrome. Oral Surg. 36:763–768, 1973.

Turk, D. C., and Rudy, T. E.: Assessment of cognitive factors in chronic pain: A worthwhile enterprise? J. Consult. Clin. Psychol. 54:760–768, 1986.

Turk, D. C., and Rudy, T. E.: Toward a comprehensive assessment of chronic pain patients. Behav. Res. Ther. 25:237–249, 1987.

van der Laan, G. J., Duinkerke, A. S., Luteijn, F. P., and van de Poel, A. C.: Relative importance of psychologic and social variables in TMJ pain dysfunction syndrome (PDS) signs. Community Dent. Oral Epidemiol. 16:117–121, 1988.

Villarosa, G. A., and Moss, R. A.: Oral behavior patterns as factors contributing to the development of head and facial pain. J. Prosthet. Dent. 54:427–430, 1985.

Wannam, A., and Agerberg, G.: Headache and dysfunction of the masticatory system in adolescents. Cephalalgia 6:247–255, 1986.

Ware, J. C., and Rugh, J. D.: Destructive bruxism: Sleep stage relationship. Sleep 11:172–181, 1988.

Wedel, A., and Carlsson, G. E.: Factors influencing the outcome of treatment in patients referred to a temporomandibular joint clinic. J. Prosthet. Dent. 54:420–426, 1985.

Westling, L.: Fingernail biting: A literature review and case reports. J. Craniomandib. Pract. 6:182–187, 1988.

Wilkinson, T. M.: Multidisciplinary approach to the treatment of craniomandibular disorders. Aust. Prosthet. J. 1:19–24, 1987.

Wolff, H. G.: Headache and Other Head Pain, Ed 2. New York, Oxford University Press, 1963.

Yemm, R.: A comparison of the electrical activity of masseter and temporal muscles of human subjects during experimental stress. Arch. Oral Biol. 16:269–273, 1971.

Yemm, R.: Neurophysiologic studies of temporomandibular joint dysfunction. Oral Sci. Rev. 1:31–53, 1976.

Zarb, G. A., and Speck, J. E.: The treatment of mandibular dysfunction. In Zarb, G. A., and Carlsson, G. E. (Eds.): Temporomandibular Joint Function and Dysfunction. Copenhagen, Munksgaard, 1979, pp. 373–396.

Zarb, G. A., and Thompson, G. W.: Assessment of clinical treatment of patients with temporomandibular joint dysfunction. J. Prosthet. Dent. 24:542–554, 1970.

21

DIAGNOSIS AND NONSURGICAL TREATMENT OF MASTICATORY MUSCLE PAIN AND DYSFUNCTION*

GLENN T. CLARK, D.D.S., M.S., and ROBERT L. MERRILL, D.D.S.

INTRODUCTION

Temporomandibular disorders (TMDs) can be broadly separated into masticatory muscle disorders and temporomandibular joint (TMJ) disorders (Clark, 1989; Eversole, 1985; Griffiths, 1983). Masticatory muscle disorders are characterized by muscle pain and tenderness, a painful limitation of normal mandibular movement, intermittent swelling of the muscles, and poor coordination of mandibular movement.

The common painful disorders of the masticatory muscles are myalgia, trismus, and myositis. The muscles of mastication are also sus-

ceptible to disorders of movement (dyskinesia, dystonia, and tremor), mobility (muscle contracture), and growth (hypertrophy, atrophy, and neoplasia). This chapter will focus only on the painful muscular disorders (for discussion of other conditions, see Chapter 23).

DIAGNOSIS OF MASTICATORY MUSCLE DISORDERS

Myalgia

Myalgia is described as a dull, aching, continuous pain that increases with function. A diagnosis of myalgia in the masticatory muscles requires (1) the presence of a subjective com-

---

*See Chapters 5, 7–9, 16, 18–20, 23, 25, and 26.

plaint of pain in the muscles and (2) the verification of tenderness by palpation of the muscle (Clark, 1981a; 1981b; 1989; Duinkerke, 1986; Farrar, 1983; Forssell, 1984; Fricton, 1989; Roy, 1988; Seligman, 1988; Solberg, 1986c). As will be discussed further on, masticatory muscle myalgia can occur as a local or regional problem due either to direct muscle tissue trauma, forceful jaw closing habits (e.g., bruxism or tooth-clenching), or prolonged protective muscle splinting secondary to a regional pain, infection, or tissue injury such as TMJ arthritis. Masticatory myalgia has also been called myofascial pain or myofascial pain-dysfunction (MPD) syndrome (see Chapters 18, 19, and 25). When myalgia presents as part of a more diffuse upper quadrant or generalized muscle pain disorder, it has been called fibromyalgia or primary fibromyalgia syndrome.

Although it is not clear whether myofascial pain and fibromyalgia are distinctly different problems, they have been differentiated by muscle pain researchers in the following way: fibromyalgia is more diffuse and involves muscle and nonmuscle sites such as the interspinous ligaments; myofascial pain, however, involves only muscle sites (Fishbain, 1989; Hench, 1989; Wolfe, 1988; Yunus, 1988). Fibromyalgia is characterized by daytime pain, which increases with stress and cold weather, nonrestorative sleep, fatigue, and morning stiffness or aching. There are multiple muscle and nonmuscle sites of tenderness (usually more than six) (Tunks, 1988), which may or may not refer pain, but often produce regional autonomic phenomena when stimulated by palpation. The tender sites in myofascial pain (usually fewer than six) only involve muscles and may or may not be associated with autonomic phenomena on palpation. The etiology of myofascial pain and fibromyalgia is not clear, but speculation includes theories of autonomic dysfunction, subclinical traumatic muscle injury, stress and anxiety, and disturbed sleep.

Palpation of the muscles of mastication for increased tenderness is the primary method of confirming myalgia regardless of its cause (Butler, 1975; Clark, 1981a; Duinkerke, 1986; Solberg, 1986a; van der Laan, 1988b). Palpation for tenderness is performed by applying a standard level of force with an index finger to the muscle site being evaluated (Fig. 21–1). The pressure level used should be between 3 and 5 lbs of force. Since this level of pressure applied to the superficial masseter, deep masseter, or anterior temporalis muscles will generally not induce pain in normal subjects, it will identify

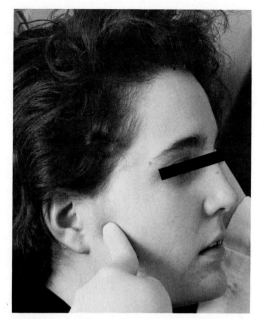

FIGURE 21–1. The masseter muscle is being digitally palpated with an index finger pressure of between 3 and 5 lbs of force. Note the examiner's opposite hand supporting the head.

patients with muscle pain. The middle and posterior temporalis muscles are usually less sensitive and therefore require 4 to 6 lbs of force to elicit pain. Other masticatory muscle sites such as the medial and lateral pterygoid and the digastric muscles are difficult to palpate and have no standardized levels of force that consistently elicit pain.

It is essential to have the patient rate the level of pain during each palpation. This can be done using a visual analog or Likert scale, or using words such as none, mild, moderate, or severe to describe the palpation-induced pain level. Pressure at each palpation site should be held for at least 2 to 3 seconds to see if the pain is localized or refers to another site in the orofacial region. Muscle swelling, enlargement, and unusual texture should also be noted during palpation of the masticatory muscles. Finally, the symmetry of muscle contraction as the mouth closes into maximum intercuspation is evaluated by palpation during a clenching effort.

Trismus

Trismus, also known as protective muscle splinting, is a restriction of mandibular movement (usually mouth opening) due to an abnormal excitation and/or inhibition of muscle activity. For example, during an opening movement the jaw closing muscles might exhibit increased activity and the jaw opening muscles might exhibit inhibition (Bell, 1982; Schwartz, 1966b; Solberg, 1986c; Yemm, 1979). Trismus is produced by a normal protective neurophysiologic process. When the condition is present, the involved muscles are attempting to avoid pain by preventing movement. Although trismus is a noninflammatory condition, the problem can develop spontaneously as a protective response secondary to regional tissue pain or articular dysfunction or, more frequently, after a regional traumatic injury or dental/surgical operative procedure. Post-traumatic trismus usually has an acute onset and there is a greater restriction of mandibular motion. Hysterically induced trismus resulting from acute psychological distress can also develop suddenly and cause a severe restriction of mandibular motion.

Myalgia is usually associated with trismus, and jaw tremor and incoordination sometimes occur when movement is attempted. Trismus is usually self-limiting when the cause is no longer present, although prolonged, unresolved trismus of any kind can produce a chronic restriction of movement. Abnormal muscle activity is usually not evident when the jaw is in rest position because it is movement that is affected by this problem. If the patient exhibits an involuntary, continuous contraction of the muscle with activity, even at rest, it is best described as muscle spasm. True jaw muscle spasm is rare.

Measuring and recording of restricted mandibular motion is essential for the diagnosis of trismus. These measurements should be completed for opening, lateral, and protrusive movements. Three vertical measurements are suggested: (1) pain-free opening, (2) full active opening, and (3) passive stretch-jaw opening ability (see pages 349 and 376). The location of any pain during an active movement or passive stretching of the jaw should also be recorded. Finally, the quality and symmetry of jaw movement should be noted. This involves assessing the patient's jaw movements for incoordination or tremor.

Myositis

Myositis describes inflammation and edema of muscle and fascial tissues. It usually occurs in conjunction with significant myalgia but may come and go even though the myalgia persists (Solberg, 1986c). Myositis, an inflammatory condition with or without swelling, is thought to be secondary to severe spasm or prolonged trismus. A diagnosis of muscle swelling is often made only from the history because the swelling is typically mild and diffuse and may not be noted on visual examination.

ETIOLOGY OF MASTICATORY MUSCLE DISORDERS

All painful muscle problems, whether they occur in the jaw, neck, back, or extremities, share common potential etiologies, namely direct trauma or muscle hyperactivity.

Muscle Hyperactivity

The onset of pain in the masticatory muscles is often associated with a reported increase in bruxism, clenching, or elevated orofacial muscle tension levels. Further, patients with masticatory muscle pain frequently have a history of recently increased emotional distress as a result of either difficulty in relationships, problems associated with employment, or other stressful life events (see Chapter 20). The exact mechanism by which emotional distress translates into a muscle pain disorder is unclear, but strong associations between these factors can be drawn from the literature (Amen, 1988; Duinkerke, 1986; Greene, 1974; Heloe, 1980; Moulton, 1966; Stegenga, 1989; van der Laan, 1988a; 1988b). Several studies using psychological inventories and interviews of patients with predominantly a masticatory muscle disorder have indicated that they are likely to have high psychosocial distress and difficulties dealing with life events.

Overall, patients with masticatory muscle pain are characterized as being more anxious, more somatically focused, and more depressed than the general population (Heiberg, 1978; Kydd, 1959; Laskin, 1969; Lupton, 1966; Marbach, 1981; Moulton, 1966; Rugh, 1987). This characterization, however, is not true for the primary TMJ patients. The probable mechanism for a transfer of emotional distress into muscle pain is via elevated levels of masticatory muscle activity. This activity could be mediated through the voluntary skeletal muscle system or via the involuntary smooth muscle (vasomotor) system.

Trauma

Direct trauma to the masticatory muscles is not common but can occur from a blow, inadvertent injection of local anesthetic agents with epinephrine, or forceful overstretching (Christiansen, 1987; Pullinger, 1985). It has also been speculated that muscle trauma may occur from a rapid stretching of the muscle during an automobile accident, although evidence for this theory is still very limited (Weinberg, 1987). Finally, masticatory muscle trauma may also occur due to the excessive forces produced during bruxism in sleep (Carlsson, 1979; Clark, 1981b; 1987; Fricton, 1989; Good, 1982; Wanman, 1986; Zarb, 1979).

DIAGNOSTIC TESTS

Masticatory muscle disorders are currently best documented by a clinical examination, which includes thorough muscle palpation, range-of-motion measurements, and a quality of motion assessment involving coordination and velocity of movement (Fig. 21–2). Additional tests described further on should be used only when they will serve to provide crucial diagnostic information not available from the clinical examination.

Passive Stretch Test (see Chapter 23)

This test should be performed on any patient with less than normal mouth opening ability. It

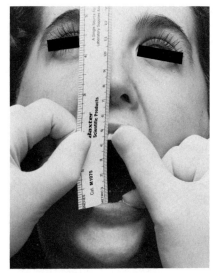

FIGURE 21–3. Passive stretch test. The jaw is stretched from the maximum voluntary opening by applying about 2 to 3 lbs of pressure to the lower and upper incisors with the middle or index finger and the thumb.

typically involves forceful stretching of the jaw in an attempt to determine whether the limitation is due to active muscle contraction (trismus) or to TMJ restriction. It is performed by applying about 2 to 3 lbs of pressure to the lower and upper incisors with the middle finger and thumb (Fig. 21–3). If the patient has too much pain to allow this manipulation, a vapocoolant spray first should be used on the skin over the masseter and temporalis muscles. This spray will generally block the pain transiently to allow for better stretching (Fig. 21–4). The

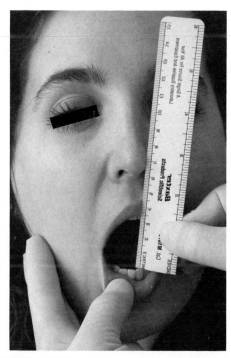

FIGURE 21–2. The voluntary pain-free opening is being measured from the mandibular incisor to the ipsilateral maxillary incisor. A measurement should also be made of the maximum voluntary opening.

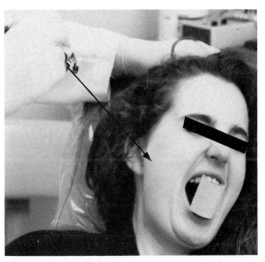

FIGURE 21–4. Vapocoolant spray is being directed, as indicated by arrow, to the superficial masseter muscle, allowing it to be stretched.

amount of resistance and the tactile feeling elicited at the most open position when applying the passive stretch test is described as *end feel*. A soft end feel exists when the patient refuses to allow much force to be applied because of pain. A hard or springy end feel exists when firm pressure is applied and no movement results.

Anesthetic Nerve and Muscle Blocking

Injection of muscles using about 1 ml of a 1 per cent solution of procaine hydrochloride without epinephrine can be done as a diagnostic test to help localize the sources of pain. For example, if palpation of a tender site elicits a change in a regional pain phenomena, anesthetic muscle blocking is then used to see if injection in the muscle tender point abolishes the pain (Bell, 1982; Fricton, 1989; Graff-Radford, 1987; Marbach, 1980; Phero, 1987; Solberg, 1986b) (Fig. 21–5). Anesthetic nerve blocking can also be done to rule out or identify the peripheral nature of an orofacial pain problem; for example, blocking the inferior alveolar nerve to rule out pain of dental origin.

Magnetic Resonance Spectroscopy

Magnetic resonance spectroscopy holds promise as a future diagnostic tool to evaluate the health of muscle tissue (Hasso, 1989; Schellhas, 1988; 1989; Westesson, 1987). At present, however, it is not useful as a clinically diagnostic tool.

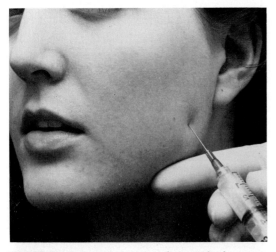

FIGURE 21–5. A trigger point in the superficial masseter that is referring pain to the temporomandibular joint is injected with a 1 per cent procaine solution without epinephrine.

Thermography

Thermography is also not currently of diagnostic utility because, at best, it only confirms the presence of altered temperature in a painful muscle, and it is many times less sensitive than palpation procedures (see page 360).

Biopsy

Excisional or needle biopsy of muscle tissue is not a routine procedure and has very little applicability for the painful disorders of the muscles of mastication (Byrne, 1986; Fricton, 1989).

Electromyography

Pain is not diagnosed with the use of electromyography (EMG). At best, EMG can detect the presence of abnormal protective muscle activity occurring with jaw movement in patients with trismus. EMG can also be used to monitor the level of jaw muscle activity during sleep to document the presence of active bruxism (Balciunas, 1987; Isberg, 1985). These uses do not replace the clinical examination procedures that are used to render the diagnosis of myalgia, trismus, and myositis.

Jaw Tracking

As with EMG, jaw tracking procedures are not diagnostic of a painful disorder of the masticatory muscles. Abnormal movements can usually be recognized clinically, and use of a millimeter ruler is a sufficiently accurate way to document the range of maximum jaw movement.

TREATMENT OF MASTICATORY MUSCLE DISORDERS

Initial Treatment Selections

If a patient has musculoskeletal pain (myalgia), trismus, or myositis in the masticatory system, one of several initial treatment options must be chosen. First, if the patient has specific muscle pain symptoms that seem related to either a bruxing or tooth-clenching habit, the primary mode of therapy will be the full arch occlusal stabilization appliance. The treatment procedures associated with this appliance are discussed later in the chapter (see page 352). In addition to myalgia, the signs that indicate bruxism-induced problems include: tooth wear, increased pain and "jaw stiffness" in the morning, mobility of the anterior teeth, and alveolar bone tenderness.

The initial treatment of trismus and myositis will involve decreasing the use of the jaw by softening the diet, avoiding tooth-to-tooth contact, and identifying and eliminating the etiologic factors as described in the next section. Rest and limited jaw movement are also recommended until the initial acute symptoms begin to abate. Muscle relaxant therapy utilizing moist heat and, for myositis, use of anti-inflammatory drugs and possibly short-term prednisone therapy to address the inflammatory condition, may be instituted for both conditions. Appliance therapy for myositis has produced mixed results.

Patients who have sustained a traumatic injury to the head, neck, or jaws may present with muscle pain, but they may also have a significant TMJ problem. Joint swelling, crepitus, loud clicking, or jaw locking will first require imaging of the TMJs (usually tomograms and/or MRI) before a definitive treatment plan can be made. Because taking of the radiographs and MRI need to be scheduled, and the construction of the appliance usually takes several days, it is important to prescribe an initial home-based therapy program that will begin the healing process.

Patient Self-Management Program

Most musculoskeletal diseases are phasic in nature, and many individuals will have a major resolution of their symptoms without an aggressive in-office therapy program (Clark, 1988; 1986; Greene, 1974; 1983; Magnusson, 1980; Mejersjo, 1983). This fact, along with the powerful effect produced by a visit to a specialist who has ruled out a life-threatening disease, can be conducive to a resolution of the acute phase of the symptoms (Magnusson, 1986; Wanman, 1986). For these reasons, the following initial treatment is recommended at the end of the first diagnostic visit. This regimen will usually result in some symptomatic relief while the patient is waiting for the tomograms or MRI to be taken or the occlusal appliance to be constructed. This initial therapy should be tried for at least two to four weeks to determine its effect. Only after this period has passed without a resolution in symptoms should more involved treatment be initiated. It may be necessary to supplement the specific symptomatic therapy with a broader program of physical and psychological therapy to improve the patient's overall

general physical and mental health. In general, all therapy should strive to provide the optimum conditions for symptomatic recovery, along with attempts to identify and eliminate the causes of the symptoms.

The specific home-based treatment measures that are recommended for a painful muscular disorder begin with the prescription of a nonnarcotic, nonsteroidal anti-inflammatory analgesic. The importance of taking this prescription contingently during the treatment period should be explained to the patient. The use of moist heat to the area of pain is also beneficial as an aid to muscular relaxation and to eventual healing and remobilization of tight muscles, ligaments, and joints. This heat should be applied at least three to four times a day no more than 20 minutes for each application.

Because of the accompanying TMJ symptoms that often occur, it is important to avoid biomechanically stressful forces. Therefore, during the acute phase of jaw pain and dysfunction, a soft diet is recommended to prevent further injury to a weakened joint system. Issuing a recommended list of foods to patients will help them follow this advice.

Resting the jaw is one of the most important aspects of conservative therapy. The patient also should be made aware of the relationship between stress and muscle tension. A complete or partial reduction of all physically and mentally stressful activity should be recommended during the conservative therapy period. Resting the mandible is often accomplished by making patients aware of their unconscious postural, swallowing, clenching, or teeth-grinding habits. Patients should be instructed to say repeatedly to themselves, "Teeth apart and jaws relaxed" to help reduce harmful oral habits.

With acute musculoskeletal pain conditions that are directly related to muscle tension from stress of recent onset, prescription of a muscle relaxant, or an antianxiety agent such as one of the benzodiazepines that induce muscle relaxation, is sometimes recommended. Antianxiety medications should be used only in small dosages taken before sleep, and only for a period of 2 to 4 weeks. Such medications have a high abuse potential and are not recommended for treatment of a chronic condition. Because longstanding stress is one of the primary factors associated with the development of musculoskeletal pain, there are alternative stress control methods that can be considered. These will be discussed further on. Finally, for the more generalized, chronic, painful muscle disorder fibromyalgia, the prescription of a tricyclic antidepressant such as amitriptyline is often very helpful.

Self-Management Therapy Alternatives

If the initial therapy is successful, the patient should then begin a series of exercises to aid in remobilizing the jaw. These include gently stretching the muscles of mastication to full length, increasing jaw coordination by practicing moving the mandible in a hinge type motion, and making specific lateral movements without protrusion (Burgess, 1988; Magnusson, 1980) (Fig. 21–6). The patient with TMJ clicking should limit jaw motion to a click-free range and chew on the side of the mouth that avoids any jaw joint noises. If there is an unstable occlusion, defined as a lack of multiple bilateral posterior tooth contacts, an occlusal stabilization appliance should also be prescribed.

If the initial home-based therapy does not resolve all of the symptoms, and they are primarily related to abnormal temporomandibular function, it will then be necessary to evaluate carefully the TMJ radiographs and the clinical findings. The symptoms that indicate chronic TMJ dysfunction include: pain on palpation of

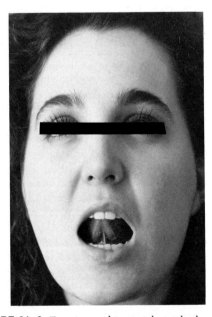

FIGURE 21–6. Exercise used to stretch gently the masticatory muscles. The patient is instructed to place the tip of the tongue on the palate immediately behind the central incisors where the letter "N" is articulated. The opening stretch should not go so far as to cause the tongue to be pulled from the palate. This limits the amount of condylar translation.

the TMJ, reduced translation of one or both joints, painful clicking, and crepitus. In addition, a very important consideration is a history of previous clicking that now has been replaced by a restriction of jaw movement. A diagnosis of a nonreducing, anteriorly displaced disc should be considered when a patient can open the mouth only 25–35 mm and feels there is a blockage in the joint that prevents wider opening.

If the muscular pain symptoms are not resolved with the initial home-based therapy program and the use of an occlusal stabilization appliance, a more involved course of physical therapy should be added, and possibly a behavioral medicine treatment program.

Occlusal Appliance Therapy

The basic approach to appliance therapy for the treatment of abnormal masticatory muscle function involves a full arch occlusal stabilization appliance (Agerberg, 1974; Clark, 1984a; 1984b; Diamond, 1987; Monteiro, 1988; Rubinoff, 1987; Zarb, 1970). This is constructed with a flat occlusal surface that is adjusted to have multiple tooth contact in an habitual comfortable jaw closure position (Fig. 21–7A and B). This appliance should be worn at all times except when eating, for 6 to 8 weeks, and should be readjusted several times to establish an optimally comfortable jaw position. The patient must be instructed not to bring the teeth together on the appliance while it is worn. Following relief of symptoms, the patient should reduce the amount of daytime wear of the appliance.

Physical Therapy

For a patient who primarily has a myogenous pain disorder that is not relieved by a home-based therapy program, a physical therapy regimen is often recommended (Clark, 1986; 1987; 1988; Fricton, 1989). This therapy can be performed by the dentist or the patient can be referred to a physical therapist. The treatment usually involves the repeated use of a vapo-coolant spray while passive stretching of the shortened jaw muscles is performed (Burgess, 1988; Campbell, 1989; Schwartz, 1966a; Solberg, 1986c; Travell, 1983). The use of other physical therapy modalities such as ice packs, heating pads, hydrocollators, electrical stimulators, or ultrasound to the tender muscles is also recommended. Another common treatment technique for myogenous pain conditions is the

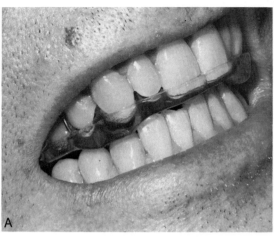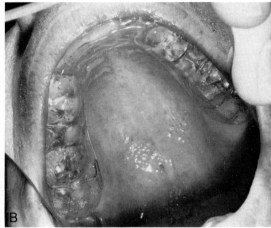

FIGURE 21–7. *A*, Flat plane maxillary stabilization appliance constructed of hard acrylic with ball clasps. The occlusal plane is flat except for increased thickness in the canine areas to provide canine guidance. *B*, Occlusal view of appliance. Note the thickened areas over the maxillary canines that provide canine guidance.

injection of a local anesthetic agent (1 per cent procaine hydrochloride solution without epinephrine) into the identified tender areas or trigger points in the muscle (Campbell, 1989; Fine, 1988; Padamsee, 1987; Travell, 1983).

If physical therapy is successful, the patient may return to normal function. This treatment program is typically limited to six to 10 visits. If the patient continues with a painful disorder, the perpetuating etiologic factors are probably not being addressed. This situation dictates prescription of a behavioral medicine program.

Behavioral Medicine Treatment

The techniques commonly used by the clinical psychologist for patients with chronic muscle pain involve stress recognition and relaxation training (Fordyce, 1978; Rugh, 1976). The specific method will vary depending on the preference of the therapist, but usually some form of cognitive behavioral therapy combined with EMG biofeedback, self-hypnosis, or progressive relaxation training is used. If the relationship between emotional distress, muscle hyperactivity, and painful muscular symptoms has been identified, the patient will usually be receptive to a referral for stress control or relaxation training.

Chronic Pain Treatment

Although chronic pain is not a clinically separate physical or organic problem, it can be a significant aspect of any painful disorder of the temporomandibular apparatus (see Chapter 25). Prolonged benign pain has as much clinical

significance to the patient's prognosis as the physical findings associated with the specifically diagnosed anatomical disorder. In a small percentage of patients, treating the pathological condition accompanied by chronic pain will not eliminate the pain. It is typical for patients having chronic pain to have a record of seeing many doctors who have pursued isolated medical therapies without benefit. Most of the treatments provided were usually indicated, but are rendered without due consideration of the chronic pain behavior. A treatment approach focusing on the psychological components of pain has been more successful. For this reason, the traditional understanding of pain and the pharmacological and surgical approaches to its treatment need to be re-evaluated. Simultaneous medical and psychological approaches, with recognition of the multidimensionality of the chronic pain experience, appear to be more beneficial (Curro, 1987).

If the patient has chronic, unrelenting pain, atypical pain, or symptoms that do not have a direct link to stressful events, referral to a chronic pain clinic is advised. Chronic pain therapies may be successful in the management of such patients even though they do not focus on the putative organic cause of the problem. Sometimes relief of unrelenting pain for a period of time is all that is necessary to begin the healing process. Treatment in a chronic pain clinic usually includes (1) transcutaneous electrical nerve stimulation (TENS), (2) diagnostic and therapeutic nerve blocks, (3) physical therapy, (4) occupational therapy, (5) acupuncture, (6) an intense behavioral medicine program, (7) a medication detoxification program, and, when appropriate, (8) a course of tricyclic antidepressant medication. These techniques provide effective relief from chronic pain but are more threatening and invasive and should be performed only after other measures have failed.

Behavioral Medicine Alternatives

If behavioral medicine therapy educates the patient to deal with stress better, and achieves muscular relaxation as well, this will often lead the way to normal function. If, however, severe chronic pain and dysfunction persist, it may not be possible to practice the specific relaxation techniques without some supportive chronic pain therapy. If the patient has involved psychological problems for which psychiatric treatment may be necessary, the psychologist will be able to aid in this evaluation and in making a referral to a psychiatrist. Psychiatric therapy may involve prolonged treatment as well as antidepressants or other appropriate psychoactive drugs.

Failure of Treatment

If the patient does not wish to see a psychologist or psychiatrist, or if the chronic pain and behavioral medicine treatments are not successful, the best recommendations that can be made are to tell the patient that: (1) at present you do not know the answer to the problem and active in-office treatment will be discontinued, (2) the daily active home-based treatment program should be continued, and (3) if there is considerable change in the symptoms, or after six months have passed, a re-evaluation will be done.

SUMMARY

In this chapter the various painful masticatory muscle disorders with which patients present have been reviewed. A step-by-step sequence of treatment of these problems has been considered. The following of this escalating sequence of conservative, yet appropriate, therapies will provide a logical plan for managing painful masticatory muscle disorders, and the majority of patients should be treated successfully.

REFERENCES

Agerberg, G., and Carlsson, G. E.: Late results of treatment of functional disorders of the masticatory system: A follow-up by questionnaire. J. Oral Rehabil. 1:309–316, 1974.

Amen, D. V., and Mostofsky, D. I.: Behavioral management of myofascial pain dysfunction syndrome. J. Roy. Soc. Health 108(3):81–82, 1988.
Balciunas, B. A., Staling, L. M., and Parente, F. J.: Quantitative electromyographic response to therapy for myo-oral facial pain: A pilot study. J. Prosthet. Dent. 58:366–369, 1987.
Bell, W. E.: Clinical Management of Temporomandibular Disorders. Chicago, Yearbook Medical Publishers, 1982, pp. 183–185.
Burgess, J. A., Sommers, E. E., Truelove, E. L., and Dworkin, S. F.: Short-term effect of two therapeutic methods on myofascial pain and dysfunction of the masticatory system. J. Prosthet. Dent. 60:606–610, 1988.
Butler, J. H., Folke, L. E., and Bandt, C. L.: A descriptive survey of signs and symptoms associated with the myofascial pain-dysfunction syndrome. J. Am. Dent. Assoc. 90:635–639, 1975.
Byrne, E., and Trounce, I.: Chronic fatigue and myalgia syndrome: Mitochondrial and glycolytic studies in skeletal muscle. J. Neurol. Neurosurg. Psychiatry 50:743–746, 1986.
Campbell, S. M.: Regional myofascial pain syndromes. Rheum. Dis. Clin. North Am. 15:31–44, 1989.
Carlsson, G. E., Kopp, S., and Oberg, T.: Arthritis and allied diseases of the temporomandibular joint. In Zarb, G. A., and Carlsson, G. E. (Eds.): Temporomandibular Joint Function and Dysfunction. Copenhagen, Munksgaard, 1979, pp. 269–320.
Christiansen, E. L., Thompson, J. R., and Hasso, A. N.: CT evaluation of trauma to the temporomandibular joint. J. Oral Maxillofac. Surg. 45:920–923, 1987.
Clark, G. T.: Management of muscular hyperactivity. Int. Dent. J. 31:216–225, 1981a.
Clark, G. T.: A critical evaluation of orthopedic interocclusal appliance therapy: Design, theory and overall effectiveness. J. Am. Dent. Assoc. 108:359–362, 1984a.
Clark, G. T.: A critical evaluation of orthopedic interocclusal appliance therapy: Effectiveness for specific symptoms. J. Am. Dent. Assoc. 108:364–368, 1984b.
Clark, G. T.: Diagnosis and treatment of painful temporomandibular disorders. Dent. Clin. North Am. 31:645–674, 1987.
Clark, G. T., Beemsterboer, P. L., and Rugh, J. D.: Nocturnal masseter muscle activity and the symptoms of masticatory dysfunction. J. Oral Rehabil. 8:279–286, 1981b.
Clark, G. T., and Lanham, F.: Multidimensional assessment of treatment outcome for 100 consecutive TMJ clinic patients (abstr.). Scottsdale, AZ, Western Pain Society, 1986.
Clark, G. T., Lanham, F., and Flack, V. F.: Treatment outcome results for consecutive TMJ clinic patients. J. Craniomandib. Disord. 2:87–95, 1988.
Clark, G. T., Seligman, D. A., Solberg, W. K., and Pullinger, A. G.: Guidelines for the examination and diagnosis of temporomandibular disorders. J. Craniomandib. Disord. 3:7–14, 1989.
Curro, F. A.: Assessing the physiologic and clinical characteristics of acute versus chronic pain (Introduction). Dent. Clin. North Am. 31:xiii–xxiii, 1987.
Diamond, M. W.: An overview of the multimodal approach to TMJ disorders. Dent. Clin. North Am. 31:695–701, 1987.
Duinkerke, A. S., Luteijn, F., Bouman, T. K., and de Jong, H. P.: Comparison of tests for dysfunction of the stomatognathic system. Community Dent. Oral Epidemiol. 14:334–337, 1986.
Eversole, L. R., and Machado, L.: Temporomandibular

joint internal derangements and associated neuromuscular disorders. J. Am. Dent. Assoc. 110:69–79, 1985.

Farrar, W. B., and McCarty, W. L. Jr.: A Clinical Outline of Temporomandibular Joint Diagnosis and Treatment. Montgomery, AL, Walker Printing, 1983.

Fine, P. G., Milano, R., and Hare, B. D.: The effects of myofascial trigger point injections are naloxone reversible. Pain 32:15–20, 1988.

Fishbain, D. A., Goldberg, M., Steele, R., and Rosomoff, H.: DSM-III diagnoses of patients with myofascial pain syndrome (fibrositis). Arch. Phys. Med. Rehabil. 70:433–438, 1989.

Fordyce, W.: Behavioral Methods for Chronic Pain and Illness. St. Louis, C. V. Mosby, 1978.

Forssell, H., and Kangasniemi, P.: Mandibular dysfunction in patients with muscle contraction headache. Proc. Finn. Dent. Soc. 80:211–216, 1984.

Fricton, J. R.: Myofascial pain syndrome. Neurol. Clin. 7:413–427, 1989.

Good, A. E., and Upton, L. G.: Acute temporomandibular arthritis in a patient with bruxism and calcium pyrophosphate deposition disease. Arthritis Rheum. 25:353–355, 1982.

Graff-Radford, S. B., Reeves, J. L., and Jaeger, B.: Management of chronic head and neck pain: Effectiveness of altering factors perpetuating myofascial pain. Headache 27:186–190, 1987.

Greene, C. S., and Laskin, D. M.: Long-term evaluation of conservative treatment for myofascial pain-dysfunction syndrome. J. Am. Dent. Assoc. 89:1365–1368, 1974.

Greene, C. S., and Laskin, D. M.: Long-term evaluation of treatment for myofascial pain-dysfunction syndrome: A comparative analysis. J. Am. Dent. Assoc. 107:235–238, 1983.

Griffiths, R. H.: Report of the president's conference on the examination, diagnosis, and management of temporomandibular disorders. J. Am. Dent. Assoc. 106:75–77, 1983.

Hasso, A. N., Christiansen, E. L., and Alder, M. E.: The temporomandibular joint. Radiol. Clin. North Am. 27:301–314, 1989.

Heiberg, A. N., Heloe, B., and Krogstad, B. S.: The myofascial pain dysfunction: Dental symptoms and psychological and muscular function. An Overview. Psychother. Psychosom. 30:81–97, 1978.

Heloe, B., and Heiberg, A. N.: A follow-up study of a group of female patients with myofascial pain-dysfunction syndrome. Acta Odontol. Scand. 38:129–134, 1980.

Hench, P. K.: Evaluation and differential diagnosis of fibromyalgia: Approach to diagnosis and management. Rheum. Dis. Clin. North Am. 15:19–29, 1989.

Isberg, A., Widmalm, S. E., and Ivarsson, R.: Clinical, radiographic, and electromyographic study of patients with internal derangement of the temporomandibular joint. Am. J. Orthod. 88:453–460, 1985.

Kydd, W. L.: Psychosomatic aspects of temporomandibular joint dysfunction. J. Am. Dent. Assoc. 59:31–44, 1959.

Laskin, D. M.: Etiology of the pain-dysfunction syndrome. J. Am. Dent. Assoc. 79:147–153, 1969.

Lupton, D. E.: A preliminary investigation of the personality of female TMJ patients. Psychother. Psychosom. 14:199, 1966.

Magnusson, T., and Carlsson, G. E.: Treatment of patients with functional disturbances in the masticatory system. A survey of 80 consecutive patients. Swed. Dent. J. 4:145–153, 1980.

Magnusson, T., Egermark-Eriksson, I., and Carlsson, G. E.: Five-year longitudinal study of signs and symptoms of mandibular dysfunction in adolescents. J. Craniomandib. Pract. 4:338–344, 1986.

Marbach, J. J., and Lund, P.: Depression, anhedonia and anxiety in temporomandibular joint and other facial pain syndromes. Pain 11:73–84, 1981.

Marbach, J. J., and Varoscak, J. R.: Treatment of TMJ and other facial pains: A critical review. NY State Dent. J. 46:181–188, 1980.

Mejersjo, C., and Carlsson, G. E.: Long-term results of treatment for temporomandibular joint pain-dysfunction. J. Prosthet. Dent. 49:809–815, 1983.

Monteiro, A. A., and Clark, G. T.: Mandibular movement feedback vs occlusal appliances in the treatment of masticatory muscle dysfunction. J. Craniomandib. Dis. Facial Oral Pain 2:41–47, 1988.

Moulton, R. E.: Emotional factors in non-organic temporomandibular joint pain. Dent. Clin. North Am. 10:609–620, 1966.

Padamsee, M., Mehta, N., and White, G. E.: Trigger point injection: A neglected modality in the treatment of TMJ dysfunction. Periodontics 12:72–92, 1987.

Phero, J. C., Raj, P. P., and McDonald, J. S.: Transcutaneous electrical nerve stimulation and myoneural injection therapy for management of chronic myofascial pain. Dent. Clin. North Am. 31:703–723, 1987.

Pullinger, A. G., Monteiro, A. A., and Liu, A.: Etiological factors associated with temporomandibular disorders (abstr). J. Dent. Res. 64:269, 1985.

Roy, E. P., and Gutmann, L.: Myalgia. Neurol. Clin. 6:621–636, 1988.

Rubinoff, M. S., Gross, A., and McCall, W. D., Jr.: Conventional and nonoccluding splint therapy compared for patients with myofascial pain dysfunction syndrome. Gen. Dent. 35:502–506, 1987.

Rugh, J. D.: Psychological components of pain. Dent. Clin. North Am. 31:579–594, 1987.

Rugh, J. D., and Solberg, W. K.: Psychological implications in temporomandibular pain and dysfunction. Oral Sci. Rev. 1:3–30, 1976.

Schellhas, K. P., Wilkes, C. H., and Bakar, C. C.: Facial pain, headache, and temporomandibular joint inflammation. Headache 29:228–231, 1989.

Schellhas, K. P., Wilkes, C. H., Omlie, M. R., et al.: The diagnosis of temporomandibular joint disease: Two-compartment arthrography and MR. Am. J. Roent. 151:341–350, 1988.

Schwartz, L.: Local anesthetics. In Schwartz, L. (Ed.): Disorders of the Temporomandibular Joint: Diagnosis, Management, Relation to Occlusion of Teeth. Philadelphia, W. B. Saunders, 1966a, pp. 232–238.

Schwartz, L.: Limitation. In Schwartz, L. (Ed.): Disorders of the Temporomandibular Joint: Diagnosis, Management, Relation to Occlusion of Teeth. Philadelphia, W. B. Saunders, 1966b, pp. 315–334.

Seligman, D. A., Pullinger, A. G., and Solberg, W. K.: Temporomandibular disorders. Part III: Occlusal and articular factors associated with muscle tenderness. J. Prosthet. Dent. 59:483–489, 1988.

Solberg, W. K.: Temporomandibular Disorders. E. T. Heron (Print) LTD, Silver End, Witham, Essex, 1986a.

Solberg, W. K.: Temporomandibular disorders: Management of problems associated with inflammation, chronic hypomobility, and deformity. Br. Dent. J. 160:421–428, 1986b.

Solberg, W. K.: Temporomandibular disorders: Masticatory myalgia and its management. Br. Dent. J. 160:351–356, 1986c.

Stegenga, B., de Bont, L. G. M., and Boering, G.: Osteoarthrosis as the cause of craniomandibular pain and dysfunction: A unifying concept. J. Oral Maxillofac. Surg. 47:249–256, 1989.

Travell, J. G., and Simons, D. G.: Myofascial Pain and

Dysfunction: The Trigger Point Manual. Baltimore, Williams & Wilkins, 1983, pp. 165–321.

Tunks, E., Crook, J., Norman, G., and Kalaher, S.: Tender points in fibromyalgia. Pain 34:11–19, 1988.

van der Laan, G. J., Duinkerke, A. S. H., Luteijn, F., and van de Poel, A. C. M.: Role of psychologic and social variables in TMJ pain dysfunction syndrome (PDS) symptoms. Community Dent. Oral Epidemiol. 16:274–277, 1988a.

van der Laan, G. J., Duinkerke, A. S. H., Luteijn, F., and van de Poel, A. C. M.: Relative importance of psychologic and social variables in TMJ pain dysfunction syndrome (PDS) signs. Community Dent. Oral Epidemiol. 16:117–121, 1988b.

Wanman, A., and Agerberg, G.: Two-year longitudinal study of signs of mandibular dysfunction in adolescents. Acta Odontol. Scand. 44:333–342, 1986.

Weinberg, S., and Lapointe, H.: Cervical extension-flexion injury (whiplash) and internal derangement of the temporomandibular joint. J. Oral Maxillofac. Surg. 45:653–656, 1987.

Westesson, P.-L., Katzberg, R. W., Tallents, R. H., et al.: Temporomandibular joint: Comparison of MR images with cryosectional anatomy. Radiology 164:59–64, 1987.

Wolfe, F.: Fibrositis, fibromyalgia, and musculoskeletal disease: The current status of the fibrositis syndrome. Arch. Phys. Rehabil. 69:527–531, 1988.

Yemm, R.: Neurophysiological studies of temporomandibular joint dysfunction. In Zarb, G. A., and Carlsson, G. E. (Eds.): Temporomandibular Joint Function and Dysfunction. Copenhagen, Munksgaard, 1979, pp. 216–237.

Yunus, M. B., Kalyan-Raman, U. P., and Kalyan-Raman, K.: Primary fibromyalgia syndrome and myofascial pain syndrome: Clinical features and muscle pathology. Arch. Phys. Med. Rehabil. 69:451–454, 1988.

Zarb, G. A., and Speck, J. E.: The treatment of mandibular dysfunction. In Zarb, G. A., and Carlsson, G. E. (Eds.): Temporomandibular Joint Function and Dysfunction. St. Louis, C. V. Mosby, 1979, pp. 373–396.

Zarb, G. A., and Thompson, G. W.: Assessment of clinical treatment of patients with temporomandibular joint dysfunction. J. Prosthet. Dent. 24:542–554, 1970.

DIAGNOSIS AND NONSURGICAL TREATMENT OF THE ARTHRITIDES*

SIGVARD KOPP, D.D.S., Odont. Dr.

INTRODUCTION

Noninfectious arthritis may involve the temporomandibular joint (TMJ) as part of systemic inflammatory joint disease (polyarthritis), local primary or secondary degenerative joint disease (osteoarthrosis, osteoarthritis), or facial trauma (traumatic arthritis).

Connective Tissue Aspects

Under normal circumstances the mineralized TMJ surfaces are covered by a fibrocartilaginous tissue; that is, a connective tissue rich in collagenous fibers, providing tensile strength, and a ground substance containing sulfated proteoglycans (Kempson, 1970). In addition, the TMJ is provided with a disc consisting of a central part composed of dense fibrous connective tissue, which contains ground substance, chondroid cells, sulfated proteoglycans (PGs), as well as collagen fibers. The PGs provide the resistance to compression characteristic of cartilage (Fig. 22–1A).

The PG molecule consists of a protein core with attached sulfated glycosaminoglycans (GAGs) and a hyaluronate binding region that combines with hyaluronate (HA), creating macromolecules of molecular weights from 10 to 20 $\times 10^6$ daltons (Hascall, 1974) (Fig. 22–1B). The sulfated GAGs provide negative charges that repel each other and bind water molecules, creating a high osmotic pressure. Fibrocarti-

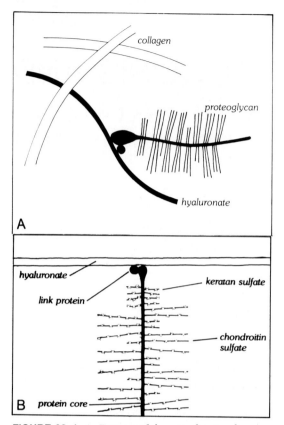

FIGURE 22–1. *A*, Diagram of the main functional components of the soft tissue articular surface. *B*, Diagram of the proteoglycan unit. The closely attached glycosaminoglycans with the negative charges repel each other, causing the entire complex to expand in solution. (Data courtesy of Pharmacia AB, Uppsala, Sweden.)

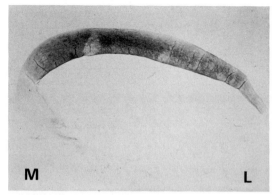

FIGURE 22–2. Photomicrograph of a frontal section from the central part of a disc showing the distribution of sulfated proteoglycans as indicated by toluidine blue staining at a pH level of 0.5. Note the staining in all parts of the section. Medial (M), lateral (L).

lage, in general, contains a high proportion of the GAG dermatan sulfate (Habuchi, 1973). The GAGs of the fibrocartilage of pooled TMJ discs from rats, rabbits, dogs, and monkeys have been found to consist mainly of HA and dermatan sulfate (Granström, 1973). In human TMJ discs sulfated GAGs are found mostly in the central dense connective tissue region (Fig. 22–2) in connection with chondroid cells as well as fibrocytes (Kopp, 1976). No difference in distribution is found between medial and lateral sides. In early stages of osteoarthrosis the sulfated GAGs in thin and disrupted regions are found in significantly lesser amounts than in corresponding normal areas, which is in agreement with what occurs in hyaline articular cartilage. The histochemical characteristics of the GAGs found in the TMJ disc correspond to those of HA, chondroitin/dermatan sulfate, and keratan sulfate, although the last is a rather infrequent finding.

The soft tissue articular surfaces of the con-

dyle and articular eminence contain more sulfated GAGs in the lateral part of the joint and less in the posterior part, i.e., the mandibular fossa and posterior surface of the condyle (Kopp, 1978). There is an even distribution between the lateral and medial sides on the anterior part of the condyle, whereas most of the sulfated GAGs are located in the lateral part of the articular eminence. The amount of sulfated GAGs is less in areas with joint surface lesions of both degenerative and inflammatory nature (Fig. 22–3). Sulfated GAGs with a pericellular location are more frequently observed in the mineralized cartilage layer than in the nonmineralized cartilage layer and are least conspicuous in the fibrous connective tissue lining on the surface.

The most likely explanation for the topographic variation of the sulfated GAGs in the

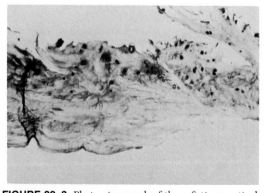

FIGURE 22–3. Photomicrograph of the soft tissue articular lining from the lateral part of an articular eminence with degenerative joint disease. The surface layers (bottom) have lost sulfated proteoglycan as shown by staining with toluidine blue at a pH of 0.5, while the deeper layers (top), including the mineralized cartilage layer, show a strong staining reaction, especially pericellularly.

TMJ is a variation in functional loading between different areas of the joint. The predilection of the sulfated GAGs for the lateral part of the eminence, the anterior part of the condyle, and the central part of the disc is in accordance with our present knowledge of the loading conditions of the TMJ. Both laterotrusive and protrusive movements in the TMJ during mastication and bruxism cause compressive forces in its lateral part (Hansson, 1977).

The synovial fluid of the joint contains HA produced by the synovial membrane, plasma dialysate, abraded synovial lining cells, macrophages, as well as a few leukocytes. Sodium HA, or hyaluronan, as it has been proposed to be called (Balazs, 1986), is a GAG composed of a linear polysaccharide formed by repeating disaccharide units consisting of N-acetyl-D-glucosamine and D-glucuronic acid. HA can be synthesized by most cells and is widely distributed in the body. High concentrations of HA are found in the vitreous body of the eye and in the umbilical cord. The HA of the synovial fluid must be of high molecular weight to be able to carry out its functions. Its main tasks are to reduce the friction between the surfaces of the soft tissues, to form a barrier that prevents blood cells with their degradative enzymes from entering the articular cavity, and to contribute to the transfer of nutritive substances from the synovial membrane to the articular cartilage.

Diagnostic Aspects

The basic structures of the TMJ are similar to those of other synovial joints and are therefore also subjected to the same disease processes; that is, degeneration and inflammation. Degenerative joint disease primarily affects the articular surface tissues, while the inflammatory joint diseases originate in the synovial lining tissues. There are several joint diseases with an inflammatory component that may involve the TMJ, e.g., degenerative joint disease (DJD, osteoarthrosis, osteoarthritis), traumatic arthritis, rheumatoid arthritis, gout, ankylosing spondylitis, psoriatic arthritis.

The most reliable but late clinical sign of structural damage of the articular surfaces of the TMJ is crepitus, and the main clinical sign of inflammatory involvement is tenderness to palpation of the joint (Franks, 1969). Both signs are nonspecific, however, and occur in several different diseases of the TMJ. Joint tenderness may also be present with primary muscular disorders.

Radiography has long been the main basis for diagnosis of organic diseases of the TMJ. However, it has been difficult to determine the abnormalities that are characteristic of individual diseases of the joint. A reduced joint space has been shown to be associated with joint crepitus as well as a higher overall frequency of radiographic changes (Kopp, 1979a). The most likely explanation is that both crepitus and radiographic changes develop as a consequence of pathologic processes in the joint and ensuing reduction in the thickness of the articular surface tissues. The combined radiographic signs of reduction of joint space, sclerosis of the subcortical bone of the condyle, and flattening of the lateral part of the condyle (Fig. 22–4) have frequently been found among patients with crepitation and pain of the TMJ due to DJD (Kopp, 1979b). Reduced joint space and subcortical bone sclerosis of the TMJ are also associated with loss of molar support and are probably the result of increased loading in the joint (Kopp, 1979a). The radiographic sign of erosion of the articular cortical layer is also frequently found in patients with TMJ crepitus but is not characteristic of DJD. It is more indicative of chronic inflammatory joint disease. Erosion of the articular cortical outline of the TMJ is frequently associated with the presence of inflammatory cells and an abnormal concentration of plasma proteins in the synovial fluid (Kopp, 1983).

Absence of radiographic changes of the TMJ does not exclude the possibility of early disease. In patients with clinical signs but without radiographic evidence of joint disease, cellular find-

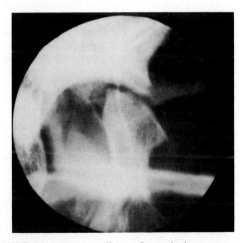

FIGURE 22–4. Transmaxillary radiograph showing signs of degenerative joint disease as indicated by a reduced joint space, sclerosis of the subcortical bone, and flattening of the lateral part of the condyle.

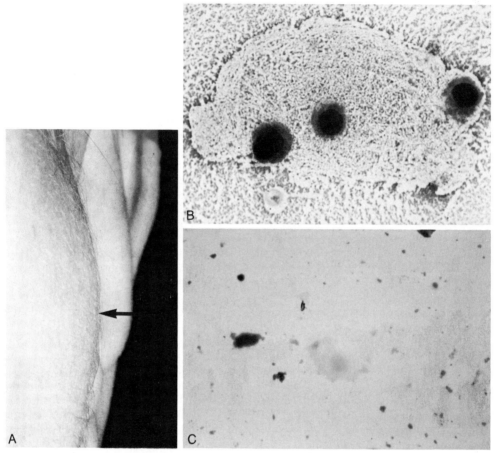

FIGURE 22–5. Patient with severe pain from arthritis of the left TMJ. *A*, There is a tender swelling (arrow) over the joint. *B*, Exudate aspirated from the joint containing mononuclear blood cells and fibrin strands. *C*, Fibrocartilage debris stained by toluidine blue at a pH of 0.5 indicates sulfated proteoglycan.

ings and abnormalities of plasma protein content, such as fibrin in the synovial fluid, are indicative of an inflammatory process. Fibrocartilage debris and corresponding high amounts of chondroitin/dermatan sulfate are also markers of fibrocartilage breakdown (Fig. 22–5). In involvement of the TMJ by the inflammatory joint diseases such as rheumatoid arthritis (RA) and ankylosing spondylitis (AS), the radiographic sign of cortical erosion is correlated with the severity of the TMJ condition and with the duration and extension of the general joint disease (Åkerman, 1988b; Wenneberg, 1983). In chronic RA and AS, tenderness to palpation and crepitus of the TMJ are the most frequent clinical findings (Tegelberg, 1987a; Wenneberg, 1982).

Thermologic techniques have been used to study both intra-articular temperature and the temperature on the skin surface overlying joints with inflammation, the latter both with infrared thermography and thermocouples in contact with the skin. Patients with unilateral tenderness to palpation of the TMJ clinically diagnosed as having nonsystemic TMJ arthritis have a higher skin surface temperature over the symptomatic joint than over the nonsymptomatic joint (Kopp, 1988) (Fig. 22–6). In RA patients with unilateral TMJ involvement and posterior joint tenderness, the skin surface temperature over the TMJ on the symptomatic side is higher than on the nonsymptomatic side, while the opposite is found for the skin surface temperature over the tender masseter muscle (Tegelberg, 1987b) (Fig. 22–7). Intra-articular temperature of the TMJ in RA increases with extension and severity of general rheumatoid disease (Åkerman, 1988a) but decreases with increasing muscle pain and tenderness. This condition reflects two subgroups of patients with acute and chronic TMJ arthritis, respectively, needing different treatment (see page 350).

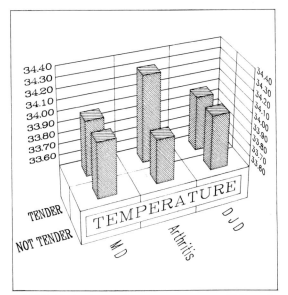

FIGURE 22–6. Skin surface temperature over TMJs with unilateral tenderness to palpation in 40 patients with muscular disorder (MD), 11 patients with TMJ arthritis, and 8 patients with TMJ degenerative joint disease (DJD). (From Kopp, S., and Haraldson, T.: Skin surface temperature over the temporomandibular joint and masseter muscle in patients with craniomandibular disorder. Swed. Dent. J. 12:63–67, 1988.)

TREATMENT OF TEMPOROMANDIBULAR JOINT ARTHRITIS

The treatment of TMJ arthritis is directed toward reducing or eliminating the inflammatory process in the joint and, if possible, its cause, as well as creating the most favorable loading condition possible for the joint and muscles.

Nonsteroidal Anti-inflammatory Drugs (NSAIDs)

There are a large variety of nonsteroidal anti-inflammatory drugs (NSAIDs) that can be used to reduce TMJ inflammation and associated pain. They should be used at an early stage before any other treatment. However, they are not a long-term remedy for TMJ arthritis.

Mode of Action

There is evidence that NSAIDs have a stabilizing effect on lysosomal membranes and an inhibitory effect on leukocyte migration. The main effect, however, is that they inhibit the

production of prostaglandins by blocking the enzyme cyclooxygenase, which explains their reduction of inflammation and pain (Adams, 1977; Dannenberg, 1979). NSAIDs are known to produce a wide variety of effects on metabolism similar to those produced by glucocorticosteroids, e.g., an antianabolic effect (Kalbhen, 1978), and their long-term use is therefore questionable.

Drugs

The oldest NSAID is acetylsalicylic acid (ASA; aspirin), which has analgesic, anti-inflammatory, and antipyretic effects. It is well known that headache, arthralgia, and muscular ache respond to ASA. Its modest anti-inflammatory effect is exerted at a relatively high dose (3 to 5 gm), which often creates gastrointestinal symptoms or bleeding (30 to 45 per cent). These side effects can be reduced by using enteric-coated preparations, but the analgesic effect will then be delayed. Indomethacin is frequently used in RA as an anti-inflammatory agent at night to prevent morning stiffness and pain. Although it is quite effective against arthritis, it may produce peptic ulcers, which limits its usefulness. Among the newer NSAIDs, naproxen and ibuprofen are well-known compounds that have been used exten-

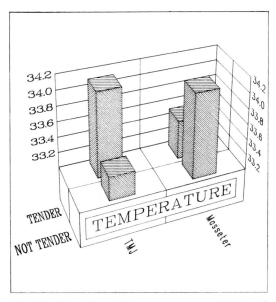

FIGURE 22–7. Skin surface temperature over TMJs with posterior tenderness and tender masseter muscles in patients with RA. Note the reciprocal relationship between joint and muscle temperature.

sively as analgesics in DJD and RA and should therefore be suitable alternatives.

Indications

The NSAIDs are indicated in patients with exacerbations of TMJ involvement with degenerative, inflammatory, or traumatic joint disease. Effort should be made, however, to find a means for further local treatment.

Intra-articular Injections

Glucocorticosteroids have been used for a long time as anti-inflammatory drugs for intra-articular use, while sodium hyaluronate has been tried more recently. Both drugs will be considered in the following sections.

Injection Technique

Before preparation for the injection begins, the joint should be thoroughly palpated during mandibular movements to locate the condyle and the mandibular fossa. The fossa is felt as a depression anterior to the tragus upon mouth opening. Hair or beard over the joint is shaved and any hair in the vicinity of the joint area is held aside with adhesive tape. A head cap can then be used to cover the hair. The skin surface 4 to 5 cm around the injection site is cleansed with benzalkonium chloride (0.1 per cent), iodine (5 per cent), and alcohol (70 per cent). The washing should be adequate to cleanse the folds of the skin and to remove microorganisms by mechanical means. A surgical cover (Steri-Drape) with a 6 cm hole in the center can be placed over the joint to maintain a clean area around it. The operator should wear rubber gloves and a face mask. A mouth prop makes opening during the injection more comfortable for the patient.

A sterile disposable 23-gauge needle 1 to 1½ inches long should be used. A smaller diameter creates a risk of bending the needle underneath the skin and a wider diameter results in a larger skin puncture than necessary. Two sterile disposable 2 ml syringes should be available, one for aspiration and one for injection of the drug. The needle is inserted into the fossa 2 to 3 mm beneath the zygomatic arch and 8 to 10 mm anterior to the anterior border of the tragus (Fig. 22–8). These landmarks may vary so palpation of the fossa is essential. The needle is directed slightly upward and backward to account for the angulation of the condyle. If resistance is felt or the needle is stuck, it might

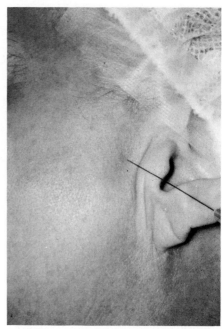

FIGURE 22–8. Site of intra-articular injection of the TMJ.

have penetrated the posterior part of the disc lying behind the condyle and not the joint space proper. This can occur in patients with restricted condylar translation. The needle should not be forced further; it should be withdrawn and the insertion tried again. The needle should penetrate 20 to 30 mm beneath the skin surface provided that no resistance is felt. Aspiration is made with the empty syringe. Clear or bloody exudate in varying amounts may be obtained; this should be saved for later analysis. The second syringe containing the drug is then connected to the needle and the therapeutic injection is given. If strong resistance is felt when injecting the drug, no force should be used; instead the needle should be relocated slightly to permit unrestrained injection. Scratching of the articular surfaces by the needle should be avoided. A volume of 1 ml is commonly injected without any difficulty. The needle is then removed and the site is covered by a dressing under light pressure for one minute. Usually, there is no need for a dressing over the injection site when the patient leaves.

Postinjection bleeding is not a common occurrence. The puncture of the joint might cause pain, however, depending on its condition. In case of acute inflammation in the joint a local anesthetic might be added to the drug suspension to be injected. Preoperative local anesthesia does not provide significant benefits because two injections instead of one have to be made. Skin surface anesthesia will block only the minute amount of pain created by the needle penetration of the skin.

If the injection is made too far anteriorly, the upper branch of the facial nerve might be affected. The blink reflex of the eye might then be impaired. This condition is usually only temporary and may be caused by either the local anesthetic agent or by trauma of the needle. Infection of the joint following intra-articular injection is extremely rare. Hollander (1969) has calculated the risk to be 1:10,000. On the contrary, puncture and aspiration of the joint might provide a diagnosis if infection is present.

Glucocorticosteroid

MODE OF ACTION

The anti-inflammatory effect of glucocorticoids on synovial tissues given systemically or intra-articularly is well documented (Hollander, 1969). Intra-articular corticosteroids have been proved useful in alleviating pain, swelling, and dysfunction in inflammatory diseases of joints and muscles, such as RA and gout, as well as in primarily noninflammatory joint diseases such as DJD. The symptomatic relief from an intra-articular injection of glucocorticoid has been reported to last between one week and 12 months (Toller, 1976), while the glucocorticoid has been found to remain in the synovial lining cells for two weeks (Zacco, 1954).

The mechanism by which glucocorticoids exert their anti-inflammatory action is not entirely understood. They have been reported to stabilize the membrane of the lysosomes of damaged cells and thereby prevent the release of proteolytic enzymes and inhibit the enzymes already released (Smith, 1987). Mast cell activity and histamine activity are also inhibited by glucocorticoids (Asboe-Hansen, 1963). The synthesis of prostaglandins is reduced by inhibition of production of arachidonic acid from cellular phospholipids (Dannenberg, 1979).

Glucocorticoid also inhibits the synthesis of proteoglycans and collagen; that is, it has an antianabolic effect and may thus impair healing processes (Dannenberg, 1979). This factor is mostly valid with prolonged use. One or only a few intra-articular injections, however, do not produce any general side effects such as iatrogenic Cushing's syndrome, osteoporosis, and inhibition of ACTH production. A single injection may have a systemic effect on general joint symptoms in patients with RA. There are many new synthetic glucocorticoids, which are more potent than cortisone and hydrocortisone, but unfortunately their side effects are also greater.

Local side effects of intra-articular injections of glucocorticoids, such as destruction of articular cartilage, infection, and progression of an already manifest joint disease, have been reported (Poswillo, 1970). The cause of these deleterious effects has not been fully explained and adequate controls are lacking. In an experimental study of intra-articular glucocorticoid treatment on induced arthritis of the guinea pig knee, the drug did not cause any macroscopic or microscopic damage on noninduced control knees (Mejersjö, 1987). In a clinical study, it was shown that intra-articular glucocorticoid injections resulted in less release of proteoglycan into the joint fluid than before treatment. Relapse of symptoms coincided with an increase of proteoglycan release (Saxne, 1985; 1986). Besides the glucocorticoid, other factors such as infection, trauma in association with the actual injection, and the suspension medium are more likely explanations of the deleterious effects, at least when a limited number of injections have been made (Brånemark, 1967; Oláh, 1976; Poswillo, 1970).

DRUGS

There are many glucocorticoid preparations available for intra-articular injection. First, there are cortisone and hydrocortisone, which rapidly diffuse out of the joint, and new synthetic steroid esters, which are poorly soluble in aqueous media and are administered as microcrystalline suspensions. The disodium phosphate ester of betamethasone (3 mg/ml), which is readily soluble and thereby has a quick effect, is used together with its acetate ester (3 mg/ml), which has a sustained release and prolonged effect (Celestone). The duration of these preparations seems to be directly related to the insolubility of the ester. Methylprednisolone acetate (Depo-medrol) has an intermediate solubility and duration, while triamcinolone acetonide (Kenacort), and especially triamcinolone hexacetonide (Lederspan), have very low solubility and long duration. The crystals of the latter are retained in the joint for up to six weeks (Bird, 1979).

The long-acting glucocorticoids may produce an acute postinjection flare due to their crystalline nature. This reaction occurs in about 2 per cent of injections and is reversible. The reaction usually begins several hours after injection and subsides spontaneously in 24 to 72 hours. Varying degrees of redness, local heat, swelling, and pain may be noted by the patient. Glucocorticoid is often injected together with a local anesthetic agent to counteract some of these local adverse effects.

CLINICAL STUDIES

Patients with long-standing local pain and dysfunction due to arthritis of the TMJ have been subjected to intra-articular glucocorticosteroid injections following failure of conservative treatment (Kopp, 1981). The results show that intra-articular injections of glucocorticosteroid combined with a local anesthetic agent have a good long-term palliative effect on subjective symptoms and clinical signs from the joint. The prognosis, however, is poor in patients with advanced radiographic signs of DJD or when there is general joint disease. Patients have been followed for eight years after glucocorticosteroid treatment of the TMJ (Wenneberg, 1989), and the subjective symptoms and the clinical signs have remained very slight or absent. TMJ clicking and crepitus, however, did not decrease significantly. Radiographic signs of erosion of the cortical outline of the joint were found in four patients (33 per cent) before treatment and in none of the patients eight years after treatment, which suggests a healing process.

In another long-term study including treatment with glucocorticoid a significant effect was found on subjective symptoms and clinical signs such as joint tenderness, maximum voluntary mouth opening, and bite force (Kopp, 1987). Neither joint crepitus nor muscle tenderness were affected by the treatment. In a recent clinical trial of methylprednisolone acetate (Depo-medrol) on RA of the TMJ this preparation had a significant short-term effect on both subjective symptoms and clinical signs that exceeded that of saline (Åkerman, 1989). The long-term effect is not yet known.

ANIMAL STUDIES

Glucocorticosteroids have a well-documented anti-inflammatory effect by reducing vasodilation, edema, and the number of leukocytes at the local site. Their antianabolic properties, however, make fibroblasts grow less (Pratt, 1978), secrete less collagenase, and produce less collagen as well as GAGs, including HA (Moscatelli, 1977) and chondroitin sulfate. Wound healing may therefore be delayed, in part, because steroids reduce the number of new capillaries and fibroblasts in the early stages of healing (Asboe-Hansen, 1958). The

latter effect is advantageous, however, in reducing pannus formation in RA (Åkerman, 1986). Repeated injections of glucocorticosteroid on induced inflammatory joint lesions in the guinea pig knee resulted in more osteophyte formation, chondrocyte necrosis, and chondrocyte cluster formation than did no treatment (Mejersjö, 1987). The response of the connective tissue to corticosteroid, therefore, seems to differ between diseased and healthy tissue (Shaw, 1973). The treatment was administered six to eight weeks after induction of arthritis, which might have been too late to influence significantly the progression of the joint lesion, or the injections may have been too few (two injections at one-week intervals) to show the potential range of effects.

INDICATIONS

Intra-articular injections of glucocorticosteroids into the TMJ have been advocated in patients with acute synovitis secondary to DJD and in patients with acute exacerbations of inflammatory joint disease (Carlsson, 1979). Their use can be recommended only when the TMJ is the primary site of disease.

ADMINISTRATION

After penetration of the joint and aspiration, 0.5 to 1.0 ml of the drug is injected, preferably into the upper joint compartment (see page 362). A long-acting preparation, methylprednisolone acetate (Depo-medrol), or a combination of betamethasone acetate and betamethasone disodium phosphate (Celestone) is preferred. The dosage of the specific drug is determined according to its individual clinical potency. An appropriate dosage of methylprednisolone is 20 mg in a 0.5 to 1.0 ml suspension, which corresponds to 3 mg of betamethasone (Haynes, 1975). A local anesthetic (0.5 ml) can be added to the steroid suspension to reduce the discomfort that may occur shortly after the injection. The concentration of the local anesthetic will be above the level for local soft tissue anesthesia for about an hour, although the palliative effect may be longer as a result of muscle relaxation (Kutscher, 1969).

If the desired therapeutic effect is not obtained, the reason might be periarticular injection or an incorrect diagnosis—that is, the condition was not of an intra-articular inflammatory nature. Nevertheless it is justifiable to repeat the injection once after four weeks if the effect was unsatisfactory; a third injection might be justified in severe cases (Wenneberg, 1978).

An interval of at least four weeks between corticosteroid injections and a maximum number of three injections in each joint have been recommended for small joints (Balch, 1977). A minimum interval of three months has also been suggested (Hunneyball, 1986). The diverging opinions are probably due to lack of knowledge of what really happens in the diseased human joint after steroid injections. The subjective and clinical short-term and long-term results for the TMJ are, however, often excellent after a series of three injections with one-week intervals (Kopp, 1981; Wenneberg, 1989). Clinical side effects of a severe nature are rare, although slight temporary stiffness or pain is reported by some patients.

It should be strongly emphasized that the patients receiving intra-articular TMJ steroid injections may also need a bite appliance or prosthetic treatment to reduce the biomechanical load on the joints and muscles created by bruxism or tooth loss, and physical exercises to revitalize the jaw musculature after the painful inflammatory process.

PROGNOSTIC FACTORS

The long-term prognosis of steroid treatment of TMJ arthritis is less favorable if severe radiographic signs of destruction of the TMJ and general joint symptoms are present (Kopp, 1981). Crepitus of the TMJ has also been found to be a negative factor in the treatment of degenerative and traumatic arthritis (Kopp, 1985). Generally the most pronounced effect is obtained in patients with severe clinical symptoms.

Sodium Hyaluronate

MODE OF ACTION

Sodium hyaluronate, which is prepared from natural high molecular weight HA, may be used as an anti-inflammatory drug. It is commonly referred to as hyaluronic acid, but at normal physiological pH the acid can occur only as a sodium salt, such as sodium hyaluronate. When dissolved in isotonic sodium chloride, the long HA molecules form random coils that become entangled with other HA molecules. At a concentration of 1 per cent its viscosity is almost 500,000 times greater than physiologic saline and at 10 per cent it becomes solid and can be formed into balls or sheets. HA is characterized by its high viscosity and elasticity. Clinical research suggests that high molecular weight and high concentration are important features

of HA with respect to its anti-inflammatory properties and its ability to enhance wound healing (Laurent, 1988).

The proposed mode of action of HA in arthritis is that it normalizes the biochemical conditions in the joint by replacing the low molecular weight HA of the inflamed joint by high molecular weight HA. It should thereby restore soft tissue lubrication, reduce friction and pain, improve joint mobility, restore the synovial barrier function (which inhibits invasion by leukocytes and enzymes), and restore the blood supply. More specific effects, both physiochemical and cell biological, are prevention of adhesions and enhancement of cellular migration during tissue repair by stimulating fibroblast proliferation. It also seems to reduce postoperative undesirable bone formation (Laurent, 1986). Intra-articularly administered HA disappears from the joint within 72 hours (Fraser, 1973), but it is reported that it stimulates the synthesis of endogenous HA by the fibroblasts of the synovial membrane of the joint (Åsheim, 1976; Smith, 1987). HA has not been shown to produce any permanent deleterious effects on joint tissues because it is a normal structural component of the connective tissue matrix (Falk, 1974).

DRUG

Hylartil is a preparation of natural high molecular weight HA produced by Pharmacia AB, (Uppsala, Sweden). It contains 1 per cent HA (10 mg/ml) dissolved in a phosphate buffer (pH 7–7.5) with added sodium chloride. It has an average molecular weight of 4.3×10^6.

CLINICAL STUDIES

Intra-articular injections of high molecular weight HA have been tried with encouraging results on patients with severe clinical signs of TMJ DJD not responding to conservative treatment (Kopp, 1979b). It had a therapeutic effect similar to that of glucocorticosteroid in this patient category (Kopp, 1985; 1987) (Fig. 22–9). Hyaluronate is therefore a therapeutic alternative to glucocorticosteroid in patients affected with TMJ inflammation caused by advanced DJD. Intra-articular administration of HA has also been tried in patients with symptomatic RA of the TMJ. In general it had less short-term effect on symptoms and signs than intra-articular glucocorticosteroid but had comparable effects if decreased intra-articular temperature was present in the injected joint. This suggests that HA has a special effect on joints with

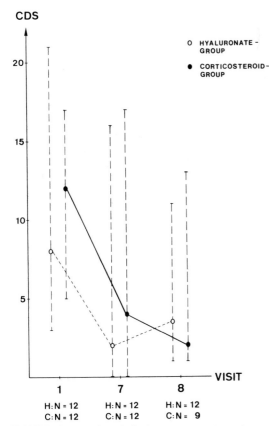

FIGURE 22–9. Clinical dysfunction sum (according to Helkimo, 1974) after hyaluronate (H) and corticosteroid (C) injections between visit 1 (pretreatment), visit 7 (one year after treatment), and visit 8 (two years after treatment). Group values expressed as median and range. (From Kopp, S., Carlsson, G. E., Haraldson, T., and Wenneberg, B.: Long-term effect of intra-articular injections of sodium hyaluronate and corticosteroid on temporomandibular joint arthritis. J. Oral Maxillofac. Surg. 45:929–935, 1987.)

decreased blood flow (Åkerman, 1989). Another interesting feature was that the abnormally low intra-articular temperature frequently was increased following HA injection. Intra-articular injections of HA also have been tried with promising results in human knee joints with DJD (Namiki, 1982; Peyron, 1974).

ANIMAL STUDIES

The therapeutic effect of HA has been ascribed to diminished granulation tissue formation and diminished formation of adhesions (Rydell, 1970), by reduction of synovitis and normalization of HA synthesis (Åsheim, 1976). High molecular weight HA was tried on experimental arthritis of knee joints of adult rabbits and was found to counteract reduction of water content of the articular cartilage (Wigren, 1978). A comparison of the effects of HA and glucocorticosteroid on papain-induced knee joint lesions in the guinea pig showed that HA had an inhibitory effect on the formation of granulation tissue and gross structural changes of the joints (Mejersjö, 1987).

INDICATIONS

HA and glucocorticosteroid administered by the intra-articular route have a similar long-term effect on chronic nonsystemic arthritis of the TMJ. Intra-articular HA might be the best alternative, however, due to the reduced risk of side effects. It is also beneficial for patients with advanced DJD for whom glucocorticosteroids seem to be less effective. The use of HA for chronic systemic arthritis, e.g., RA, must be investigated further.

ADMINISTRATION

HA in a concentration of 1 per cent can be injected intra-articularly with a 23-gauge needle. At least two injections with a two-week interval should be given for arthritis of the TMJ. Because HA acts by restoring the physiological environment in the joint, this preparation should be used as early as possible.

PROGNOSTIC FACTORS

Advanced age is a negative prognostic factor for the outcome of this treatment on nonsystemic monoarthritis (DJD, traumatic arthritis) of the TMJ (Kopp, 1985), which again emphasizes the importance of early treatment.

Physical Therapy

Background

Restricted mouth opening due to the painful synovitis and intra-articular effusion is a frequent finding associated with acute arthritis of the TMJ. Healing of traumatic arthritis and inflammatory joint disease involves a fibrin network created by the inflammatory process, and there is a risk for development of fibrous adhesions between the joint components (Fig. 22–10). Restricted mandibular mobility is a common finding also in chronic RA (Tegelberg, 1987a) and AS (Wenneberg, 1982), and is mainly due to restricted translation in the joint.

The jaw muscles are often affected by TMJ arthritis. They may develop tension due to the articular pain, as in DJD, or may be more directly involved by the inflammatory process as in RA. In painful chronic rheumatoid TMJ arthritis there is a decreased temperature on

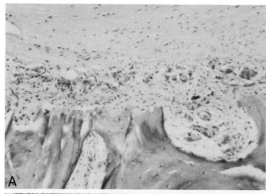

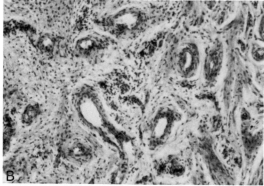

FIGURE 22–10. Photomicrograph of RA of the temporomandibular joint. *A,* Cell-rich, well-vascularized tissue (pannus) replacing the temporomandibular disc and resorbing the bone of the superior aspect of the condyle, causing adhesions between the articular surface. *B,* Close-up of the pannus.

the skin surface over the joint (Tegelberg, 1987b) as well as over the origin of the masseter muscle (Tegelberg, 1988a) that is most likely explained by a decreased muscular blood flow (Fig. 22–11). The intra-articular temperature is also frequently reduced at this stage which, like the decreased skin surface temperature, is associated with palpatory tenderness of the jaw muscles (Åkerman, 1988a). These findings show that the muscles play a substantial role in the symptoms of acute and especially chronic arthritis of the TMJ. The cause of the decreased temperature might be disuse atrophy of the muscles (Brooke, 1972; Isenberg, 1984), a sympathetic vasoconstrictive response due to pain (Engel, 1984; Schmitt, 1984; Uematsu, 1984), or increased muscular tension (Möller, 1979; 1981; Pochaczevsky, 1984). Muscular weakness and atrophy are early and prominent features in all stages of RA (Edström, 1974; Tiselius, 1969).

Irrespective of whether reduced mandibular mobility is caused by intra-articular restriction or by muscular dysfunction, physical exercises

are beneficial to prevent or lessen the formation of intra-articular adhesions and to increase the blood flow and strength of the jaw muscles. Physical therapy is therefore a valuable adjunct to other treatments in TMJ arthritis aimed at a more normal functional capability of the craniomandibular system.

Effect of Physical Therapy

The short-term effects of a self-administered physical training program on craniomandibular disorders in RA and AS have been compared with the effects of no treatment (Tegelberg, 1988b). All patients, including those not subjected to local physical training, reported reduced severity of symptoms at follow-up. Clinically, however, only those who performed physical exercises showed decreased dysfunction (Fig. 22–12). In patients with RA, the reduction in the degree of dysfunction was greatest among those with initial restriction in TMJ translatory mobility. They showed a significant increase in maximum voluntary mouth opening (Fig. 22–13). None of the patients reported an impaired condition at follow-up. In patients with AS, the reduction in clinical dys-

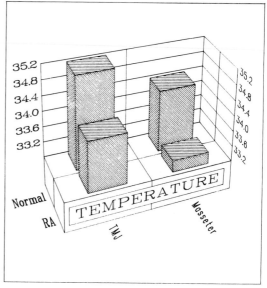

FIGURE 22–11. Distribution of skin surface temperature over the TMJ and masseter muscle in individuals with chronic rheumatoid arthritis (n = 71) and individuals without general joint symptoms (Normal; n = 52). (From Tegelberg, Å., and Kopp, S.: Skin surface temperature over the temporomandibular and metacarpophalangeal joints in individuals with rheumatoid arthritis. Acta Odontol. Scand. 45:329–336, 1987b; Tegelberg, Å., and Kopp, S.: Skin surface temperature over the masseter muscle in individuals with rheumatoid arthritis. Acta Odontol. Scand. 46:151–158, 1988a.)

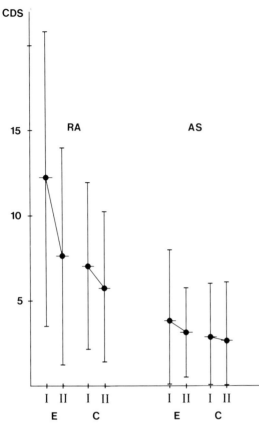

FIGURE 22–12. Mean clinical dysfunction score (CDS) (according to Helkimo, 1974) at two examinations (I, II) 3 weeks apart in patients with rheumatoid arthritis (RA) and ankylosing spondylitis (AS). Mean values are indicated by dots and ranges by vertical bars. (E = patients subjected to physical training, and C = control patients subjected to no treatment.) (From Tegelberg, Å., and Kopp, S.: Short-term effect of physical training on temporomandibular joint disorders in individuals with rheumatoid arthritis and ankylosing spondylitis. Acta Odontol. Scand. 46:49–56, 1988b.)

function was greatest among those with severe disease reflected by high values of the serum concentration of C-reactive protein and a high degree of craniomandibular disorder. Another interesting finding was that lack of occlusal support was a negative prognostic factor.

Indications

Physical therapy is indicated in all forms of arthritis of the TMJ (DJD, inflammatory joint disease, traumatic joint disease) when the acute inflammatory process has subsided, to mobilize the joint and prevent adhesions, and to establish normal muscle function and blood circulation, thereby restoring the bite force. Especially in chronic arthritides, continued exercises are val-

uable to maintain an acceptable function in the craniomandibular system.

Technique

The self-administered physical training program is a modification of exercises described earlier (Schwartz, 1959) and one that has evolved in many clinics throughout the world. The exercises (mouth opening, laterotrusion, and protrusion) are first performed without resistance (exercises 1 through 4 below) and then, if allowed with respect to pain or other discomfort, against resistance to recruit the highest possible number of muscular motor units (exercises 5 through 7 below). The last part of the program is especially indicated to restore mus-

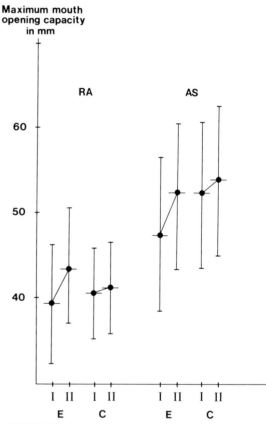

FIGURE 22–13. Mean maximum voluntary mouth opening capacity at two examinations (I, II) 3 weeks apart in patients with rheumatoid arthritis (RA) and ankylosing spondylitis (AS). Mean values are indicated by dots and ranges by vertical bars. (E = patients subjected to physical training, and C = control patients subjected to no treatment.) (From Tegelberg, Å, and Kopp, S.: Short-term effect of physical training on temporomandibular joint disorders in individuals with rheumatoid arthritis and ankylosing spondylitis. Acta Odontol. Scand. 46:49–56, 1988b.)

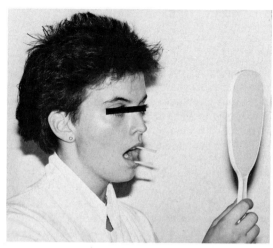

FIGURE 22–14. Physical exercise in front of a mirror. Toothpicks between the central incisors in the upper and lower jaw used to show deviations in movement.

cular strength in atrophied muscles. It is most important that the patient receives a thorough explanation and a practical demonstration of the exercise program. To ensure full cooperation, which is essential, the aims and goals of the treatment must also be explained. During the demonstration and while the patient is exercising, the use of a mirror is valuable to give feedback about the movements performed (Fig. 22–14). The physical therapy program is as follows:

1. Relax and lower your shoulders.
2. Let your lower jaw relax and say the "M" sound. Make sure that the teeth do not contact. Relax your tongue.
3. Make small, relaxed up and down and side to side movements without tooth contact to warm up the muscles.
4. Open and close your mouth as much as you can without pain or discomfort. Move your jaw as far as possible forward and then back again. Make similar movements toward both sides and then relax.
5. Make the same movements as in exercise 4 but against resistance with your hand, e.g., push your fist below the jaw during opening and push your thumb against your chin during forward movement and against the right and left side of your chin during side movements. Keep your jaw at the extreme point of movement for a few seconds.
6. Open your mouth as wide as possible, then try to close while you resist this movement by pushing downward against your lower front teeth with your fingers. Hold the jaw in this position for a few seconds.

7. Open your mouth as wide as you can, then stretch further by pushing your fingers against the front teeth of the upper and lower jaw. Relax.
8. While looking in the mirror, try to move your lower jaw straight up and down. Avoid deviations as well as movements that produce clicking or locking of the jaw.
9. End the exercise program by resting on your back for five to 10 minutes.

Each exercise should be performed about 10 times and the whole training program should be performed twice a day, unless otherwise prescribed. Movements that cause pain should be avoided. Application of heat locally over the TMJs and cheeks for not more than 10 to 15 minutes at a time often makes the exercises easier and more comfortable to perform due to increased elasticity of the tissues and increased local blood circulation.

It is important to evaluate the effects of the program at follow-up; to reinstruct and motivate, if necessary; and to check for improvement in symptoms and signs and maximum mandibular movement capacity.

Prognostic Factors

The prognosis is quite good when physical therapy is used in patients with TMJ arthritis. Persistent pain and locking, however, are factors that might reduce the applicability of jaw exercises. In advanced cases of TMJ arthritis with complete or partial ankylosis (e.g., in RA and psoriatic arthritis) hardly any improvement in mandibular mobility can be expected.

Occlusal Treatment

The loss of occlusal support has a negative effect on muscle and joint function as well as on the joint tissues proper. Muscular hyperfunction or occlusal trauma might be the primary cause of traumatic arthritis and DJD, while these factors might be detrimental and accelerate tissue destruction in the case of systemic inflammatory involvement of the TMJ. Patients with TMJ arthritis frequently respond better clinically to intra-articular injections of glucocorticosteroid than to occlusal treatment (occlusal appliances, occlusal grinding, and occlusal correction with complete dentures) (Kopp, 1981). The difference in treatment effect, however, is most pronounced in the young and middle-aged, and less pronounced in the elderly. The effect of glucocorticosteroid on clinical dysfunction seems to decline with age and the effectiveness of occlusal treatment increases. A partial explanation for this observation is that tooth loss produces a permanent unfavorable biomechanical condition in the joint. Clinically, the conclusions are that intra-articular treatment with glucocorticosteroid should be followed or preceded by occlusal rehabilitation to prevent overloading of the diseased joint and also that occlusal treatment alone might be the best choice of treatment in the elderly patient with nonsystemic arthritis of the TMJ and extensive loss of occlusal support. Lack of occlusal support may otherwise act as a chronic cause of TMJ arthritis leading to relapse of symptoms when the pharmacodynamic effect of the glucocorticosteroid has ceased.

SUMMARY

Noninfectious arthritis may involve the temporomandibular joint (TMJ) in systemic inflammatory joint disease (polyarthritis), local primary or secondary degenerative joint disease (osteoarthritis), or after facial trauma (traumatic arthritis). The basic structures of the TMJ are similar to those of other synovial joints and therefore subjected to the same disease processes. An inflammation in the synovial membrane of the TMJ affects the synovial fluid, the constituents of the articular fibrocartilage, and later the underlying bone. An early accurate diagnosis is important to make early effective treatment possible.

The nonsurgical treatment of TMJ arthritis aims at reducing the local inflammatory process, providing the best possible functional conditions for the joint and restoring satisfactory muscle function.

Nonsteroidal anti-inflammatory drugs can be used to reduce the inflammation and pain associated with TMJ arthritis by their inhibitory effect on prostaglandin production. They should be used preferably at an early stage, however, before any other measures are taken, and are not a long-term remedy for TMJ arthritis.

Intra-articular injections of the TMJ can be done safely provided that an appropriate technique is used. Glucocorticosteroids are the most well-documented anti-inflammatory drugs for intra-articular use. Their anti-inflammatory effect is mainly due to inhibition of prostaglandin production. They also have an effect on pannus formation by reducing proliferation of fibroblasts and ingrowth of capillaries. There are many synthetic glucocorticoids available with differing potency. They are indicated in patients with acute arthritis due to degenerative and inflammatory joint disease.

Sodium hyaluronate has been tried with promising results as an intra-articular anti-inflammatory agent. It restores the synovial barrier function, which inhibits invasion by leukocytes and enzymes. It also prevents formation of adhesions between joint surfaces. Because HA and glucocorticosteroid seem to have a similar long-term effect on nonsystemic chronic arthritis of the TMJ, HA is the better alternative due to reduced risk for side effects.

Physical therapy is an important adjunct in the treatment of TMJ arthritis because the jaw muscles are also frequently affected. Restricted mouth opening is a common finding in both acute and chronic arthritis and there is a risk for development of fibrous adhesions between the joint surfaces that might produce a permanent restriction of joint translation. Physical therapy is indicated in all forms of arthritis when the acute inflammatory process has subsided.

Loss of occlusal support has a negative influence on TMJ function and during arthritis the joint is especially vulnerable to overloading. Another factor of importance with respect to TMJ loading is bruxism (muscular hyperactivity). It should also be kept at a low level during arthritis. Occlusal appliances, occlusal adjustment, and prosthetic treatment can reduce these problems for a patient with chronic TMJ arthritis.

The choice of treatment for TMJ arthritis depends on many factors such as disease activity (acute or chronic), stage (early or late), and whether permanent joint damage already is present. The various treatments described can be used to permit most patients to function well in a relatively pain-free manner.

REFERENCES

Adams, S. S.: The mode of action of non-steroidal anti-inflammatory agents. In Olhagen, B., and Gullberg, R. (Eds.): Nordiskt Symposium. Kronisk Artrit. Nottingham, England, The Boots Company, LTD, 1977, pp. 129–136.

Åkerman, S., and Kopp, S.: Intra-articular and skin surface temperature of the temporomandibular joint in patients with rheumatoid arthritis. Acta Odontol. Scand. 46:41–48, 1988a.

Åkerman, S., Kopp, S., Nilner, M., et al.: Relationship between clinical and radiologic findings of the temporomandibular joint in rheumatoid arthritis. Oral Surg. Oral Med. Oral Pathol. 66:639–643, 1988b.

Åkerman, S., Kopp, S., and Nilner, M.: Short term trial of intra-articular sodium-hyaluronate, glucocorticoid and saline injections on rheumatoid arthritis of the temporomandibular joint. J. Craniomand. Disorders (in press.)

Åkerman, S., Kopp, S., and Rohlin, M.: Histological changes in temporomandibular joints from elderly individuals. An autopsy study. Acta Odontol. Scand. 44:231–239, 1986.

Asboe-Hansen, G.: Hormonal effects on connective tissue. Physiol. Rev. 38:446–462, 1958.

Asboe-Hansen, G.: The hormonal control of connective tissue. Int. Rev. Connect. Tissue Res. 1:29–61, 1963.

Åsheim, Å., and Lindblad, G.: Intra-articular treatment of arthritis in race horses with sodium-hyaluronate. Acta Vet. Scand. 17:379–394, 1976.

Balazs, E. A., Laurent, T. C., and Jeanloz, R. W.: Nomenclature of hyaluronic acid. Biochem. J. 235:903, 1986.

Balch, H. W., Gibson, J. M. C., El-Ghobarey, A. F., et al.: Repeated corticosteroid injections into knee joints. Rheumatology and Rehabilitation, 16:137–140, 1977.

Bird, H. A., Ring, E. F. J., and Bacon, P. A.: A thermographic and clinical comparison of three intra-articular steroid preparations in rheumatoid arthritis. Ann. Rheum. Dis. 38:36–39, 1979.

Brånemark, P-I., Goldie, I., and Lindström, J.: Observations on the action of intra-articularly administered prednisolone tertiary butyl acetate (Codelcortone TBA) and methylprednisolone acetate (Depomedrone) in the normal rabbit knee joint. Acta Orthop. Scand. 38:247–248, 1967.

Brooke, M. H., and Kaplan, H.: Muscle pathology in rheumatoid arthritis, polymyalgia rheumatica and polymyositis. Arch. Pathol. 94:101–118, 1972.

Carlsson, G. E., Kopp, S., and Öberg, T.: Arthritis and allied diseases. In Zarb, G. A., and Carlsson, G. E. (Eds.): Temporomandibular Joint. Function and Dysfunction. Copenhagen, Munksgaard, St. Louis, C. V. Mosby, 1979, pp. 269–320.

Dannenberg, A. M.: The anti-inflammatory effects of glucocorticosteroids—A brief review of the literature. Inflammation 3:329–343, 1979.

Edström, L., and Nordemar, R.: Differential changes in type I and type II muscle fibres in rheumatoid arthritis. Scand. J. Rheumatol. 3:155–160, 1974.

Engel, J. M.: Thermography in rheumatology. In Francis, E., Ring, J., and Philips, B. (Eds.): Recent Advances in Medical Thermology. New York, Plenum Press, 1984, pp. 425–427.

Falk, J.: Repeated injections of sodium-hyaluronate into the knee joints of dogs. Internal Report, Pharmacia AB, Sweden. Report L 287 C 8, 1974.

Franks, A. S. T.: Temporomandibular joint in adult rheumatoid arthritis. A comparative evaluation of 100 cases. Ann. Rheum. Dis. 28:139–145, 1969.

Fraser, J. R. E., Antonas, K. N., and Muirden, K. D.: Distribution of biologically labelled radioactive hyaluronic acid injected into joints. Ann. Rheum. Dis. 32:103–111, 1973.

Granström, G., and Linde, A.: Glycosaminoglycans of temporomandibular articular discs. Scand. J. Dent. Res. 81:461–466, 1973.

Habuchi, H., Ymagata, T., Iwata, H., and Suzuki, S.: The occurrence of a wide variety of dermatan sulfate-chondroitin sulfate copolymers in fibrous cartilage. J. Biol. Chem. 248:6019–6028, 1973.

Hansson, T., and Öberg, T.: Arthrosis and deviation in form in the temporomandibular joint. A macroscopic study on a human autopsy material. Acta Odontol. Scand. 35:167–174, 1977.

Hascall, V. C., and Heinegård, D.: Aggregation of cartilage proteoglycans. I. The role of hyaluronic acid. J. Biol. Chem. 249:4232–4241, 1974.

Haynes, R., and Larner, J.: Adrenocorticotrophic hormone; adrenocortical steroids and their synthetic analogs; inhibitors of adrenocortical steroid biosynthesis. In Goodman, L. S., and Gilman, A. (Eds.): The Pharmacological Basis of Therapeutics. New York, Macmillan, 1975, p. 1472.

Helkimo, M.: Studies on function and dysfunction of the masticatory system. II. Index for anamnestic and clinical dysfunction and occlusal state. Swed. Dent. J. 67:101–121, 1974.

Hollander, J. L.: Arthritis and Allied Conditions, 7th ed. Philadelphia, Lea & Febiger, 1969, pp. 381–398, 889–890, 935–936.

Hunneyball, I. M.: Intra-articular administration of drugs. Pharmacy International 5:118–122, 1986.

Isenberg, D.: Myositis in other connective tissue disorders. Clin. Rheum. Dis. 10:156–157, 1984.

Kalbhen, D. A., Schauer, M., and Wentsche, B.: Tierexperimentelle Untersuchungen uber den Einfluss intraartikulär applizierter Antiphlogistika auf den Gelenkknorpel in vivo. Z. Rheumatol. 37:380–394, 1978.

Kempson, G. E., Muir, H., Swanson, S. A. V., and Freeman, M. A. R.: Correlations between stiffness and the chemical constituents of cartilage on the human femoral head. Biochem. et Biophys. Acta 215:70–77, 1970.

Kopp, S.: Topographical distribution of sulphated glycosaminoglycans in human temporomandibular joint disks— A histochemical study of an autopsy material. J. Oral Pathol. 5:265–276, 1976.

Kopp, S.: Topographical distribution of sulphated glycosaminoglycans in the surface layers of the human temporomandibular joint. A histochemical study of an autopsy material. J. Oral Pathol. 7:283–294, 1978.

Kopp, S., Carlsson, G. E., Haraldson, T., and Wenneberg, B.: Long-term effect of intra-articular injections of sodium hyaluronate and corticosteroid on temporomandibular joint arthritis. J. Oral Maxillofac. Surg. 45:929–935, 1987.

Kopp, S., and Haraldson, T.: Skin surface temperature over the temporomandibular joint and masseter muscle in patients with craniomandibular disorder. Swed. Dent. J. 12:63–67, 1988.

Kopp, S., and Rockler, B.: Relationship between clinical and radiographic findings in patients with mandibular pain-dysfunction. Acta Radiol. 20:465–477, 1979a.

Kopp, S., and Rockler, B.: Relationship between radiographic signs in the temporomandibular joint and hand joints. Acta Odontol. Scand. 37:169–175, 1979b.

Kopp, S., and Wenneberg, B.: Injection of Healonid in the temporomandibular joint—A preliminary report. Report Series, Department of Stomatognathic Physiology, Göteborg University. Nov. 22, 1979c.

Kopp, S., and Wenneberg, B.: Effects of occlusal treatment and intraarticular injections on temporomandibular joint pain and dysfunction. Acta Odontol. Scand. 39:87–96, 1981.

Kopp, S., Wenneberg, B., and Clemensson, E.: Clinical, microscopical and biochemical investigation of synovial fluid from temporomandibular joints. Scand. J. Dent. Res. 91:33–41, 1983.

Kopp, S., Wenneberg, B., Haraldson, R., and Carlsson, G. E.: Short-term effect of intra-articular injections of sodium hyaluronate and corticosteroid on temporomandibular joint pain and dysfunction. J. Oral Maxillofac. Surg. 43:429–435, 1985.

Kutscher, A., Zegarelli, E., and Lamont-Havers, R.: Pharmacologic methods. In Schwartz, L., and Chayes, C.M. (Eds.): Facial Pain and Mandibular Dysfunction. Philadelphia, W. B. Saunders, 1969, pp. 315–317.

Laurent, C., Hellström, S., and Stenfors, L-E.: Hyaluronic acid reduces connective tissue formation in middle ears filled with absorbable gelatin sponge: An experimental study. Am. J. Otolaryngol. 7:181–186, 1986.

Laurent, C., Hellström, S., and Fellenius, E.: Hyaluronan improves the healing of experimental tympanic membrane perforations—A comparison of preparations with different rheological properties. Arch. Otolaryngol. 114:1435–1441, 1988.

Mejersjö, C., and Kopp, S.: Effect of corticosteroid and sodium hyaluronate on induced joint lesions in the guinea-pig knee. Int. J. Oral Maxillofac. Surg. 16:194–201, 1987.

Möller, E.: The myogenic factor in headache and facial pain. In Kawamura, Y., and Dubner, R. (Eds.): Oral-facial Sensory and Motor Functions. Chicago, Quintessence, 1981, pp. 225–239.

Möller, E., Collin-Rasmussen, O., and Bonde-Petersen, F.: Mechanism of ischemic pain in human muscles of mastication. Intra-muscular pressure, EMG, force and blood flow of the temporal and masseter muscles during biting. Adv. Pain Res. Ther. 3:271–281, 1979.

Moscatelli, D., and Rubin, H.: Hormonal control of hyaluronic acid production in fibroblasts and its relation to nucleic acid and protein synthesis. J. Cell Physiol. 91:79–88, 1977.

Namiki, O., Toyoshima, H., and Morisaki, N.: Therapeutic effect of intra-articular injection of high molecular weight hyaluronic acid on osteoarthritis of the knee. Int. J. Clin. Pharmacol. Ther. Toxicol. 20:501–507, 1982.

Olah, E. H., and Kostenszky, K. S.: Effect of loading and prednisolone treatment on the glycosaminoglycans content of articular cartilage in dogs. Scand. J. Rheumatol. 5:49–52, 1976.

Peyron, J. G., and Balazs, E. A.: Preliminary clinical assessment of Na-hyaluronate injection into human arthritic joints. Pathol. Biol. 22:731–736, 1974.

Pochaczevsky, R., Wexler, C. E., Meyers, P. H., et al.: Liquid crystal thermography of the spine and extremities—Its value in the diagnosis of spinal root syndrome. In Francis, E., Ring, J., and Philips, B. (Eds.): Recent Advances in Medical Thermology. New York, Plenum Press, 1984, pp. 493–501.

Poswillo, D.: Experimental investigation of the effects of intra-articular hydrocortisone and high condylectomy on the mandibular condyle. Oral Surg. 30:161–173, 1970.

Pratt, W. B.: The mechanism of glucocorticoid effects in fibroblasts. J. Invest. Dermatol. 71:24–35, 1978.

Rydell, N.: Decreased granulation tissue reaction after installment of hyaluronic acid. Acta Orthop. Scand. 41:307–311, 1970.

Saxne, T., Heinegård, D., and Wollheim, F. A.: Proteoglycans in synovial fluid: The effect of intra-articular corticosteroid injections. Br. J. Rheumatol. 24:221, 1985.

Saxne, T., Heinegård, D., and Wollheim, F. A.: Therapeutic effects on cartilage metabolism in arthritis as measured by release of proteoglycan structures into the synovial fluid. Ann. Rheum. Dis. 45:491–497, 1986.

Schmitt, M., and Guillot, M.: Thermography and muscular injuries in sports medicine. In Francis, E., Ring, J., and Philips, B. (Eds.): Recent Advances in Medical Thermology. New York, Plenum Press, 1984, pp. 439–445.

Schwartz, L.: Disorders of the Temporomandibular Joint. Philadelphia, W. B. Saunders, 1959, pp. 223–231.

Shaw, N. E., and Lacey, E.: The influence of corticosteroids on normal and papain-treated articular cartilage in the rabbit. J. Bone Joint Surg. 55B:197–205, 1973.

Smith, M. M., and Ghosh, P.: The synthesis of hyaluronic acid by human synovial fibroblasts is influenced by the nature of the hyaluronate in the extracellular environment. Rheumatol. Int. 7:113–122, 1987.

Tegelberg, Å., and Kopp, S.: Clinical findings in the stomatognathic system in individuals with rheumatoid arthritis and osteoarthrosis. Acta Odontol. Scand. 45:65–75, 1987a.

Tegelberg, Å., and Kopp, S.: Skin surface temperature over the temporomandibular and metacarpophalangeal joints in individuals with rheumatoid arthritis. Acta Odontol. Scand. 45:329–336, 1987b.

Tegelberg, Å., and Kopp, S.: Short-term effect of physical training on temporomandibular joint disorders in individuals with rheumatoid arthritis and ankylosing spondylitis. Acta Odontol. Scand. 46:49–56, 1988b.

Tegelberg, Å., and Kopp, S.: Skin surface temperature over the masseter muscle in individuals with rheumatoid arthritis. Acta Odontol. Scand. 46:151–158, 1988a.

Tiselius, P.: Studies on joint temperature, joint stiffness and muscle weakness in rheumatoid arthritis—An experimental and clinical investigation. Thesis. University of Uppsala, 1969.

Toller, P.: Non-surgical treatment of dysfunctions of the temporomandibular joint. Oral Sci. Rev. 7:70–85, 1976.

Uematsu, S.: Telethermography in the diagnosis of reflex sympathetic dystrophy. In Francis, E., Ring, J., and Philips, B. (Eds.): Recent Advances in Medical Thermology. New York, Plenum Press, 1984, pp. 379–395.

Wenneberg, B., Hollender, L., and Kopp, S.: Radiographic changes in the temporomandibular joint in ankylosing spondylitis. Dentomaxillofac. Radiol. 12:25–30, 1983.

Wenneberg, B., and Kopp, S.: Short term effect of intra-articular injections of a corticosteroid on temporomandibular joint pain and dysfunction. Swed. Dent. J. 2:189–196, 1978.

Wenneberg, B., and Kopp, S.: Clinical findings in the stomatognathic system in ankylosing spondylitis. Scand. J. Dent. Res. 90:373–381, 1982.

Wenneberg, B., Kopp, S., and Gröndahl, H-G.: Long term effect of intra-articular injections of glucocorticoids into the temporomandibular joint. A clinical and radiographic 8 year follow-up. Journal of Craniomandibular Disorders: Facial & Oral Pain (in press).

Wigren, A., Falk, J., and Wik, O.: The healing of cartilage injuries under the influence of joint immobilization and repeated hyaluronic acid injections—An experimental study. Acta Orthop. Scand. 49:121–133, 1978.

Zacco, M., Richardson, E. M., Crittenden, I. O., et al.: Disposition of intra-articularly injected hydrocortisone acetate, hydrocortisone and cortisone acetate in arthritis. J. Clin. Endocrinol. 14:711–718, 1954.

DIAGNOSIS AND NONSURGICAL TREATMENT OF INTERNAL DERANGEMENTS*

GLENN T. CLARK, D.D.S., M.S., and ROBERT L. MERRILL, D.D.S.

INTRODUCTION

The term internal derangement implies an anatomic disturbance in the relationship of the components of the disc-condyle complex with consequent changes in the smooth movement of the joint such as clicking, popping, momentary catching, or locking, with or without associated pain and muscular disturbance (Anderson, 1989; Annandale, 1887; Blaschke, 1980b; Carlsson, 1985; Clark, 1987; 1989a; Greene, 1988; Hasso, 1989; Helkimo, 1987; Katzberg, 1980; Lewis, 1987; Lundh, 1987; Magnusson, 1986; Norgaard, 1944; Petersen, 1987a; Pullinger, 1989; Solberg, 1986b; Stegenga, 1989; Wabeke, 1989; Wanman, 1986). It also broadly describes a subgroup of temporomandibular joint (TMJ) disorders that can be differentiated into the following three related problems with clinically distinguishable features: (1) disc-condyle incoordination, (2) restricted translation of the condyle, and (3) condyle subluxation or dislocation (Agerberg, 1974; Carlsson, 1985; Clark, 1987; 1989a; Pullinger, 1988a; 1988b; Seligman, 1988b; Solberg, 1986d). This chapter will focus on the diagnosis and nonsurgical treatment of these conditions.

DIAGNOSIS OF INTERNAL DERANGEMENT

Disc-Condyle Incoordination

Disc-condyle incoordination is manifested clinically as a brief interference with the jaw opening movement that usually has an associated distinct joint sound or click. If the inter-

*See Chapters 5, 6, 8, 9, 16–21, 24, and 25.

ference with movement is severe, the patient may describe the problem as a momentary or intermittent locking of the jaw joint. The proposed anatomic mechanisms that produce this joint movement disturbance are (1) an articular surface abnormality, such as flattening with subsequent disc deformation, (2) displacement of the disc from its ideal relationship with the condyle, (3) disc-articular surface adherence and adhesions, and (4) disc perforation (Anderson, 1989; Bell, 1982; Clark, 1989a; Dolwick, 1983; Farrar, 1978; 1979; Lundh, 1987; McCarty, 1980).

Some combination of these disc and articular surface abnormalities leads to a momentary increased friction or a jamming between the disc and the articulating surfaces of the joint. Although this momentary impedance in movement usually results in a clicking or popping sound when it releases, the disc-condyle incoordination may simply manifest itself as a brief, lateral shift in jaw movement rather than as a joint sound (Clark, 1984a; 1988; Greene, 1988; Lundh, 1987; Wabeke, 1989).

Achievement of full condylar translation after the click implies either a release or a reduction of the jammed disc. This allows the disc to continue its normal rotational movement around the condyle during opening. During closure the disc will return to its original starting position relative to the condyle, usually after producing a less noticeable reciprocal or closing click just before full intercuspation (Lundh, 1987). In some patients the opening movement produces a less noticeable click while the closing movement produces a severe jamming and loud click.

To confirm that there is a disc-condyle incoordination, the TMJs are palpated bilaterally with very light pressure while the patient opens the mouth widely and closes several times. Any significant joint movement interference (especially if sound is produced) will be palpable. To document the problem, the timing of the joint movement interference relative to the degree of mouth opening is measured with a millimeter ruler. Many varied patterns of disc-condyle interference exist. Unfortunately, based on these various patterns of joint sound or movement interference, no definitive statement can be made regarding the severity, prognosis, or even the specific nature of the anatomic deformity.

Restricted Translation of the Condyle

Restricted translation of the condyle is sometimes described as closed locking, but more accurately it is defined as a restricted translation or partial hypomobility of the condyle (Clark, 1988; Farrar, 1983; Katzberg, 1980; McCarty, 1980; Nielsen, 1989; Pedersen, 1987b; Solberg, 1986b; Wilkes, 1978). The mechanism of this condylar movement restriction is thought to be either condyle or disc deformation, disc-articular surface adhesion, disc displacement, or disc perforation. If the disc does not fully rotate from an anterior to a posterior position relative to the condyle during mandibular movement, a clear restriction of mouth opening will result. To confirm that a true condylar restriction exists, maximum active mouth opening is measured with a millimeter ruler. Confirmation can also be obtained by palpating the lateral pole of the condyle during opening. Movement anterior to the crest of the articular eminence will not be felt if a restriction exists. Finally, a passive stretch manipulation of the jaw by the examiner will not produce normal opening.

When associated pain occurs, it often results secondarily from a protective jaw closing muscle trismus (splinting) response (Clark, 1984c). This trismus response is an attempt to prevent either pinching or stretching of the disc tissue, or impingement on the vascular, highly innervated disc attachment tissues that are sometimes drawn into an area of articular loading. The latter is also a frequent source of pain. Of course, the pain could also be from a primary masticatory muscle disorder or any number of other orofacial pain conditions (see Chapters 8, 21, and 25).

Because full, friction-free movement of the disc does not occur, this condition can eventually lead to either a perforation of the disc or retrodiscal tissue or, more likely, to fibrosis of the disc-attachment tissues. In either case, there is usually a subsequent osseous remodeling (flattening) of the condyle and articular eminence (see Chapter 6) (Axelsson, 1987; Carlsson, 1979; Hansson, 1977; Moffett, 1964; Solberg, 1986c). These changes are essentially adaptive attempts to restore increased movement in a highly frictional joint. The incoordination phase, and even the restriction phase of an internal derangement, are usually not accompanied by obvious radiographic osseous change during the first six months.

Condylar Subluxation or Dislocation

Subluxation occurs when the mouth is in an open position and there is a momentary inability to close the mouth. Dislocation is a long-lasting inability to close the mouth. The cause may be due to either (1) jamming of the disc-condyle complex in a position anterior to the crest of the articular eminence; (2) a true hyperextension of the disc-condyle complex well beyond its normal maximum translation, with resultant muscle trismus; or (3) a disc rotation problem that prevents closing of the mouth. In the case of a disc rotation problem, the disc has difficulty returning to its usual more anterior position relative to the condyle. A subluxation is self-reducing by the patient; a dislocation requires manual manipulation of the mandible by the doctor to achieve reduction.

Subluxation of the condyle may be the initial feature of TMJ symptoms in some patients. The onset is often associated with excessively wide yawning. Precipitation of a transient subluxation also is not uncommon after extended mouth opening in a dentist's office. In the absence of pain, infrequent momentary subluxation or dislocation upon wide opening is not a serious clinical problem for most patients. Differential diagnosis of a true condylar hyperextension versus a disc-condyle rotation or jamming problem requires actual examination of the jaw position during the event. Measurement of mouth opening, palpation of the position of the condyles relative to the articular eminences, and radiographic examination and MRI of the TMJs in the open-mouth position will usually distinguish between these problems.

ETIOLOGY OF INTERNAL DERANGEMENTS

In common with general orthopedic problems, the etiology of internal derangements is often multifactorial and difficult to determine. Nevertheless, the four major causes that are most likely to be involved are macrotrauma, microtrauma, arthritic disease, and abnormal biomechanical loading.

Macrotrauma

Macrotrauma to the temporomandibular apparatus can occur from either impact or overstretching (Clark, 1987; Pullinger, 1987; 1985; Zarb, 1979). The predominant causes are blows to the jaw, iatrogenic stretching during dental and surgical treatment, or an impact to the jaw sustained during a motor vehicle accident. These conditions produce bruising or joint tissue lacerations with resultant inflammation. This can lead to impaired function, altered articular surfaces, and eventually to an internal derangement and osteoarthritis. Patients who

report to a TMJ and facial pain clinic are more likely to have a history of major trauma (30 per cent) than a nonpatient population of individuals with varying observed TMJ symptoms (13 per cent) (Christiansen, 1987; Pullinger, 1985; 1989; Weinberg, 1987).

Microtrauma

Microtrauma to the temporomandibular articulation can occur from repetitive behaviors such as tooth grinding (bruxism), chronic clenching, or atypical chewing habits such as chronic gum chewing. These behaviors can be highly injurious and produce painful TMJ and masticatory muscle disorders (Carlsson, 1979; Clark, 1981; Good, 1982; Helkimo, 1987; Lund, 1989; Ogus, 1979; Rugh, 1984; Seligman, 1988a; Stegenga, 1989; Zarb, 1979). Repetitive overloading of joint tissues causes deformative and degenerative changes to occur in the disc, flattening the anterior or more commonly the posterior bands, and predisposing to disc displacement.

Arthritis

Arthritis in its degenerative and inflammatory forms is a factor in many patients. Rapid arthritic breakdown of the TMJ structures produces painful articular symptoms as well as secondary masticatory muscle symptoms (Akerman, 1988a; 1988b; Axelsson, 1987; Carlsson, 1979; Clark, 1987; Good, 1982; Kononen, 1987; Larheim, 1982; Marbach, 1979; Murakami, 1984; Ogus, 1979; Tegelberg, 1987a; 1987b; Toller, 1973). As a result of the tissue-synovial fluid changes and erosion of the articulating surfaces, the articulating parts no longer slide smoothly over each other during translatory movements, which leads to momentary sticking or catching of the disc. The sticking events, during closure, encourage disc-condyle incoordination as the condyle rides over the posterior rim of the immobile disc.

Abnormal Biomechanical Loading

Abnormal biomechanical loading of the TMJ can occur any time the dental-occlusal structures develop abnormally or undergo deterioration as a result of tooth or tooth structure loss, or are inadvertently forced into an abnormal relationship due to dental occlusal therapy (Carlsson, 1979; Clark, 1987; Ogus, 1979; Radin, 1972; Stegenga, 1989). Abnormal loading in the TMJ encourages disc sticking as the forces cause the synovial secretions to be expressed from the functional areas of the joint. With decreased lubrication of the areas subject to the most stress, the disc can act like a suction cup, sticking to or hesitating on the articular eminence, bringing about an internal derangement.

DIAGNOSTIC TESTS

Even though internal derangements involve specific pathologic conditions, identifying the probable etiology of the problem is not always straightforward. This is especially true for intracapsular condyle restrictions that are easily mimicked by jaw muscle pain and stiffness problems.

Factors such as the onset, duration, character, and location of the jaw dysfunction, and their relationship to pain in the region, are important in the diagnostic process. When taken into consideration along with physical signs such as joint noises, abnormal jaw movement patterns and restrictions, and the results of the passive stretch and joint manipulation tests when indicated, they are of greater clinical significance than any other diagnostic modalities, including radiographs, in establishing a differential diagnosis (Anderson, 1989; Clark, 1987; 1989a; Dolwick, 1983; McCarty, 1980; Mejersjo, 1987; Pullinger, 1987; Solberg, 1986a). These factors are currently best determined and documented by a thorough history and clinical examination. Additional diagnostic tests should only be ordered if they will either confirm or rule out specific recognized pathologic entities suspected from the clinical findings. Furthermore, these tests should only be requested when they will definitely influence the diagnostic, prognostic, or treatment decision process.

Passive Stretch and Joint Manipulation Tests

The differentiation between a muscular cause of limited jaw movement and a true intracapsular restriction may require two diagnostic tests, passive stretch and joint manipulation. The passive stretch test is performed by first spraying the masseter and temporalis muscles with a vapocoolant spray (usually fluoromethane) to help transiently block the protective muscle trismus response that prevents opening (see Chapter 21). The examiner then immediately attempts to increase mouth opening by applying a mild force between the maxillary and mandibular teeth with the fingers (see Fig.

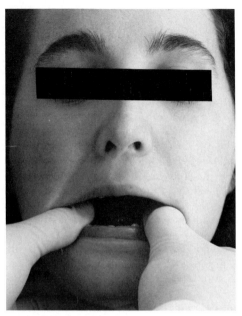

FIGURE 23–1. Joint manipulation involves the manual inferior distraction of the condyle, followed by a mildly forced, slow translation of the restricted condyle in a forward and medial direction.

21–3). If a muscular induced limitation is present, mouth opening will increase to a relatively normal distance (Solberg, 1986a).

If the passive stretch test fails to yield full translation of a restricted joint, the next test involves joint manipulation. This manipulation is most successful in patients with acute (less than two weeks) restriction who have a previous history of disc-condyle incoordination. The test first involves the manual inferior distraction of the condyle, followed by a mildly forced, slow translation of the restricted condyle in a forward and medial direction (Schwartz, 1966b; Solberg, 1986a; Zarb, 1979) (Fig. 23–1). This is followed by a slow seating of the condyle/disc complex in the glenoid fossa. Prior to the manipulation, some clinicians will infuse about 0.5 to 1 ml of a 1 per cent solution of lidocaine without epinephrine into the superior joint space and relax the jaw muscles with hot packs. If this maneuver is successful, the condyle will be reseated into the displaced disc and normal translation will be reestablished.

Radiographs

Except when associated with osteoarthritis, patients with TMJ internal derangements are usually free of overt radiographic signs. As previously mentioned, radiographs should be made only when indicated by the clinical examination. Clinical signs such as severe joint tenderness, repeatable joint noises, crepitation, or a progressive deterioration of TMJ movement indicate a need for radiographs of the TMJ (see Chapter 16). These radiographs might include a panoramic view of the jaws, transcranial TMJ films, tomograms, computerized tomography (CT), or arthrographic films (Katzberg, 1980; Oberg, 1980; Pullinger, 1986) (see Chapter 16). When available, axially corrected lateral tomographic projections are preferred over transcranial projections for imaging the bony structures of the TMJ. While CT scans have merit, at this time they are not superior to the conventional tomographic radiography techniques for hard tissue imaging of the TMJ structures and are inferior to magnetic resonance imaging (MRI) or arthrography for soft tissue imaging.

Arthrography, which is accomplished by injecting a radiopaque contrast medium in the joint compartments prior to fluoroscopic examination and the taking of radiographs, provides visualization of the disc profile and can reliably evaluate the dynamic function of the disc (Anderson, 1989; Bibb, 1989; Blaschke, 1980a; 1980b; Lewis, 1987; Schellhas, 1988).

Magnetic Resonance Imaging

Magnetic resonance imaging (MRI) is rapidly becoming the technique of choice for visualizing the intra-articular soft tissues because it is not invasive, does not involve ionizing radiation, and does not cause distortion of the intra-articular structures as occurs with arthrography (see Chapter 16). This procedure has essentially replaced the invasive arthrographic disc imaging procedure. Arthrography was previously the only way to view dynamically the disc during movement, but now multiple MRI images at different jaw openings can be linked to give a more dynamic view of TMJ and disc function (Hasso, 1989; Schellhas, 1988; 1989; Westesson, 1987).

Diagnostic Arthroscopy

Another new diagnostic technique is direct visualization of the joint with an arthroscope. Several excellent investigations have been made in testing the diagnostic value of this technique (McCain, 1989; Murakami, 1989). Another advantage of arthroscopy for TMJ derangements is its therapeutic use (Clark, 1989b). Arthroscopic surgery is being used for separation of persistent disc-articular surface adherence, and lysis and lavage of fibrotic adhesions in the

treatment of TMJ movement restrictions (see Chapter 17).

Anesthetic Nerve Blocks

Anesthetic nerve blocks with lidocaine (no epinephrine) is a standard and underutilized procedure that has value in the differentiation of pain sources (Bell, 1982; Phero, 1987; Schwartz, 1966a; Zarb, 1979).

Comprehensive Medical and Psychologic Evaluations

Some patients may need more comprehensive medical and psychologic evaluations and should be referred to the appropriate specialists for these evaluations (see Chapter 20).

Additional Documentation Procedures

Optoelectric or magnetic jaw tracking procedures, joint sound recording procedures, and even electromyographic recordings of the jaw muscle contraction patterns associated with mandibular movement have been used in an attempt to provide additional documentation of the patient's condition. These procedures, however, do not have a recognized diagnostic value above and beyond information that can be gathered during a clinical examination and are not to be considered as the standard of practice (Balciunas, 1987; Ciancaglini, 1987; Dao, 1988; Greene, 1990; Lund, 1989; Widmer, 1990).

TREATMENT OF INTERNAL DERANGEMENTS

Anti-inflammatory Therapy

If the patient exhibits joint pain (arthralgia) to any significant degree, a course of nonsteroidal anti-inflammatory drug therapy is appropriate (Marbach, 1980). In addition, there should be voluntary limitation of jaw movement, the elimination of all hard or chewy foods from the diet, and the application of a small ice pack on the involved joint several times a day for not more than 20 minutes at a time if there is obvious swelling. If the temporalis and masseter muscles are tight and tender to palpation, the application of moist heat three or more times a day for not more than 20 minutes is also recommended (Carlsson, 1979; 1985; Clark, 1987; Farrar, 1983; Kopp, 1985; 1987; Mejersjo, 1987; Solberg, 1986c; Toller, 1973).

There is usually a reduction of joint inflammation and pain after two to three weeks of anti-inflammatory treatment. If patients experience relief from pain and have a reasonably stable occlusal relationship (multiple bilateral posterior tooth contacts), a series of jaw movement exercises can be recommended for remobilization of the jaw joint (see Chapter 21). If the occlusion is unstable, occlusal appliance therapy may be necessary to keep the joint from excessive loading during function. These cases may eventually require occlusal therapy (orthodontics, prosthetics, or occlusal adjustment) to provide a reasonably stable posterior occlusion. However, definitive evaluation of the occlusion during the acute phase should not be done because the intracapsular swelling may cause a dramatic occlusal change, which will return to normal only after the inflammation subsides.

Occlusal Appliance Therapy

For patients with any type of internal derangement, those who exhibit evidence of dental attrition suggestive of bruxism, or those who give a history of chronic clenching, occlusal appliance therapy should be considered. There are two basic approaches to occlusal appliance therapy for the treatment of internal derangements. If the patient has a tender, painful, or inflamed joint due to bruxism, a full arch occlusal stabilization appliance is the treatment of choice (Agerberg, 1974; Clark, 1984b; 1984c; Diamond, 1987; Dolwick, 1983; McCarty, 1980; Monteiro, 1988). This appliance has a flat occlusal surface, which is adjusted to have multiple tooth contacts in an habitual, comfortable jaw closure position. The appliance should be worn at all times, except when the patient eats, for the first six to eight weeks, while being adjusted several times to establish a comfortable jaw position.

The purpose of the appliance is not to discover a new therapeutic jaw position or to recapture the disc, but to serve as a behavioral feedback device that makes the patient conscious of any oral parafunction. The patient must, therefore, be instructed not to bring the teeth together on the appliance while it is worn. After the patient experiences relief of the symptoms, the amount of daytime wear of the appliance should be reduced. Continued use of the appliance at night is indicated only if there is evidence of ongoing wear of its occlusal surface indicating a strong, continuing clenching or bruxing habit.

If the patient has symptoms of a significant, painful TMJ internal derangement of the incoordination type (clicking), use of a mandibular anterior repositioning appliance is a treatment option (Clark, 1984a; 1986; 1988) Diamond, 1987; Okeson, 1988; Solberg, 1986b). The purpose of this appliance is similar to the stabilization appliance in that it serves as a good behavioral modification device to alter oral habits. Additionally, it assists the patient with avoidance of the disc-condyle incoordination. It should not be used, however, to re-align or reposition the jaw permanently. The appliance is similar to the flat plane stabilization appliance with, however, a significant difference in the occlusal surface. Fossae in the appliance surface guide the condyle into a predetermined anterior position that has been found, by trial, to eliminate the clicking (Fig. 23–2). As the mandible is anteriorly positioned, with the condyle slightly forward on the eminence, the posterior teeth will not be touching if this position is maintained with the splint removed. This type of appliance is used only if a small anterior positional change in the mandible stops the clicking during repeated mouth opening and closing.

Once inserted, this appliance will need constant monitoring to make sure the altered jaw position keeps the disc-condyle incoordination event from occurring when it is in place. It is suggested that the repositioning appliance be worn for 24 hours a day for at least eight to 10 weeks, except that it should always be removed while eating. Removal of the appliance to eat is important because this will ensure that the patient does not have a permanent occlusal position change. The patient should eat only soft, nonchewy foods. Eventually, after the clin-

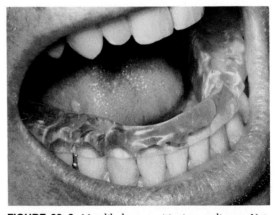

FIGURE 23–2. Mandibular repositioning appliance. Note the fossae in the occlusal surface of the appliance that guide the mandible into a forward position recapturing the dislocated disc and eliminating the click.

ical symptoms have lessened, the patient should decrease the amount of time the appliance is used during the day. Even though the jaw joint may still catch or click to some extent when the appliance is out, most patients can avoid this by eating soft foods and limiting their mouth opening.

Use of the repositioning appliance has been unsuccessful at stopping joint sounds over a long period of time in a large percentage of patients (Clark, 1984a). The goal of the part-time repositioning appliance procedure is not to stop the sounds but merely to reduce the frequency of the sounds and the pain associated with the joint incoordination. If successful, the patient should have a decreased tendency for the TMJ to lock and the painful articular and muscular aspects of the disc-condyle incoordination should dissipate.

Limited Function Protocol

The patient may not be expected to function normally again if (1) the anti-inflammatory therapy does not successfully resolve the inflammation because of chronic bruxism or because a polyarthritic inflammatory joint condition exists, (2) the occlusal repositioning appliance is unsuccessful at resolving the disc-condyle incoordination and the patient declines the arthroscopic or disc repair surgery, or (3) there are chronic osteoarthritic joint changes. If any of these situations are present, a discussion with the patient about expected limitations with regard to jaw function is in order. These recommendations include (1) placing the patient on a periodic recall for monitoring of further joint and/or occlusal changes, (2) advising the patient about continued exercises and occlusal appliance use at night to slow down any degenerative processes, (3) prescribing an anti-inflammatory non-narcotic analgesic agent to be taken as needed, (4) consultation with a rheumatologist as needed, (5) explanation of necessary dietary limitations, and (6) explanation of the possible long-term occlusal effects of progressive joint remodeling and adaptation.

SUMMARY

Evaluating a patient's TMJ function by history, clinical examination, and with tomograms, arthrograms, MRI, or by direct visualization with an arthroscope, as necessary, may reveal important findings that need to be treated. Nonsurgical treatment involves anti-inflammatory therapy, occlusal appliance therapy, and rehabilitation of function. TMJ surgery, whether it is arthroscopic or an open procedure, should be recommended only when it is definitely indicated by the findings and when appropriate nonsurgical therapy has failed. Because of the occurrence of scar tissue in the joint that can limit jaw motion after open surgery, and the malocclusion that often occurs secondary to condyle-articular arthroplasty, open TMJ surgery must be recommended cautiously to the patient.

REFERENCES

Agerberg, G., and Carlsson, G. E.: Late results of treatment of functional disorders of the masticatory system: A follow-up by questionnaire. J. Oral Rehabil. 1:309–316, 1974.
Akerman, S., and Kopp, S.: Intra-articular and skin surface temperature of the temporomandibular joint in patients with rheumatoid arthritis. Acta Odontol. Scand. 46:41–48, 1988a.
Akerman, S., Kopp, S., and Rohlin, M.: Macroscopic and microscopic appearance of radiologic findings in temporomandibular joints from elderly individuals. An autopsy study. Int. J. Oral Maxillofac. Surg. 17:58–63, 1988b.
Anderson, G. C., Schiffman, E. L., Schellhas, K. P., and Fricton, J. R.: Clinical vs. arthrographic diagnosis of TMJ internal derangement. J. Dent. Res. 68:826–829, 1989.
Annandale, T.: Displacement of the inter-articular cartilage of the lower jaw, and its treatment by operation. Lancet 1:411, 1887.
Axelsson, S., Fitins, D., Hellsing, G., and Holmlund, A.: Arthrotic changes and deviation in form of the temporomandibular joint—An autopsy study. Swed. Dent. J. 11:195–200, 1987.
Balciunas, B. A., Staling, L. M., and Parente, F. J.: Quantitative electromyographic response to therapy for myo-oral facial pain: A pilot study. J. Prosthet. Dent. 58:366–369, 1987.
Bell, W. E.: Clinical Management of Temporomandibular Disorders. Chicago, Yearbook Medical, 1982, pp. 183–185.
Bibb, C. A., Pullinger, A. G., Baldioceda, F., et al.: Comparative imaging study. In Sanders, B., Murakami, K., and Clark, G. T. (Eds.): Diagnostic and Surgical Arthroscopy of the Temporomandibular Joint. Philadelphia, W. B. Saunders, 1989, pp. 143–157.
Blaschke, D. D.: Arthrography of the temporomandibular joint. In Solberg, W. K., and Clark, G. T. (Eds.): Temporomandibular Joint Problems, Biologic Diagnosis and Treatment. Chicago, Quintessence, 1980a, pp. 69–86.
Blaschke, D., Solberg, W. K., and Sanders, B.: Arthrography of the temporomandibular joint: Review of current status. J. Am. Dent. Assoc. 100:388–395, 1980b.
Burman, D. D., and Sinberg, S. E.: Condylar movement in the study of internal derangement of the temporomandibular joint. J. Bone Joint Surg. 28:351–371, 1946.
Carlsson, G. E.: Long-term effects of treatment of craniomandibular disorders. J. Craniomandib. Pract. 3:337–342, 1985.
Carlsson, G. E., Kopp, S., and Oberg, T.: Arthritis and allied diseases of the temporomandibular joint. In Zarb, G. A., Carlsson, G. E. (Eds.): Temporomandibular Joint

Function and Dysfunction. Copenhagen, Munksgaard, 1979, pp. 269–320.

Christiansen, E. L., Thompson, J. R., and Hasso, A. N.: CT evaluation of trauma to the temporomandibular joint. J. Oral Maxillofac. Surg. 45:920–923, 1987.

Ciancaglini, R., Sorini, M., De Cicco, L., and Brodoloni, F.: Digital phonoarthrometry of temporomandibular joint sounds: A preliminary report. J. Oral Rehabil. 14:385–392, 1987.

Clark, G. T.: Treatment of jaw clicking with temporomandibular repositioning: Analysis of 25 cases. J. Craniomandib. Pract. 2:263–270, 1984a.

Clark, G. T.: A critical evaluation of orthopedic interocclusal appliance therapy: Design, theory and overall effectiveness. J. Am. Dent. Assoc. 108:359–362, 1984b.

Clark, G. T.: A critical evaluation of orthopedic interocclusal appliance therapy: Effectiveness for specific symptoms. J. Am. Dent. Assoc. 108:364–368, 1984c.

Clark, G. T.: The TMJ repositioning appliance: A technique for construction, insertion, and adjustment. J. Craniomandib. Pract. 4:37–46, 1986.

Clark, G. T.: Diagnosis and treatment of painful temporomandibular disorders. Dent. Clin. North Am. 31:645–674, 1987.

Clark, G. T., Beemsterboer, P. L., and Rugh, J. D.: Nocturnal masseter muscle activity and the symptoms of masticatory dysfunction. J. Oral Rehabil. 8:279–286, 1981.

Clark, G. T., Lanham, F., and Flack, V. F.: Treatment outcome results for consecutive TMJ clinic patients. J. Craniomandib. Disord. Facial Oral Pain 2:87–95, 1988.

Clark, G. T., Seligman, D. A., Solberg, W. K., and Pullinger, A. G.: Guidelines for the examination and diagnosis of temporomandibular disorders. J. Craniomandib. Disord. 3:7–14, 1989a.

Clark, G. T., Moody, D. G., and Sanders, B.: Analysis of arthroscopically treated TMJ derangement and locking. In Sanders, B., Murakami, K., and Clark, G. T. (Eds.): Diagnostic and Surgical Arthroscopy of the Temporomandibular Joint. Philadelphia, W. B. Saunders, 1989b.

Dao, T. T. T., Feine, J. S., and Lund, J. P.: Can electrical stimulation be used to establish a physiologic occlusal position? J. Prosthet. Dent. 60:509–514, 1988.

Diamond, M. W.: An overview of the multimodal approach to TMJ disorders. Dent. Clin. North Am. 31:695–701, 1987.

Dolwick, M. F., and Riggs, R. R.: Diagnosis and treatment of internal derangements of the temporomandibular joint. Dent. Clin. North Am. 27:561–572, 1983.

Farrar, W. B.: Characteristics of the condylar path in internal derangements of the TMJ. J. Prosthet. Dent. 39:147–153, 1978.

Farrar, W. B., and McCarty, W. L. Jr.: Inferior joint space arthrography and characteristics of condylar paths in internal derangements of the TMJ. J. Prosthet. Dent. 41:548–555, 1979.

Farrar, W. B., and McCarty, W. L. Jr.: A Clinical Outline of Temporomandibular Joint Diagnosis and Treatment. Montgomery, AL, Walker Printing, 1983.

Good, A. E., and Upton, L. G.: Acute temporomandibular arthritis in a patient with bruxism and calcium pyrophosphate deposition disease. Arthritis Rheum. 25:353–355, 1982.

Greene, C. S.: Can technology enhance TM disorder diagnosis? J. Cal. Dent. Assoc. 18:21–24, 1990.

Greene, C. S., and Laskin, D. M.: Long-term status of TMJ clicking in patients with myofascial pain and dysfunction. J. Am. Dent. Assoc. 117:461–465, 1988.

Hansson, T., and Oberg, T.: Arthrosis and deviation in form in the temporomandibular joint. A macroscopic study on a human autopsy material. Acta Odontol. Scand. 35:167–174, 1977.

Hasso, A. N., Christiansen, E. L., and Alder, M. E.: The temporomandibular joint. Radiology Clin. North Am. 27:301–314, 1989.

Helkimo, E., and Westling, L.: History, clinical findings, and outcome of treatment of patients with anterior disk displacement. J. Craniomandib. Pract. 5:269–276, 1987.

Katzberg, R. W., Dolwick, M. F., Helms, C. A., et al.: Arthrotomography of the temporomandibular joint. Am. J. Roentgenol. 134:995–1003, 1980.

Kononen, M.: Clinical signs of craniomandibular disorders and patients with psoriatic arthritis. Scand. J. Dent. Res. 95:340–346, 1987.

Kopp, S., Carlsson, G. E., Haraldson, T., and Wenneberg, B.: Long-term effect of intra-articular injections of sodium hyaluronate and corticosteroid on temporomandibular joint arthritis. J. Oral Maxillofac. Surg. 45:929–935, 1987.

Kopp, S., Wenneberg, B., Haraldson, T., and Carlsson, G. E.: The short-term effect of intra-articular injections of sodium hyaluronate and corticosteroid on temporomandibular joint pain and dysfunction. J. Oral Maxillofac. Surg. 43:429–435, 1985.

Larheim, T. A., Hoyeraal, H. M., Stabrun, A. E., and Haanaes, H. R.: The temporomandibular joint in juvenile rheumatoid arthritis. Scand. J. Rheumatol. 11:5–12, 1982.

Lewis, T. C.: A radiologic and anatomic study of internal derangements of the temporomandibular joint. Oral Surg. 64:638–644, 1987.

Lund, P., and Widmer, C. G.: An evaluation of the use of surface electromyography in the diagnosis, documentation, and treatment of dental patients. J. Craniomandib. Disord. Facial Oral Pain 3:125–137, 1989.

Lundh, H., Westesson, P-L., and Kopp, S.: A three-year follow-up of patients with reciprocal temporomandibular joint clicking. Oral Surg. 63:530–533, 1987.

Magnusson, T., and Carlsson, G. E.: Treatment of patients with functional disturbances in the masticatory system. A survey of 80 consecutive patients. Swed. Dent. J. 4:145–153, 1980.

Magnusson, T., Egermark-Eriksson, I., and Carlsson, G. E.: Five-year longitudinal study of signs and symptoms of mandibular dysfunction in adolescents. J. Craniomandib. Pract. 4:338–344, 1986.

Marbach, J. J.: Arthritis of the temporomandibular joints. Am. Fam. Physician 19:131–139, 1979.

Marbach, J. J., and Varoscak, J. R.: Treatment of TMJ and other facial pains: A critical review. NY Dent. J. 46:181–188, 1980.

McCain, J. P., de la Rua, H., and Le Blanc, W. G.: Correlation of clinical, radiographic, and arthroscopic findings in internal derangements of the TMJ. J. Oral Maxillofac. Surg. 47:913–921, 1989.

McCarty, W.: Diagnosis and treatment of internal derangements of the articular disc and mandibular condyle. In Solberg, W. K., and Clark, G. T. (Eds.): Temporomandibular Joint Problems, Biologic Diagnosis and Treatment. Chicago, Quintessence, 1980, pp. 145–164.

Mejersjo, C.: Therapeutic and prognostic considerations in TMJ osteoarthrosis: A literature review and a long-term study in 11 subjects. J. Craniomandib. Pract. 5:70–78, 1987.

Moffett, B. C., Johnson, L. C., McCabe, J. B., and Askew, H. C.: Articular remodeling in the adult human temporomandibular joint. Am. J. Anat. 115:119–142, 1964.

Monteiro, A. A., and Clark, G. T.: Mandibular movement feedback vs occlusal appliances in the treatment of masticatory muscle dysfunction. J. Craniomandib. Disord. Facial Oral Pain 2:41–47, 1988.

Murakami, K.: Diagnostic arthroscopy. In Sanders, B., Murakami, K., and Clark, G. T. (Eds.): Diagnostic and Surgical Arthroscopy of the Temporomandibular Joint. Philadelphia, W. B. Saunders, 1989, pp. 73–94.

Murakami, K., Matsumoto, K., and Iizuka, T.: Suppurative arthritis of the temporomandibular joint. Report of a case with special reference to arthroscopic observations. J. Maxillofac. Surg. 12:41–45, 1984.

Nielsen, L., Melsen, B., and Terp, S.: Prevalence, interrelation, and severity of signs of dysfunction from masticatory system in 14–16-year-old Danish children. Community Dent. Oral Epidemiol. 17:91–96, 1989.

Norgaard, F.: Arthrography of the mandibular joint. Acta Radiol. 25:679–685, 1944.

Oberg, T.: Radiology of the temporomandibular joint. In Solberg, W. K., and Clark, G. T. (Eds.): Temporomandibular Joint Problems, Biologic Diagnosis and Treatment. Chicago, Quintessence, 1980, pp. 49–63.

Ogus, H.: Degenerative disease of the temporomandibular joints in young persons. Br. J. Oral Surg. 17:17–26, 1979.

Okeson, J. P.: Long-term treatment of disk-interference disorders of the temporomandibular joint with anterior repositioning occlusal splints. J. Prosthet. Dent. 60:611–616, 1988.

Pedersen, A., and Hansen, H. J.: Internal derangement of the temporomandibular joint in 211 patients: Symptoms and treatment. Community Dent. Oral Epidemiol. 15:339–343, 1987a.

Pedersen, A., and Hansen, H. J.: Long-term evaluation of 211 patients with internal derangement of the temporomandibular joint. Community Dent. Oral Epidemiol. 15:344–347, 1987b.

Phero, J. C., Raj, P. P., and McDonald, J. S.: Transcutaneous electrical nerve stimulation and myoneural injection therapy for management of chronic myofascial pain. Dent. Clin. North Am. 31:703–723, 1987.

Pullinger, A. G.: Natural history and pathologic progression of internal derangements with persistent closed lock. In Sanders, B., Murakami, K., and Clark, G. T. (Eds.): Diagnostic and Surgical Arthroscopy of the Temporomandibular Joint. Philadelphia, W. B. Saunders, 1989, pp. 158–189.

Pullinger, A. G., Monteiro, A. A., and Liu, A.: Etiological factors associated with temporomandibular disorders (abstract). J. Dent. Res. 64:269, 1985.

Pullinger, A. G., and Seligman, D. A.: TMJ osteoarthrosis: A differentiation of diagnostic subgroups by symptom history and demographics. J. Craniomandib. Disord. Facial Oral Pain 1:251–256, 1987.

Pullinger, A. G., Seligman, D. A., and Solberg, W. K.: Temporomandibular disorders. Part I: Functional status, dentomorphologic features, and sex differences in a nonpatient population. J. Prosthet. Dent. 59:228–235, 1988a.

Pullinger, A. G., Seligman, D. A., and Solberg, W. K.: Temporomandibular disorders. Part II: Occlusal factors associated with temporomandibular joint tenderness and dysfunction. J. Prosthet. Dent. 59:363–367, 1988b.

Pullinger, A. G., Solberg, W. K., Hollender, L., and Guichet, D.: Tomographic analysis of mandibular condyle position in diagnostic subgroups of temporomandibular disorders. J. Prosthet. Dent. 55:723–729, 1986.

Radin, E. L., Paul, I. L., and Rose, R. M.: Role of mechanical factors in pathogenesis of primary osteoarthritis. Lancet 1:519–522, 1972.

Rugh, J. D., Barghi, N., and Drago, C. J.: Experimental occlusal discrepancies and nocturnal bruxism. J. Prosthet. Dent. 51:548–553, 1984.

Schellhas, K. P., Wilkes, C. H., and Bakar, C. C.: Facial pain, headache, and temporomandibular joint inflammation. Headache 29:228–231, 1989.

Schellhas, K. P., Wilkes, C. H., Omlie, M. R., et al.: The diagnosis of temporomandibular joint disease: Two-compartment arthrography and MR. Am. J. Roent. 151:341–350, 1988.

Schwartz, L.: Local anesthetics. In Schwartz, L. (Ed.): Disorders of the Temporomandibular Joint: Diagnosis, Management, Relation to Occlusion of Teeth. Philadelphia, W. B. Saunders, 1966a, pp. 232–238.

Schwartz, L.: Limitation. In Schwartz, L. (Ed.): Disorders of the Temporomandibular Joint: Diagnosis, Management, Relation to Occlusion of Teeth. Philadelphia, W. B. Saunders, 1966b, pp. 315–334.

Seligman, D. A., Pullinger, A. G., and Solberg, W. K.: The prevalence of dental attrition and its association with factors of age, gender, occlusion and TMJ symptomatology. J. Dent. Res. 67:1323–1333, 1988a.

Seligman, D. A., Pullinger, A. G., and Solberg, W. K.: Temporomandibular disorders. Part III: Occlusal and articular factors associated with muscle tenderness. J. Prosthet. Dent. 59:483–489, 1988b.

Solberg, W. K.: Temporomandibular Disorders. Silver End, Witham, Essex, E T Heron Ltd, 1986a.

Solberg, W. K.: Temporomandibular disorders: Management of internal derangement. Br. Dent. J. 160:379–385, 1986b.

Solberg, W. K.: Temporomandibular disorders: Management of problems associated with inflammation, chronic hypomobility, and deformity. Br. Dent. J. 160:421–428, 1986c.

Solberg, W. K.: Temporomandibular disorders: Masticatory myalgia and its management. Br. Dent. J. 160:351–356, 1986d.

Stegenga, B., de Bont, L. G. M., and Boering, G.: Osteoarthrosis as the cause of craniomandibular pain and dysfunction: A unifying concept. J. Oral Maxillofac. Surg. 47:249–256, 1989.

Tegelberg, A., and Kopp, S.: Subjective symptoms from the stomatognathic system in individuals with rheumatoid arthritis and osteoarthrosis. Swed. Dent. J. 11:11–22, 1987a.

Tegelberg, A., Kopp, S., Huddenius, K., and Forssman, L.: Relationship between disorder in the stomatognathic system and general joint involvement in individuals with rheumatoid arthritis. Acta Odontol. Scand. 45:391–398, 1987b.

Toller, P. A.: Osteoarthrosis of the mandibular condyle. Br. Dent. J. 134:223–231, 1973.

Wabeke, K. B., Hansson, T. L., Hoogstraten, J., and van der Kuy, P.: Temporomandibular joint clicking: A literature overview. J. Craniomandib. Disord. Facial Oral Pain 3:163–173, 1989.

Wanman, A., and Agerberg, G.: Two-year longitudinal study of signs of mandibular dysfunction in adolescents. Acta Odontol. Scand. 44:333–342, 1986.

Weinberg, S., and Lapointe, H.: Cervical extension-flexion injury (whiplash) and internal derangement of the temporomandibular joint. J. Oral Maxillofac. Surg. 45:653–656, 1987.

Westesson, P-L., Katzberg, R. W., Tallents, R. H., et al.: Temporomandibular joint: Comparison of MR images with cryosectional anatomy. Radiology 164:59–64, 1987.

Widmer, C. G., Lund, J. P., and Feine, J. S.: Evaluation of diagnostic tests for TMD. J. Cal. Dent. Assoc. 18:53–60, 1990.

Wilkes, C. H.: Arthrography of the temporomandibular joint in patients with the TMJ pain-dysfunction syndrome. Minn. Med. 61:645–652, 1978.

Zarb, G. A., and Speck, J. E.: The treatment of mandibular dysfunction. In Zarb, G. A., and Carlsson, G. E. (Eds.): Temporomandibular Joint Function and Dysfunction. St. Louis, C. V. Mosby, 1979, pp. 373–396.

24

SURGICAL CONSIDERATIONS*†

*BERNARD G. SARNAT, M.D., M.S., D.D.S.,
and DANIEL M. LASKIN, D.D.S., M.S.*

INTRODUCTION

There is considerable literature in regard to the management of temporomandibular joint (TMJ) disturbances. The variety of surgical procedures often recommended for the same condition, however, attests to the difficulty still encountered in the treatment of certain problems. In some instances this may be one of inaccurate preoperative diagnosis. Regrettably, there have been too few adequate studies correlating the clinical signs and symptoms with the actual pathologic changes in the joint. Other times, treatment may be unsuccessful because

confusion in the descriptive terminology used in the literature leads to the improper choice of surgical procedures. In still other instances, poor results may occur because the treatment was directed toward relief of symptoms rather than removal of the etiologic agent. Finally, difficulties can also arise when surgery may not be the preferred treatment for certain joint conditions. Because of these existing complex problems, there is an increasing need for a critical examination of the surgical considerations of the TMJ and related structures.

This chapter is not intended to be a detailed review but to serve as a basis for further study. General principles of therapy rather than specific techniques are presented. More detailed information can be found in the extensive list of references included.

*Revision principally by Daniel M. Laskin, D.D.S., M.S.
†See Chapters 3–5, 7, 8, 10–13, 16, 17, 19, 21–23, and 26

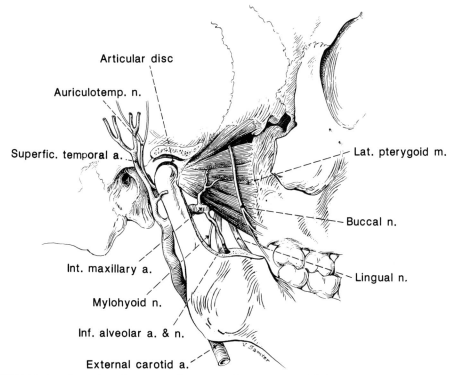

FIGURE 24–1. Relationship of arteries and nerves to the temporomandibular joint region. (From Zimmermann, A.A.: An evaluation of Costen's syndrome from an anatomic point of view. *In* Sarnat, B.G. (Ed.): The Temporomandibular Joint. Springfield, IL, Charles C Thomas, 1951.)

SURGICAL ANATOMY

The detailed morphology of the temporomandibular joint (TMJ) has been described in Chapter 5. Among the anatomic structures in the region of the TMJ that can lead to complications if damaged during a surgical procedure are the parotid gland, facial nerve, internal maxillary artery, superficial temporal artery and vein, and the auriculotemporal nerve (Fig. 24–1). The major hazard is the possibility of injury to one or more branches of the facial nerve, with resultant paralysis of portions of the facial musculature. To lessen this risk, five main surgical approaches to the joint have been used, namely, the preauricular, endaural, postauricular, retromandibular, and submandibular (Kreutziger, 1984) (Fig. 24–2). Of these, the preauricular and retromandibular procedures are preferred. An intraoral approach also has been described (Sear, 1972), but it provides limited access and its use has been restricted to condylectomy and open reduction of some subcondylar fractures (Jeter, 1988).

In the preauricular approach an incision is made vertically in front of the ear or, for better cosmetic results, either entirely along the curvature of the anterior border of the auricle to the level of the lobule or partially behind the tragus (Nishioka, 1987). For additional exposure below the ear, the incision is extended only through the skin. A deep incision in this region may sever the main trunk of the facial nerve where it enters the posterior aspect of the parotid gland. For greater accessibility, the superior end of the vertical incision can be brought obliquely forward, parallel to the temporal branch of the facial nerve. Although some surgeons prefer to arc the incision forward about 2.5 centimeters in front of the upper attachment of the ear, this modification provides no appreciable improvement in access. When this incision is used, the anterior end should be made only through the skin to avoid cutting the temporal branch of the facial nerve.

Once the skin incision is made, the superior end is deepened to the level of the temporalis fascia. This establishes the plane for further dissection. The dissection is kept close to the ear cartilage to avoid injury to the auriculotemporal nerve, branches of the facial nerve, and the superficial temporal artery and vein (see Fig. 24–1). When the incision has been deepened properly, the superior pole of the parotid gland, the superficial temporal artery and vein, and the auriculotemporal nerve are bluntly

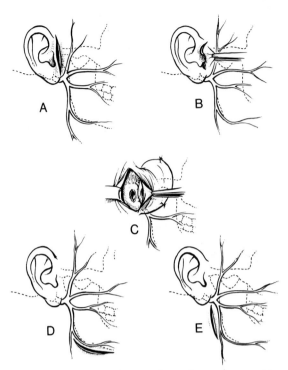

FIGURE 24–2. Surgical approaches to the temporomandibular joint. *A,* Preauricular. *B,* Endaural. *C,* Postauricular. *D,* Submandibular. *E,* Retromandibular. These incisions are designed to avoid injury to the facial nerve. (From Laskin, D.M.: Surgical management of diseases of the temporomandibular joint. *In* Hayward, J. (Ed.): Oral Surgery. Springfield, IL, Charles C Thomas, 1976.)

pushed forward with a periosteal elevator to expose fully the temporalis fascia and the deep layer of the parotideomasseteric fascia overlying the TMJ.

Next, an incision about 2 centimeters long is made through the superficial layer of the temporalis fascia at a 45-degree angle extending to the root of the zygomatic arch (Fig. 24–3). From there it is carried vertically to the inferior aspect of the wound. Sharp and blunt dissection is then used to create a flap that is reflected downward and forward to expose the region of the TMJ. This modification of the procedure described by Al-Kayat (1980) provides the same protection for the frontal branch of the facial nerve without the need for the extensive incision. The fascial flap also enables the upper joint space to be closed adequately when there is insufficient capsular tissue.

In the endaural procedure (see Fig. 24–2B) an incision is made above the level of the zygomatic arch and extended downward and backward in the intercartilaginous cleft between the tragus and the helix. From there it is directed inward along the roof of the auditory

meatus for about a centimeter and then continued in the sagittal plane around the anterior half of the meatal circumference at the junction of the cartilaginous and bony canals (Davidson, 1956). Rongetti (1954) prefers to extend the lower end of this incision in a straight line anteroinferiorly in the incisura intertragica, cutting through the cartilage in that area. In either case, the anterior meatal wall is then reflected forward exposing the TMJ as well as the neck of the condyloid process. This approach can be used for discectomy and condylectomy, but its use is restricted in the reduction of a medially displaced, fractured condyloid process owing to the limited access. A further disadvantage of the method is the possibility of meatal stenosis.

The postauricular approach to the TMJ, as first described by Bockenheimer (1920) and modified by Axhausen (1931), entails an incision behind the ear, followed by division of the cartilaginous auditory canal and reflection of the entire auricle (see Fig. 24–2C). The articulation is then exposed from behind by reflecting the parotid gland forward. The cosmetic results of this method are excellent. The disadvantages of the procedure are the possibility of infection and necrosis of the ear cartilage, stenosis of the auditory canal, and anesthesia of the auricle (Husted, 1946). Moreover, one must still encounter the parotid gland and facial nerve in approaching the articulation.

Use of either the submandibular or retromandibular approach is generally limited to procedures in the subcondylar and ramal regions, although the latter approach also can be used effectively for TMJ surgery in the child. In the

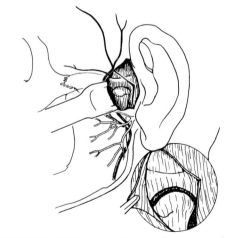

FIGURE 24–3. Diagram of flap used to expose the temporomandibular joint. Insert shows flap retracted and incision of upper joint space.

submandibular approach (Risdon, 1934) an incision is made starting at least 1 centimeter below the angle of the mandible and extended forward parallel to the lower border avoiding the marginal mandibular branch of the facial nerve above and the cervical branch below (see Fig. 24–2D). After the attachment of the masseter muscle is freed from the lateral surface of the ramus, the TMJ is exposed by upward retraction of the overlying tissues. Because the entire parotid gland and facial nerve are reflected in the tissue flap, the possibility of permanent facial nerve damage is slight.

The retromandibular approach (see Fig. 24–2E) has several advantages over the submandibular for the performance of a subcondylar surgical procedure. Perhaps the major advantage is the more direct access and better visibility. The incision is also shorter and less conspicuous. Moreover, the amount of tissue disruption is less, and complete detachment of the masseter muscle and ligation of major vessels are not required. Finally, there is less chance of damage to the facial nerve since the dissection is in front of the main trunk and between the widely spaced buccal and marginal mandibular branches rather than directly in the region of the latter branch.

The retromandibular incision is usually about 2 centimeters long and starts slightly below the lobule of the ear. It is made parallel with, and slightly behind, the posterior border of the ramus. The initial cut extends through the skin and subcutaneous tissues to the level of the parotideomasseteric fascia. The overlying tissues are then undermined anteriorly in all directions to permit free movement over the surgical site. Next, the parotideomasseteric fascia is split vertically, anterior to the lower pole of the parotid, and that portion of the gland is undermined and retracted posteriorly to expose the masseter muscle. The masseter is incised along the posterior border of the ramus and then elevated to expose the underlying bone. Although the initial site of exposure is in the subcondylar region, the entire ramus can be visualized, when necessary, by shifting the overlying tissues either superiorly or inferiorly. In a child, the shorter ramus height also permits access to the TMJ.

The proximity of the internal maxillary artery to the medial aspect of the neck of the condyloid process makes this vessel particularly vulnerable during subcondylar surgery (see Fig. 24–1). Because of inaccessibility, it is difficult to clamp and tie the artery when it is either torn or cut and there can be considerable blood loss. If the bleeding is not controlled by temporary packing, the wound can be packed with a gauze strip that is gradually withdrawn over a period of several days.

The parotid gland is encountered in both the preauricular and retromandibular approaches, and injury to it can result in extravasation of saliva and formation of a sialocele. This can occasionally be difficult to eradicate. For this reason, in either approach, it is preferable to retract the gland rather than dissect through it bluntly.

TREATMENT OF GROWTH DISTURBANCES

Knowledge of the normal growth pattern of the mandible is essential to a better understanding of growth disturbances and their treatment (Sarnat, 1986). There are various unilateral and bilateral growth disturbances of the condyloid process and related structures. They range from underdevelopment or overdevelopment of only one condyle to underdevelopment or overdevelopment of the entire face, and may have a variety of causes (see Chapters 4, 10, 12, and 24).

Absent or Diminished Growth
(Table 24–1)

The method of treatment of growth deficiencies of the TMJ depends on the age of the patient. In the adult, correction of the deformity is concerned only with establishment of normal jaw relations, function, and appearance since continued growth deficiency is no longer a problem. In a young individual, establishment of proper jaw relations and replacement of the deficient condylar growth site are both necessary because otherwise a deformity may recur as the child becomes older. Early surgical correction is very important in the child, more so with a unilateral than with a bilateral growth deficiency, because the former leads to progressive asymmetry of the mandible. This is much more difficult to treat from a cosmetic and occlusal standpoint than the symmetrically underdeveloped mandible. In both instances, insufficient autogenous tissue and the possibility of surgical trauma to the growing and erupting permanent tooth buds are other factors of concern.

TABLE 24–1. Causes of Underdevelopment of the Temporomandibular Joint and Mandible

I. Unilateral
 A. Prenatal growth disturbance: condylar aplasia or hypoplasia
 B. Postnatal growth disturbance
  1. Trauma
  2. Infection
  3. Radiation
  4. Idiopathic: progressive hemifacial atrophy
II. Bilateral
 A. Prenatal growth disturbance
  1. Hereditary
   a. Chromosomal anomalies
    (1) Edward's syndrome (trisomy 18)
    (2) Triploidy syndrome
    (3) Turner's syndrome
   b. Achondroplasia
   c. Nanocephalic dwarfism
   d. Mandibulofacial dysostosis
   e. Oculomandibulodyscephaly
   f. Progeria
   g. Hanhart's syndrome
   h. Larsen's syndrome
   i. Ullrich-Feichtiger syndrome
  2. Nonhereditary
   a. Robin anomal
   b. Möbius syndrome
   c. Arthromyodysplasia congenita
   d. Radiation of fetus
 B. Postnatal growth disturbance
  1. Endocrine
   a. Hypothyroidism
   b. Pituitary dysfunction
  2. Dietary deficiency: vitamin D
  3. Idiopathic: rheumatoid arthritis

Condylar Agenesis (Otomandibular Dysostosis, Hemifacial Microsomia)

Although this condition is usually unilateral, it may sometimes be bilateral (see Chapter 12). In addition, anomalies are frequently found in other parts of the body. The articular fossa, the eminence, the condyloid and coronoid processes, the lower ramus, and part or even all of the mandibular body (and teeth) may be rudimentary or absent. Other facial structures also may be affected in different combinations. There may be macrostomia, and the external ear may be abnormal in configuration, size, and position, or totally absent (Fig. 24–4). The external opening of the auditory canal is sometimes unexposed, and the canal, middle and inner ears, temporal bone, zygoma, and maxilla may be deficient. When the facial nerve is partially absent, there is corresponding weakness of the facial musculature. The etiologic background may be genetic or environmental and is related to maldevelopment of the first and second branchial arches (see Chapters 3 and 12).

Correction of condylar agenesis is directed toward improvement of ramal height and the addition of a surrogate growing condyle on the affected side to lessen further mandibular deformation. Both autogenous metatarsal and rib (costochondral junction) grafts have been suggested and used for the latter purpose (Choukas, 1971; Glahn, 1967; Roy, 1956; Stuteville, 1955; Ware, 1966; 1970). Of the two tissues, costochondral junction grafts seem to give more consistent results (Poswillo, 1974; 1987; Ware, 1980; 1981). A second procedure may be necessary several years later to obtain better symmetry of the mandible. If growth of the relatively normal side has ceased by that time, the final reconstruction can be done with tibia, metatarsal, or bone from the iliac crest. Otherwise, rib should be used again.

Besides restoration of ramal height and addition of a condylar growth site, orthodontic therapy, orthognathic surgery, genioplasty, soft tissue and cartilage grafts, implants for facial augmentation, and otoplasty are often necessary (Ware, 1980). Certain aspects of treatment may be undertaken when the patient is still growing, but the final result cannot be attained until growth of the face and jaws has ceased.

Condylar Hypoplasia

Although congenital hypoplasia of the mandibular condyle can occur, most often underdevelopment is a result of postnatal causes (see Table 24–1). Any local interference (trauma, infection, or radiation) that affects the condyle will alter the orderly progression of development and result in some type of TMJ and mandibular deformity (Fig. 24–5). Trauma is the most common etiologic factor. Growth arrest and deformity of the facial skeleton may result from birth trauma (improper application of obstetric forceps or breech delivery) directly to the TMJ region or transmitted from another part of the mandible. Although some degree of facial paralysis may be noted at the time of injury, the skeletal deformity usually is not discovered for months. Later in life, trauma sustained either directly to the joint or indirectly from a blow to the chin (a scar may be noted), with or without a fracture of the condyloid process, also may result in an altered TMJ and underdeveloped mandible. The extent of the deformity will be determined not only by the severity and duration of the injury but also by the particular time of occurrence. Thus,

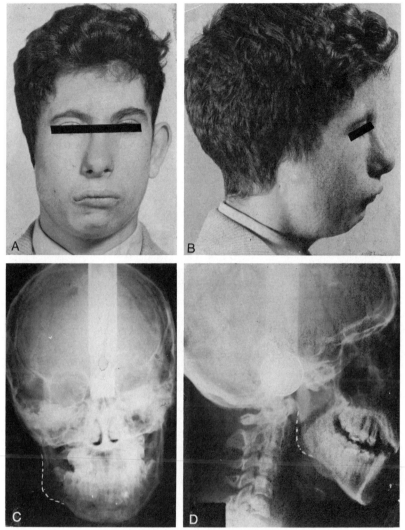

FIGURE 24–4. *A*, Frontal and *B*, lateral view photographs and *C*, posteroanterior and *D*, lateral view radiographs of a patient born with hemifacial microsomia. Note absence of the right external ear and the macrostomia. In the radiographs, note the lack of development of the angle of the mandible on the right side.

the effect will be more extreme early in life when condylar growth activity is greatest, and considerably less later in life when growth activity has decreased and the mandible has nearly assumed its adult size and shape.

Inflammation on an infectious basis is another cause of changes in the TMJ and underdevelopment of the mandible. Primary infection involving the TMJ and the condylar cartilage is uncommon. More frequent is the spread of regional infection. In the past, otitis media, as a result of an upper respiratory infection or scarlet fever, was a frequent antecedent to suppuration in the TMJ region (Fig. 24–6). With the advent of antibiotics, this complication is now seldom seen. Growth arrest may also

result secondary to the spread of a dental infection to the regional tissues and the joint. Primary osteomyelitis of the TMJ is rare.

Radiation therapy for tumors in the region of the growing condyle may not only destroy the tumor but also affect the condyle and the TMJ. This can result in an asymmetrical mandible and ankylosis. The radiation-damaged tissue may be subject to osteomyelitis, sequestration, dermatitis and, after 10 to 15 years, development of a malignancy.

There are also a number of systemic conditions that can cause postnatal condylar hypoplasia and retarded mandibular growth. These may be inflammatory, dietary, or endocrine in origin. Rheumatoid arthritis in children is associ-

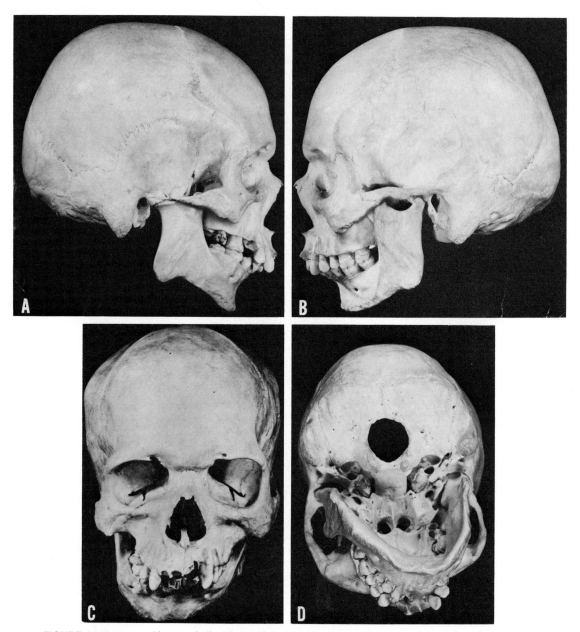

FIGURE 24–5. Views of human skull with an ankylosis of the temporomandibular joint and an interference with condylar and mandibular growth on the right side. The ramus is shorter and wider on the right side, there is antegonial notching, and the mandible is skewed to the right. (Courtesy of E. Lloyd DuBrul, D.D.S., M.S., Ph.D.)

ated with mandibular underdevelopment (Fig. 24–7). The TMJ at times is the first to manifest clinical symptoms of this disease. The condylar cartilage is damaged or destroyed in much the same manner as in joints elsewhere in the body (see Chapters 11 and 22).

Hematogenous spread of infection from distant sources can also involve the TMJ. For example, the organism responsible for osteomyelitis in a long bone may pass to the jaw

joint and set up a new focus with possible growth arrest and ankylosis (Fig. 24–8). Systemic infections, although rare, can also affect the TMJ and result in growth retardation or arrest. These include gonorrhea, syphilis, tuberculosis, typhoid fever, dysentery, pneumonia, influenza, scarlet fever, and measles.

Because a lack of vitamin D has a systemic effect, the manifestations seen in the condylar cartilage are only part of the total picture. In

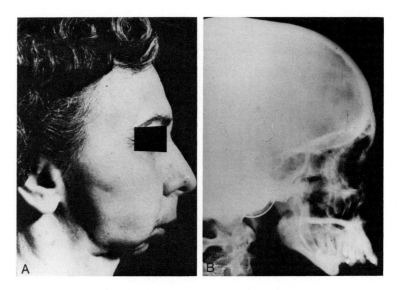

FIGURE 24–6. *A*, Lateral view photograph and *B*, radiograph of a patient who had scarlet fever and bilateral otitis media as an infant, which spread to both temporomandibular joints. Note the relatively normal-sized maxilla and the extremely underdeveloped mandible. (From Sarnat, B.G.: Developmental facial abnormalities and the temporomandibular joint. Dent. Clin. North Am. 587–600, Nov. 1966.)

rachitic children the reduced cartilaginous growth not only produces shorter extremities, but also results in facial disharmony. Delayed eruption and malpositioning of the teeth occur because the intermaxillary space required for eruption is decreased as a result of the short ramus. In addition, the anterior border of the ramus fails to resorb at the time the posterior teeth are about to erupt (see Chapters 4 and 13).

Both hypothyroidism and hypopituitarism can affect the growing mandible as well as other parts of the skeleton. The severe and striking results of hypothyroidism are manifested in understature and disproportion. Studies of cretins reveal a generalized retardation of growth

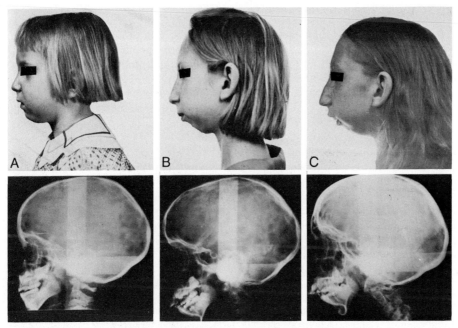

FIGURE 24–7. Lateral photographs and radiographs of a patient with rheumatoid arthritis of the temporomandibular joints. These illustrate the progressive bilateral deformity that occurred over a number of years. *A*, 4 years, 6 months; *B*, 12 years, 6 months; and *C*, 15 years, 9 months. (From Engel, M.B., Richmond, J., and Brodie, A.G.: Mandibular growth disturbance in rheumatoid arthritis of childhood. Am. J. Dis. Child. 78:728–743, 1949. Copyright 1949 American Medical Association.)

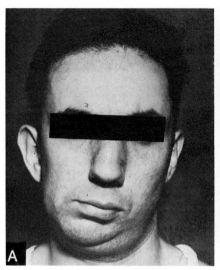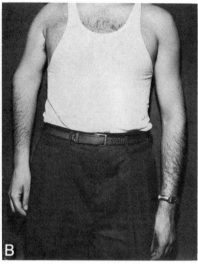

FIGURE 24–8. Unilateral growth arrest and ankylosis of the right side of the mandible after an infection in the temporomandibular joint during infancy. *A,* Note the flatness of the face on the unaffected side. *B,* Right arm of same patient showing growth arrest and deformity after osteomyelitis. The involvement of the temporomandibular joint was secondary to the hematogenous spread of this infection. (From Sarnat, B.G., and Robinson, I.B.: Surgery of the mandible: Some clinical and experimental considerations. Plast. Reconstr. Surg. *17:*27–57, 1956.)

within the facial area, with the cranial skeleton being relatively larger (Engel, 1941). The teeth are retarded in development and in eruption, but their size is not affected. Therefore, the teeth and the alveolar processes seem overly large for the smaller body of the maxilla and mandible. In hypopituitarism, facial growth is decreased proportionately so that the jaws, though small, are in proper relationship.

The characteristic clinical and radiographic observations on the human mandible following an arrest of growth of one condyle are as follows: (1) on the side of injury, there is a short wide condyloid process and ramus in a more anterior position than its opposite; a relatively longer, heavier, and posteriorly directed coronoid process; a shallow mandibular notch; a short body; an exaggerated antegonial notch; unerupted and impacted molars; and fullness of the face; (2) on the opposite uninjured side, there is elongation of the body of the mandible and a flat appearance of the face; and (3) malocclusion occurs, with the mandible skewed toward the side of the affected condyle (see Figs. 24–5, 24–8) (see Table 24–1).

With a bilateral condylar growth arrest there is usually a symmetrical underdevelopment of the mandible (micrognathia) (see Fig. 24–7). This is characterized by a short mandible, with the chin retruded to about the level of the hyoid bone (see Table 24–1). Occasionally associated with this may be hypoventilation (Valero, 1965) and hypersomnolence (Conway, 1977). Increased antegonial notching is present bilaterally.

Tooth eruption is considerably dependent upon mandibular growth. Therefore, patients with inadequate condylar growth and retarded mandibular development may have disturbances in the eruption and the position of teeth, particularly in the region of the affected ramus. This is true for at least two reasons. First, the mandibular ramus does not increase in height sufficiently to open the space between the upper and lower jaws into which the teeth erupt. Second, posterior growth of the ramus is less, so that mandibular body length is also less. As a result the last molars are left within the ramus.

The surgical treatment of condylar hypoplasia depends on the age of the patient when the condition is recognized. Because the facial deformity usually develops slowly, patients in whom there is no associated jaw dysfunction generally are at an age when growth has stopped or nearly stopped before concern about their appearance causes them to seek care. For these individuals, various forms of orthognathic surgery are used to correct the malocclusion and facial deformity. In cases of unilateral hypoplasia, the normal side may be shortened or the abnormal side lengthened, depending upon the existing occlusal relationship and the predicted esthetic effect. In bilateral cases, the mandible is lengthened. To achieve a good functional occlusion orthodontic treatment often is necessary before surgical repositioning of the jaw. In addition, genioplasty and facial augmentation grafts may be needed to provide a better esthetic result (Sarnat, 1959). In patients with severe condylar hypoplasia presenting for treatment during the growth period, restoration of normal ramal height and replacement of the deficient condyle with an autogenous costochondral graft is recommended to prevent progressive deformity (Lindqvist, 1988; Obeid, 1988; Ware, 1980) (see Chapter 13). Treatment of those individuals with associated limitation of jaw movement is discussed under ankylosis (see page 408).

Extrinsic factors also can affect the growing condyle and mandible. In torticollis, or wry neck, the shortened sternomastoid muscle alters the normal position of the head and an asymmetry results with lesser development of not only the mandible but also the entire skull on the affected side (Fig. 24–9) (Peresson, 1950; Sarnat, 1956). The maxillary alveolar process is also less developed on the affected side. These findings may be a result of pressure on the ramus, and particularly the condyle, thereby causing decreased growth. The hyoid group of muscles may also play a role. Early correction of the torticollis is important to avoid severe deformities. Another extrinsic factor, scar contracture of the neck from a burn, can cause mandibular deformity (Sarnat, 1959).

The conditions resulting from condylar hy-poplasia should be differentiated from progressive hemifacial atrophy in which both the bony structures (including the condyle) and the soft tissues on one side of the face in the region of the distribution of the trigeminal nerve regress on possibly a neurotrophic or traumatic basis (Fig. 24–10). There is a progressive atrophy of the skin, subcutaneous fat, connective tissue proper, muscle, cartilage, and bone. In addition to the face, the tongue and soft palate are affected. No specific etiology for this problem is known (Sarnat, 1971a). The condition usually begins before puberty and continues into adulthood.

Treatment usually is surgical and involves many considerations. Because the skin is atrophic and thin, it must be supplemented with a large skin flap that includes subcutaneous fat. Regions of bony loss, chiefly around the orbit, can be built out with grafts. Finally, a dental prosthesis may be constructed to compensate for some of the facial and dental irregularities.

Increased Growth

There are various conditions in which there is unilateral or bilateral overdevelopment of the TMJ and mandible (Table 24–2). While some are directly related to excessive growth of the condyle, others are the result of more general-

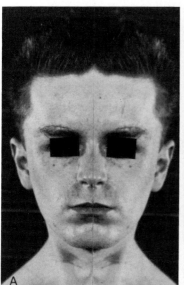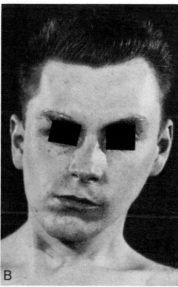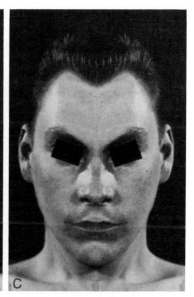

FIGURE 24–9. Asymmetry of face after torticollis for many years. *A,* Two right (smaller) halves of face (one reversed) to illustrate asymmetry. *B,* Note lesser development of right side of face; also note neck scar after correction of torticollis. *C,* Two left (larger) halves of face (one reversed) to illustrate asymmetry. (From Sarnat, B.G., and Robinson, I.B.: Surgery of the mandible: Some clinical and experimental considerations. Plast. Reconstr. Surg. *17*:27–57, 1956.)

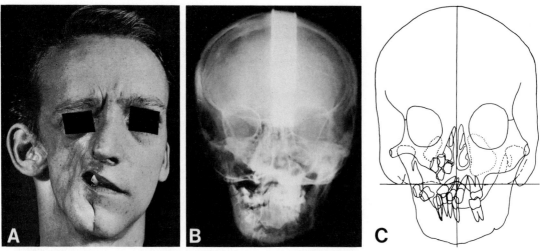

FIGURE 24–10. *A*, Photograph, *B*, cephalometric radiograph, and *C*, tracing of the cephalometric radiograph of a patient with right progressive hemifacial atrophy. Note gross asymmetry of the face. The size and shape of the upper and lower jaw and facial structures on the two sides are different as indicated by the size of the zygomatic-frontal buttresses, condyles, rami, orbits, and maxillary sinuses. Also note the lesser developed and unerupted teeth in the right maxilla and mandible. (From Sarnat, B.G.: Clinical and experimental considerations in facial bone biology: Growth, remodeling and repair. J. Am. Dent. Assoc. 82:876–889, 1971a.) (See also Figure 12–20.)

ized overgrowth or tumor formation. One cause of unilateral facial enlargement is prenatal hemifacial hypertrophy (Fig. 24–11). Not only the TMJ, facial bones, orbit, jaws, and teeth, but also the soft tissue structures including the tongue, palate, and ear are enlarged on one side. The enlarged teeth help differentiate this from other deformities of mandibular overgrowth in which the size of the teeth is normal. Sometimes, other regions of the body are involved (see Chapter 12). Unilateral enlargement

of the facial bones is also caused by various fibro-osseous tumors. This is seldom related to the condyle. In addition, the face may be enlarged because of lymphangiomatous tissue or masseter muscle hypertrophy.

TABLE 24–2. Causes of Overdevelopment of the Temporomandibular Joint and Mandible

I. Unilateral
   A. Developmental
      1. Condylar hyperplasia
      2. Hemifacial hypertrophy
   B. Neoplastic
      1. Chondroma, osteochondroma, or osteoma of condyle
      2. Fibrous dysplasia
   C. Idiopathic
II. Bilateral
   A. Hereditary
      1. Klinefelter's syndrome
      2. Angiokeratoma corporis diffusum syndrome
   B. Developmental: true prognathism
   C. Endocrine (pituitary)
      1. Giantism
      2. Acromegaly
   D. Idiopathic

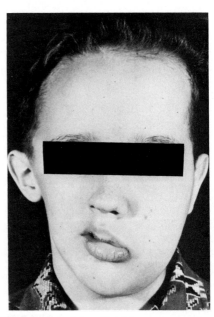

FIGURE 24–11. Left hemifacial hypertrophy. The condition was evident at birth. (From Sarnat, B.G., and Robinson, I.B.: Surgery of the mandible: Some clinical and experimental considerations. Plast. Reconstr. Surg. 17:27–57, 1956.) (See also Figure 12–21.)

Unilateral Hyperplasia of the Mandibular Condyle

This condition is generally characterized by a slowly developing, progressive, unilateral, symmetrical enlargement of the condyle and elongation of the mandibular neck causing facial asymmetry and shifting of the midline of the chin to the unaffected side resulting in a crossbite malocclusion (Obwegeser, 1986). In some instances, however, unilateral overgrowth of the mandible occurs without either clinical or radiographic evidence of enlargement of the condyle (Fig. 24–12). The ramus and the body of the mandible are longer and larger on the affected side giving a prognathic appearance. In contrast to unilateral hypoplasia, there is a compensatory eruption of the maxillary teeth and downward growth of the maxillary alveolar bone in an attempt to maintain occlusion. There is also compensatory eruption of the mandibular teeth resulting in increased alveolar height and a bowing effect on the inferior border of the mandible.

The discrepancy between the two sides of the mandible usually first becomes apparent during the second decade of life when, for reasons unknown, one condyle becomes more active than the other. In some cases trauma has been suspected as the cause (Lineaweaver, 1989). Rushton (1951) relates enlargement of the condyle to abnormally rapid chondrogenesis with subsequent ossification. Since the histologic picture is relatively normal, and the condition is self-limiting, it is not a truly neoplastic process. A chondroma, osteochondroma, or osteoma (Fig. 24–13) can produce a similar mandibular deformity but can usually be distin-

guished by the less regular shape and greater enlargement of the condyloid process, as well as by the more varied histologic pattern.

The treatment of unilateral condylar hyperplasia will depend on whether the condyle is still growing (Hampf, 1985). This can be determined by scintigraphy or by comparison of serial cephalometric radiographs taken at about six-month intervals. Condylectomy is the preferred treatment if there is still active growth (Sear, 1972). Sufficient tissue is removed to eradicate the growth site and permit simultaneous correction of the deviation. When a large shift of the mandible is necessary to re-establish a proper jaw relationship, a subcondylar osteotomy or an oblique osteotomy of the ramus should be done on the opposite side to limit rotation of that condyle and prevent postsurgical joint pain and dysfunction. Differential impaction of the maxilla at the Le Fort I level may also be necessary if there is a severe occlusal cant. Although considerable improvement is obtained, preoperative and postoperative orthodontic treatment is usually necessary to produce an exact occlusion. A genioplasty may help to correct the asymmetry of the chin. Minimal fullness of the face due to appositional growth of the lower border of the mandible on the affected side generally will lessen as a result of postsurgical remodeling. In severe cases, however, the excessive bone will have to be removed surgically. This can be done at the same time that the jaw is repositioned or, in borderline cases, as a secondary operation. The procedure can be accomplished via either an intraoral or extraoral approach.

If scintigraphy and/or serial radiographs show

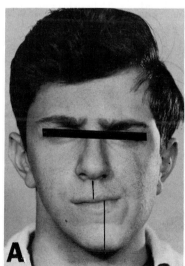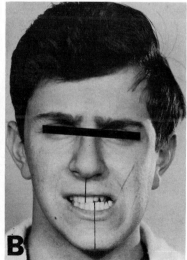

FIGURE 24–12. Unilateral overgrowth of the right mandible without clinical or radiographic evidence of condylar enlargement. The facial deformity was not discovered until the patient was in his early teens. (From Sarnat, B.G., and Robinson, I.B.: Surgery of the mandible: Some clinical and experimental considerations. Plast. Reconstr. Surg. *17*:27–57, 1956.)

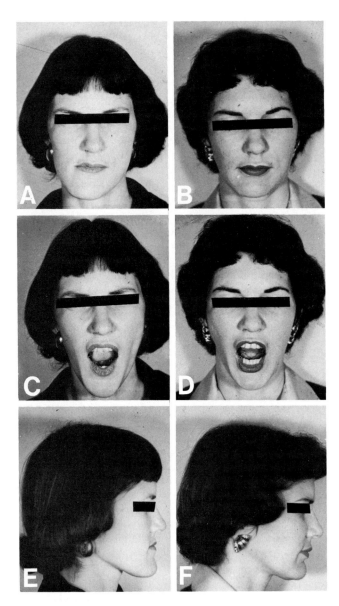

FIGURE 24–13. *A, C, E,* Preoperative and *B, D, F,* postoperative photographs of a patient with a left unilateral condylar osteoma resulting in increased length of the left side of the mandible and a crossbite malocclusion. Note in the preoperative photograph with the jaws in occlusion *(A)* that the middle of the chin deviates to the patient's right and with the mouth open *(C)* that the chin is in the midline (see Figure 24–30 and Table 24–2.)

that growth of the condyle has ceased, the facial deformity is corrected by shortening the affected side of the mandible. This is accomplished by either a subcondylar osteotomy or an oblique osteotomy of the ramus. For the same reason stated earlier, a subcondylar or oblique osteotomy is generally done on the opposite side. However, if the normal side is advanced as well as rotated, a sagittal ramus osteotomy is used. Maxillary surgery, genioplasty, and reduction of the inferior mandibular border may also be needed.

Mandibular Prognathism

The prognathic mandible is larger and in a more forward position than the maxilla so that the chin is unduly prominent. In addition, the normal maxillomandibular relationship between the teeth is disturbed so that the mandibular teeth are more anterior to the comparable ones in the maxilla. No definite etiologic factors have been implicated in true mandibular prognathism. It is possible that the prognathism may be a genetic problem that proceeds to unfold with growth.

While there may be considerable morphologic variation within the group of prognathic mandibles, they have the following common characteristic features: (1) the mandibular angle tends to be more obtuse than is normal, (2) the mandibular notch forms the arc of a larger circle, (3) the condyle is not enlarged, (4) the mandibular neck is longer and relatively nar-

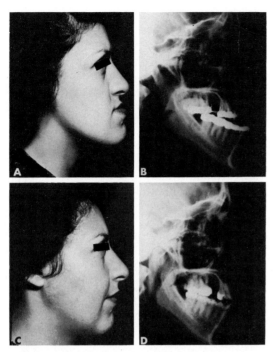

FIGURE 24–14. *A, C,* Preoperative and *B, D,* postoperative lateral photographs and radiographs of a patient with extreme bilateral mandibular prognathism of unknown etiology. Note the improved appearance of the profile after surgery was performed and the mandible was repositioned. Masticatory function was also considerably improved. (From Sarnat, B.G., and Robinson, I.B.: Surgery of the mandible: Some clinical and experimental considerations. Plast. Reconstr. Surg. *17:*27–57, 1956.)

rower than normal, (5) the linear distance between the superior aspect of the condyle and gnathion (lowest anterior point of the chin) is greater than in the normal mandible, and (6) impaction of the third molars generally does not occur because of the unusual length of the mandibular body. Less frequently seen is a unilateral mandibular prognathism with a crossbite malocclusion (see Fig. 24–12). The patient with a prognathic mandible presents for improvement of impaired masticatory function as well as cosmetic treatment (Fig. 24–14). The deformity may also be the cause of personality changes.

DIFFERENTIAL DIAGNOSIS

There are other conditions that give the appearance of mandibular prognathism that must be differentiated from the true type of prognathism previously mentioned. Hyperpituitarism (giantism, acromegaly) leads to an overgrowth and characteristic prognathism (see Fig. 24–16). A normal-sized lower jaw also may appear prominent because of a forward shift due to malposed teeth. Bilateral chronic anterior dis-

location also gives the appearance of prognathism (Fig. 24–15). In certain patients with cleft palate or achondroplasia the mandible is relatively prominent in comparison with an underdeveloped maxilla.

INDICATIONS AND CONTRAINDICATIONS FOR TREATMENT

The primary indications for surgical treatment of the prognathic mandible are the improvement of mastication and esthetics. Surgery is generally contraindicated, however, in individuals who are still growing. Recurrence of the prognathism is likely to develop when such patients are treated by means of a ramus cut or excision of part of the mandibular body because of continued growth in the condylar region. If growth of the mandible is altered by surgical treatment and maxillary growth still continues, a relative maxillary prognathism, which is possibly worse than the original deformity, may

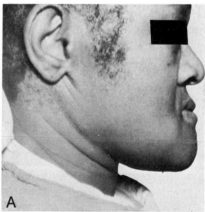

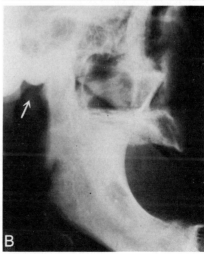

FIGURE 24–15. *A,* Lateral photograph and *B,* radiograph of a patient with a chronic bilateral anterior dislocation of the mandible. The arrow indicates the articular eminence.

appear some years later. Therefore, unless there are psychologic or other overriding reasons for earlier treatment, usually all surgical procedures should be postponed until the patient has attained, or nearly attained, adulthood. Radiographs of the wrists, as well as serial cephalometric radiographs, are helpful in determining the extent of the growth period since there appears to be a correlation between closure of the metacarpal epiphyses and cessation of mandibular growth. Scintigraphy can also be used. When surgery is performed during adolescence, the deformity should be overcorrected to allow for some adjustment to continued growth.

Medical contraindications to surgical treatment should also be considered. Moreover, patients with systemic conditions causing mandibular prognathism, such as hyperpituitarism, should not be treated for this local manifestation without full consideration of the larger problem (Fig. 24–16).

TREATMENT

Many different surgical procedures have been used for retroposition of the prognathic mandi-

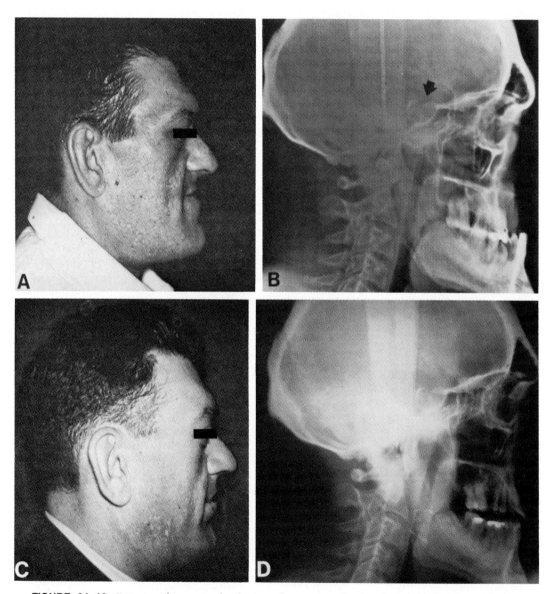

FIGURE 24–16. Patient with acromegaly showing characteristic facial and skeletal features, including mandibular prognathism. *A*, Lateral profile view preoperatively. *B*, Presurgical radiograph showing enlarged mandible and sella turcica (arrow). *C*, *D*, Postoperative result. Surgery was not done until treatment of the pituitary dysfunction had been accomplished and growth had ceased.

ble (Bell, 1980; Epker, 1986). In an endeavor to find the best surgical approach practically every portion of the mandible has been sectioned. Generally, however, the cuts can be classified into those concerned with the body, ramal, or subcondylar regions.

Although at one time the procedures used to treat mandibular prognathism were generally done from an extraoral approach, currently mainly intraoral techniques are used. The most common surgical operations are the sagittal ramus osteotomy and the oblique and vertical ramus osteotomies. The sagittal ramus osteotomy has the advantage of allowing the use of rigid fixation, thereby permitting the patient to open the mouth postoperatively. The disadvantage is the relatively high incidence of temporary inferior alveolar nerve paresthesia or anesthesia, with the occasional possibility that it can be permanent.

Surgical and orthodontic treatment complement each other in correction of the prognathic mandible. The former treatment permits extensive repositioning of the mandible, while the latter serves to eliminate tooth interference that might prevent a comfortable balanced occlusion. Postoperatively, moreover, the orthodontic appliance provides a positive means of controlling the jaw relations with the use of maxillomandibular rubber bands or wires.

Pituitary Dysfunction

Overactivity of the eosinophilic cells of the anterior lobe of the pituitary gland associated with giantism and acromegaly frequently affects growth of the mandible. In giantism, or hyperpituitarism of the adolescent, there is a proportionate overdevelopment of the osseous system because the epiphyses are still open. Sometimes massiveness and protrusion of the mandible are also noted. There is considerable disproportion between the size of the crowns of the teeth, which show no enlargement, and the large size of the jaw bones. In contrast to giantism, acromegaly or hyperpituitarism of the adult is characterized by the development of striking disharmonies of the body. Statural growth is basically not affected because the onset of the disease begins after the epiphyses have closed. The skeleton, however, shows increased density and overgrowth of osteophytic prominences due to subperiosteal bone deposition.

The central feature of the acromegalic changes in the skull is the enormous enlargement of the mandible (see Fig. 24–16). This is a result of the latent epiphyseal-like growth

potential of the cartilage of the mandibular condyle. Although the growth hormone stimulates periosteal appositional growth of the other facial bones, this does not keep pace with the excessive endochondral condylar growth. As a result, the mandible grows out of proportion to the maxilla. The tongue also becomes greatly enlarged and is responsible for compensatory bone apposition along the anterior surface of the mandible and spacing between the teeth. Correction of the mandibular prognathism should not be undertaken until overactivity of the pituitary is controlled. The patient can then be treated as any other case of prognathism (see Fig. 24–16).

ARTHRITIS (see Chapters 11 and 22)

Infectious

Infectious arthritis of the TMJ may be part of a generalized systemic disease, resulting either from localization of blood-borne organisms from a distant infection, or arise from direct extension of an adjacent infection. It is characterized by inflammation, pain, and limited mandibular movement. When systemic in origin, there will also be the symptoms of the associated disease. If suppuration is present, aspiration of the joint may confirm the diagnosis and identify the causative organism(s). The findings on the radiographs are usually negative in the early stages, but several weeks later may show evidence of bone destruction.

The management of infectious arthritis includes specific antibiotic therapy, application of moist heat, proper diet and hydration, control of pain, and restriction of motion. Early treatment will result either in resolution of the infection or in a localized accumulation of suppurative material within the joint. In the latter instance, aspiration or incision and drainage through a preauricular incision is indicated. Extensive bone necrosis requires removal of the devitalized bone. If the condyloid process is involved, sequestrectomy is usually synonymous with condylectomy. When the destructive process has also extended to the ramus, a submandibular approach offers greater accessibility than a preauricular exposure for removal of the necrotic bone and drainage.

Once the infection has been controlled, exercising the mandible will usually bring about a normal range of motion when there is only a minimal amount of tissue damage. The intra-articular injection of hyaluronidase or cortisone is sometimes used to soften scar tissue. In other instances, active gentle stretching by mechanical devices may be of some aid in overcoming the resultant fibrosis (Connole, 1988). Appliances must be used with extreme caution because rapid expansion can tear tissue, cause hemorrhage and edema, and ultimately result in increased scarring. When either extreme limitation of motion or complete ankylosis has occurred, surgical intervention is generally necessary. When the condyloid process and portions of the ramus have been destroyed due to associated osteomyelitis, the TMJ may need to be reconstructed. In the child, a rib transplant is used to provide a new growth site. In the adult, rib, iliac crest, or an alloplast can be used to replace the lost tissue.

Traumatic

Traumatic arthritis can be caused by an acute injury or excessive opening of the mouth such as occurs with wide yawning, posterior tooth extraction, or endotracheal intubation. There is pain, joint tenderness, and limitation of jaw movement. The radiographs are usually noncontributory except when there is a widening of the joint space due to intra-articular edema or hemorrhage.

In cases of traumatic arthritis uncomplicated by the presence of a fracture, the treatment consists of the use of an analgesic, the application of moist heat for 20 to 30 minutes four times a day, and restriction of mandibular activity. Restriction of mandibular activity may be accomplished by using a head-chin strap or maxillomandibular fixation. Generally, however, the patient voluntarily tends to limit motion because of the associated muscle spasm, pain, and tenderness. A soft, nonchewy diet also enables the patient to restrict joint movement.

When the injury has been mild, the symptoms will gradually disappear leaving no residual disability. When the damage has been more severe, the morphological and functional disturbances in the joint may ultimately lead to symptoms and articular changes resembling those found in secondary degenerative arthritis. Arthroplasty or high condylectomy may sometimes be necessary in such cases. In the child, injury to the cartilaginous growth site in the condyle may subsequently also be manifested by severe facial deformity, which requires surgical correction (see section on condylar hypoplasia). Parents should be informed of this possibility and the patient should be followed by the use of serial cephalometric radiographs to identify early changes.

Rheumatoid

Involvement of the TMJ is a relatively frequent finding in patients with rheumatoid arthritis (Franks, 1969). Both children (see Fig. 24–7) and adults are affected. In the child, destruction of the condylar growth site can result in facial deformity.

The treatment of rheumatoid arthritis of the TMJ is similar to that for other joints in the body (Zide, 1986). During the acute stage, nonsteroidal anti-inflammatory drugs are used, along with a soft diet, moist heat, and limitation of jaw function. In severe cases, second-line drugs such as hydroxychloroquine, gold, and penicillamine may be used to control the pain and inflammation. As the symptoms subside, mild jaw exercises may help prevent loss of motion. In some patients the disease progresses to ankylosis despite any form of therapy. For these patients, surgical intervention, when the disease process is no longer active, is usually the only treatment offering any measure of assistance (see section on ankylosis, page 408). In those patients with facial deformity and/or an anteriorly opened bite, orthodontics and orthognathic surgery can be used to help correct these conditions.

Degenerative (Osteoarthritis, Osteoarthrosis)

Degenerative arthritis of the TMJ takes two forms—primary and secondary. Although the pathologic changes are similar, the etiologic factors differ. Primary degenerative arthritis is caused by the normal wear and tear associated with aging and usually begins around the fifth decade. Severe malocclusion or a mutilated dentition can contribute to the process and hasten its appearance.

The onset of primary degenerative arthritis is usually insidious and the symptoms are relatively mild. Generally, they consist of slight cracking or crepitation on jaw movement. Pain is an infrequent symptom. Radiographically, there is usually evidence of some subcondylar sclerosis, condylar flattening, and lipping in both joints. Patients seldom complain about the condition. Treatment, if necessary, consists of mild analgesics when pain is present, and correction of any dental impairment that may be contributing to jaw dysfunction.

Secondary degenerative arthritis usually occurs in the 20- to 40-year age group and produces more severe symptoms than primary degenerative arthritis. It is generally a sequel to chronic myofascial pain-dysfunction (MPD) syndrome (see Chapter 19); therefore, the symptoms relate to both conditions. Trauma may also be a causative factor. Pain in the TMJ, masticatory muscle pain and tenderness, crepitus, and limited jaw movement are the usual symptoms. Subcondylar sclerosis, condylar flattening, lipping of bone on the anterior aspect of the condyle, and spur formation or erosions on the articular surface are frequently seen in the radiographs. Most often, the condition involves only one joint.

Treatment is directed toward relief of the pain and improving function. This is accomplished by the appropriate application of moist heat or diathermy to the joint region as well as the involved muscles, use of a soft, nonchewy diet, and restricted jaw motion. Use of a nonsteroidal anti-inflammatory analgesic such as aspirin or ibuprofen, as well as a drug with muscle-relaxing properties such as diazepam, also helps relieve joint and muscle pain. Since psychological stress is usually a contributing factor to MPD syndrome, diazepam serves a double function when this condition is also present. The use of a bite plate is also beneficial in lessening masticatory muscle spasm and pain. Once the acute symptoms are controlled in patients in whom the arthritis is associated with MPD syndrome, further efforts must be directed toward elimination of this condition to halt the progress of the arthritic process (see Chapter 21).

In the early stages of secondary degenerative arthritis, there are no indications for surgical intervention. Although the pathologic changes that occur in the TMJ may not be completely reversible, conservative treatment can result in complete subsidence of both joint and muscle

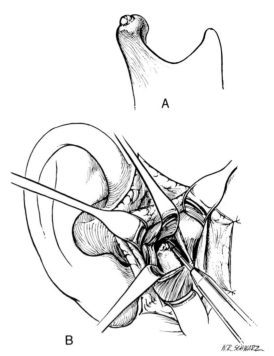

FIGURE 24-17. Diagram showing temporomandibular joint arthroplasty. This procedure is used when there are minimal bony changes in the condyle. A, Exostosis on articular surface. B, Smoothing of articular surface with a bur. (From Laskin, D.M.: Surgical management of diseases of the temporomandibular joint. In Hayward, J. (Ed.): Oral Surgery. Springfield, IL, Charles C Thomas, 1976.)

symptoms with little or no impairment of function (Greene, 1976). Even in the later stages, with proper care, the degenerating surfaces of the articulating bones may readjust to each other and the patient will have relative comfort. When the degenerative changes are so ad-

FIGURE 24-18. Diagram showing high condylectomy performed from a preauricular approach. A, Level of osteotomy. B, Cut made above attachment of lateral pterygoid muscle preserving function. C, Appearance of remaining portion of condyle after recontouring. (From Laskin, D.M.: Surgical management of diseases of the temporomandibular joint. In Hayward, J. (Ed.): Oral Surgery. Springfield, IL, Charles C Thomas, 1976.)

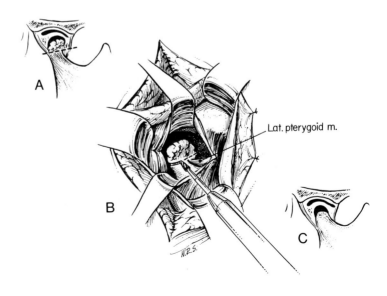

vanced that conservative treatment gives little or no relief of pain, surgical management is indicated. Such treatment consists of either an arthroplasty to smooth bony irregularities (Fig. 24–17) or a high condylectomy to eliminate any eroded areas and still preserve the attachment of the lateral pterygoid muscle (James, 1971) (Fig. 24–18).

SUBLUXATION

Subluxation is usually defined as a self-reducing, partial dislocation of a joint. When referring to the TMJ this definition implies that the condyle passes anterior to the articular eminence during the opening movement. Tomographic analysis of the range of mandibular motion has shown, however, that in many individuals the condyle normally may be located as much as 5 millimeters anterior to the summit of the eminence when the mouth is in a wide-open position. This condition can, therefore, be termed subluxation only if other symptoms such as pain, temporary locking, or popping noises accompany the anterior positioning of the condyle.

Subluxation, a symptom complex rather than a disease, results from an abnormal looseness of the capsule. This may follow unrestrained yawning, acute trauma such as a blow, dislocation of the mandible, convulsions, or excessive manipulation of the jaw during such procedures as endotracheal intubation or dental extraction, particularly when the patient is under general anesthesia. It also occurs in Parkinson's disease (Merrill, 1968) and Ehlers-Danlos syndrome, a disorder of connective tissue characterized by hyperextensibility of the joints (Goodman, 1969). Looseness of the capsule also may follow the chronic degenerative changes of prolonged osteoarthritis.

Since subluxation is associated with wide mouth opening, conscious limitation of movement can eliminate the problem in many instances. Such actions as unrestrained yawning or taking large bites of food should be avoided. The patient should be trained to open synchronously, with only a hinge movement, and any unilateral chewing habit should be corrected. Isometric exercises to strengthen the jaw closing muscles are also beneficial in preventing subluxation. In addition to these measures, attention must be given to correction or treatment of any existing etiologic conditions.

Most patients can be managed successfully by these methods. In those patients with extreme laxity of the capsule and ligaments who continue to have popping and locking, injection of a sclerosing solution can be used to produce fibrosis of the capsule and thereby restrict excessive motion (see next section on dislocation). Surgery is generally not indicated for the treatment of subluxation.

DISLOCATION

A dislocation may be defined as a derangement between the articulating components of a joint that is not self-reducing. Dislocation of the TMJ may occur as a result of: (1) external trauma, especially when the mouth is open, (2) sudden wide opening, as while yawning or during an epileptic seizure, (3) prolonged wide opening of the mouth during dental, oral, and pharyngeal procedures, (4) extreme capsular laxity associated with chronic subluxation, and (5) muscular discoordination from drugs (Kraak, 1967) or neurological disorders. The dislocation may be unilateral or bilateral. In some instances, the patient may have a history of recurrent dislocations.

Although the TMJ is capable of an extreme range of motion, dislocation is generally limited to an anterior direction. Because of the posterior and superior bony boundaries of the glenoid fossa, dislocation in these directions is possible only when the external force applied to the mandible is so extreme as to cause a fracture of the temporal bone. Since the mandible is a single bone and both TMJs function as a unit, the medial boundary of one side also serves to limit lateral displacement on the other side. Thus, lateral dislocation can occur only when associated with a contralateral fracture of the neck of the condyloid process.

In an anterior dislocation, the condyle is displaced in front of, and superior to, the articular eminence (see Fig. 24–15). When bilaterally dislocated, the mandible is held in an open position with only the posterior maxillary and mandibular teeth, if present, contacting (Fig. 24–19), (Table 24–3). In unilateral dislocation there is also an open bite, but the midline of the chin is deviated toward the normal side (Fig. 24–20) (Table 24–3).

Dislocations should be reduced as soon as possible before there is severe muscle spasm. Reduction can be accomplished by manually pressing the mandible downward to stretch the spastic elevator muscles and then backward to relocate the condyle within the fossa. If done early, the procedure generally can be accom-

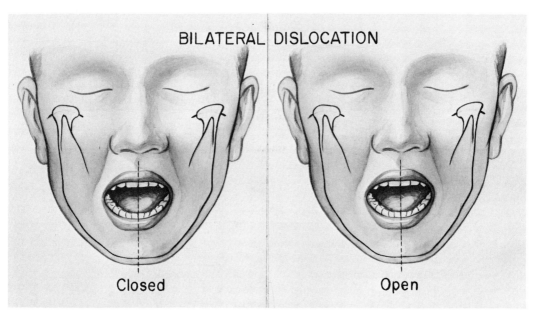

FIGURE 24–19. Diagrammatic illustration of the clinical features in a patient with a bilateral anterior dislocation of the condyloid process. The jaws are held in a wide-open position and there is relatively little change when an attempt is made to close the mouth (see Table 24–3).

plished without the aid of anesthesia. In delayed reductions, the use of either a local anesthetic injected into the joint and lateral pterygoid muscle (Johnson, 1958), or the administration of intravenous diazepam and a narcotic to relieve the muscular spasm and lessen the pain may be beneficial. When ineffective, general anesthesia can be used to provide adequate relaxation. Once reduction has been accomplished, the mandible should be immobilized for several days by means of a head-chin strap or maxillomandibular fixation. This facilitates repair of the capsule and readjustment of muscular balance, and prevents a redislocation

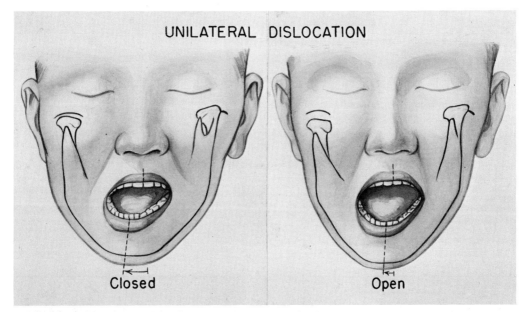

FIGURE 24–20. Diagrammatic illustration of the clinical features in a patient with a unilateral anterior dislocation of the left condyloid process. The jaws are held in an open position with the midline of the chin deviated to the normal side. Upon attempted further opening, the midline shifts to a more central position (see Table 24–3).

TABLE 24–3. The Position of the Midline of the Chin and Other Clinical Findings

Condition	MIDLINE OF CHIN		Facial Deformity
	Mouth Closed	Mouth Open	
NORMAL	No deviation	No deviation	None
ANTERIOR DISLOCATION (UNILATERAL) (FIG. 24–20)	Deviation to unaffected side	Deviation is decreased	Prominence of chin on the unaffected side
ANTERIOR DISLOCATION (BILATERAL) (FIG. 24–19)	No deviation	No deviation	Symmetrical prominence of chin
FRACTURED DISLOCATED CONDYLOID PROCESS (UNILATERAL) (FIGS. 24–22, 24–24)	No deviation	Deviation to affected side	May have swelling in associated areas of trauma or fracture
FRACTURED DISLOCATED CONDYLOID PROCESS (BILATERAL) (FIG. 24–23)	No deviation	No deviation	Retropositioning of mandible
PARTIAL ANKYLOSIS WITHOUT GROWTH ARREST (UNILATERAL)	No deviation	Deviation to affected side	None
PARTIAL ANKYLOSIS WITH GROWTH ARREST (UNILATERAL) (FIGS. 24–8, 24–26)	Deviation to affected side	Deviation is increased	Unaffected side flat; chin appears prominent on affected side
TUMOR OF CONDYLE (FIGS. 24–13, 24–30)	Deviation to unaffected side	Deviation is decreased	Chin appears prominent on unaffected side
GROWTH ARREST (UNILATERAL)	Deviation to affected side	Deviation is increased	Unaffected side flat; chin appears prominent on affected side
GROWTH ARREST (BILATERAL) (FIG. 24–7)	No deviation	No deviation	Symmetrical underdevelopment of chin and mandible

in the Differential Diagnosis of Temporomandibular Joint Conditions

| | CONDYLAR MOTION | | |
Occlusion	Unaffected Side	Affected Side	Degree of Opening
Normal	Hinge and glide	Hinge and glide	Normal
Mandibular teeth buccal to maxillary on unaffected side	Hinge and glide	Slight hinge and rotation	Limited by muscle spasm on affected side
Premature molar contact and anteriorly opened bite	—	Slight hinge	Mandible fixed in limited open position
Usually unchanged	Hinge and glide	None	Limited
Premature molar contact and anteriorly opened bite	—	None	Very limited
Usually unchanged	Hinge and glide	Slight hinge	Limited
Distal positioning of mandibular teeth on affected side; often lingual occlusion on unaffected side	Hinge and glide	Slight hinge	Limited
Mandibular teeth buccal to maxillary on unaffected side (crossbite)	Hinge and glide	Hinge or hinge and glide	Relatively normal
Distal positioning of mandibular teeth on affected side; often lingual occlusion on unaffected side	Hinge and glide	Hinge and glide	Relatively normal
Retropositioning of mandibular teeth	—	Hinge and glide	Relatively normal

while the tissues are still lax. If the joint was normal at the time that dislocation occurred, this treatment should be adequate to restore proper function. In instances where dislocation followed extreme capsular laxity, however, there may be a tendency toward repeated episodes. Under such circumstances, more definitive treatment is usually indicated.

Treatment of recurrent dislocation with the intra-articular injection of a sclerosing solution, such as tincture of iodine, was first recommended by Hartisch in 1883. Sodium psylliate, sodium morrhuate, sodium sotradecel, and eucupine or intracaine in oil have been used to produce fibrosis of the capsule, and thereby restrict excessive motion (Schultz, 1956). It has been claimed, on the basis of certain animal experiments, that these materials cause no histologically demonstrable changes in any of the other structures of the joint (Moose, 1941; Schultz, 1956). Some, however, believe that an agent that can produce sclerosis of the capsule may very likely also affect the blood vessels in the posterior aspect of the joint and the synovial membrane, and thus ultimately lead to further degenerative changes (Bellinger, 1948). To avoid this possibility, the sclerosing solution should be injected into the capsular tissue surrounding the condyloid process rather than directly into the joint space (Gerry, 1947). Despite its seeming simplicity, complications can follow the misapplication or excessive use of sclerosing solutions (Schwartz, 1968).

Five basic surgical methods have been recommended for the correction of recurrent dislocation of the TMJ: (1) mechanical tightening of the capsule, (2) fastening parts of the joint or mandible to adjacent fixed structures, (3) creating mechanical interferences in the condylar path, (4) elimination of interference with the condylar path, and (5) reduction of muscle pull. The exact way in which these objectives have been accomplished varies considerably.

Tightening of the capsule by excision of the redundant tissue is perhaps the simplest of the surgical techniques (Perthes, 1907). This procedure is usually somewhat more effective than simple plication. Limitation of motion has also been produced by fastening the coronoid process to the zygomatic arch with wire, catgut suture, or mersaline tape (Blake, 1918; Merrill, 1968); suturing fascia from the temporal or mastoid region to the lateral aspect of the capsule (Link, 1933; Nieden, 1923) or through the condyle (Gordon, 1955); or by sewing the disc to the periosteum of the glenoid fossa or to the capsule (Annandale, 1887). Mechanical

blocks in the condylar path have been created by placing the articular disc in a vertical position anterior to the condyle (Konjetzny, 1921), by increasing the height of the articular eminence (Lindemann, 1925), by placing bone (zygomatic, tibial) or cartilage (rib) implants between the condyle and the eminence (Mayer, 1933), by using metal implants (Buckley, 1988), and by in-fracturing of the zygomatic arch (Gosserez, 1967; LeClerc, 1943). Conversely, eminectomy has been done to eliminate interference with the condylar path (Myrhaug, 1951).

A relatively good success rate has been reported with most of the surgical procedures except those that attempt to produce limitation by anchoring the mandible to adjacent structures. The reason for such diverse methods being effective appears to be related to one common factor: all of the procedures are intra-articular operations that obviously produce capsular scarring. When the etiologic factors originally leading to laxity of the capsule and ligaments are no longer active, such scarring is sufficient to obtain improvement. Since similar effects can be produced more easily and safely, however, with proper injection of a sclerosing solution, this is preferable to surgery in most cases (Laskin, 1976).

The reason that the sclerosing technique and the surgical procedures described sometimes fail is related to a persistence of the factors causing looseness of the capsule and ligaments. As an example, the patient with uncontrollable epilepsy or severe parkinsonism will continue to stretch these structures and eventually dislocation will recur. For such individuals, if one or two attempts at sclerosis fail, a permanent cure can be achieved by bilateral lateral pterygoid myotomy (Laskin, 1972; Miller, 1976; Sindet-Pedersen, 1988). Detachment of these muscles limits anterior translation of the condyles and thereby confines them to the glenoid fossae.

There have been cases reported (Chin, 1988; Gottlieb, 1952; Hayward, 1965; Topazian, 1967; Watanabe, 1950) in which acute dislocations were not reduced immediately and in which simple manual reduction eventually became impossible either due to contracture of the spastic musculature, severe fibrosis, or bony remodeling changes in both the condyle and fossa (see Fig. 24–15). Such cases of protracted dislocation often can be treated by manual manipulation aided by downward traction using transosseous wires placed through the angles of the mandible (Hayward, 1965). If this procedure fails, temporalis myotomy performed through an intraoral vertical incision over the anterior border of the ramus is generally effective (Laskin, 1972). As a last resort, direct open manipulation of the condyle, subcondylar osteotomy, or condylectomy have been recommended (Topazian, 1967).

FRACTURES

Although trauma to the mandible may result in only transitory injury to the soft tissue components of the TMJ, it may also produce a fracture of the condyloid process. In adults, the most common causes are manual blows, automobile accidents, or industrial mishaps. In children, fractures are most often due to a fall. Improper application of obstetrical forceps during breech delivery occasionally results in fractures in the newborn infant. Frequently this is associated with varying degrees of facial paralysis, fractures of the clavicle, and bruising of the overlying tissues. A battered infant also may sustain a fracture of the condyloid process (Fig. 24–21).

Fractures of the condyloid process are commonly referred to as condylar fractures. Although some fractures involve the intracapsular portion and are therefore true condylar fractures, most often the fracture occurs across the mandibular neck, which is the thinnest part of the condyloid process. Such fractures are more correctly termed subcondylar or condyloid process fractures. Fractures beginning in the mandibular notch and extending downward and backward are oblique fractures of the ramus rather than subcondylar fractures since the con-

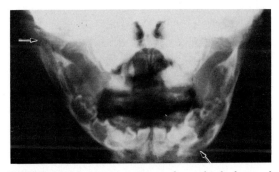

FIGURE 24–21. Anteroposterior radiograph of a battered seven-week-old infant. Note fracture and dislocation of right condyloid process and displaced fragments of left body of mandible (arrows). The fracture of the left body was treated with a splint and circumferential wiring. The condyloid fracture was not treated. A deformity developed subsequently. (From Sarnat, B.G.: Experimental and clinical postnatal craniofacial changes. Surg. Gynecol. Obstet. *148*:659–669, 1979. By permission of Surgery, Gynecology & Obstetrics.)

dyloid process remains intact. In those oblique fractures occurring high on the ramus, however, the condyle may sometimes be dislocated from the fossa.

Fractures of the condyloid process may be unilateral or bilateral. Bilateral fractures generally occur when the force is applied directly to the chin. When the blow has been directed to the side of the mandible, usually only the contralateral condyloid process is fractured. There are exceptions, however, in both instances. Unilateral fracture of the condyloid process is often combined with a fracture of the body of the mandible in the region of the mental foramen on the opposite side.

More important than the level of the fracture is the amount of displacement or dislocation. The degree and direction of displacement will not only depend upon the location of the fracture, but also on the direction of force causing it, the position of the jaw at the time the force was applied (mouth open or closed), the pull of the lateral pterygoid muscle, and the presence of associated fractures in the body or ramus. There are a great variety of positions that the fractured condyloid process may assume. Most commonly, however, there is a medial or anteromedial tipping or dislocation. Lateral displacement is next in frequency of occurrence.

Diagnosis

The recognition of fractures of the condyloid process depends upon the history, clinical examination, and interpretation of the radiographs. One should always consider the possibility of such a fracture when there is a history of a blow to the chin or clinical evidence of trauma in that region. In a unilateral fracture, lateral excursion to the normal side is generally limited and the chin deviates to the affected side during the opening movement (Fig. 24–22) (see Table 24–3). In a bilateral fracture there is frequently an anteriorly opened bite. Lateral excursion and protrusion cannot be performed and there may be difficulty in opening the mouth (Fig. 24–23) (see Table 24–3).

In addition to the condyloid process, the roof of the glenoid fossa or the tympanic plate can also be fractured. The presence of blood in the external auditory canal may be a sign of involvement of the tympanic plate and/or an associated fracture of the base of the skull.

The final diagnosis of a fracture of the condyloid process will depend upon the radiographic findings. For proper interpretation, a minimum of a panoramic radiograph and lateral

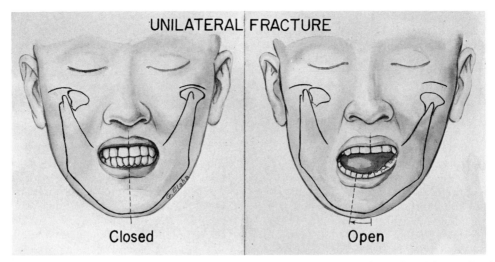

FIGURE 24–22. Diagrammatic illustration of the clinical features in a patient with a unilateral fractured and dislocated right condyloid process. When the mouth is closed, there may be malocclusion with deviation of the mandible toward the fractured side. When the mouth is opened, the chin deviates further to the affected side (see Table 24–3).

oblique and posteroanterior views of the mandible are necessary. Use of a single projection often gives a false impression of the position of the condyloid process. Only by tomography or by comparing radiographs taken at about right angles to each other can the exact location be determined (see Chapter 16).

Treatment

Fractures of the condyloid process can be treated by: (1) closed reduction and maxillo-

mandibular fixation, or (2) open reduction and fixation with transosseous wires, metallic plates, or pins. In the closed method, although an attempt can be made to accomplish reduction by manipulation of the mandible or by placing a block between the upper and lower posterior teeth, most often such procedures are unsuccessful. In actuality, therefore, the closed method principally refers to immobilization of the jaws in occlusion and allowing the condyloid process to remain in its displaced position.

When there is minimal or no displacement,

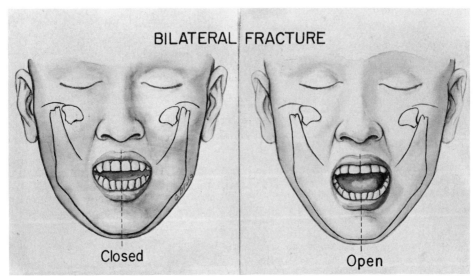

FIGURE 24–23. Diagrammatic illustration of the clinical features in a patient with bilaterally fractured and dislocated condyloid processes. When the teeth are occluded, there is a premature molar contact and a resulting anteriorly opened bite. The ability to open the mouth is limited. When opening is attempted, the midline of the chin does not deviate (see Table 24–3).

fractures of the condyloid process can be satisfactorily treated by closed reduction and maxillomandibular fixation. There are divided opinions, however, concerning the management of the fractured, dislocated condyloid process. Some surgeons believe that these should be treated by the closed method as well (Lyons, 1947; Dessner, 1958; MacLennan, 1965). In favor of this concept is both clinical and experimental evidence that relatively normal function can be maintained even after subcondylar osteotomy (Spilka, 1956; Verne, 1957) or condylectomy (Gonzalez-Ulloa, 1956; Sarnat, 1971b; Swanson, 1959). Those who favor open reduction argue that patients with unreduced, fractured, displaced condyloid processes sometimes develop degenerative arthritis, open bite, or even ankylosis (Richardson, 1953; Thoma, 1945; Wassmund, 1934; Zide, 1983). They emphasize, moreover, the fact that in young individuals normal facial growth and muscle balance will not take place if there is failure of the condyloid process to unite with the rest of the mandible, or if union occurs but the alignment is abnormal (Jarabak, 1954) (Fig. 24–24). Nevertheless, some consideration must also be given to the possibility that condylar damage and retarded

growth can result from both the injury and the surgery. Moreover, in some cases, an overgrowth on the side of condylar fracture has been reported (Lineaweaver, 1989; Lund, 1974).

The most rational approach to the treatment of the fractured, displaced condyloid process seems to be based upon the following factors: (1) the age of the patient, (2) whether the fracture is unilateral or bilateral, (3) whether the patient has adequate teeth for fixation, (4) the level at which the condyloid process is fractured, (5) whether or not the fragments are in contact, and (6) whether the condyle is within the glenoid fossa. Consideration must also be given to the general condition of the patient and to the time that has elapsed since the injury.

A fractured, severely dislocated condyloid process in a young actively growing individual, whether unilateral or bilateral, should generally be treated by open reduction to lessen the possibility of subsequent facial deformity (Laskin, 1976). There is, however, no unanimity of opinion (Amaratunga, 1988; Gilhuus-Moe, 1969) (see Fig. 24–24). Leake (1971) did not suggest even immobilization of the mandible.

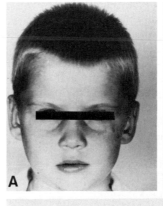
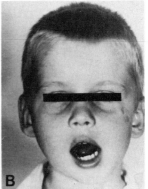
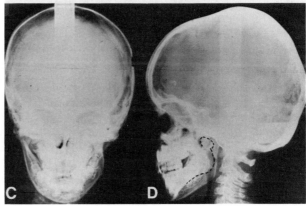

FIGURE 24–24. View of child with a history of severe fracture and dislocation of the left mandibular condyloid process. *A*, Closed-mouth view and *B*, open-mouth view of same child. Note the accentuation of the deformity. *C*, *D*, Radiographs showing short, wide condyloid process and short ramus on the side of injury. Note in *C* the vertical direction of the ramus on the side of injury compared with the oblique inclination of the ramus on the uninjured side. (From Sarnat, B.G.: Normal and abnormal craniofacial growth. Angle Orthod. 53:263–289, 1983.)

Others, including the authors, do not concur (MacLennan, 1969).

In patients who have attained maximal facial development, open reduction is seldom indicated, with the following possible exceptions: when the malpositioned condyloid process may interfere with motion of the jaw; in the case of a unilaterally dislocated condyloid process with no occluding teeth on the involved side; or when the condyloid processes are bilaterally fractured and dislocated. Even in the last instance some surgeons believe that if sufficient teeth are present, the use of maxillomandibular fixation alone will allow for the reorganization of the tissue between the ramus and the glenoid fossa so that an open bite will not result. In edentulous patients, their artificial dentures, in conjunction with a head-chin strap or skeletal suspension and interdental fixation, may be used to maintain the maxillomandibular relationship.

Open reduction of a fractured condyloid process is accomplished best by use of a retromandibular incision. Such an approach provides direct access to the fracture site, does not require extensive muscle detachment, and permits holes to be drilled without difficulty for transosseous wires or for the insertion of plates and screws. The reduction of a medially dislocated condyloid process can be facilitated by using a muscle relaxant such as succinylcholine. Downward traction on the mandible by means of a wire inserted through the bone at the angle may also be helpful in providing better access.

Maxillomandibular fixation following either open or closed reduction of a fracture of the condyloid process is maintained for a shorter period than with fractures in other parts of the jaw. In children, gentle active motion is generally encouraged after an interval of two to three weeks. In the adult, fixation is maintained for three to four weeks. This procedure is used to lessen the possibility of ankylosis during the reparative process. After treatment of the fracture has been completed, any minor discrepancies in the occlusion should be corrected by judicious grinding of the teeth. This decreases the chance for the development of postoperative degenerative arthritis in the joints. Although alignment of the fractured condyloid process may not be anatomically correct, function is generally quite satisfactory and, with time, bone remodeling usually occurs (Lindahl, 1977).

ANKYLOSIS

Ankylosis may be defined as a chronic limitation of motion in a joint (see Chapter 10). It

TABLE 24–4. Causes of Ankylosis of the Mandible

I. Congenital
II. Traumatic (direct and indirect; local and regional)
    A. At birth
    B. Later
        1. Accidental (fractures, including displaced fracture of zygomatic arch; hemarthrosis)
        2. Surgical (scarring)
III. Inflammatory
    A. Local
    B. Regional
        1. Otitis media and mastoiditis
        2. Osteomyelitis of mandible, dental and parotid abscesses, etc.
        3. Radionecrosis (soft tissue and bone)
        4. Noma
    C. Hematogenous
        1. Osteomyelitis
        2. Scarlet fever
        3. Gonorrhea
IV. Neoplastic
    A. Local
    B. Regional, including osteochondroma of coronoid process
V. Idiopathic, including rheumatoid arthritis and enlarged coronoid processes

may be partial or complete, fibrous or bony, intra-articular (true) or extra-articular (false), and unilateral or bilateral. Combinations of these occur. If left untreated, ankylosis interferes with ingestion, mastication, oral hygiene, and speech. Frequently, but not always, associated with ankylosis is a deformity of the mandible (Blair, 1928) (see Figs. 24–5 and 24–8).

Etiology

There are many causes of ankylosis of the TMJ (Table 24–4). Ankylosis on a prenatal basis is not common and may be related to abnormalities of the joint, ramus, or temporal and zygomatic bone complex. Since the condition is usually not discovered until some months after birth, there is often difficulty in determining whether it was prenatal or postnatal in origin.

Most frequently, ankylosis results from trauma. Injury to the joint structures, associated muscles, and adjacent soft tissues causes hemorrhage and inflammation. The subsequent fibrosis and/or bone formation can produce permanent limitation of motion. At birth, trauma may be caused by forces sustained directly to the joint region or transmitted from another part of the mandible during forceps or breech delivery. Some degree of facial paresis or paralysis may be noted immediately after the injury.

Trauma occurring later in life can also produce ankylosis. Often the injury to the joint occurs indirectly from a blow on the chin. An extra-articular ankylosis may result from trauma to the coronoid process, a depressed zygomatic arch, scarring associated with a burn (Schwartz, 1976), or with the use of cautery in the treatment of intraoral carcinoma.

Inflammation on an infectious basis is another important cause of ankylosis. Primary infection of the TMJ is uncommon. The local spread of a regional infection to the joint is more frequent. In the past, otitis media often led to suppurative infections in the TMJ. Since the advent of antibiotics, this complication is seldom seen.

Ankylosis may also result secondary to the spread of a dental infection. In this instance the extra-articular tissues rather than the joint itself may be involved. A similar sequence of events may occur subsequent to the noninfectious inflammation in patients (young and old) who have received radiation for benign or malignant tumors in the region. In the preceding conditions, generally only one joint is directly involved.

Unilateral or bilateral intra-articular ankylosis can also be caused by the hematogenous spread of infection and by certain general inflammatory joint involvements. The acute nonsuppurative polyarthritis of rheumatic fever may include the TMJs and there may be some limitation of joint movement both early and late. This is also true of the suppurative arthritis of gonococcal origin. The organisms responsible for osteomyelitis at a distant site may spread via the blood stream to the TMJ and set up a new focus with resulting ankylosis and growth arrest (see Fig. 24–8). Rheumatoid arthritis is another cause of ankylosis (see Chapters 10 and 11).

Neoplasms are an infrequent primary cause of ankylosis of the TMJ. They seldom arise within the joint. More often, a tumor, such as an osteochondroma or an enlargement of the coronoid process (Fig. 24–25), may cause limitation of motion because of impingement on the zygomatic arch (Lyon, 1963). A double condyle has also been reported as a cause of ankylosis (Stadnicki, 1971; To, 1989). Spread of benign or malignant lesions from regions adjacent to the mandible will also produce limited jaw movement.

Findings

Generally no facial asymmetry will be noted in patients with ankylosis of the TMJ unassociated with condylar growth arrest or loss of tissue (see Table 24–3). In a unilateral partial ankylosis, however, there may be a slight shifting of the midline of the chin to the affected side when an attempt is made to open the mouth. This is a direct result of the condyle gliding downward and forward on the unaffected side and remaining relatively immobile on the affected side. Palpation of the condyles by inserting a finger into each external auditory canal or by placing a finger just anterior to the tragus of the ear may reveal whether there is motion when the patient opens and closes the mouth. Radiographic studies will usually disclose changes in the TMJ, with obliteration of the normal landmarks and often a large radiopaque area in the region normally occupied by the condyle and the articular space. The bony enlargement may extend to include the region of the mandibular neck, the mandibular notch, the coronoid process, and the zygomatic arch.

When ankylosis is associated with either a growth arrest (see Table 24–3) or loss of tissue, the resultant deformity is quite apparent. If the patient is able to open the mouth slightly, the deviation of the mandible to the affected side may be exaggerated even further (Fig. 24–26). Ankylosis and facial deformity, however, need not occur together. In patients who demonstrate an almost complete inability to open the mouth, but in whom condylar growth has not been affected, such as in a false or extra-articular ankylosis, there is no deformity of the mandible. In addition, when the TMJ has been affected on only one side by condylar growth arrest and ankylosis, the characteristic findings are not seen on the opposite nonankylosed side of the mandible, which has only a limitation of motion (see Figs. 24–5 and 24–8). On the other hand, a child may have a middle ear infection that spreads to the TMJ and affects both the condylar growth site and joint function. As a result, both ankylosis and growth deformity occur, although the latter is not apparent until later.

Treatment

Because of the slow progress of the condition, the patient with ankylosis may not be seen by the doctor for months or even years after the onset. In those few instances in which there is minimal scarring and one has decided to attempt dilation of the jaws, use of a constant mild force repeated at intervals is preferable to a short-acting powerful one such as use of a mouth prop under general anesthesia. The mild force may stretch the scar, whereas the powerful sudden one will tear the scar causing hemorrhage, producing more scar, and making

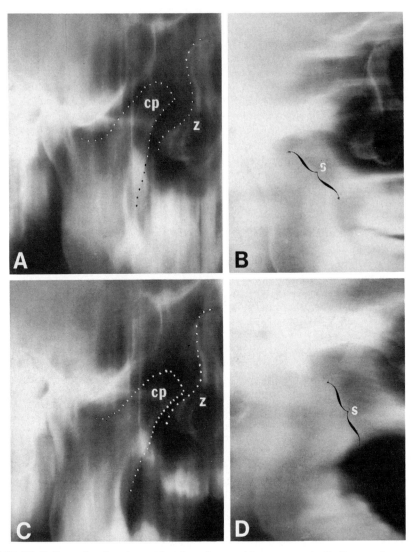

FIGURE 24–25. Radiographs of patient with enlarged coronoid processes. *A, C,* Preoperative and *B, D,* postoperative lateral cephalometric tomograms taken with teeth in occlusion *(A, B)* and with maximum opening of mouth *(C, D).* Note greatly enlarged coronoid process in *A* and *C* (cp) impinging on zygomatic bone (z) and limiting opening of mouth. Note in *B* and *D* the site of resection (s) after removal of the enlarged coronoid process and the increased opening of the mouth in *D.* (From Lyon, L., and Sarnat, B.G.: Limited opening of the mouth due to enlarged coronoid processes. Report of a case. J. Am. Dent. Assoc. 67:644–650, 1963.)

the ankylosis worse. Moreover, excessive force may permanently damage the teeth and their supporting structures. Various types of intraoral mechanical dilators have been used, such as the reversed spring clothespin, fitted trays with intraoral springs, and extraoral extensions and elastics. All of these are of limited value.

In instances where dilation has failed or is not indicated, one must resort to surgical treatment to mobilize the mandible. There are three basic principles involved in the surgical treatment of true ankylosis (Laskin, 1976). First, corrective surgery should be instituted as early as feasible so as to prevent severe facial deformity (Moss, 1968; Rowe, 1972). Second, the new joint should be established at the most superior part of the ramus so as to maintain maximal ramal height. This will minimize postoperative shift of the mandible as well as lessen the chance for an open bite to develop. In a young individual, consideration should not only be given to maintenance of ramal height but also to replacement of the growth site (Politis, 1987). The third principle concerns interposition of a relatively inert material in the new joint space to prevent fusion of the parts.

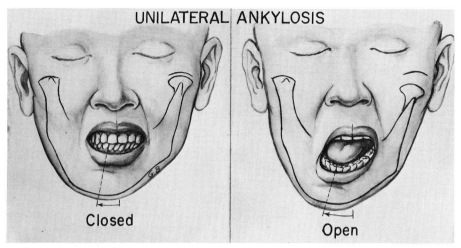

UNILATERAL ANKYLOSIS

Closed   Open

FIGURE 24–26. Diagrammatic illustration of the clinical features in a patient with a unilateral partial ankylosis of the right temporomandibular joint and lessened growth of the mandible. When the teeth are occluded, the chin appears prominent on the affected side. Upon attempted opening, there is increased deviation in that direction (see Table 24–3).

In the adult, a preauricular approach is used for any surgical procedure in the joint region and a retromandibular or submandibular incision for ramal surgery (see Fig. 24–2). In a child, both areas can be exposed adequately from a retromandibular approach. In addition to the extraoral approaches, an intraoral approach is sometimes used for the coronoid process (Brown, 1946; Lyon, 1963).

When the ankylosis is intra-articular, an arthroplasty or condylectomy may suffice to re-establish movement (Fig. 24–27). The higher the cut, the greater the chance for preserving the lateral pterygoid muscle and the less chance of inducing facial deformity due to ramal shortening. When there has been a fracture of the condyloid process leading to ankylosis, the fusion is usually between the stump of the mandibular neck and the glenoid fossa or zygomatic arch, and a condylectomy must be performed. In instances where the bony fusion involves both the condyloid and coronoid processes, an ostectomy of the ramus is usually the procedure of choice. If no material is added to the site, or gap, after the ostectomy, the procedure is known as a gap arthroplasty. If material is added to lessen the possibility of recurrence of the ankylosis, the procedure is known as an interpositional arthroplasty. The purpose of the interposed material is to establish a false joint, maintain ramal height, and lessen the possibility of an opening of the bite. After freeing the ankylosed joint, it is important to determine that the entire mandible is adequately mobilized. Sometimes an unsuspected ankylosis of the other joint is discovered.

In the adult, when only an arthroplasty is done, Silastic is generally the preferred material for placement over the stump of the condyloid process to prevent fusion and maintain height of the ramus (see Fig. 24–27). Autogenous muscle, fascia lata, and cartilage, as well as tantalum foil, zirconium, and many other materials also have been used with varying degrees of success. Most of these materials, however, lack adequate bulk to replace the lost condylar height. When a condylectomy is performed, an alloplastic condyle and fossa can be used to reconstruct the TMJ (Kent, 1983; 1986) (Fig. 24–28). Silastic block is used to prevent union when an ostectomy is performed in the upper part of the ramus.

Because lack of the condyle in a growing child will result in facial deformity, it is essential not only to restore ramal height but also, if possible, to insert a new growth site (Fig. 24–29). An autogenous costochondral graft is used for this purpose (Bowerman, 1987; Obeid, 1988). Because it has a cartilaginous surface, there is little possibility of fusion with the glenoid fossa.

An important aspect of the treatment of ankylosis is postsurgical physical therapy. Failure to exercise the jaw properly and prevent scarring can result in failure to re-establish a normal degree of opening. The patient should begin to exercise immediately after surgery and continue daily for at least six to eight weeks. Various types of screw, wedge, or spring devices can be used (Connole, 1988). Measurements should be made to note the degree of change. With proper effort on the part of the patient, at least

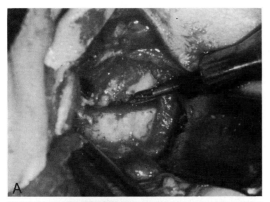

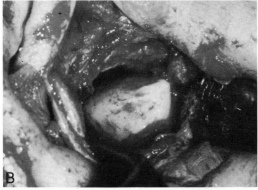

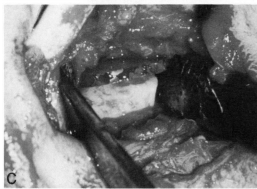

FIGURE 24–27. Temporomandibular joint arthroplasty for ankylosis. *A*, Osteotomy to separate ankylosed part of condyle from remainder of mandible. *B*, Arthroplasty completed and bony stump recontoured. *C*, Silastic inserted between mandible and fossa to maintain ramal height and prevent recurrence of ankylosis. The Silastic can be wired either to the mandible or to the lateral aspect of the glenoid fossa.

onlay grafts and osteotomies can be used to improve the facial appearance. Orthodontic treatment during the growth period is also helpful in correcting occlusal problems. In the adult, the damage to the condylar growth site often has been present for so long that a permanent deformity has been produced. Even though this may not be progressive, it is not self-correcting and there is no way to compensate for the lost or retarded growth. Orthodontic treatment and surgical procedures, however, do give functional and cosmetic improvement. Consequently, it is important not only to treat the ankylosis but also to improve the appearance of these abnormalities. Cartilage and bone grafts can be transplanted to build up the flat, relatively unaffected side of the mandible in the asymmetries when one condyle has been affected, or to the mental region when there has been a symmetrical growth arrest. In the latter instance, an advancement genioplasty can also be done. The position of the jaw can be altered by osteotomies in different parts of the mandible.

INTERNAL DERANGEMENTS

Although some patients with internal derangements of the TMJ can be successfully treated by nonsurgical means (see Chapter 23),

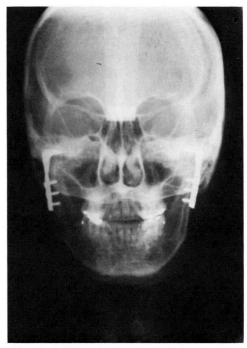

FIGURE 24–28. Radiograph of patient who had placement of bilateral condylar and fossa prostheses to correct an ankylosis resulting from rheumatoid arthritis.

three-quarters of the opening gained at surgery should be maintained permanently.

The problem of treating the growth deformity associated with ankylosis is a difficult one. In the child, minimal deformities may correct themselves as a result of functional remodeling and growth, and placement of a costochondral graft will limit subsequent changes. Otherwise, when full growth potential has been achieved,

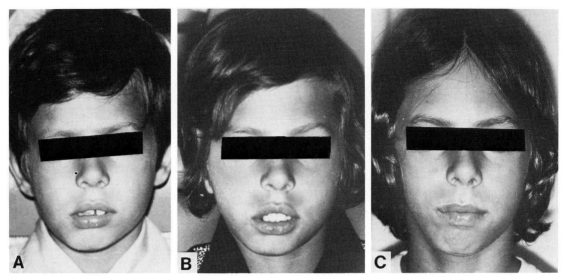

FIGURE 24–29. Six-year-old child with ankylosis of the mandible treated by insertion of a costochondral graft. *A,* Preoperative view showing facial asymmetry. *B,* View of patient one year after surgery showing decreased asymmetry. *C,* View of patient three years after surgery. Note the maintenance of facial growth and improvement in facial symmetry.

those who do not respond favorably to such therapy can often be helped by surgical treatment. There are three indications for surgery. First, it should be considered in any patient with TMJ clicking who also has uncontrollable pain and/or dysfunction (inability to open and close the mouth without manually or functionally manipulating the mandible). Second, it is indicated in any patient with inability to open the mouth adequately because of an anteriorly displaced, nonreducing intra-articular disc. Postponing surgery in such patients can lead to further damage to the disc and the possibility that instead of it being amenable to anatomic repositioning it will have to be removed and replaced. Because there is currently no replacement that has given consistently good results, it is advisable to make an early attempt to salvage the patient's own disc. The final indication for surgery is the presence of a loud clicking or popping sound, unassociated with TMJ pain and dysfunction, but which the patient finds socially unacceptable. This represents only a small group of patients, since most find their joint noise more acceptable than the thought of undergoing an operation.

There are basically two operations used on patients with displaced discs: discoplasty (meniscoplasty) and discectomy (meniscectomy). Although the intra-articular aspects of the two procedures differ, the initial surgical approach to the TMJ is the same in both (see section on surgical anatomy, page 383). After the TMJ region has been exposed and the position of the

condyle has been determined, an incision is made into the upper joint space and any adhesions between the disc and the eminence are detached. The superior surface of the disc is then inspected for irregularities, degenerative changes, or perforations. If the decision is made that the disc can be retained, the lower joint space is opened, the disc is anatomically repositioned, and a sufficient wedge of retrodiscal tissue is excised so that when the edges are sutured the disc maintains its normal position. If the disc cannot be retained, because there has been sufficient destruction to prevent its surgical repositioning, or because it has an unrepairable perforation, discectomy is performed.

Although some surgeons do not replace the disc (Eriksson, 1985), most believe that replacement is necessary to prevent bone-to-bone contact and the development of degenerative joint changes. Silicone rubber sheet (Silastic) is currently the most satisfactory alloplastic material, provided that it is of sufficient thickness, that it completely covers the fossa and eminence, that it is adequately stabilized, and that there is about a millimeter of clearance between the condyle and the implant. It should not be reinforced with Dacron because reinforced Silastic has been shown to crack along the threads (Eriksson, 1986). Rather than place a permanent Silastic implant, some surgeons insert a temporary Silastic implant and rely on the fibrous capsule that forms to serve as the disc replacement (Hall, 1985). Because of the foreign body reaction that sometimes occurs with perma-

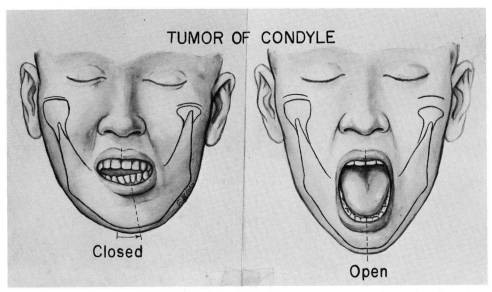

FIGURE 24–30. Diagrammatic illustration of the clinical features in a patient with a unilateral neoplastic enlargement of the right mandibular condyle. When the mouth is closed, the teeth on the affected side do not occlude properly and the chin deviates to the normal side with a resultant crossbite malocclusion. Upon opening the mouth, the unaffected condyle moves forward and the facial deformity tends to be corrected as the chin assumes a more normal midline relationship (see Figure 24–13 and Table 24–3).

nently placed Silastic (Dolwick, 1985), dermis (Meyer, 1988), auricular cartilage (Ioannides, 1988; Matukas, 1990; Witsenburg, 1984) and a pedicled temporalis muscle-pericranial flap (Feinberg, 1989) have also been used as disc replacements.

The precise role of arthroscopic surgery in the management of internal derangements of

the TMJ has still not been determined (see Chapter 17). The procedures currently being attempted range from lysis of adhesions and lavage of the joint (Sanders, 1986) to anterior release of the displaced disc and attempts to fix it in a normal position by suturing or scarification of the retrodiscal tissue (Tarro, 1989). All these procedures seem to have in common the

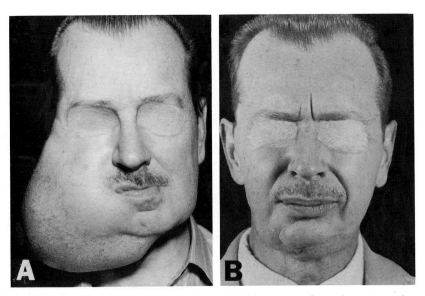

FIGURE 24–31. *A*, Photograph of a patient with an ameloblastoma involving the entire right mandible including the condyloid and coronoid processes for nearly 30 years. *B*, After hemiresection of the mandible. (From Byars, L.T., and Sarnat, B.G.: Surgery of the mandible: The ameloblastoma. Surg. Gynecol. Obstet. *81*:575–584, 1945. By permission of Surgery, Gynecology & Obstetrics.)

creation of improved disc mobility. This may explain why early reports seem to indicate that the greatest success is achieved in the treatment of anteriorly displaced, nonreducing discs that are mobilized by the elimination of adhesions (Gabler, 1989; Indresano, 1989).

NEOPLASMS

Tumors originating primarily in the TMJ are rare. Enlargements of the condyle because of a chondroma, osteochondroma, or osteoma constitute by far the largest group (see Figs. 24–13, 24–30) (see Chapter 10). There are apparently only a few reports of synovialoma, myxoma, giant cell tumor, fibrous dysplasia, chondroblastoma, osteoblastoma, and synovial hemangioma.

Malignant tumors are even rarer, with reports of multiple myeloma, fibrosarcoma of the joint capsule, and osteogenic sarcoma and chondrosarcoma of the condyle. Regional tumors, however, such as adenocarcinoma of the parotid

FIGURE 24–32. *A*, Photograph and *B*, radiograph of the tumor and mandible that were resected from the patient in Figure 24–31A. In *B*, note the distortion of the condyle, ramus, and angle of mandible and absence of coronoid process (From Byars, L.T., and Sarnat, B.G.: Surgery of the mandible: The ameloblastoma. Surg. Gynecol. Obstet. *81:* 575–584, 1945. By permission of Surgery, Gynecology & Obstetrics.)

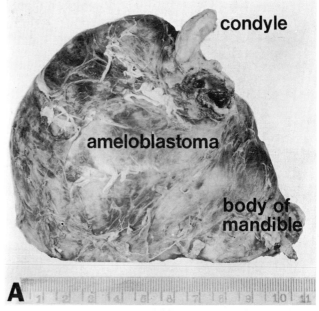
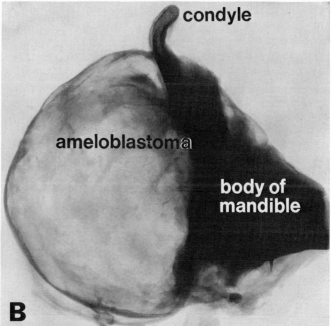

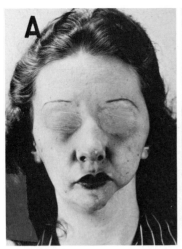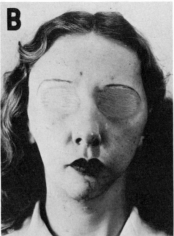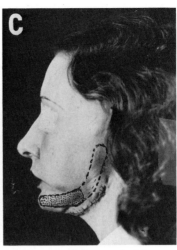

FIGURE 24–33. *A*, Preoperative and *B*, *C*, postoperative views of patient who had a surgical removal of the entire left half of the mandible. Bony and cartilaginous portions of autogenous rib were used to restore the missing segment and improve facial contour. The bony part (stippled area) was attached to the remaining mandible and the cartilaginous end (clear area) was inserted into the region of the glenoid fossa (From Byars, L.T., and Sarnat, B.G.: Surgery of the mandible: The ameloblastoma. Surg. Gynecol. Obstet. *81:*575–584, 1945. By permission of Surgery, Gynecology & Obstetrics.)

gland, carcinoma of the cheek, or ameloblastoma (Figs. 24–31, 24–32) (Byars, 1945) can involve the joint secondarily. Metastasis to the condyloid process from tumors at distant sites also occurs occasionally (see Fig. 25–2).

When a neoplasm involves the condyle or invades the fossa, the patient may frequently develop dysfunction (Bavitz, 1990) and have pain, difficulty in occluding the teeth, and deviation of the chin to the unaffected side (see Figs. 24–13 and 24–30). When the mouth is opened, the deviation generally tends to diminish. If the tumor is slow growing, the teeth may ultimately supraerupt and achieve some contact to compensate for the mandibular displacement. Often a crossbite relationship will exist (see Table 24–3).

When it is necessary to resect the condyloid process, ramus, and portions of the body of the mandible for treatment of a neoplasm, a bone-cartilage rib graft is sometimes used to maintain the integrity of the mandible. The cartilage end of the graft is trimmed to serve as a false joint in the region of the glenoid fossa and the bone end of the graft is attached to the remaining portion of the mandible (Fig. 24–33). A more anatomical reconstruction, however, can be obtained by the use of a composite graft consisting of a hollowed out allogeneic mandible filled with autogenous cancellous bone and marrow (Marx, 1986). Alloplastic materials, metallic (tantalum, Vitallium) and synthetic (acrylic), have also been implanted with varying degrees of success.

SUMMARY

The TMJ is a delicately balanced structure that depends upon the normal relations and actions of the rest of the masticatory apparatus for its functional integrity. Although anatomically the left and right joints are considered separately, functionally both joints work as a unit so that alterations on one side ultimately can affect the other. This is an essential consideration in planning surgical procedures for the TMJ.

The mandibular condyle, in addition to its role in function of the joint, also serves as an important site of growth of the mandible. This too must be considered in surgical planning and particularly in selection of reconstructive procedures. Finally, the unique situation caused by the presence of teeth, which must function in harmony with the TMJs, needs to be considered.

Most disturbances of the TMJ are similar to those involving other joints of the body, being mainly developmental, inflammatory, degenerative, traumatic, or neoplastic. The clinical differences are generally not related to histopathologic variations but rather to anatomic and physiologic variations between the TMJ and most other joints. The correct diagnosis and proper treatment of these conditions are dependent upon an understanding of the normal structure and function as well as pathophysiology of this region. Surgical management may be of real benefit in carefully selected patients.

In other instances, an operative procedure is undertaken with no apparent lasting improvement. Before an adequate answer can be provided to many of these difficult problems, there is a great need for further careful basic animal and clinical research.

REFERENCES

Al-Kayat, A., and Bramley, P.: A modified pre-auricular approach to the temporomandibular joint and malar arch. Br. J. Oral Surg. 17:91–103, 1980.

Amaratunga, N. A. deS.: Mandibular fractures in children—A study of clinical aspects, treatment, needs and complications. J. Oral Maxillofac. Surg. 46:637–640, 1988.

Annandale, T.: On the displacement of the inter-articular cartilage of the lower jaw and its treatment by operation. Lancet 1:411–412, 1887.

Axhausen, G.: Die operative Freilegung des Kiefergelenks. Chirurg. 3:713–716, 1931.

Bavitz, J. B., and Chewning, L. C.: Malignant disease as temporomandibular joint dysfunction: Review of the literature and report of a case. J. Am. Dent. Assoc. 120:163–166, 1990.

Bell, W. H., Profitt, W. R., and White, R. P. Jr.: Surgical Correction of Dentofacial Deformities, vol. I. Philadelphia, W. B. Saunders, 1980.

Bellinger, D. H.: Present status of arthrosis of the temporomandibular joint. J. Oral Surg. 6:9–16, 1948.

Blair, V. P.: The consideration of contour as well as function in operations for organic ankylosis of the lower jaw. Surg. Gynecol. Obstet. 46:167–179, 1928.

Blake, J. B.: Recurrent dislocation of the lower jaw. Ann. Surg. 68:141–145, 1918.

Bockenheimer, P.: Eine neue Methode zur Freilegung der Kiefergelenke ohne sichtbare Narben und ohne Verletzung des Nervus Facialis. Zentralbl. f. Chir. 47:1560–1562, 1920.

Bowerman, J.: Reconstruction of the temporomandibular joint for acquired and congenital malformation. Br. J. Oral Maxillofac. Surg. 25:100–104, 1987.

Brown, J. B., Peterson, L., Cannon, B., and Lischer, C.: Ankylosis of the coronoid process of the mandible and associated scar limitation of jaw function. Plast. Reconstr. Surg. 1:277–283, 1946.

Buckley, M. J., and Terry, B. C.: Use of bone plates to manage chronic mandibular dislocation: Report of cases. J. Oral Maxillofac. Surg. 46:998–1002, 1988.

Byars, L. T., and Sarnat, B. G.: Surgery of the mandible: The ameloblastoma. Surg. Gynecol. Obstet. 81:575–584, 1945.

Chin, R. S., Gropp, H., and Beirne, O. R.: Long-standing mandibular dislocation: Report of a case. J. Oral Maxillofac. Surg. 46:693–696, 1988.

Choukas, N. C., Toto, P. D., and Shukes, R. C.: Metatarsal transplantations following unilateral mandibular condylectomies in Macaca mulatta monkeys. J. Oral Surg. 29:171–177, 1971.

Connole, P. W., and Obeid, G.: A simple appliance for continuous jaw exercise. J. Oral Maxillofac. Surg. 46:520–521, 1988.

Conway, W. A., Bower, G. C., and Barnes, M. E.: Hypersomnolence and intermittent upper airway obstruction. JAMA 237:2740–2742, 1977.

Davidson, A. S.: Endaural condylectomy. Br. J. Plast. Surg. 8:64–67, 1956.

Dessner, L., and Olov, F. H.: Fracture dislocations of the mandibular condyle in children. Svensk. tandlak. Tskr. 51:57–68, 1958.

Dolwick, M. F., and Aufdemorte, T. B.: Silicone-induced foreign body reaction after temporomandibular joint arthroplasty. Oral Surg. 59:449–452, 1985.

Engel, M. B., Bronstein, I. P., Brodie, A. G., and Wesoke, P. H.: A roentgenographic cephalometric appraisal of untreated and treated hypothyroidism. Am. J. Dis. Child. 61:1193–1198, 1941.

Engel, M. B., Richmond, J., and Brodie, A. G.: Mandibular growth disturbance in rheumatoid arthritis of childhood. Am. J. Dis. Child. 78:728–743, 1949.

Epker, B. N., and Fish, L. C.: Dentofacial Deformities, vol. I. St. Louis, C. V. Mosby, 1986.

Eriksson, L., and Westesson, P-L.: Long-term evaluation of meniscectomy of the temporomandibular joint. J. Oral Maxillofac. Surg. 43:263–269, 1985.

Eriksson, L., and Westesson, P-L.: Deterioration of temporary silicone implant in the temporomandibular joint: A clinical and arthroscopic follow-up study. Oral Surg. 62:2–6, 1986.

Feinberg, S. E., and Larson, P. E.: The use of pedicled temporalis muscle-pericranial flap for replacement of the TMJ disc. J. Oral Maxillofac. Surg. 47:142–146, 1989.

Franks, A. S. T.: Temporomandibular joint in adult rheumatoid arthritis: A comparative evaluation of 100 cases. Ann. Rheum. Dis. 28:139–145, 1969.

Gabler, M. J., Greene, C. S., Palacios, E., and Perry, H. T.: Effect of arthroscopic temporomandibular joint surgery on articular disc position. J. Craniomandib. Disord. Facial Oral Pain 3:191–202, 1989.

Gerry, R. G.: The clinical problems of the temporomandibular articulation. J. Am. Dent. Assoc. 34:261–269, 1947.

Gilhuus-Moe, O.: Fractures of the Mandibular Condyle in the Growth Period. Oslo, Universitetsforlaget, 1969.

Glahn, M., and Winther, J. E.: Metatarsal transplants as replacement for lost mandibular condyle. Scand. J. Plast. Reconstr. Surg. 1:97–100, 1967.

Gonzalez-Ulloa, M.: Late results in the treatment of prognathism by double condylectomy. Plast. Reconstr. Surg. 18:50–64, 1956.

Goodman, R. M., and Allison, M. L.: Chronic temporomandibular joint subluxation in Ehlers-Danlos syndrome: Report of case. J. Oral Surg. 28:659–661, 1969.

Gordon, S.: Subluxation of the temporomandibular joint. Plast. Reconstr. Surg. 16:57–69, 1955.

Gosserez, M., and Dautrey, J.: Osteoplastic bearing for the treatment of temporo-mandibular luxations. In, Husted, E., and Hjorting-Hansen, E. (Eds.): Transactions of the 2nd International Conference on Oral Surgery. Copenhagen, Munksgaard, 1967, p. 261.

Gottlieb, O.: Long-standing dislocation of the jaw. J. Oral Surg. 10:25–32, 1952.

Greene, C. S., and Markovic, M.: Response of temporomandibular joint patients with positive radiographic findings to nonsurgical treatment. J. Oral Surg. 34:692–697, 1976.

Hall, H. D.: Meniscectomy for damaged discs of the temporomandibular joint. South. Med. J. 78:569–572, 1985.

Hampf, G., Tasanen, A., and Nordling, S.: Surgery in mandibular condylar hyperplasia. J. Maxillofac. Surg. 13:74–78, 1985.

Hartisch, J.: Ueber Kasuistik und Therapie der habituellen Schulter—und Unterkieferluxation. Unpublished Diss. Friedrichs-Universität, Halle-Wittenberg, 1883.

Hayward, J. R.: Prolonged dislocation of the mandible. J. Oral Surg. 23:585–594, 1965.

Husted, E.: Surgical diseases of the temporomandibular joint. Acta Ondontol. Scand. *14*:119–151, 1946.

Indresano, A. T.: Arthroscopic surgery of the temporomandibular joint: Report of 64 patients with long-term follow-up. J. Oral Maxillofac. Surg. *47*:439–441, 1989.

Ioannides, C., and Freihofer, H. P. M.: Replacement of the pathological temporomandibular articular disc using autogenous cartilage of the external ear. Int. J. Oral Surg. *13*:401–405, 1984.

James, P.: The surgical treatment of mandibular joint disorders. Ann. R. Coll. Surg. *49*:310–328, 1971.

Jarabak, J. K.: Subcondylar fractures of the mandible: Research and treatment. Am. J. Orthodont. *40*:729–755, 1954.

Jeter, T. S., VanSickels, J. E., and Nishioka, G. J.: Intraoral open reduction with rigid fixation of mandibular subcondylar fractures. J. Oral Maxillofac. Surg. *46*:113–116, 1988.

Johnson, W. B.: New method for reduction of acute dislocation of the temporomandibular articulations. J. Oral Surg. *16*:501–504, 1958.

Kent, J. N., Misiek, D. J., Akin, R. K., et al.: Temporomandibular joint condylar prosthesis: A ten-year report. J. Oral Maxillofac. Surg. *41*:245–254, 1983.

Kent, J. N., Block, M. S., Homsy, C. A., et al.: Experience with a polymer glenoid fossa prosthesis for partial or total temporomandibular joint reconstruction. J. Oral Maxillofac. Surg. *44*:520–533, 1986.

Konjetzny, G. E.: Die operative Behandlung der habituellen Unterkieferluxation. Arch. f. klin. chir. *116*:681–692, 1921.

Kraak, J. G.: A drug-initiated dislocation of the temporomandibular joint. J. Am. Dent. Assoc. *74*:1247–1249, 1967.

Kreutziger, K. L.: Surgery of the temporomandibular joint. Oral Surg. *58*:637–646, 1984.

Laskin, D. M.: Myotomy for the management of recurrent and protracted mandibular dislocation. *In* Kay, L. (Ed.): Oral Surgery. Copenhagen, Munksgaard, 1972.

Laskin, D. M.: Surgical management of diseases of the temporomandibular joint. *In*, Hayward, J. (Ed.): Oral Surgery. Springfield, IL, Charles C Thomas, 1976.

Leake, D., Doykos, J., Habal, M., and Murray, J.: Long-term follow-up of fractures of the mandibular condyle in children. Plast. Reconstr. Surg. *47*:127–131, 1971.

LeClerc, G., and Girard, G.: Un nouveau procede de butee dans le traitement chirurgical de la luvation recidivante de la manchoire inferieure. Mem. Acad. Chir. *69*:457–459, 1943.

Lindahl, L. A., and Hollender, L.: Condylar fractures of the mandible. A radiographic study of remodelling processes in the temporomandibular joint. Int. J. Oral Surg. *6*:153–165, 1977.

Lindemann, A.: Die chirurgische Behandlung der Erkrankungen des Kiefergelenks. Zschr. Stomatol. *23*:395–406, 1925.

Lindqvist, C., Jokinen, J., Paukku, P., and Tasanen, A.: Adaptation of autogenous costochondral grafts used for temporomandibular joint reconstruction: A long-term clinical and radiologic follow-up. J. Oral Maxillofac. Surg. *48*:465–470, 1988.

Lineaweaver, W., Vargervik, K., Tomer, B. S., and Ousterhout, O. K.: Posttraumatic condylar hyperplasia. Ann. Plast. Surg. *22*:163–172, 1989.

Link, K.: Zur operativen Behandlung der gewohnheitsmassign Verrenkung des Unterkiefers. Vierteljahrschr. Zahnheilk. *4*:395–404, 1933.

Lund, K.: Mandibular growth and remodelling processes after condylar fracture. A longitudinal roentgencephalo-metric study. Acta Odontol. Scand. *32*(Suppl. 64):1–117, 1974.

Lyon, L., and Sarnat, B. G.: Limited opening of the mouth due to enlarged coronoid processes. Report of a case. J. Am. Dent. Assoc. *67*:644–650, 1963.

Lyons, Chalmers J Club: Fractures involving the mandibular condyle: Post-treatment survey of 120 cases. J. Oral Surg. *5*:45–73, 1947.

MacLennan, W. D.: Fractures of the mandibular condylar process. Br. J. Oral Surg. *7*:311–339, 1969.

MacLennan, W. D., and Simpson, W.: Treatment of fractured mandibular processes in children. Br. J. Plast. Surg. *18*:423–427, 1965.

Marx, R. E., and Saunders, T. R.: Reconstruction and rehabilitation of cancer patients. *In* Fonseca, R. J., and Davis, W. H.: Reconstructive Preprosthetic Oral and Maxillofacial Surgery. Philadelphia, W. B. Saunders, 1986.

Matukas, V. J., and Lachner, J.: The use of autologous auricular cartilage for temporomandibular joint disc replacement: A preliminary report. J. Oral Maxillofac. Surg. *48*:348–353, 1990.

Mayer, L.: Recurrent dislocation of the jaw. J. Bone Joint Surg. *15*:880–896, 1933.

Meyer, R. A.: The autogenous dermal graft in temporomandibular joint disc surgery. J. Oral Maxillofac. Surg. *46*:948–954, 1988.

Merrill, R. G.: Habitual subluxation and recurrent dislocation in a patient with Parkinson's disease. J. Oral Surg. *26*:473–477, 1968.

Miller, G. A., and Murphy, E. J.: External pterygoid myotomy for recurrent mandibular dislocation. Oral Surg. *42*:705–716, 1976.

Moose, S. M.: Experimental injections of fibrosing solutions into the temporomandibular joints of monkeys. J. Am. Dent. Assoc. *28*:761–765, 1941.

Moss, M. L., and Rankow, R. M.: The role of the functional matrix in mandibular growth. Angle Orthod. *38*:95–103, 1968.

Myrhaug, H.: A new method of operation for habitual dislocation of the mandible—Review of former methods of treatment. Acta Odontol. Scand. *9*:247–261, 1951.

Nieden, H.: Ueber operative Behandlung habitueller Kieferluxationen. Deutsche Zschr. Chir. *183*:358–363, 1923.

Nishioka, G. J., and VanSickels, J. E.: Modified endaural incision for surgical access to the temporomandibular joint. J. Oral Maxillofac. Surg. *45*:1080–1081, 1987.

Obeid, G., Guttenberg, S. A., and Connole, P. W.: Costochondral grafting in condylar replacement and mandibular reconstruction. J. Oral Maxillofac. Surg. *48*:177–182, 1988.

Obwegeser, H. L., and Makek, M. S.: Hemimandibular hyperplasia—Hemimandibular elongation. J. Maxillofac. Surg. *14*:183–208, 1986.

Peresson, A.: Changes of the masticatory apparatus in myogenic torticollis. Surg. Gynecol. Obstet. *92*:122, 1950.

Perthes, G.: Die Verletzungen und Krankheiten der Kiefer. Deut. Chir. *33a*:40–60, 1907.

Politis, C., Fossion, E., and Bossuyt, M.: The use of costochondrial grafts in arthroplasty of the temporomandibular joint. J. Craniomaxillofac. Surg. *15*:345–354, 1987.

Poswillo, D. E.: Biological reconstruction of the mandibular condyle. Br. J. Oral Maxillofac. Surg. *25*:149–160, 1987.

Poswillo, D. E.: Surgery of the temporomandibular joint. Oral Sci. Rev. *6*:87–118, 1974.

Richardson, F. H., and Cohen, B. M.: Fractures of the mandibular condyle. Oral Surg. *6*:1149–1164, 1953.

Risdon, F.: Ankylosis of the temporomandibular joint. J. Am. Dent. Assoc. *21*:1933–1937, 1934.

Rongetti, J. R.: Meniscectomy. A new approach to the temporomandibular joint. Arch. Otolaryngol. *60*:566–572, 1954.

Rowe, N. L.: Surgery of the temporomandibular joint. Proc. R. Soc. Med. Engl. *65*:383–388, 1972.

Roy, E. W., and Sarnat, B. G.: Growth in length of rabbit ribs at the costochondral junction. Surg. Gynecol. Obstet. *103*:481–486, 1956.

Rushton, M. A.: Unilateral hyperplasia of the jaws in the young. Int. Dent. J. *2*:41–76, 1951.

Sanders, B.: Arthroscopic surgery of the temporomandibular joint: Treatment of internal derangement with persistent closed lock. Oral Surg. *62*:361–372, 1986.

Sarnat, B. G.: Plastic surgery: Its scope and possibilities. J. Natl. Med. Assoc. *51*:350–359, 1959.

Sarnat, B. G.: Developmental facial abnormalities and the temporomandibular joint. Dent. Clin. North Am. 587–600, Nov. 1966.

Sarnat, B. G.: Clinical and experimental considerations in facial bone biology: Growth, remodeling and repair. J. Am. Dent. Assoc. *82*:876–889, 1971a.

Sarnat, B. G., and Muchnic, H.: Facial skeletal changes after mandibular condylectomy in growing and adult monkeys. Am. J. Orthod. *60*:33–45, 1971b.

Sarnat, B. G.: Experimental and clinical postnatal craniofacial changes. Surg. Gynecol. Obstet. *148*:659–669, 1979.

Sarnat, B. G., and Robinson, I. B.: Surgery of the mandible: Some clinical and experimental considerations. Plast. Reconstr. Surg. *17*:27–57, 1956.

Schultz, L. W.: Twenty years' experience in treating hypermobility of the temporomandibular joints. Am. J. Surg. *92*:925–928, 1956.

Schwartz, E. E., Weiss, W., and Plotkin, R.: Ankylosis of the temporomandibular joint following burn. JAMA *235*:1477–1478, 1976.

Schwartz, L., and Chayes, C. M.: Facial Pain and Mandibular Dysfunction. Philadelphia, W. B. Saunders, 1968.

Sear, A. J.: Intra-oral condylectomy applied to unilateral condylar hyperplasia. Br. J. Oral Surg. *10*:143–153, 1972.

Sindet-Pedersen, S.: Intraoral myotomy of the lateral pterygoid muscle for treatment of recurrent dislocation of the mandibular condyle. J. Oral Maxillofac. Surg. *46*:445–449, 1988.

Spilka, C. J.: Surgical correction of mandibular prognathism. Oral Surg. *9*:1255–1266, 1956.

Stadnicki, G.: Congenital double condyle of the mandible causing temporomandibular joint ankylosis. J. Oral Surg. *29*:208–211, 1971.

Stuteville, O. H., and Lanfranchi, R. P.: Surgical reconstruction of the temporomandibular joint. Am. J. Surg. *90*:940–950, 1955.

Swanson, A. E.: Mandibular condylectomy for temporomandibular joint ankylosis—postoperative evaluation. J. Can. Dent. Assoc. *25*:129–138, 1959.

Tarro, A. W.: Arthroscopic treatment of anterior disc displacement: A preliminary report. J. Oral Maxillofac. Surg. *47*:353–358, 1989.

Thoma, K. H.: Functional disturbances following fractures of the mandibular condyle and their treatment. Am. J. Orthod. *31*:575–596, 1945.

To, E. W. H.: Mandibular ankylosis associated with a bifid condyle. J. Craniomaxillofac. Surg. *17*:326–328, 1989.

Topazian, R. G., and Costich, E. R.: Management of protracted dislocation of the mandible. Trauma *7*:257–264, 1967.

Valero, A., and Alroy, H.: Hypoventilation in acquired micrognathia. Arch. Intern. Med. *115*:307–310, 1965.

Verne, D., Polachek, R., and Shapiro, D. M.: Osteotomy of the condylar neck for the correction of prognathism: A study of fifty-two cases. J. Oral Surg. *15*:183–191, 1957.

Ware, W. H.: Growth centre transplantation in temporomandibular joint surgery. *In* Transactions of the 3rd International Conference on Oral Surgery. R. V. Walker, ed. London, E & S Livingstone, 1970, pp. 148–157.

Ware, W. H.: Management of skeletal and occlusal deformities of hemifacial microsomia. *In* Bell, W. H., Proffit, W. R., and White, R. P. Jr. (Eds.): Surgical Correction of Dentofacial Deformities. Philadelphia, W. B. Saunders, 1980.

Ware, W. H., and Brown, S. L.: Growth center transplantation to replace mandibular condyles. J. Maxillofac. Surg. *9*:50–58, 1981.

Ware, W. H., and Taylor, R. C.: Cartilaginous growth centers transplanted to replace mandibular condyles in monkeys. J. Oral Surg. *24*:33–43, 1966.

Wassmund, M.: Uber Luxationsfrakturen des Kiefergelenk. Deut. Kieferchir. *1*:27–54, 1934.

Watanabe, Y., and Otake, M.: Unreduced dislocation of the mandibular joint following eclampsia: Report of a surgically treated case. Oral Surg. *3*:1010–1017, 1950.

Witsenburg, B., and Friehofer, H. P. M.: Replacement of the pathological temporomandibular articular disc using autogenous cartilage of the external ear. Int. J. Oral Surg. *13*:401–405, 1984.

Zide, M. F., and Kent, J. H.: Indications for open reduction of mandibular condyle fractures. J. Oral Maxillofac. Surg. *41*:89–98, 1983.

Zide, M., Carlton, D., and Kent, J. H.: Rheumatoid arthritis and related arthropathies: Systemic findings, medical therapy, and peripheral joint surgery. Oral Surg. *61*:119–125, 1986.

25

DIFFERENTIAL DIAGNOSIS OF CRANIOFACIAL-CERVICAL PAIN*

SANFORD L. BLOCK, D.D.S., LL.B.

---

*See Chapters 5, 7–11, and 18–24

INTRODUCTION

In the practice of both dentistry and medicine, one of the most compelling symptoms for which the patient seeks assistance is what has been called the puzzle of pain (Melzack, 1973). It is pain that the patient interprets as a cardinal sign of illness. The word pain is derived from the Greek word for penalty, which has an association with punishment and suffering. It may be defined as an unpleasant sensation that is induced by the presence of a real, threatened, or imagined injury. An individual's perception of pain is symptomatic of multiple interrelationships of noxious stimuli and disturbed physiology and is encompassed by psychological and subjective components.

In attempting a logical approach to diagnosis, the clinician must endeavor to question with an open mind. Moreover, one's special area of interest should not inadvertently narrow pursuit of the problem. Whether one is a dentist, otolaryngologist, or an internist, one must remember that a dental abscess, acute otitis media, or arteritis may all cause pain in the same location. Pain is certainly the great "masquerader" until properly diagnosed.

The purpose of this chapter is to consider those painful conditions that directly or indirectly relate to masticatory dysfunction. However, it will also emphasize the diagnosis of those pain states and conditions that are without temporomandibular joint (TMJ) or other masticatory system components but that have closely related pain referral patterns.

CRANIOFACIAL PAIN

Craniofacial pain, excluding that of oropharyngeal origin, is mediated mainly through the trigeminal system. The vagus, oculomotor, trochlear, and abducens nerves, as well as the second and third cervical nerves that innervate the region of the angle of the mandible, play a minor role.

Primary Superficial Pain

Superficial facial pain of cutaneous origin is well localized and usually has a "double pain" quality. Because it is readily discernable, its location and possible cause can usually be determined without difficulty. Local anesthetic agents used topically (mucosa) or by superficial infiltration (skin), or extreme cooling with an ethyl chloride spray, will usually obtund the perception of superficial pain. Pain that will not respond to this approach must be considered as referred from a deeper source.

Inflammatory

In the differential diagnosis of localized sharp or burning pain in the facial region, one should consider the superficial inflammatory processes that may affect the skin and hairline areas. Furuncles, carbuncles, and folliculitis may cause acute inflammatory reactions accompanied by pronounced pain, tenderness, and visible cellulitis. The infecting organism is usually *Staphylococcus aureus*. Secondary spasm and subsequent tenderness can occur in the deeper surrounding masticatory muscles.

External otitis, a diffuse inflammation of the skin lining the external auditory canal caused by bacterial or mycotic infection, is also characterized by sharp, local pain. Furunculosis of the ear canal will cause an intense localized aching pain involving the pinna as well. With chronicity, the auricular muscles, along with the masseter and temporalis, become tender. Mandibular function or swallowing may intensify the pain, which will sometimes outlast the infection.

Neoplasia

Benign and malignant cutaneous lesions may lead to significant pain due to pressure necrosis or invasion of adjacent tissues, including nerves. Overproduction of the neuroglia or supporting tissue within the cutaneous nerves, with the loss of insulating periaxonal myelin, disturbs nerve transmission, which causes unpleasant skin sensations from any stimulus. By ephaptic transmission, tactile and sympathetic cutaneous efferent impulses may short circuit to pain fibers, which gives rise to symptomatic causalgia. Significant destruction or reduction in A-type fibers by neoplastic invasion may also cause loss of normal sensory inhibition and leave disagreeable forms of sensation (gate mechanism).

Trauma

Superficial pain following facial trauma may persist for months because of local entrapment of a cutaneous nerve. A laceration of the parietal area may lead to a trigeminal nerve neuroma. Similar neuroma formation may involve the postauricular and greater occipital nerves, leading to pain in or around the ear. Scarring of injured tissue may also cause pain due to traction upon a nerve during head and neck movements.

Secondary Superficial Pain

Superficial polyneuritic facial pains result from metabolic or toxic conditions that cause noninflammatory degeneration of peripheral nerves.

Polyneuritis

Polyneuritic pain is not as common in cutaneous areas of the face as in the deeper structures and the extremities. These pains are classified as secondary pains because they are initiated by a primary disturbance. Metabolic disorders occur from alcohol-induced vitamin or dietary deficiency states (beriberi, pellagra, and chronic malnutrition), cachexia of wasting diseases (tuberculosis and cancer), infectious diseases, uremia, endocrine disturbances (diabetes mellitus), amyloidosis, and sarcoidosis. Numerous toxic chemicals used in both medicine and industry are also responsible for nerve damage. Metabolic interference occurs with the administration of certain drugs such as isoniazid or hydralazine, which inhibit the utilization of pyridoxine and result in polyneuritis.

Polyneuritis may occur at any age, but is most common in young adults and middle-aged individuals. The clinical picture varies from mild to severe depending on the degree of nerve damage. Mild pain is usually accompanied by a sensation of either numbness or tingling (paresthesia) without loss of deep sensation or muscle weakness. In more extreme cases there is loss of both vibratory sensation and tendon reflexes as well as cutaneous tingling, numbness, or burning sensations. The skin may become extremely sensitive to external stimuli such as touch and pressure. In severe instances there can be paralysis of facial, palatal, and pharyngeal muscles, and an absence of all tendon and skin reflexes. In an evaluation of 26 patients with infectious polyneuritis, Merritt (1975) frequently found paralysis of the cranial nerves. Eighty-five per cent had facial paralysis, 50 per cent had dysphagia and dysarthria, and 20 per cent had paralysis of the spinal accessory nerve. Muscle tenderness developed in a majority of cases, although paralysis of the jaw muscles was infrequent (Merritt, 1975).

Hyperalgesia

Among other secondary neurogenic sources of cutaneous or superficial pain are the hyperalgesias, or areas of excessive pain sensitivity. Since hyperalgesia may be of superficial or deep origin, local or referred, careful evaluation of its distribution and tissue locus should be undertaken.

Cutaneous hyperalgesia accompanies injury or inflammation of the skin. Local lesions such as furuncles, cellulitis, abrasions, and neoplasia may bring about an increased pain reaction to touch, pinprick, pressure, or thermal changes. Distant lesions producing cervical nerve root compression, herpes zoster of the trigeminal nerve, or pain from an abscess of the hard or soft tissues may all cause cutaneous hyperalgesia. The more superficial hyperalgesias will produce increased pain response to pinprick while the deeper subcutaneous tissues respond to pinching a fold of skin. Muscle spasm or rigidity may accompany or cause persistent hyperalgesia. Frequently, the superficial hyperalgesia will mask the deep tenderness.

Deep Craniofacial Pain

Primary Masticatory Muscle Pain

MYOFASCIAL PAIN-DYSFUNCTION SYNDROME

Myofascial pain-dysfunction (MPD) syndrome represents the most common myogenic

disorder of the face. It is primarily a psychophysiological disease (Laskin, 1969; 1986) that is characterized by emotional repression and perpetuated by anxiety and frustration. This leads to somatized translation of stress into hyperactivity in the masticatory musculature (Reuben, 1977). Many patients who develop the syndrome may have pre-existing emotional disturbances and also stress-related habit patterns such as night grinding or clenching of the teeth. Other perpetuating factors that aggravate the involved muscles are physical factors such as trauma, malocclusion from alteration in the vertical dimension or skeletal asymmetry (Bush, 1985), and dental irritation. Systemic factors include chronic infections and metabolic disease. In addition to the psychological factors previously mentioned, depression and fatigue can play a role.

The pain is described as a dull to sharp ache in the region of the TMJ, preauricular and postauricular areas, and at the angle of the mandible. The pain may remain localized or be referred to other parts of the head and neck. It may vary from a maximum intensity early in the morning upon awakening to minimal morning pain and a gradual increase as the day progresses, with exacerbations during eating and excessive mandibular function. There is tenderness to palpation over all or part of one or more of the masticatory muscles as well as the suprahyoid, infrahyoid, and cervical muscles. Usually this tenderness is unilateral. Joint sounds may be an associated finding or may develop later in chronic states due to incoordination of the lateral pterygoid muscle and stretching of the retrodiscal ligament. There is also functional limitation and deviation of the mandible upon opening and limited lateral excursions. Ear stuffiness can also accompany the syndrome and may be precipitated by pressure from the medial pterygoid muscle upon the tensor veli palatini muscle preventing eustachian tube dilation (Block, 1976). This symptom has also been attributed to spasm of the tensor tympani muscle (Principato, 1978). Other ear symptoms such as tinnitus have been mentioned, but a definitive physiological correlation has not been shown (Bush, 1986).

Referred pain in distant parts of the face arises from trigger points in the involved muscles. Trigger points are manifestations of abnormal functioning muscle spindles, and present as hyperirritable spots within a taut band of voluntary muscle or fascia. They may elicit pain on compression and also cause referred pain, tenderness, and autonomic signs and symptoms. The pain referral pattern tends to be consistent. The pain pattern, however, varies with the muscle involved. The masseter muscle will refer pain to the preauricular and postauricular region and mandibular body; the temporalis muscle to the side of the head, masseter region, orbit, and maxillary teeth; the medial pterygoid to the retromandibular region; and the lateral pterygoid to the ear and the TMJ (Fig. 25–1). The sternocleidomastoid muscle refers pain to the ear, mastoid, and anterior cervical region. Although these patterns are predictable to a certain extent, they may also involve other areas as a result of their referral

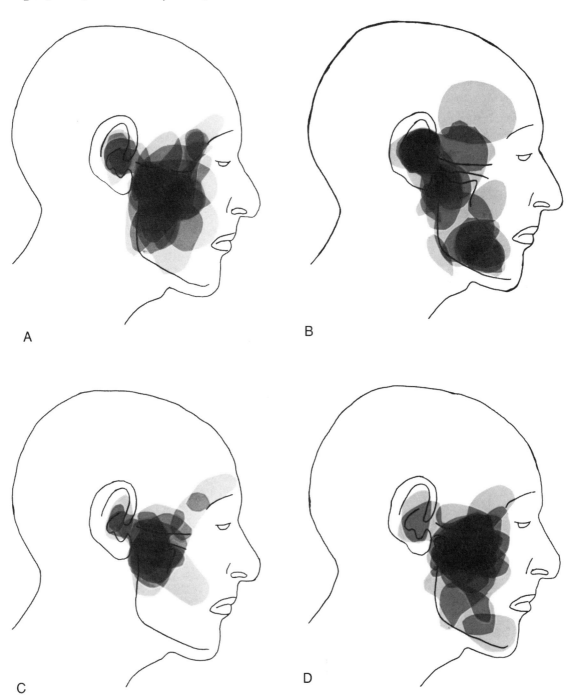

A

B

C

D

FIGURE 25–1. Extraoral sites of referred pain from the primary masticatory muscles initiated by injection of hypertonic saline solution. The darker areas are more frequent sites of referral. *A*, Lateral pterygoid. *B*, Medial pterygoid. *C*, Masseter. *D*, Temporalis. (Courtesy of B. Bobofchak, D.D.S., and D. Laskin, D.D.S.)

pattern and central excitation. Careful palpation of the muscles will locate these tender areas, inciting a wincing reaction from the patient. Infiltration of a local anesthetic agent without a vasoconstrictor into the trigger area, as well as the use of a vapocoolant spray over the tender region followed by gradual stretch, will reduce or eliminate the painful spasm (Zohn, 1976).

Muscle tenderness may also exist without the presence of trigger areas. A muscle may develop protective spasm in response to tension caused by trigger points in a parallel muscle, such as masseter spasm responding to a trigger point in the temporalis muscle (Travell, 1983). Further discussion of myofascial pain-dysfunction syndrome can be found in Chapters 18, 19, and 20.

MASSETER AND TEMPORALIS TENDINITIS

A sudden injury or strain, as well as persistent MPD syndrome, can result in a tendon tear or traction periostitis and create inflammation and pain. The muscle attachments also become inflamed, yielding a combined tendon-muscle trigger point. Repeated contraction with function creates a chronically inflamed scar (Cyriax, 1979).

With masseteric tendinitis, pain is referred to the adjacent alveolar ridge and midcheek, which causes a steady ache or sinus-type pain exacerbated by biting or active resistance. Masseter tendinitis can also result in pain referral to the adjacent maxillary molars (Travell, 1983) and has in many cases been the cause of root canal treatment being performed unnecessarily. Bidigital palpation at the anterior border of the zygomatic arch will trigger pain in the adjacent alveolar ridge followed by a residual ache (Friedman, 1985). The active resistance test of holding down the mandible while the patient attempts to close the mouth will provoke pain and aid in differentiating masseter tendinitis from dental pain, sinusitis, primary joint inflammation, and parotitis.

Inflammation of the tendinous coronoid attachment of the temporalis muscle can also cause referred pain. Trauma, bruxism, clenching, prolonged dental treatment, or dental extractions may create trigger points in the tendinous insertion or cause a traction periostitis. Biting and traction may only provoke pain intermittently. Palpation will refer pain to the adjacent alveolar ridge and teeth (Travell, 1983). A history of dental pain of unexplainable origin should alert the practitioner to the possibility of this condition. Injection of a local anesthetic agent into the involved attachment will reduce or eliminate the pain and triggering. Dental radiographs, dental pulp testing, tomography, computed tomography (CT) scans, an erythrocyte sedimentation rate, measurement of serum amylase, and a complete blood count (CBC) are helpful in differentiating tendinitis from dental disease, sinus disease, parotid disease, temporal arteritis, and TMJ inflammation.

TRAUMATIC MYOSITIS

Traumatically induced muscle pain is seen quite frequently. In addition to the pain, there is tenderness and limitation of mandibular function. The pain is usually severe initially, but gradually dissipates with time. The injury generally involves either the temporalis or masseter muscle and is the result of a blunt or sharp blow creating tissue tearing and hemorrhage. Injury to the adjacent bone and periosteum also may occur. Swelling may be visualized or palpated. Organization of the hematoma will follow, with eventual scar formation within the muscle. Calcified regions may also develop in the organizing tissue. A diagnosis can sometimes be made by injection of a local anesthetic agent into the involved muscle. In myositis the pain is augmented rather than relieved (Solberg, 1981). No abnormality in serum calcium, phosphorus, or alkaline phosphatase has been demonstrated, although creatine kinase and the erythrocyte sedimentation rate may be elevated (Wallach, 1986).

The muscle pain and spasm that may follow trauma can reflexly involve other muscles of mastication, adding further to the masticatory dysfunction. With long-standing dysfunction, cervical muscles may also become involved. These patients frequently complain of temporal headaches and exacerbation of pain upon palpation of locally involved areas or from mandibular function. When the anterior temporalis muscle is the site of injury, the patient will complain of pain and pressure within the eye or in the orbital region.

INFECTIOUS MYOSITIS

Bacterial or viral infection may occur within muscle, usually through introduction of organisms from a penetrating wound, dental infection, or other surrounding tissue infection. Abscess formation in muscle is uncommon because it does not provide a suitable medium for growth of bacteria. Pain, limitation of mandibular function, swelling, and tenderness are observed, as in traumatic myositis. In addition, there may be fever, chills, and sweating. If infectious myositis is not treated early, severe scarring may occur and eventually lead to non-painful muscle contraction and possible ankylosis.

Viral myositis may be seen in some patients who present with a recent history of upper respiratory infection. It is unclear if viral myositis is a postinfection immune phenomenon caused by the virus or a true infection of the muscle. Viral-like particles have been found in muscle, and biopsy reveals fiber necrosis and degeneration. Urine tests reveal myoglobin, especially with influenza and infection with the herpes group virus. Other viruses implicated are coxsackievirus, hepatitis B, and ECHO virus (Lerner, 1980). The activity of myofascial trigger areas tends to increase during a viral illness, so that MPD syndrome patients will experience exacerbations of muscle pain for several weeks to months. Differentiation of infectious myositis from MPD syndrome and traumatic myositis, as well as adjacent tissue disease, can be made by a careful history, examination, serum chemistry, and radiographs. With the former, there is an elevation of serum muscle enzymes, especially creatine phosphokinase, lactic dehydrogenase, and serum glutamic oxalic transaminase. The erythrocyte sedimentation rate and C-reactive protein may also be elevated, and the CBC and white cell count are abnormal. A soft tissue Gallium 67 scan may be helpful in locating any infection.

NEOPLASIA

Benign and malignant tumors of the masticatory muscles are an uncommon source of facial pain. With benign neoplasms or cysts, pain is generally precipitated by pressure, irritation, or infection. Malignant neoplasia is rarely found in the facial and masticatory muscles; more frequently, there is direct invasion from an adjacent primary growth. Infection of the neoplasm is usually the cause of facial pain. A CT scan, magnetic resonance imaging (MRI), and serum muscle enzyme determinations will usually differentiate any neoplastic swellings from an infective process.

Secondary Masticatory Muscle Pain

Noxious stimuli from various sources, in addition to causing pain, also establish a hyperexcitable state within the central nervous system at segmental and suprasegmental levels causing reflex muscle spasm. Local tissue reactions causing stimulation of nerve, muscle, and gland activity accompany this state. Prolonged noxious stimulation will perpetuate skeletal muscle contraction and be a persistent source of spasm and pain. This may lead to masticatory muscle dysfunction. The development of focal areas of hyperirritability in muscle following prolonged pain and dysfunction may lead to development of trigger points. These focally hyperirritable regions may cause additional sensory, motor, and autonomic alterations, such as referred pain, spasm, and vasomotor responses (Travell, 1983).

TEMPOROMANDIBULAR JOINT AND VASCULAR PAIN

Secondary muscle spasm pain can be reflexly induced through various noxious sources. Osteoarthritis and rheumatoid arthritis of the TMJ, an anteriorly displaced, nonreducing disc in the TMJ, trauma, or neoplasia may be primarily responsible for surrounding muscle spasm. Vascular pains such as migraine and cluster headache, if severe and chronic, may also precipitate secondary muscle spasm. Panoramic and transcranial radiographs, corrected tomography, a CT scan, arthrography, and MRI (Katzberg, 1986; Schellhas, 1988) will aid in diagnosing TMJ causes.

CERVICAL PAIN

Cervical spine disease can cause secondary facial pain by inducing muscle guarding and referred pain. Primary cervical pain of myofascial origin, or from traumatic cervical strain, degenerative or inflammatory spinal disease, and neoplasia, may also be accompanied by pain referred cephalad to the facial area (Dalessio, 1987). Rarely does true referred pain of facial origin have posterior cervical or caudad reference patterns. Pain that is experienced at the base of the neck is seldom due to the central excitatory effects of noxious stimulation of the trigeminal nerve. In certain instances of acute masseter and posterior digastric muscle pain, however, posterior reference to the mastoid bone and sternocleidomastoid muscles may occur, recruiting a guarding or splinting reaction of the cervical muscles through reflex contraction. Paradoxically, trigger points in the sternocleidomastoid and trapezius muscles may cause pain in an otherwise normal masseter muscle (Travell, 1983). Examination of the cervical muscles will elicit tenderness of these trigger points, with referral to the ipsilateral masticatory muscle.

SINUS DISEASE AS A SECONDARY SOURCE

Acute inflammatory disease of the maxillary, ethmoid, frontal, and sphenoid sinuses may cause pain in the head, neck, shoulder, and face. Frontal sinus pain is usually localized over the forehead. Reflex contraction pain is not commonly seen with this locally involved area. Sphenoid and ethmoid sinus disease may refer deep pain to the pharynx, vertex of the skull, eye, and maxillary teeth. The possibility of secondary muscle contraction pain from these conditions also exists; lateral pterygoid and masseter muscle involvement are most common. Maxillary sinus disease evokes pain in the ipsilateral eye, zygoma, maxillary teeth, infraorbital region, nose, and ear. Nasal structures acutely involved also may create secondary myogenic reflex contraction. Pain from the nose may be referred to the zygoma, vertex, frontal region, maxillary teeth, and eyes. Headache associated with nasal and paranasal pain can be due to prolonged contraction of cervical and head muscles.

EAR DISEASE

Prolonged external ear furunculosis may cause secondary involvement of the temporalis and masseter muscles. Middle ear infection will also cause reflex spasm in the sternocleidomastoid and occipital muscles, as well as in the masticatory muscles. Pain from the masticatory muscles is intensified by mandibular motion such as talking or chewing.

NEUROGENIC DISORDERS

Severe or chronic neurogenic disorders, as with other head pains, can lead to secondary muscle contraction. Trigeminal pain due to facial trauma, or dental or other infection, is usually well localized but may cause masticatory muscle spasm and referred pain due to secondary excitatory effects. The muscle pain may be of greater intensity and more diffuse than that of MPD syndrome. Neuritic pains of facial, glossopharyngeal, and vagus nerve origin usually induce secondary muscle involvement of a lesser degree.

Trigeminal and glossopharyngeal neuralgia may be mistaken for pain from masticatory dysfunction, but the pain is generally more paroxysmal and intense. Masticatory pain is of a more constant, dull, aching quality, with exacerbation upon mandibular function. In neuralgia, the pain may be induced by light touch, as compared with deep palpation with masti-catory muscle or TMJ involvement. Glossopharyngeal neuralgia may be triggered by jaw function or tongue and throat movement. Stabilization of the mandible while attempting to apply a stimulus to the tongue or throat will differentiate the source. As with other attempts in determining the pain source, local anesthetic infiltration or block along the nerve distribution may aid in differentiating nerve from muscle pain.

INTRACRANIAL LESIONS

When head pain is long-standing, with accompanying dysesthesia, muscle weakness or incoordination, and nausea and vomiting, one must question the presence of an intracranial lesion (Rushton, 1962). Intracranial lesions generally will not cause secondary muscle contraction unless there is an intense afferent spread from a portion of the cranium, creating excitatory effects within the brain stem and upper spinal cord (Dalessio, 1987). Sensations of vise-like or band-like tightness occur. Patients with a cerebellar or cerebellopontine angle tumor may develop pain in the face, neck, and occipital, frontal, and temporal regions, in part resulting from unilateral muscle contraction.

Skeletal Pain: Craniofacial Origin

INFLAMMATORY DISEASE

Inflammatory disease or osteomyelitis of the facial bones most often is secondary to infections of dental or paranasal sinus origin or results from fractures or gunshot wounds. The most common organisms involved are *Staphylococcus aureus* and *Staphylococcus albus*, and less frequently streptococci. Syphilis, actinomycosis, and tuberculosis are least common.

Acute infections from sinus, nasal, and ear disease may initially have an insidious onset. Pain may be referred to the orbit, ear, and temporal and nasal regions. Local tenderness and hyperalgesia over the frontal and malar bones are common in nasal and paranasal disease. Injuries present the more apparent symptoms of pain, deformity, and elevation of temperature and can easily be diagnosed from the history, visible local signs, and radiographs.

Osteomyelitis causes deep somatic pain and extreme tenderness over the bony structures. The pain is intense, constant, localized, and is primarily due to the accompanying periostitis. Generally, cranial bones are relatively insensitive; it is the sudden expansion, stretching, or irritation of the periosteum that results in the relatively high degree of pain. Mastoid, cranial base, and frontal sinus infections, which are below the hairline, produce more severe pain than those above the hairline because of the more complex innervation and pain referral patterns.

In general, infection and inflammation of the face will be accompanied by systemic as well as local signs and symptoms. Elevation of temperature; extreme local tenderness and swelling; headache and local pain that is increased with head movement, walking, or bending; erythema; lymphadenopathy; and purulent discharge are some of these signs. Masticatory muscles may become secondarily involved either through constant central reflex contraction leading to spasm, or by direct spread of the infection. A three-phase bone scan (nucleotide angiogram, blood pool scan, and regular bone scan) will help distinguish osteomyelitis from cellulitis (Waldvogel, 1980).

METABOLIC SKELETAL DISEASE

Metabolic diseases of bone must be differentiated from facial neuralgias, degenerative joint disease, MPD syndrome, and CNS disorders only in rare instances because they are usually painless conditions.

Osteitis Fibrosa Cystica (Hyperparathyroidism). This results from parathyroid gland hyperplasia or neoplasia. Symptoms are associated with increased mobilization of calcium and general demineralization of the skeleton. Cystic tumors occur in the jaws and long bones (Rosenberg, 1962). There is a loss of bone trabeculation, with thinning of the cortex, and the bone marrow is replaced by fibrous tissue.

Pain arising from these osteolytic lesions is usually due to secondary infection or expansion of the periosteum. Tenderness of the masticatory muscles and hypotonia may also be present. In most instances, skeletal pain of metabolic origin occurs only after the condition is quite advanced. When the periosteum is involved, the pain is sharp. Exacerbation of pain occurs with pressure against the periosteum or endosteum.

Other systemic diseases that involve the periosteum and cause pain are Paget's disease, hyperthyroidism, metastatic carcinoma, osteomalacia, multiple myeloma, vitamin D deficiency, metabolic amino acid disturbances, and osteogenesis imperfecta cystica. Differentiation of these diseases from other conditions that produce lytic lesions is aided by blood serum determinations. In hyperparathyroidism the serum calcium, alkaline phosphatase, and parathormone levels are elevated, and serum phosphorus is low or normal. Examination of radiographs reveals endosteal and periosteal resorption, and the biopsy shows tunneling resorption and osteitis fibrosa cystica.

Osteomalacia. This metabolic disease is characterized by structural alteration and weakening of bone resulting from inadequate mineralization of the osteoid matrix. Clinically, osteoporosis accompanies osteomalacia. It occurs in both adults and children, and is called rickets in the latter. Inadequate dietary intake of calcium and vitamin D is one of the initiating factors. Pain, aggravated by motion, is usually present in the porotic bony areas. Due to a decrease in serum calcium there is muscle irritability and hypotonia (Smith, 1969). Percussing the main branch of the facial nerve in the preauricular area as it exits from the stylomastoid foramen may yield tetanic-like facial contractions (Chvostek's sign). Radiographic evaluation reveals pseudofractures; biopsy shows wide osteoid segments and delayed mineralization; and blood chemistry studies show low serum calcium and phosphorus and high alkaline phosphatase. Osteomyelitis, multiple myeloma, and metastatic malignancy should be considered in the differential diagnosis.

Hyperuricemia (Gout). This results from a purine metabolism disorder or the abnormal excretion of uric acid. Joint inflammation associated with the accumulation of urate crystals in the synovial fluid is present in 85 per cent of all gout patients (Kelly, 1980). In 70 per cent of the cases at least one joint is involved, the most common being the first metatarsophalangeal joint. Ear tophi, once commonly associated with the disease, are not as common now due to effective drug control of the disorder. Gout is aggravated by an ingestion of foods high in purine, such as red meats and glandular organs.

Muscle tissue may become irritable, with the onset of myofascial trigger points and associated stiffness. Involvement of the TMJ is not common (Cacioppi, 1968; Chun, 1973; Kleinman, 1969). TMJ inflammation will cause secondary periarticular and masticatory muscle tenderness as well as limitation of mandibular opening. Radiographs may reveal articular erosion and spurs in the TMJ and other joints, as well as periarticular soft tissue swelling. Polarizing microscopy of the synovial fluid reveals the urate crystals. Biochemical studies show an elevated serum uric acid in 90 per cent of gout patients.

If there is renal involvement, creatinine and blood urea nitrogen are elevated (Wallach, 1986). These tests will help differentiate this disorder from osteoarthritis, rheumatoid arthritis, and septic arthritis.

Paget's Disease. This occurs after 40 years of age. Evidence is accumulating that it may be a response to a slow virus infection (Wallach, 1979). Symptoms begin slowly, with initial complaints of bone pain, and progress to severe headaches, deafness (bony impingement on the eighth nerve and auditory ossicle involvement), blindness, facial paralysis, dizziness, and weakness due to cranial base involvement and pressure on cranial nerves (secondary occipital and trigeminal neuralgia are possible). There is slow expansion of the maxilla, with spacing of the teeth and inability to wear artificial dentures. There is also an increase in hat size due to enlargement of the skull. Radiographs of the skull show a ground glass appearance, a prominent calvarium, and reduced maxillary sinus size. The serum phosphorus, alkaline phosphatase, and 24-hour urinary hydroxyproline levels are elevated. The laboratory tests and radiographs will differentiate this disease from metastatic carcinoma, hemangioma of bone, Caffey's disease, and hyperparathyroidism.

SKELETAL TRAUMA

Injuries to the facial bones generally present obvious physical signs, which are readily diagnosed. The history, clinical examination, and radiographic evaluation will reveal the existence of fractures. Local tenderness, malocclusion, crepitation of bony fragments, pain and tenderness with mandibular function, facial asymmetry, swelling, and ecchymosis are some of the signs and symptoms. Malunion or secondary infection are detectable through clinical examination and radiographs.

Obscure midface or basilar skull fractures may be easily missed and a cause of chronic pain may be overlooked. The pain resulting from skull fractures has been described as sharp, aching, or throbbing. Palpation over the site of injury may produce exquisite tenderness. Pain is usually due to traction and displacement of periosteal attachments, as well as soft tissue edema (Symonds, 1960). Linear fractures of the temporal bone produce symptoms of middle and inner ear involvement. Complete deafness, equilibrium disturbances, and facial nerve paralysis are possible. Scar formation in the scalp and other superficial areas may subsequently result in neuroma formation, with hypersensi-

tive nerve endings. These areas have discrete tenderness, which may be eliminated temporarily by injection of a local anesthetic agent.

Hyperactive muscle contraction of the scalp, neck, and masticatory muscles may occur after skeletal trauma (Youmans, 1973). Painfully chronic involvement of the temporalis muscle leads to masticatory pain and dysfunction. The pain referral pattern of these head injuries to the temple, posterior cranium, and occipital areas is also due to muscle contraction.

Depressed fractures of the zygomatic arch or fracture of the zygomatic complex may cause mandibular dysfunction either due to impingement of the fractured segment against the coronoid process or from possible fibrous adhesions between the coronoid process and the zygomatic arch. Limitation of mandibular motion and pain may occur if the problem is not corrected.

NEOPLASIA

Facial pain from skeletal neoplasia may be caused by the expansive or inflammatory effects on the periosteum (Fig. 25–2). Slowly expanding bony lesions do not create pain as a rule.

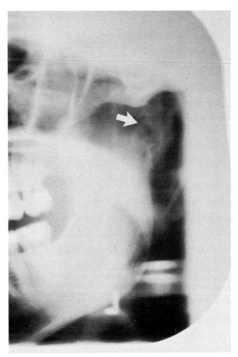

FIGURE 25–2. Radiograph of metastatic carcinoma from the breast to the left TMJ (arrow) producing an open bite deformity, facial asymmetry, pain in the TMJ, and limited mandibular opening. Before the onset of the pain the patient noticed a change in her bite, being unable to bring her upper and lower front teeth together.

Metastatic lesions that involve the facial skeleton produce pain of varying intensity depending upon the site and rate of growth. Pain in the chin from metastasis to the mandible is not uncommon.

TEMPOROMANDIBULAR JOINT ARTHROPATHY

TMJ arthropathy—arthritis, subluxation, dislocation, fracture, ankylosis—are important conditions to include in the differentiation of facial pains (see Chapters 7, 8, 21, and 24).

Vascular Pain

PRIMARY VASCULAR PAIN

Primary craniofacial pain of vascular origin involves pathologic changes such as obstruction, inflammation, or necrosis of the vascular bed, with secondary effects on nerve and muscle. These changes may be part of a general disease process, but only the facial pain will be considered in this discussion.

Temporal and Cranial Arteritis (Giant Cell Arteritis). This is a relatively benign variant of polyarteritis (Hollander, 1974) that is associated with a muscle and joint disorder of older age groups called polymyalgia rheumatica in 60 per cent of the patients (Fauchald, 1977; Hamilton, 1971). It is found predominantly in women over the age of 55. Characteristically, one or more branches of the carotid artery are involved. The patient complains of unilateral or possibly bilateral deep, boring headache combined with short, sharp, pin-stabbing, painful areas along the distribution of a prominent, pulseless, tortuous, tender, and inflamed temporal artery (Healy, 1979). The artery has a ropy feel and texture. The preauricular location of the pain leads to confusion with pain of TMJ etiology. Similar symptoms may be found in the postauricular and occipital arteries. Although jaw claudication has been reported (Desser, 1969), it is not common.

Secondary reflex contraction pain may occur in the masseter and temporalis muscles leading to mandibular dysfunction, especially when eating. A low-grade fever may occur early in the illness. Glossodynia may be present with lingual artery involvement. Visual loss may be rapid, sometimes within one or two days, due to changes in the ophthalmic artery. Eye pain, photophobia, and diplopia may also occur. Intracranial arteries may become involved, causing symptoms of confusion, convulsions, hemiparesis, and coma due to unilateral cerebral ischemia. It may be difficult to diagnose arteritis using carotid and cerebral arteriography because of the pre-existence of arteriosclerosis in many of the older patients. Laboratory tests show an elevated erythrocyte sedimentation rate and abnormal liver function tests in most patients, especially alkaline phosphatase. Diagnosis is generally confirmed by biopsy of the temporal artery. Because of the high incidence of debilitating cranial infarcts associated with temporal arteritis, and the potential for rapid blindness and CNS damage, expedient diagnosis is essential (Bengtsson, 1982).

Internal Carotid Artery Occlusion. This is another vascular impairment causing unilateral head and face pain in over 50 per cent of such patients. The pain is a poorly localized, steady ache of moderate intensity, without throbbing, in the temporal, occipital, and orbital regions. Pain in the orbital and retrobulbar region may be accompanied by transient or permanent unilateral blindness. The latter results from dislodged atherosclerotic plaques from the internal carotid artery becoming emboli and entering the ophthalmic and central retinal arteries. Platelet and fibrin or cholesterol emboli can sometimes be seen in the retina. When transient attacks of blindness occur it is called amaurosis fugax. Transient hemiparesis and aphasia may also occur. Weak or absent pulsation of the internal carotid artery may be found on the involved side. Care must be taken in examination of this vessel when occlusive disease is thought to exist so as not to dislodge an existing thrombus or plaque. Ultrasound and magnetic resonance angiography are valuable diagnostic aids.

Congenital Aneurysm. A congenital aneurysm of the internal carotid or one of the other intracranial arteries may also produce intermittent head and face pain. Many aneurysms remain symptomless until their enlargement causes pressure upon neural structures. Aneurysm of the posterior communicating artery may cause severe, sharp pain in and behind the eye. The pain is usually unilateral and associated with unequal pupils, possible paralysis of the extraocular muscles, and diminished sensation in the frontal region.

Arteriovenous and venous sinus aneurysms also cause severe recurrent head pain that may be increased with exertion. These patients often have a previous history of migraine-like pains and recurrent epileptic seizures along with sensory or motor deficits. Other types of aneurysm are associated with hypertension, arteriosclerosis, infection, and collagen disorders.

SECONDARY VASCULAR PAIN

Secondary vascular disease may also be a source of deep craniofacial pain. The most common initiating mechanism is vasodilation associated with inflammation around the vessels. Initially, specific inciting factors such as injury, bacterial or chemical toxins, and stress lead to a vasospasm of local arteries. The resulting vasoconstriction produces a local reduction in blood flow with secondary metabolic acidosis and anoxia. The noninnervated vascular bed, which depends on normal metabolic balance to maintain its tone, then dilates. The alteration in vascular tone can be both intracranial and extracranial. Release of vasoactive substances into the arterial walls and surrounding tissues produces sterile inflammation and edema. The chemotoxins released affect the surrounding perivascular pain fibers. Secondary effects upon vessels causing pain within the head and face are exemplified by conditions such as migraine, cluster headache, and hypertensive vascular pain states.

Migraine Headache. This is one of the most common headaches, occurring in over 12 million Americans. Two basic forms exist—the classic form, which has a prodromal phase, and the common form, which has no prodrome. Migraine is a recurrent, unilateral (80 per cent of cases), throbbing head and face pain with associated emotional irritability, nausea, and visual and constitutional changes. It has a familial basis, is more common in women than men, and may begin in childhood, most commonly before 40 years of age. Hormonal factors (Selby, 1960), stress, hot and humid climate, bright light, dietary factors, hunger, and vasoactive medications are some of the external triggering mechanisms. Other possible triggers are menstruation, physical and mental exhaustion, sleep (occurs during or immediately after REM sleep), and hypertension. Oral habit patterns tend to be more frequent in common migraine patients than in nonheadache patients (Moss, 1988).

There are four phases of migraine—the preheadache phase (prodrome), reversible head pain phase (vasodilation), the intractable pain phase (extracranial edema), and the postheadache phase (vascular stabilization) (Dalessio, 1985). Classic migraine may show prodromal (present in 85 per cent of migraine attacks) and preheadache warnings, such as restlessness, hunger, and wakefulness followed by profound sleep, that last about 20 minutes. Visual disturbances, when present, are manifested as blind spots, zigzag patterns, flashing lights, color dis-

tortion, and other hallucinations, which may be the result of a sudden epileptiform discharge across the surface of the brain. These phenomena may be associated with cerebral vasoconstriction and ischemia. Unilateral paresthesia of the face and scalp and vertigo may also occur. With onset of the attack there is a deep, diffuse, throbbing pain, which may become steady. Pain may be localized in the occipital, temporal, frontal, supraorbital, postauricular, and retrobulbar regions.

Facial pain occurs in the malar region, maxilla, mandible, base of the nose, and medial wall of the orbit, and may be mistaken for masticatory muscle pain. Attacks may be bilateral or alternate from side to side. The pain is often increased by lying down, physical effort, bright lights, and loud noises and decreased by compression of the common carotid and scalp vessels and with use of ergot or other vasoconstrictors. The attacks may last from a few minutes to several days, but most commonly last about a day. Lambert (1984) found that painful discharges from the trigeminal nerve created a diminished resistance in the carotid blood flow followed by increased extracranial blood flow leading to a migrainous type pain (Goadsby, 1985; Moskowitz, 1984). This response is called the trigeminovascular reflex and may account for vascular changes accompanying painful conditions such as MPD syndrome and severe dental pain. Dalessio (1972) found that sustained reflex contraction of the masticatory and facial muscles during attacks of migraine led to residual tenderness of the muscles of the head and neck. Masticatory muscle dysfunction is not a common feature in migraine, although some muscle tenderness is present in over 65 per cent of migraine patients. Dietary factors such as alcohol, chocolate, tyramine-containing foods (aged cheeses, cured meats, bananas, lima beans), and caffeine may precipitate an attack or provoke an increase in pain due to the presence of chemically vasoactive substances. A 70 per cent familial relationship is found in migraine patients. Mitral valve prolapse has been reported in 15 per cent of migraine cases (Spence, 1984). Diagnostic tests such as a CBC, erythrocyte sedimentation rate, EEG, digital subtraction angiography, a CT scan, and MRI of the head will help rule out inflammatory disease, aneurysm, and neoplasia.

Cluster Headache (Histaminic Cephalgia). This is another secondary unilateral vascular condition causing painful clustered attacks in the face associated with concurrent autonomic symptoms. The episodes occur one to three times per day for about 30 to 60 minutes. Three forms of cluster headache are recognized—classical form, chronic paroxysmal hemicrania, and atypical cluster headache. Males are more commonly affected than females. There are no visual prodromes as in migraine, and the intensity of the pain is severe to excruciating, occurring most frequently at night. The pain is a sudden, sharp, burning, and boring type located in the eye, retro-orbit, temple, face, and neck, and may be referred to the teeth. The attacks last a few minutes to an hour or longer and come on suddenly, often awakening the sleeping person (cluster headache often occurs during REM sleep). Patients feel better after rising and walking around as opposed to migraine patients who feel better lying down. The attacks tend to occur in groups or clusters for a period of several weeks to months. After a remission for years, the attacks tend to recur. A family history is much less frequent in cluster headache patients than in those with migraine. During the attack, there may be recurrences in response to vasodilating substances such as alcohol and nitroglycerin. Heavy smoking has also been reported as a trigger in chronic cluster headache patients (Kudrow, 1980). Characteristic facial (Graham, 1972) and other physical features (Schele, 1978) have been noted in patients with cluster headache.

Classic cluster headache can be divided into upper and lower syndromes. The lower syndrome has associated infraorbital pain and may show signs of Horner's syndrome (ptosis, miosis, facial flushing, anhidrosis, and rhinorrhea). The upper syndrome is related to dilation of the external carotid, while the lower is related to dilation of the internal carotid artery (Diamond, 1986).

Chronic paroxysmal hemicrania produces attacks similar to the classic form of cluster headache, but without periods of remission. It is more common in women. A typical cluster headache is associated with migraine or vertigo.

One of the mechanisms in the onset of cluster headache may be a defect in the hypothalamic oscillator center, which predisposes to the elevation of such vasoactive compounds as serotonin, sympathomimetics, histamine, and prostaglandins (Eversole, 1987). Contraction pain in the masticatory muscles is not a common finding, although there may be some residual muscle tenderness. Similar tests as those used in migraine and a good descriptive history will help differentiate cluster headache from trigeminal neuralgia, temporal arteritis, pheochromocytoma, and neoplastic disease.

Hormonal Headache. This is similar to migraine and is commonly associated with the menstrual cycle, occurring in over 60 per cent of female migraine patients (Selby, 1960). It results from vasodilatory effects upon the branches of the external carotid and cranial vessels. The headache is throbbing, unilateral or bilateral, lasting hours to 1 to 2 days, and may be associated with nausea, vomiting, and prodromal effects. The headaches occur at any time during, or just after, the menstrual cycle. Oral contraceptives have resulted in an increase in such headaches even in those who have been migraine-free (Desrosiers, 1973). The effects upon the masticatory muscles are the same as in migraine, with some associated tenderness and referred odontalgia.

Arterial Hypertension. Hypertension is another possible cause of secondary vascular pain in the face. These headaches, like migraine, are characterized by a throbbing pain in the frontal, orbital, temporal, and/or occipital regions. The pain may be unilateral or bilateral, and may increase in intensity during the night and be present in the morning upon awakening. The headache may be increased by effort, stooping, or by sudden jolts to the head. Stiffness of the neck, pulsatile tinnitus, and nausea may be symptoms (Round, 1988). Carotid compression decreases or eliminates the pain by suppressing the pulsatile effect of the distended intracranial arteries. The hypertension itself is not necessarily sufficient to produce pain; the relation between smooth muscle tone of the cranial arteries and the degree of pressure is more important. Thus, when arterial wall tone is low and there is a sudden rise in blood pressure, the tendency for throbbing pain is initiated. Patients with constantly elevated diastolic blood pressure above 110 mm Hg are also candidates for this pain. Neck rigidity and muscle tenderness are at times coexistent with hypertensive headache that is persistently painful. Masticatory dysfunction is not a common finding.

Neurogenic Sources of Craniofacial Pain

Neurogenic causes of deep somatic pain present a difficult problem in differential diagnosis due to the complexity of the craniofacial region. The terms *primary neuropathy* or *neuritis* have been used interchangeably to describe a prolonged disorder of sensation. Wechsler (1938) classifies neuropathy as a lesion characterized by parenchymal nerve degeneration, while neuritis is inflammatory in origin. Since degenerative changes may lead to inflammatory conditions, neuropathy may include all conditions of peripheral nerves that have a prolonged disorder of sensation and that may be accompanied by paresthesia, muscle wasting, loss of normal motor reflexes, and vasomotor changes.

NEUROPATHY (NEURITIS)

Trigeminal Neuropathy or Neuritis. Trigeminal neuropathy or neuritis symptomatically consists of a constant, deep, aching pain accompanied by characteristic burning, tingling, boring, pulling, or drawing sensations. The discomfort may remain for hours, days, or weeks. If associated motor nerve injury exists, flaccid masticatory muscle paralysis, wasting, and loss of reflexes may occur. Various factors such as surgery (dental and nondental), trauma, drug administration, nerve compression from a mandibular denture, and infection may lead to trigeminal neuropathy.

Oral surgical procedures, such as removal of impacted third molars, and injury to the inferior alveolar nerve during injection of anesthetic agents, are the most common causes of trigeminal neuropathy. The proximity of the inferior alveolar nerve to the roots makes it vulnerable during extraction of teeth. Periapical and periodontal infections, restorative dental procedures, and root canal therapy may also lead to mandibular and maxillary nerve damage.

Neuropathy can also be caused by artificial dentures that compress the inferior alveolar or mental nerve. This problem is seen with old dentures that have settled due to bone resorption, or with construction of a new denture upon an atrophic alveolar ridge in which there is a dehiscence of the mandibular canal or the mental foramen is near the crest. Constant aching pain is experienced in the jaw, mental foramen region, or along the buccal vestibule. There may also be associated numbness of the lip and chin.

Drug neuropathy, although not common, has been reported after the use of stilbamadine in the treatment of blastomycosis and trigeminal neuralgia (Goldstein, 1963). In such cases, the antiprotozoal agent produces bilateral trigeminal neuropathy.

Postherpetic trigeminal neuropathy due to the varicella zoster virus (VZV) involves the gasserian ganglion and the trigeminal nucleus in the dorsal column of the spinal cord (Hines, 1988). In one study of 72 patients with postherpetic neuropathy, 20 per cent were afflicted with trigeminal involvement. The severity of the infectivity of the VZV can be determined by the level of antibody titer to the virus, except in immune-deficient patients. This is more important than the age of the patient. A high antibody titer, however, does not ensure faster recovery from the illness (Kazuo, 1988). Generalized malaise and elevation of temperature may be seen several days before the onset of the neuropathy. There are vesicular eruptions on both the skin and mucosa innervated by the involved division of the nerve. Infections of the first division may include painful corneal ulcers. Maxillary division involvement may result in oral ulcerations along the palatal branch. The mandibular division may show painful crusting lesions on the face, especially in the mental area, although herpetiform lesions may not always be present. The pain is usually unilateral; steady, aching, or burning; and may be precipitated by peripheral stimulation. It may persist from three weeks to several months after the infective eruptions and erythema have subsided. Hypesthesia and paresthesia of the face may also remain for some time. Scars and skin pigmentation are seen following healing of the vesicular eruption. Trigeminal nerve herpes zoster may cause weakness of the masticatory muscles because of involvement of the motor root.

Facial Nerve Neuropathy. Facial nerve neuropathy may occur separately from trigeminal neuropathy from either previous trauma or infection. It presents initially as a steady aching pain, deep to the ear, and may involve the zygoma, nose, mandible, and pharynx. The pain may be followed by facial paralysis, and taste may be absent on the involved side. This condition may be confused with glossopharyngeal neuritis, which presents as a constant, burning pain deep in the ear and pharynx. A local anesthetic agent injected at the jugular foramen blocking the glossopharyngeal nerve will reduce pain due to this nerve but not pain due to involvement of the geniculate ganglion of the facial nerve (Finneson, 1969). Bell's palsy, one form of facial neuropathy, may occur due to inflammation or edema of the nerve within the mastoid canal. Transient to permanent facial paralysis may occur unilaterally. There may be accompanying symptoms of aching or burning pain deep to the ear on the involved side. Alterations in taste may also follow. Masticatory involvement due to motor nerve infection by the varicella zoster virus may lead to muscle weakness, dysfunction, and pain (Adour, 1975).

Glossopharyngeal Neuropathy. Glossopharyngeal neuropathy is an uncommon cause of facial pain. It is usually due to an inflammatory process. There is continuous burning or aching pain deep in the throat, base of the tongue, and ear. The patient may complain of difficulty in swallowing and a decrease in taste perception. A local anesthetic block of this nerve, as described earlier, will stop the pain and aid in the diagnosis.

Causalgia or Reflex Sympathetic Dystrophy. Causalgia or reflex sympathetic dystrophy is characterized by a continuous hot, throbbing, burning pain, associated with vasomotor phenomena and exacerbated by light touch or other stimuli. This entity is not found as frequently in the facial area as in other peripheral locations. The condition usually follows traumatic injury, cervical osteoarthritis, carcinoma, or surgery. In addition to the pain, there are associated symptoms of sweating and coldness or warm and dry areas because of variation in the vasomotor response. The skin may become atrophic. Occurrence around peripheral joints results in limitation of motion. Three phases of causalgia have been described: the vasoconstrictive phase; the spinal tract nociception or vasodilation phase, in which peripheral and autonomic nerve blocks have no effect on stopping the pain due to the facilitation and firing of second order sensory neurons; and the thalamic reflex phase in which minor stimuli result in exaggerated autonomic outbursts (Markoff, 1986).

The theory behind the clinical findings in causalgia states that synapses of the unmyelinated postganglionic sympathetic nerves, which are normally active in the maintenance of sympathetic tone, affect adjacent unmyelinated or poorly myelinated nociceptor afferent nerves. Also, if the injury has produced damage to the thick myelinated afferent fibers, the nociceptive small fiber activity is unopposed, with the resulting pain and associated sympathetic phenomena. Recent studies provide experimental evidence that primary afferent nociceptive C fibers can modify the response properties of the dorsal horn neurons, including the ascending second order neuron pool. Trauma or surgery cause an increased rate of firing of the larger, wide-dynamic range nociceptive neurons, resulting in pain. Sensitization of these neurons remains for a long time (Cook, 1987; Roberts, 1986). Additional findings support the theory that sympathetically maintained pain is mediated by myelinated mechanoreceptors acting on sensitized wide-dynamic range neurons causing an alpha-adrenergic mechanism in the skin (Roberts, 1988).

The ability of the autonomic nervous system to produce pain has not been completely clarified. The autonomic afferents contribute many thin myelinated and unmyelinated fibers to the substantia gelatinosa of the spinal cord, and the regional gate control can be affected by variations of input from these small fibers in the primary phase. Sympathetic blocks, such as those of the stellate ganglion, may be effective in the first phase of causalgia because increased activity is reduced, allowing normal input of large fiber activity to close the spinal gate. As the condition becomes chronic, however, sensitization of the second neuron pool becomes the source of nociception and only spinal or general anesthesia will block the pain.

In the trigeminal system, constant burning pain usually occurs without associated vasomotor changes and skin dystrophy. This effect has been seen after extraction of teeth or other surgery close to the nerve bundle. Injury to the surrounding nerves permits interaction between sympathetic and sensory fibers. Breakdown of the myelin sheath also allows nonuniform spread to adjacent neurons. Destruction of larger inhibitory fibers may cause remaining smaller C fibers to maintain solo sensory activity in the region, yielding a burning pain. This constant burning pain, localized and exacerbated by touch, is not a classic causalgia because of the lack of visible vasomotor changes.

Burning pain may have other causes besides injury, ranging from systemic factors such as B_{12} complex deficiency or anemias to local factors such as food, drug, or artificial denture allergies. New denture wearers have also developed this type of chronic pain. It is theorized that diminished sensory input caused by the denture covering the touch receptors allows an imbalance of small fiber activity to create the burning sensation. This condition may be diagnosed by removing the denture and having the patient eat and drink to determine if the pain is relieved or exacerbated. With systemic or local neuropathic conditions, the pain is worse. With the neural imbalance, the pain may be relieved (Harris, 1974).

Anesthesia Dolorosa. Anesthesia dolorosa is a denervation injury following trauma or a surgical procedure (Stookey, 1969). The area involved usually has complete or almost complete anesthesia followed by the onset of aching and burning pain. The process usually occurs when large nerve trunks or several nerve roots are injured. In the face, anesthesia may follow an injury to the mandible, maxilla, or orbit that severs a branch of the second or third division of the trigeminal nerve. Denervation may also follow neurosurgical procedures to remove cranial lesions that necessitate sacrificing a branch of the trigeminal nerve, causing a "painfully anesthetized" region in the face. Injury to the inferior alveolar nerve during dental extraction or excision of a lesion in the mandible may also cause complete anesthesia followed by anesthesia dolorosa.

Recent theories propose that denervation pain is caused by neuronal hypersensitivity affecting the reticulothalamic pathway, the conscious awareness of which is achieved by its projection upon the somatosensory cortex (Tasker, 1983b). The importance of considering this condition when anesthesia is apparent lies in the practitioner's approach to ruling out painful conditions from other tissue sources, such as the temporomandibular apparatus, which may be causing referred pain. Local anesthetic infiltration or nerve block will have no effect on pain reduction. Masticatory function is usually not affected and the muscles are nontender. Evaluation of the maxillary sinus, ear, and teeth in the opposing arch, and the elimination of possible ipsilateral neuropathy, vascular sources, and psychogenic factors, may help in diagnosing this most puzzling phenomenon.

NEURALGIA

Trigeminal Neuralgia. Trigeminal neuralgia is a recurrent, paroxysmal, unilateral facial pain occurring over the distribution of one or more branches of the fifth cranial nerve. The incidence in men is 2.7/100,000, and in women 5.0/100,000. The second division of the trigeminal nerve is most frequently involved, with the third division next in frequency, and the first division least often involved. The quality and temporal characteristics of this pain differ from that of the trigeminal neuropathies.

Trigeminal neuralgia presents in two forms, idiopathic and pathologic. Idiopathic trigeminal neuralgia, or tic douloureux, is characterized by brief episodes of severe pain, triggered by innocuous or gentle mechanical stimuli, and separated by pain-free periods. Idiopathic trigeminal neuralgia exhibits multiple trigger zones that change over time and involve all three divisions. It is thought that structural and functional changes in the trigeminal system result in an alteration in the receptive field organization of dynamic range neurons. There is an expansion of touch receptive fields and a change in the inhibitory mechanism around these large mechanoreceptors. This results in touch stimuli producing pain that under normal conditions would not occur (Dubner, 1987). The onset is

usually seen in patients 50 years of age or older. The condition is more frequent on the right side and rarely is bilateral (Rothman, 1974). Other causes have been attributed to demyelination of the ganglion or pressure from an aberrant branch of the superior cerebellar artery looping over the gasserian ganglion (Jannetta, 1968), producing arcing or lateral ephapses of nerve impulses to adjacent fibers. Arteriosclerosis causing inadequate blood supply to the ganglion may also be an etiologic factor. About 10 per cent of idiopathic trigeminal neuralgia may have been misdiagnosed as having dental causes (Mumford, 1987).

Experimentally induced central degeneration of regions within the spinal nucleus due to a chronic peripheral lesion has been studied by Black (1974). He created a unilateral pain response by performing dental pulpectomies in cats. Within two to three weeks, central hyperactive lesions were found in the descending trigeminal nucleus, triggering the ongoing hyperactivity and sending distorted afferent signals to the thalamus. A similar study was undertaken by Gobel (1977) in which tooth pulp extirpation resulted in degenerative changes in the medullary region.

Idiopathic trigeminal neuralgia characteristically has focal areas of hypersensitivity called trigger zones. These occur in numerous locations: lateral nasal, lateral labial, mental, lateral lingual, and gingival regions. The trigger zones are stimulated by touch, mandibular or facial movements, cold air, washing the face, blowing the nose, or other tactile stimuli. The quality of pain is a sharp jab or stabbing for seconds to a minute, followed again in minutes by another stabbing pain. A low-intensity ache may exist between episodes. Anesthetic infiltration or nerve block will temporarily relieve the pain.

The pain may last episodically for months, go into remission for a year or more, and return. Some patients have related a seasonal recurrence in early spring and fall. Pain during sleep is not common. Facial twitches or tics due to involuntary muscle contraction are rare; tearing and rhinorrhea may occur. Neurologic evaluation reveals no abnormal findings such as diminished or absent corneal reflex, anesthesia, paresthesia, muscle wasting, or atrophy. Ten to 20 per cent of these patients may have cranial lesions (Alling, 1977; Youmans, 1973). The most frequent is the cerebellopontine angle tumor, especially in persons below 50 years of age.

Pathologic or secondary trigeminal neuralgia is due to CNS lesions, neurologic disease, vascular lesions, and trauma. The pain symptoms are similar to those with idiopathic neuralgia, but there are also one or more atypical features such as diminished corneal reflex, masseter muscle weakness, facial muscle weakness, or hypoesthesia (sensory changes). Multiple sclerosis, basilar artery aneurysm, posterior fossa tumor, cerebellopontine angle tumors, facial fractures, orthognathic surgery, and removal of impacted teeth have all been attributed as causes of secondary trigeminal neuralgia. Brainstem disease from stroke and expanding lesions also may cause deafferentiation of the trigeminal nucleus or its descending tract producing episodic, lancinating, and burning facial pain that is not controlled by conventional medication or surgery (Clarke, 1988). History, physical examination, CT scan, MRI, blood serum chemistry, and cerebrospinal fluid (CSF) evaluation for demyelinating disease will help differentiate this painful disorder from masticatory dysfunction (Table 25–1).

Glossopharyngeal Neuralgia. Glossopharyngeal neuralgia is a rare disorder that has similarities to trigeminal neuralgia, producing severe, paroxysmal, stabbing pain in the throat, base of the tongue, ear, angle of the mandible, and neck. The pain lasts 20 to 30 seconds and is often followed by burning pain for two to three minutes. Ear pain alone may exist and is thought to be related to the tympanic branch of the glossopharyngeal nerve. Syncope and cardiac arrest have been described with this form of neuralgia (Riley, 1942).

Trigger areas are found in the tonsillar fossa and posterolateral tongue. They are stimulated by swallowing, chewing, talking, and coughing. Infiltration of the trigger area with an anesthetic agent or topical application may bring relief. A glossopharyngeal nerve block at the jugular foramen will also stop the pain. Glossopharyngeal neuralgia must be differentiated from the pain caused by nasopharyngeal lesions, medial and lateral pterygoid muscle pain, stylohyoid syndrome, pharyngeal myalgia, dental pain, and geniculate ganglion neuralgia. The incidence of cerebellopontine and nasopharyngeal tumors may be as high as 25 per cent in previously diagnosed cases of glossopharyngeal neuralgia.

Geniculate Neuralgia. Geniculate neuralgia is relatively uncommon. It was first described by Hunt (1937) as a result of his investigations of herpetic inflammation of this ganglion. Pain is felt deep to the ear and is referred to the retro-orbital, posterior nasal, malar, and palatal regions of the face. The pain may be constant, or paroxysmal and lancinating. It ranges from mild to severe, and there may be trigger points in front of or within the ear and in the tonsillar fossa. There is also an associated loss of taste. Application of a topical anesthetic in the tonsillar region, or infiltration of an anesthetic agent into the auricular trigger areas, will relieve the pain.

The pain is due to inflammation of the nervus intermedius, the sensory root of the seventh nerve. There are two forms, idiopathic and secondary to herpes zoster (Ramsay Hunt syndrome). In Ramsay Hunt syndrome, vesicular eruptions occur on the tympanic membrane and external auditory canal. If other portions of the facial nerve are involved, peripheral palsy is seen. Glossopharyngeal neuralgia, otitis media, TMJ disease, MPD syndrome, atypical vascular pain, nasopharyngeal lesions, and dental disorders must be ruled out in the differential diagnosis.

Postherpetic Neuralgia. Postherpetic neuralgia is an inflammatory process produced by the varicella zoster virus (VZV) affecting the fifth, seventh, and ninth cranial nerves and resulting in partial degeneration of these sensory fibers. The virus lies dormant in the ganglion cell bodies after initial exposure to the virus in childhood. It occurs in about 10 per cent of patients infected with the VZV (Peter, 1988). Affected adults (60 per cent) are usually over 45 years of age. Reactivation of the latent virus can be due to re-exposure, stress and fatigue, immunosuppression, and Hodgkin's disease. The nerve damage can result in paroxysmal pain as well as a more continuous neuritic pain. The first symptom encountered by the patient is a severe burning pain in the involved area followed by the characteristic cutaneous eruption of small inflamed vesicles. Severe, sharp, stabbing pains are associated with paresthesia. Between attacks, burning or itching may persist. Tactile stimulation may increase the pain, and examination may reveal hyperalgesia. Residual scars, which appear as glossy, hyperemic, atrophic areas in the skin, may remain in the sites of prior vesicular eruptions. Weakness of the masseter and pterygoid muscles on the affected side has been described, as well as paralysis of the facial muscles. Painful sensations can be referred to the orbit and sinuses. Corneal eruptions have occurred in 50 per cent of the cases with involvement of the first division of the trigeminal nerve. One of the earliest ocular signs is conjunctival congestion on the affected side. It has been theorized that destruction of large inhibitory fibers opens the spinal gate, allowing small fiber input to cause the painful episodes (Watson, 1988).

TABLE 25–1. Differential Diagnosis of Pain of Vascular, Neuralgic, Neuritic, and Temporomandibular Origin

TYPE OF PAIN	QUALITY AND DURATION	ANATOMIC LOCATION	AGE	PROVOKING AND ETIOLOGIC FACTORS	ASSOCIATED CHARACTERISTICS	DIAGNOSTIC TESTS	DIAGNOSTIC FINDINGS
Vascular	Sharp and throbbing, hours to days	Orbit, maxilla, temple, ear, neck	All ages, usually 20–50 years of age, most common in females	Stress, alcohol, dietary, hormonal, familial factors, hypertension	Autonomic effects (proptosis, miosis, lacrimation, facial flushing, rhinorrhea), aura associated with classic migraine, blindness with arteritis	Local anesthetic, CT scan, blood tests, skull radiographs, vasodilator test (with caution)	No response to local anesthetic, no lesions or A-V malformations, pain provoked with vasodilator medication
Neuralgic	Paroxysmal, intense, sharp, possible trigger point or zone, aching or burning between attacks, lasts seconds to minutes	Midface, lower lip, mandible, orbit, tongue, throat	Usually over 40 years of age, more common in females	Touch, thermal change, mandibular motion, emotional factors, seasonal, surgical, metabolic and CNS factors, zoster virus infection, neoplasia	Trigger zone guarding, hyperalgesia, central excitatory effects, poor hygiene in trigger area, skin or oral lesions from VZV (herpes zoster), diminished or absent corneal reflex, masticatory muscle weakness with CNS pathology	CT scan, skull and dental radiographs, blood tests, blink reflex, nerve conduction test, antibody titer to VZV (herpes zoster), local anesthetic blocks, peripheral trigger points	Rule out CNS lesions and A-V malformations, nerve conduction is delayed with CNS lesions and not delayed in idiopathic trigeminal neuralgia, rise in VZV titer with herpes zoster
Neuropathy (Neuritis)	Dull, aching, pulling, drawing, tingling, pins and needles, lasts hours to days	Cranial nerves V, VII, occipital nerve	Usually older age, but can occur in the young	Surgery, infection, metabolic disease, drugs, psychological factors, trauma, neoplasia	Aggravated by peripheral stimulus, paresthesia, hyperalgesia, taste alterations, seventh nerve paralysis, vasomotor effects, metabolic causes, may cross midline, scarring from herpes zoster	CT scan, skull and dental radiographs, blood tests, nerve conduction test, VZV antibody test, local anesthetic blocks	Decreased nerve conduction, positive blood test for metabolic or connective tissue disease, elevated VZV titer
TM dysfunction	Dull, steady ache provoked by function	Preauricular, lateral temple, mandible, zygoma, dental arch, mastoid, ear, orbit	18–40 years of age, more common in females	Stress, oral habits, altered occlusion, trauma, TMJ pathology	Masticatory muscles tender, mandibular limitation and deviation, with or without TMJ sounds, early morning jaw stiffness, with or without pain, mandibular locking	EMG of masticatory muscles, TMJ radiographs, tomography, CT, MRI	Trigger points show increased activity (may not indicate degree of dysfunction), radiographic lesions, disc displacement

437

Remission of the pain may occur spontaneously or gradually diminish over a period of months. Degeneration ceases about nine months after eruption of the rash. With herpetic neuropathy the degree of severity of the illness is determined by the level of antibody titer to the varicella zoster virus and not by the age of the patient (Kazuo, 1988).

Many differences exist between the findings with idiopathic trigeminal neuralgia and postherpetic trigeminal neuralgia (PHTN). Patients with PHTN have an average age of 74 years, while those with idiopathic trigeminal neuralgia (ITN) have an average age of 59 years. ITN is more prevalent in females (68 per cent as opposed to 53 per cent in PHTN). PHTN occurs most frequently in the first division, whereas ITN occurs most frequently in the second and third division. The symptoms of pain differ in that patients with PHTN have itching associated with painful points, dysesthesia, sympathetic signs, skin lesions, and no specific trigger zone (Valade, 1987). Differentiation from MPD syndrome, sinus disease, oral manifestations of vitamin deficiency, multiple sclerosis, central brain lesions, and eye lesions must be made.

Atypical Facial Neuralgia. As a category of pain, atypical facial neuralgia has become a nonspecific collection of those neuralgias of unknown origin that do not follow a normal anatomic pathway or respond to conventional treatments. Various investigators have attempted to describe the cause of this condition. Characteristically the pain is not limited to the distribution of the fifth or ninth cranial nerves and has cervical reference. Sectioning the fifth or ninth cranial nerves does not relieve the pain, which is a steady diffuse ache lasting for hours or days with no trigger zones present. This unremitting pain does not interfere with sleep. It is found more often in younger women than are major neuralgias and is not provoked by mechanical, thermal, or sensory stimuli.

Sphenopalatine ganglion neuralgia was first described by Sluder in 1908 as a unilateral aching pain in the lower half of the face. The pain involves the orbit, base of nose, and mastoid areas, and spreads to the regions supplied by the cervical nerves in the neck and shoulder. The pain is paroxysmal, recurrent, and lasts from minutes to hours. It generally occurs in persons between 30 to 50 years of age and more commonly in women. The pain is frequently referred to the maxilla or mandible and is associated with autonomic symptoms of rhinorrhea and lacrimation. Inflammation of the sphenopalatine ganglion was believed to be the

cause. Sluder recommended the use of topical cocaine or a phenol injection of the ganglion.

Vail (1932) described vidian neuralgia, a syndrome similar to sphenopalatine ganglion neuralgia. He believed that the syndrome was due to inflammation of the vidian nerve secondary to infection of the sphenoid sinus. Pain was located at the base of the nose and in the eye, ear, occipital, and shoulder regions, was paroxysmal, occurred at night, and was associated with nasal congestion. Eagle (1942) stated that the syndrome was due to a septal spur or deviation that irritated the sphenopalatine ganglion. He treated it by submucous resection of the nasal septum.

The previously mentioned atypical pains reported by Sluder (1908), Vail (1932), and Eagle (1942) were subsequently studied by others repeating the methods of treatment. There was only marginal success in attempting to control these pains. It is now theorized that these pains are probably the result of a vascular response of the internal maxillary artery, and especially that portion that supplies the sphenopalatine region. Thus a vascular etiology should be considered when unilateral pain occurs in the nasal, infraorbital, preauricular, occipital, neck, and shoulder regions that is not limited to the distribution of the fifth and ninth cranial nerves and is uncharacteristic of neuralgia. Success in treatment, however, is still limited by our lack of knowledge about a precise cause. Patients who fail to respond to specific therapies should be evaluated for psychosocial problems. The practitioner should be alerted by highly metaphorical descriptions of the pain, as well as by the acute crisis the patient with such a longstanding history presents. These patients use of denial of psychological conflict and a somatic preoccupation helps them to contain and cope with their internal psychological problems (Baile, 1986).

Multiple Sclerosis. Multiple sclerosis, or disseminated sclerosis, is a chronic disease characterized by numerous areas of demyelination of the central nervous system. Its etiology is unknown, although viral infection, allergy, heredity, and an autoimmune reaction to a slow virus (Chandrasoma, 1986; Dubois-Delcq, 1973) are all factors under investigation. The disease is found mainly in young women. The incidence is higher in cold and temperate climates and is rare in Japan (Alter, 1968; Merritt, 1975). The initial attack of multiple sclerosis may follow an acute infection, trauma, fatigue, vaccination, or pregnancy. The most frequent presenting symptoms are paresthesias of one or more extremities, the trunk, or on one side of the face; pain behind one eye (retrobulbar neuritis), diplopia, partial blindness or dim vision; weakness of one or more extremities; and motor deficits. About 1.5 per cent of the patients with multiple sclerosis have a form of trigeminal neuralgia. Areas of demyelination vary from small, pinhead-sized lesions to those encompassing a cross section of the entire spinal cord or a cerebellar lobe. Demyelinating plaques may be found at the point of entry of the trigeminal root, on the main sensory nucleus, the descending trigeminal root and gasserian ganglion, and on the facial nerve nucleus, the last producing facial weakness and continuous rhythmic fascicular contractions called facial myokymia.

The signs and symptoms related to the face are due to involvement of the descending trigeminal root. Because of the diversity of signs and symptoms that this disease causes, findings may vary. There is paroxysmal pain that may be indistinguishable from that of tic douloureux (Alling, 1977), loss or decrease of the corneal reflex, and paresthesia. In contrast to tic douloureux, multiple sclerosis occurs at an earlier age and is more often bilateral (Moulin, 1988). With spinal cord involvement, flexion of the neck may yield a sensation described by the patient as electricity (Lhermitte's sign). Weakness of the facial muscles occurs unilaterally in the lower half of the face. Complete paralysis never occurs. The pupils are irregular and partially constricted. There is partial loss of the light reflex and loss of visual acuity. Charcot's triad occurs with cerebellar involvement, which includes intention tremors, scanning speech due to incoordination of the palatal and labial muscles, and dysphagia.

When pain of undiagnosed origin occurs in women and men between 20 and 40 years of age, one must investigate the possibility of this disease. MRI techniques may reveal numerous plaques in the craniocervical region (Young, 1981). CT scans enhanced with contrast medium will also show visible lesions. CSF studies are abnormal in over 55 per cent of the patients, and agarose electrophoresis is abnormal in 90 per cent of the patients, with the presence of IgG bands and an elevated CSF IgG concentration. Differential diagnosis should include cerebellopontine angle tumors, brain stem lesions, trigeminal neuralgia, neurosyphilis, dental and sinus disease, systemic lupus erythematosus (SLE), cervical arthritis, and Bell's palsy.

Neurogenic Neoplasia. Neoplasia of the brain, spinal cord, or peripheral nerves must be ruled out on a presumptive basis in all patients with pain. Between 10 and 15 per cent of all patients with trigeminal neuralgia may have intracranial lesions. Patients with intracranial tumors frequently report a primary symptom of unilateral head pain of a steady, deep, aching quality (Rushton, 1962). Exercise, fatigue, change in posture, or exertion may increase the pain. Other general signs and symptoms, such as seizures, changes in state of consciousness, altered mental function, and visual disturbances (diplopia and blurred vision) may indicate the possible existence of a central lesion.

The incidence of head pain in patients with brain tumors may be as high as 90 per cent. Lesions that lie in the superior portion of the cranial cavity above the tentorium cerebelli (as high as 70 per cent of adult brain lesions) transmit pain via the trigeminal nerve to the anterior half of the head (the temporal and orbital regions). Most of these lesions involve the motor and sensory systems. Focal seizures, slowing of mental function, inexplicable headaches, and a slow progressive weakness are some of the initial symptoms.

Lesions that stimulate pain-sensitive structures below the tentorium cerebelli result in pain over the posterior portion of the head that is transmitted via the ninth and tenth cranial nerves and upper three cervical nerves. This type of lesion begins more commonly in childhood. The pain is initiated by traction or direct pressure on the dura, cranial nerves, cervical nerves, arteries, and venous sinuses. Because of this compressive growth, no lesion is clinically benign.

The most common lesions creating central compression and traction are the meningioma, craniopharyngioma, glioblastoma, acoustic neuroma, and pituitary adenoma. The cerebellopontine angle may contain tumors from the acoustic or trigeminal nerve and produce symptoms of paresthesia or pain in the orbital and maxillary regions as well as hearing loss, tinnitus, and loss of balance. When there is a slow rate of growth, symptoms may not occur until an advanced stage is reached. Unless a tumor or a cyst occupies a strategic position along the line of the cerebrospinal fluid ventricular pathway, it may reach considerable size before causing headache (Fulton, 1969). Generally, masticatory dysfunction does not occur unless there is compression of the trigeminal third division and its motor component.

Cerebellar or posterior fossa lesions compressing the cerebellum may cause pain associated with unilateral muscle contraction, especially in the neck and occipital regions.

Occipital pain may subsequently cause frontal and temporal pain as a result of temporalis muscle splinting; this may lead to secondary mandibular dysfunction. Sustained muscle contraction pain occurs additionally from the central excitatory effects of the noxious stimuli upon the brain stem (Dalessio, 1972). Complaints of tightness and vise-like and hatband sensations are described.

Metastatic lesions to the brain are one of the more common sources of adult intracranial tumors. They constitute between four and 20 per cent (Zulch, 1965). Recent cases have been reported in which right facial pain, diplopia, and abducens nerve paralysis occurred following parasellar metastasis of primary liver and stomach carcinoma (Bitoh, 1985). Symptoms are similar to those of histologically benign lesions but occur more rapidly. The cerebral metastasis is often the first symptom of the primary disease. Involvement of the gasserian ganglion will create paresthesia, neuralgic-like pain, changes in the corneal reflex, and possible weakness of the masticatory muscles.

Primary neurofibroma of the fifth cranial nerve is relatively uncommon. When the lesion occurs in the gasserian ganglion or middle cranial fossa, loss of sensation occurs locally, with or without paroxysmal pain. Paralysis and atrophy of the muscles of mastication may be present. Radiographs may show erosion of the foramen ovale.

NEUROGENIC SOURCE-REFERRED CRANIOFACIAL PAIN

Referred pain is perceived in a portion of one's body that is not primarily involved pathologically. In the facial area, the pattern of reference largely depends upon the afferent or efferent nerve branch being stimulated. Orbital pathology will refer pain to the temporal and maxillary regions via the first division of the trigeminal nerve. Middle ear infections may refer pain to the mandible, throat, postauricular, and occipital regions via the trigeminal, glossopharyngeal, greater auricular, and lesser occipital nerves, respectively.

In contrast, mandibular pain of dental origin will be referred via the third division to the auriculotemporal branch that innervates the external auditory meatus, auricle, and tympanic membrane. Referred ear pain frequently occurs in MPD syndrome and with TMJ dysfunction. When the source of ear pain cannot be localized in the masseter muscle or TMJ, evaluation of the lateral pterygoid muscle by palpation and

diagnostic infiltration with a local anesthetic agent should be attempted.

The sternocleidomastoid muscle frequently becomes involved in MPD syndrome and may be a source of pain referred to the ear. The area of segmental innervation for this pain pattern is cervical nerves two and three. Involvement of the nasal and paranasal structures may initially cause a localized deep pain. However, if the noxious stimulus persists, spread of the pain may follow and referred pain may occur at a distant site in the same segment, such as the zygoma, or it may ultimately spread to adjacent divisions involving the temporal, preauricular, and supraorbital regions.

Referred pain of cardiac origin is not common. During anginal attacks, pain may be referred to the neck and mandible as well as to the left arm. Rare instances of pain to the midface also have occurred. This symptom usually follows exertional effort. Coronary artery thrombosis, myocardial ischemia, and infarction may all produce the same referred pain pattern as angina pectoris.

The quality of referred pain of cardiac origin has been described as a pressure, squeezing, aching, or tightness. The intensity will vary from mild to severe. The attacks usually last only a few minutes and cause the patient to cease all voluntary activity. Mandibular dysfunction does not occur as a result of this pain, and associated jaw muscle tenderness is not found. A trial of nitroglycerin medication, under the supervision of the patient's physician, may be used to confirm the diagnosis.

Pain from Associated Tissue Systems

OPHTHALMIC PAIN (GLAUCOMA)

Glaucoma causes a continuous or intermittent rise in intraocular pressure accompanied by changes in the visual field and optic disc. Acute glaucoma is responsible for 15 per cent of all blindness in the United States. The increased intraocular pressure may create localized eye pain that radiates to the frontal, temporal, and vertex regions, ears, sinuses, and teeth. As the pressure increases, the orbital pain may become excruciating and associated with nausea, vomiting, and lethargy. The pain, a moderate to intense ache, follows the basic distribution of the first division of the trigeminal nerve. The patient will complain of dimness of vision, the appearance of halos around lights, and a fogginess of the visual field (Dalessio, 1972). Manual pressure over the eye may elicit tenderness and accentuate the pain. The cornea may have a ground glass appearance. The pupil may become oval, mid-dilated, and fixed. Photophobia, nausea, and vomiting may be present. Inflammation of the iris and ciliary body may cause similar symptoms, with associated pain in the temporal region that worsens in the morning and awakens the patient. Suspicion of glaucoma should alert the practitioner to recommend measurement of intraocular pressure. Pain will be relieved within one to two hours after treatment. Although mandibular dysfunction is usually not characteristic, prolonged symptoms of pain may lead to tenderness of the temporalis muscle.

AURAL PAIN

The ear is unique by virtue of having multiple neural innervations; therefore, the diagnosis of otalgia may at times be complex. The auriculotemporal branch of the trigeminal nerve, sensory branch of the facial, tympanic branch of the glossopharyngeal, auricular branch of the vagus, and the lesser occipital and greater auricular branches of the second and third cervical nerves all supply this organ. Primary ear disease therefore may refer pain to the teeth, tongue, pharynx, temporomandibular joint (TMJ), surrounding muscles, mastoid process, and neck via its numerous innervations. The TMJ may also refer pain to the ear; TMJ disorders should be considered whenever otalgia occurs without evidence of primary pathology within the ear.

Bullous myringitis, a viral infection of the tympanic membrane, can lead to constant ear pain, which may be referred to the TMJ and surrounding muscles. When there is elevation of temperature and conductive deafness, one may infer associated middle ear involvement. The pain may be sudden in onset or follow an upper respiratory or influenza infection. Hemorrhagic blebs may be seen on the drum. The otalgia may be followed by rupture of the tympanic membrane and drainage from the ear, with relief of pain.

Traumatic injuries to the eardrum from a blow may sometimes be undiagnosed for a long time. This is especially true when the TMJ is also involved. Associated symptoms of transient vertigo followed by tinnitus and hearing loss should alert the practitioner to the possibility of primary ear disease.

Middle ear infections have at times confused both the dentist and physician who have initiated treatment for a TMJ disorder, tonsillitis, or dental problem. Acute otitis media frequently follows an upper respiratory infection; the most common causes are viruses, streptococci, pneumococci, and staphylococci. The associated ear and preauricular pain is of constant intensity, usually unilateral, and is not exacerbated with mandibular function. There may be hearing impairment, ear stuffiness, nasal and postnasal discharge, vertigo, tinnitus, sore throat, cough, and fever. The pain may spread to the malar eminence, temporal and frontal regions, the vertex, and occiput. If some drainage occurs, the pain will become dull or throbbing. The high-intensity pain may create brainstem excitation, reflex muscle contraction, and spasm of the muscles of the head and neck. Masseter, sternocleidomastoid, and temporalis muscle involvement may follow, along with pain, tenderness, and concurrent mandibular dysfunction. The muscles thus become a secondary source of pain due to their sustained contraction.

Eliminating the possibility of any ear problem becomes important in diagnosing and treating TMJ and other facial pains. One must be familiar with this possibility and with the proper use of the otoscope. In acute otitis, hyperemia, retraction or bulging of the eardrum, and a loss of the normal light reflex may be observed. A straw-colored or reddish tinge to the tympanic membrane is evidence of a fluid level within the middle ear. The intensity of the initial ear pain is usually indicative of the degree of inflammation. Laboratory tests may show an elevated white blood cell count, with a shift to the left. CT scans with contrast or angiography may demonstrate a lesion. Tomographic and conventional radiographs may demonstrate bone destruction.

Mastoid sinus disease, which is less common now, may be responsible for persistent throbbing pain behind the ear. It is usually a complication of a middle ear infection that has spread into the mastoid air cells. Initially, the pain is intense and localized and there is exquisite tenderness over the mastoid bone. If swelling is present, it may cause anterior protrusion of the auricle and extension down the sternocleidomastoid sheath (Bezold's sign). Further extension may occur into the fascial spaces of the neck. The area circumscribing the mastoid process may be hyperalgesic. Again, as with other middle ear disease, central excitation and reflex muscle contraction can occur leading to sternocleidomastoid, masseter, and temporalis muscle spasms that, if persistent, become an encompassing source of secondary pain and mandibular dysfunction. Elevated temperature and pulse rate, malaise, nausea, vomiting, deafness, and delirium dramatize the severity of this illness. Radiographs show clouding of the mastoid air cells. If misdiagnosed and left untreated, middle ear disease may lead to meningitis, extradural abscess, facial paralysis, lateral sinus thrombosis, brain abscess, and death (Foxen, 1972).

NASAL AND PARANASAL PAIN

Diseases of the nasal and paranasal structures, either inflammatory or neoplastic, may produce pain of varying location and intensity. The ostia, turbinates, and nasofrontal duct are the most sensitive structures; the frontal, maxillary, ethmoid, and sphenoid sinuses are less sensitive. Innervation of these structures is primarily from the first and second division of the trigeminal nerve, which helps to explain the patterns of pain referral.

Infection of the mucosa of the superior nasal vestibule may lead to frontal and vertex pain. Pain is referred to the zygoma, temporal region, maxillary teeth, and jaws if the infection is located in the middle or inferior vestibule. Inflammation of the turbinates may create moderate to severe burning pain that will vary in referral pattern. Aching pain may be felt in the upper teeth, infraorbital area, zygoma, temporal region, and ear. In ethmoid sinus disease, pain will be referred to the frontal bone and bridge of the nose. The duct leading from the frontal sinus to the nasal cavity is exceedingly sensitive to pain. Pain from this structure is referred to the eye, infraorbital region, zygoma, temple, and posterior maxillary teeth. Pain from the sphenoid sinus may be referred to the pharynx, vertex, and maxillary teeth. Chronic recurrent frontal headaches associated with intermittent throbbing and lateral nasal pain radiating retrorbitally have been attributed to a posterior nasal spur from the vomer bone (Eagle, 1942; Gerbe, 1984).

The maxillary sinus, largest of the paranasal sinuses, may present diagnostic problems because of its close proximity to structures such as the teeth, pharynx, orbit, and nose. With partial involvement of the maxillary sinus there may be referred pain to the nasopharynx, posterior teeth, zygoma, and temple. A deep, aching pain in the pharynx may also occur. Pressure in the sinus from a mucocele may not be painful. Paradoxically, increased pressure within the maxillary antrum associated with inflammation of the turbinates usually is painful. The maxillary sinus is most commonly involved by inflammatory or neoplastic disease. Acute maxillary sinusitis is usually caused by streptococci, staphylococci, and anaerobic organisms. If the ostium becomes obstructed, the antrum fills with purulence under pressure. Moderate to intense aching or throbbing supraorbital and infraorbital pain occurs on the involved side. The pain is exacerbated by bending, walking, running, or sudden head movements. The nose is usually obstructed, but there may not be discharge if the maxillary ostium is blocked. Pain is decreased when lying down. Complete loss of smell occurs if there is bilateral disease. Postnasal discharge of unpleasant purulent drainage into the pharynx leads to laryngeal pain and hoarseness. Tenderness over the antrum may be present, and the temperature is usually elevated. Swelling of the cheek is less common in maxillary sinusitis than in infections of dental origin. Swelling overlying the antrum may also be indicative of neoplasia. When there is rapid onset of severe orbital pain, periorbital edema, nasal rhinorrhea, conjunctival engorgement, and elevated temperature, orbital cellulitis should be suspected as a complication of the maxillary sinusitis (Schramm, 1982). Maxillary sinus disease may also spread to other sinuses or the middle ear, or extend via branches of the facial vein into the cavernous sinus leading to cavernous sinus thrombosis, rapid blindness, meningitis, and even death.

Pain from sinus disease can lead to central brain stem excitation and reflex masticatory and neck muscle contraction. Prolonged contraction of the temporalis and masseter muscles will lead to pain and tenderness, as well as mandibular dysfunction. Long-standing intense pain of paranasal or nasal origin will also cause prolonged contraction of the cervical muscles, which become a secondary source of noxious stimuli.

Neoplasia of the maxillary sinus, especially carcinoma, may not be diagnosed until it has spread to the surrounding tissues. Pain may not be an initial symptom. Blood-stained nasal discharge and nasal obstruction associated with swelling of the cheek, buccal sulcus, or palate, and loosening of the upper molars may be the first signs. Ulceration may also appear in these areas. Proptosis and diplopia occur due to orbital floor involvement. Pain occurs in the late stages due to irritation and inflammation of the second division of the trigeminal nerve. The pain is aching or throbbing and may become progressively more severe, with reference to the ear, temple, and mandible. Clinical examination, a good history, radiographic evaluation, a CT scan, evaluation of the eye, and transillumination of the antrum will help in differentiating a sinus neoplasm from other causes of facial pain.

SALIVARY GLAND PAIN (see page 464)

Salivary gland pain, particularly parotid, may at times masquerade as either a TMJ disorder or MPD syndrome. The pain is usually sharp and localized, and its intensity varies with the degree of salivary secretion, swelling, inflammation, or obstruction. The pain generally increases upon thought, sight, or intake of food. With prolonged swelling of the gland there may be decreased secretion. Ductal stricture, a sialolith, or sialectasia may be responsible for recurrent swelling.

Inflammatory. Inflammation of the major salivary glands (sialadenitis) is usually due to staphylococcal, hemolytic streptococcal, and viral infections. These organisms travel retrograde in the duct. Sialadenitis is generally unilateral and occurs more frequently in older men in whom dehydration and debilitation are more common. The submandibular and parotid glands are involved more often than the sublingual gland. The infection fulminates within the gland, creating acinar and periacinar necrosis and abscess formation. There is elevated temperature, and swelling and tenderness of the gland. Masseter pain and spasm and mandibular dysfunction with limitation of opening and deviation to the affected side may occur in acute parotitis. The lobe of the ear may be elevated. In addition to the other presenting symptoms, the presence of suppuration from the duct, along with an elevated white blood cell count and sedimentation rate, aid in establishing the diagnosis of sialadenitis.

Chronic parotitis may be more difficult to diagnose than acute parotitis. Often recurrent inflammation of the parotid may not cause remarkable swelling and there are usually no signs of systemic infection. Fever is not characteristic. The preauricular and parotid areas may be tender to palpation, and intermittent to constant pain may be present. Increase in intensity of the pain is correlated with exacerbation of the infection. The ductal orifice may be erythematous, edematous, and milking the gland may produce an exudate. Elevation of the ear lobe may be noted. Salivary flow is reduced and the saliva is thick and tenacious. Culture of the exudate, a white blood cell count, and sialography are essential in establishing the diagnosis. Chronic recurrent parotitis may lead to mas-

seter muscle involvement, with associated pain and spasm. There may be limitation of opening of the mouth and deviation of the midline of the chin to the affected side. Secondary TMJ infection is possible through either hematogenous or direct spread.

Mumps, a viral inflammation of the parotid gland caused by a member of the paramyxovirus group, also presents as a lateral facial swelling. Pain may begin before the onset of swelling and is usually accompanied by fever. The nonpurulent swelling may be bilateral. Elevation of the ear lobe is characteristically seen. The blood count may show a decrease in neutrophils and a lymphocytosis, whereas in suppurative parotitis the number of neutrophils is usually elevated. Elevation of temperature, increased serum amylase (95 per cent of patients with epidemic parotitis), lack of suppuration (duct orifices are swollen but clear saliva is expressed), and short duration are findings that aid in the recognition of this disease. The pancreas and testicles may also be involved.

Obstructive. Sialolithiasis, a calculus within the salivary gland or duct, is more common in the submandibular gland (75 per cent) than in the parotid gland (20 per cent). Clinically, there may be continuous or intermittent swelling and pain. Painful symptoms intensify with increased swelling. A history of recurrent pain and swelling during eating, palpation of painful areas within the gland, and radiographic evidence of a sialolith are helpful in diagnosing this condition. Nonradiopaque obstruction should also be ruled out. Mandibular dysfunction is not a common finding unless painful enlargement of the parotid gland causes the patient to limit mandibular movement.

Neoplastic. Sudden acceleration of growth in an existing mass, fixation of the overlying skin, and sensations of tension and pain overlying the masseter muscle may all be symptoms of malignancy. Malignant lesions involving the parotid gland represent 18 per cent of all salivary gland tumors. They may cause facial paralysis or paresis in 20 to 30 per cent of the cases. Absence of such changes, however, does not indicate that the lesion is benign.

Pain in the parotid gland may be constant and vary in intensity. Pressure and pain can lead to reflex involvement of the underlying masseter muscle. There also may be direct invasion by the tumor. Mandibular dysfunction, with limitation of mandibular opening and deviation to the affected side, will then occur.

Pain in the submandibular gland is a prominent symptom associated with malignancy or a rapidly growing benign lesion. Again, if the pain is chronic and severe, reflex suprahyoid and masticatory muscle involvement can occur. Differentiation from masticatory involvement can be made by the history, palpation, contrast-enhanced CT scanning, technetium isotope scan, and biopsy.

LYMPHADENITIS

Enlargement of regional lymph nodes may be a significant manifestation of underlying inflammation or neoplasia. The texture of the node, its size, and the presence of tenderness, fixation, or mobility are all important signs and symptoms that help to determine the origin and nature of the etiologic factor. Pain from lymphadenitis is usually dull and diffuse. Knowledge of the regional distribution of the lymph node groups is essential in determining the possible causes of lymphadenitis. The groups of primary concern in evaluating the masticatory system are the preauricular and postauricular, parotid, tonsillar, superficial cervical, submandibular, and occipital nodes.

The preauricular, masseteric, and postauricular nodes are the primary groups concerned with pain and local tenderness in the region adjacent to the TMJ and masseter muscle. Careful palpation will discern these more superficial swellings. Preauricular nodes may need to be differentiated from the lateral condylar pole, which moves when the patient opens and closes the mouth.

OROPHARYNGEAL PAIN

Superficial Oropharyngeal Pain

General and Local Mucosal Pain

Innervation of the oral cavity is primarily by the trigeminal nerve, but there is some overlap with the seventh, ninth, and tenth cranial nerves. Persistent pain in the superficial tissues overlying the masticatory muscles can sometimes bring on secondary muscle pain. Nutritional deficiencies may also lead to generalized pain and inflammation of the oral mucosa. Iron deficiency anemia and vitamin B–complex deficiency produce a neuritic type of pain that is characteristically constant, burning, or tingling. The predominant symptoms are frequently found in the tongue. The pain is accompanied by atrophy of papillae, change in color, and ulceration with secondary infection. Due to the superficial locus, the pain is more pronounced in the movable tissues such as the tongue and mucobuccal folds.

Mucosal pain may produce a characteristic hyperalgesia and affect larger areas than the primary lesion. In general, mucosal pain is of a superficial character, similar to cutaneous pain. It is usually well localized and may have a stinging, burning, or itching quality. Generalized mucosal pain from inflammation may vary in intensity and, if severe enough, may induce headache. There may be an associated burning sensation, which also varies in intensity. Traumatic or chemical injuries, infections, allergies, nutritional deficiencies, and psychogenic factors may all be responsible for the initiation of generalized mucosal pain. Infection may compound the initial cause of mucosal pain by producing ulceration and regional lymphadenopathy.

Generalized gingival pain such as that caused by acute necrotizing ulcerative gingivitis may, if severe enough, also induce headache. It may be associated with malaise, low-grade fever, regional lymphadenopathy, and extreme difficulty in eating. There are no specific reflex patterns associated with generalized superficial somatic pain that affect the masticatory apparatus. However, alteration in the masticatory pattern may occur in long-standing cases due to the difficulty in tolerating the pain associated with chewing.

Localized raw, intense mucosal pain, as in aphthous ulceration occurring high in the mucobuccal fold opposite the masseter muscle, may induce painful reflex contraction of the masseter with a subsequent functional disturbance on the associated side. This will usually last for only a few days.

With superficial somatic pain, either topical application or local infiltration of an anesthetic agent will alleviate the symptom and aid in the differential diagnosis. Areas of hyperalgesia without visible mucosal alterations may be of deeper origin and will not be affected by this treatment. Referred pains also will not be affected by topical or local anesthesia. However, mucosal trigger areas, as seen in glossopharyngeal and trigeminal neuralgia, are temporarily blocked by the effect of topical anesthesia.

A sensation of constant burning in the palate, alveolar ridge, and tongue may be found in patients with new or existing artificial dentures. In many such instances there may be allergic, psychogenic, nutritional, or traumatic factors associated with altered occlusion or denture instability. When these conditions do not exist, it has been hypothesized that the dentures interfere with normal sensation by obtunding large sensory fiber input and reducing the modulating influence on small fiber activity, thereby leading to burning sensations. This can be verified by having the patient eat and drink without the artificial dentures. If no neuropathy is present, this will alleviate the pain. There is no definitive masticatory dysfunction.

Excessive mandibular ridge resorption may result in the mandibular canal or mental foramen being exposed on the superior portion of the mandibular ridge. Inferior alveolar or mental nerve compression may thus occur in patients wearing a lower denture. Localized pain and paresthesia result with function, and the pain may radiate to the posterior body of the mandible. Numbness of the lower lip and chin also may occur. Mandibular dysfunction may result because of an avoidance pattern. Radiographs, infiltration of a local anesthetic, and denture evaluation will differentiate this from other neuritic pains.

Glossodynia

Pain in the tongue may be an initiating source of masticatory dysfunction when the intensity is severe enough to produce a guarded chewing pattern. Trauma during mastication is one of the most common causes and may be secondarily initiated by poor dental occlusion, ill-fitting dentures and bridges, and fractured teeth. Oral surgery as well as other dental procedures may become an iatrogenic source of lingual pain. Most pain of traumatic origin is well localized, severe, and produces a constant ache that gradually subsides over a few days to a week. Other factors that may cause glossodynia are deficiency states (pernicious anemia), metabolic disease (diabetes mellitus), candidiasis, xerostomia, allergy, periodontal disease, arterial insufficiency to the tongue, psychogenic disturbances, spicy foods, and tobacco (Hall, 1987). Patients with less pain, as in pernicious anemia, diabetes, and psychogenic disturbances, complain of a constant burning, itching, or tingling.

Ulcerative viral, traumatic, and neoplastic lesions, in addition to being a primary source of lingual pain, also refer pain to the ear and pharynx. Although lingual pain is well localized, referred pain and altered chewing patterns that result from glossodynia must be ruled out in evaluation of masticatory dysfunction. A thorough workup, including serum B$_{12}$, hemoglobin and glucose levels, fungal cultures, dietary factors, and psychological evaluation, will help in isolating a possible cause.

Pharyngitis

Pharyngitis is commonly associated with upper respiratory infections, especially of viral origin. It is often accompanied by nasal infection, dysphagia, fever, and malaise. The pain is constant and burning. The patient may complain of a lumpy feeling in the throat, which is exacerbated upon swallowing. Mandibular dysfunction is generally not found, although the pharyngeal tenderness may be mistaken for posterior digastric muscle involvement. Pain may be referred to the ear via the ninth and tenth cranial nerves. If the ear pain persists, and there is increasing dysphagia, neoplasia of the throat should be considered.

Tonsillitis

Tonsillitis is a common entity that causes referred pain to the ear and throat. Pain related to chronic tonsillitis should be considered in the differential diagnosis of masticatory dysfunction. With the former, sore throat, dysphagia, earache, and malaise usually are present. Cervical lymphadenopathy may be mistaken for sternocleidomastoid muscle tenderness. Ear stuffiness, as occurs in MPD syndrome, is commonly found. The patient may relate a history of pain followed by a gradual limitation of opening of the mouth. Middle ear infection is a frequent complication that, if painfully chronic, may lead to associated pain and spasm of the temporalis, masseter, and pterygoid muscles. Examination of the pharynx will reveal enlarged hyperemic tonsils. When there is an associated middle ear infection, the tympanic membrane may show erythema, bulging, or retraction, and there may be a fluid level in the middle ear.

Deep Oropharyngeal Pain

Odontogenic Pain

The most common source of orofacial pain is the teeth. At times, because of vague localization, variability in intensity, and distant referral patterns, diagnosis becomes difficult. Further involvement of the masticatory apparatus produces greater pain and discomfort, and the ensuing cycle confuses the diagnostic picture. Fortunately this is uncommon. Although the majority of unlocalized pains of dental origin do become isolated with time, the delay of care by the proper specialist leads to further confusion, improper diagnosis, and treatment.

Careful clinical and radiographic evaluation of all teeth and supporting tissues must be made. Percussion, electrical and thermal pulpal vitality tests, and localized occlusal compression for the recognition of fractured (obvious or not) teeth or inadequate restorations are helpful in arriving at a timely diagnosis. The history of the onset and inciting factors is also important. The quality and the intensity of the pain are significant, as well as the effects of changing posture, such as occurs with a pulpitis, an acute periapical abscess, or a maxillary sinusitis. The most significant diagnostic aid is the use of a topical or local anesthetic agent to test for the source and alleviation of the pain.

Difficulty in localizing odontogenic pain is generally due to the multiple tissues involved. Recent findings indicate that there is a notable scarcity of neurons that receive afferent input exclusively from one dental pulp, making localization of a specific noxious dental problem difficult. Convergent properties of afferents from other tissues into the same trigeminal nucleus also makes odontogenic pain localization difficult and may explain the spread of dental pain to other teeth and tissues. An acute or chronic pulpitis also may be difficult to localize because it can produce a referred pain pattern in the opposite arch or in other areas within the same arch. As a rule, pain referred to the opposite arch generally follows the same tooth relationship—premolars refer to premolars and molars to molars. Periodontal pain is usually more easily localized than pulpal pain due to the proprioceptive periodontal fibers. Pain from a periapical abscess will be well localized for the same reason.

The quality and severity of the pain depend greatly on the tissue involved. Pulpitis may produce a constant ache and a periapical abscess will cause a consistent throbbing pain that is exacerbated by function and percussion.

Pain associated with a prolonged toothache may be referred to a remote site. Such referred pain is usually of a dual nature. One type of referred pain is the result of a central excitatory effect directed toward tissues supplied by the same or adjacent divisions of the trigeminal nerve. The second is pain experienced from sustained contraction of the masticatory and neck muscles (Dalessio, 1972).

Pain of severe intensity experienced in the maxillary teeth initially may become localized within the general area of the involved tooth and then, as a result of central excitatory effects, may be followed by a more diffuse type of pain radiating to all teeth in the second division of the affected side. Subsequent referral to the eye, orbital rim, and temple, as well as associated autonomic effects and scleritis, may be found on the side of the associated dental pain and infection.

Intense pain associated with the mandibular teeth, if prolonged, will radiate to the ear, maxilla, and even to the first division of the trigeminal nerve. Associated hyperalgesia of the temple, cheek, and ear may also occur. There may also be tenderness of the temporal and auricular tissues, edema of the eyelids, nasal congestion, and lacrimation. With long-standing pain, the muscles of mastication become involved. Sensations of tightness and pressure may be felt in the temporal region, and tenderness may be elicited in the temporalis muscle. The masseter muscle will also become hyperactive and develop sustained contraction, with the possible onset of trismus. Occipital muscles may be recruited due to sustained contraction, and the total barrage of pain becomes a self-perpetuating noxious experience.

Infiltration or nerve block with a local anesthetic will aid in localization and temporary pain remission, although the neck and masticatory muscle pain may still persist. Such a situation is sometimes seen in patients with MPD syndrome. The inciting factor can be a severe, prolonged pain of dental origin, which is eliminated by treatment of the offending tooth. However, the secondary source of pain, the muscles of mastication, remains.

Transient, sharp pains occur in the split-tooth syndrome (Cameron, 1976; Goose, 1981). Difficulty in diagnosing the source is often due to noncontributory radiographs and poor localization of the pain by the patient. Thermal sensitivity may or may not be present. If present, it is localized to two or three teeth. The condition must be differentiated from a fractured filling, apical periodontitis, lateral periodontal abscess, masticatory tendinitis (especially anterior superior masseter and coronoid attachment of the temporalis), and MPD syndrome. Localization of the tooth can be attempted by having the patient bite against a fine wooden stick interposed between each cusp; percussing each cusp of the suspected tooth at different angles; probing the margins and fissures of each tooth and filling; and applying thermal stimuli to the suspected tooth.

There are numerous other dental problems associated with pain that have no definitive effect on masticatory function. Generally these conditions are more apparent and, consequently, treated before secondary effects occur. These include erupting teeth; sensitivity due to attrition, abrasion, or erosion; subacute pulpitis due to caries; fractured restorations and fractured teeth; gingival recession; galvanism; traumatic occlusion leading to apical periodontitis; and malposed, impacted third molars.

Periodontal disease generally causes pain of a more moderate nature than pulpal disease. Localization is more accurate due to the proprioceptive fibers in the periodontal ligament. The intensity of pain is generally less than that seen in acute periapical infections, although the presence of a lateral periodontal abscess may cause severe pain of similar intensity to a pulpitis. Radiographic evaluation, thermal and electrical vitality testing, percussion, and the use of a local anesthetic agent will enable the clinician to locate the source of the variable pain.

Several areas of pain referral associated with MPD syndrome simulate alveolar or dental pain. Tendinitis or traction periostitis at the coronoid attachment caused by spasm of the temporalis muscle and spasm in the anterior superior portion of the masseter muscle will refer pain to the adjacent maxillary alveolar process (Friedman, 1985). The inferior portion of the masseter muscle may refer pain to the mandibular molars on the affected side. Painful spasm of the lateral pterygoid muscle may also produce the sensation of the pain in the maxillary second and third molar and tuberosity regions. The patients may not always have severe symptoms, and localization is accomplished through careful palpation and infiltration of local anesthetics. Infiltration of an anesthetic adjacent to the dental alveolus will not alleviate muscle pain, especially upon function. On the other hand, local infiltration in the suspected areas of the lateral pterygoid, temporalis, or masseter muscles will produce remission of the pain.

Myogenic Pain

Pain from the oropharyngeal muscles is not as common as from the major muscles of mastication. Pharyngeal myalgia (Williams, 1942), which may be associated with muscle pain in other areas of the head, is characterized by soreness in the throat and pain on swallowing. The pain may be unilateral or bilateral. There is a lack of visible inflammation of the throat and there may be occasional hoarseness, although the vocal cords appear normal. Pain referred to the ear is felt upon swallowing. Examination may reveal tenderness of the posterior digastric, mylohyoid, stylohyoid, and infrahyoid muscles. The etiology is obscure, although exposure of the neck to extreme cold has been suspected. This condition may last for a few weeks to more than a year.

STYLOID-STYLOHYOID SYNDROME (EAGLE'S SYNDROME)

Calcification or ossification of the stylohyoid ligament is fairly common and generally has no clinical significance. When it results in excessive length of the styloid process, however, there is occasional associated pain. Stylohyoid pain syndromes have followed tonsillectomy, with subsequent scarring of the tonsillar fossa. There are two distinct forms: the classic syndrome and the carotid artery syndrome (Gossman, 1977). The classic syndrome, which occurs after tonsillectomy and may last for long periods, consists of pain associated with speech or swallowing (Eagle, 1938). The pain is paroxysmal, stabbing, and radiates to the ear, throat, tongue, neck, temple, and TMJ region. This syndrome is misdiagnosed many times as glossopharyngeal neuralgia. Mechanical stimulation of the glossopharyngeal nerve as it is pulled across the elongated styloid process during swallowing has been considered to be the cause of the pain.

The second variant, carotid artery syndrome, does not depend on a previous history of tonsillectomy. Constant pain in the neck, pain with turning the head, regional carotidynia, and tenderness of the cervical lymph nodes may be present. Internal carotid artery compression may also occur, with subsequent decreased blood flow to the brain. Tightness in the neck and pain referred to the clavicular region also have been noted. No direct correlation of styloid process length and presenting symptoms has been found.

A styloid process, longer than 7 cm, can be palpated in the region of the tonsillar fossa posterior and parallel to the occlusal plane. Palpation may elicit the pain, and infiltration of a local anesthetic agent may eliminate it. Panoramic radiography will aid in determining the presence of an elongated styloid process and the degree of calcification. The differential diagnosis should include dental pathology; TMJ disorders; cluster headache; atypical neuralgia; glossopharyngeal and geniculate ganglion neuralgia; inflammatory disease of the base of the tongue, pharynx, and larynx; as well as early carcinoma (Archer, 1975). When Eagle's syndrome is suspected, psychological evaluation is recommended prior to surgery to rule out psychosocial disturbances seen in other atypical facial pain patients (Hampf, 1986).

MYOFASCIAL PAIN-DYSFUNCTION SYNDROME

Pharyngeal pain as it relates to muscle involvement by MPD syndrome is not a common symptom. Patients with spasm of the medial pterygoid muscle may complain of pain in the throat. Occasionally, spasm in the posterior belly of the digastric muscle may also be found. This can be associated with tenderness below and behind the angle of the mandible and pain that is exacerbated upon opening of the mouth. Tenderness in the floor of the mouth due to anterior digastric, mylohyoid, and geniohyoid muscle spasm and strong contraction of the infrahyoids and platysma muscles may also occur. The resultant muscle fatigue and spasm lead to difficulty in attempts to depress the mandible. Careful oral and neurologic evaluation, plus the use of radiographs, will aid in differentiation of this condition from salivary gland disease, glossopharyngeal neuralgia, and central motor involvement.

Skeletal Pain

INFLAMMATORY: ACUTE OSTEOMYELITIS

Mandibular and, especially, maxillary osteomyelitis are uncommon despite the high incidence of odontogenic infections. The pain is usually localized, steady, and moderate to severe. Numbness of the lower lip on the affected side may follow spread of infection into the inferior alveolar canal. Lymphadenopathy may also occur. The teeth become extremely sensitive to percussion and eventually may become hypermobile. There is generally an elevation of temperature. When localization and drainage occur, the acute symptoms begin to subside, with a decrease in the pain and fever. Mandibular dysfunction and reflex contraction of the masticatory muscles occur from central excitatory effects. There may also be trismus from direct involvement of adjacent muscles. The history, radiographs, use of anesthetic blocks, and biopsy will aid in differentiation of osteomyelitis from primary neuritis, ear disease, and TMJ or masticatory muscle pain. As with many acute orofacial pains, however, blocking the primary source may still leave secondary muscle pain and tenderness.

METABOLIC DISEASE: DIABETES MELLITUS

The effects of diabetes mellitus upon the jaw bone and periodontium are not always evident. Hypoinsulinism may be responsible for impaired circulation in the nutrient vessels supplying the bone and the associated sensory nerves. Continuous or intermittent burning pain may occur, with exacerbations, and hyperesthesia of the tongue and mucosa can be present. Loss of alveolar bone and periodontal abscesses may also occur. Xerostomia, polyphagia, polydipsia, and polyuria are associated symptoms. Masticatory muscle dysfunction is not common.

FRACTURES

Undiagnosed fractures of the jaw may be a cause of pain that is exacerbated by mandibular function. Mandibular dysfunction and masticatory muscle pain are concurrent due to a reflex guarding pattern, central excitation, and referred pain. Crepitus, displacement of fragments, asymmetry, malocclusion, and tooth mobility are all diagnostic features.

Pain referred to the zygoma and orbital rim may be present with maxillary fractures. Depressed zygomatic arch fractures may at times obstruct the movement of the coronoid process, producing pain and limited opening of the mouth. This may be mistakenly attributed solely to trismus. Even after proper reduction of the fracture, hemorrhage and ensuing fibrosis and scarring may reduce mandibular mobility.

NEOPLASIA

Benign bone lesions of the mandible and maxilla are generally pain-free. Secondary infection, encroachment on nerves, or massive expansion, however, can produce pain and mandibular dysfunction (Figs. 24–31 and 24–32). Restricted jaw motion occurs from lesions of the coronoid process (Fig. 24–25) or the condylar region.

Malignant lesions (fibrosarcoma, osteogenic sarcoma, Ewing's tumor, and metastatic tumors), due to their invasive nature, usually cause more pain than benign tumors. Metastatic carcinoma to the mandible will also cause paresthesia and anesthesia as a result of pressure on the mandibular nerve. The degree of mandibular dysfunction associated with neoplastic disease is related to the size and location of the lesion and the severity of the pain.

Neurogenic Pain: Traumatic Neuroma

Traumatic, or amputation neuroma, is a non-neoplastic proliferation of peripheral nerves at a site of injury. It is an attempt by transected nerve endings to re-establish innervation. In the oral cavity, amputation neuroma may develop secondary to jaw fracture, tooth extraction, chronic mucosal ulceration, and surgery. The mandible, buccal mucosa, lip, tongue, and floor of the mouth are sites commonly involved.

In more superficial lesions, both pain and exquisite tenderness are found. The pain is usually well localized. However, stimulation of the area of hypersensitivity may cause severe pain to radiate in the involved division. Infiltration with a local anesthetic agent will localize and temporarily alleviate the pain. Mandibular dysfunction may or may not be found, depending on the severity of pain. Due to difficulty in diagnosing neural involvement, masticatory dysfunction often has been inadvertently attributed as the source of the pain.

CERVICAL PAIN

Cervical pain is an important consideration in the production of masticatory dysfunction. Acute or long-term chronic pain brings about brain stem excitation and secondary cervical muscle hyperactivity. Cervical muscle triggering, with patterns of cephalad reference, as well as entrapment of cervical nerves two and three, will create pain patterns involving the region of the TMJ and surrounding tissues.

Superficial Cervical Pain

Superficial cervical pain is well localized, readily discernible, and is obtunded by anesthetic agents. Inflammatory conditions such as furuncles, carbuncles, and folliculitis result in relatively severe, acute, localized pain and tenderness. Along with this there is a central excitatory effect, muscle splinting, and secondary spasm in the surrounding cervical muscles. Other inflammatory conditions, such as dermatitis of the neck, usually cause primary erythema, itching, scaling, and crust formation; pain and secondary infection may follow. Herpes zoster appears as a vesicular eruption along the course of the cervical nerves. This is normally heralded by tingling or pain a few days prior to onset of the lesions. Postherpetic neuralgia may last for months or years after the eruption has subsided. The pain is sharp, persistent, and shooting, and the skin is sensitive to touch. This viral disease occurs frequently in connection with systemic infections and localized spine or nerve root lesions (syphilis, Hodgkin's disease, blood dyscrasias, metastatic carcinoma, and trauma).

Neoplasia of the skin may cause pressure on underlying structures, or there may be secondary infection leading to superficial pain. The pain is generally polyneuritic, mild, and sharp or burning. There may be associated areas of paresthesia or sensory loss and muscle weakness. The clinical examination is helpful in differentiating pain caused by neoplasms from other sources of superficial pain, because it may reveal a localized lesion or enlarged regional lymph nodes.

A disease of peripheral nerve origin and distribution, neurofibromatosis (von Recklinghausen's), is an inherited benign condition associated with the presence of superficial and deep, internal and external plexiform neuromas. When these neuromas are subjected to pressure they can cause paresthesia and neuralgia. They may also cause destruction of bone.

Superficial lesions of traumatic origin, from abrasions, burns, and contusions, tend to produce consistent sharp to burning pain of varying intensity. The injury leads to an inflammatory reaction with eventual increased vascular permeability and edema. A lowered pain threshold due to neural irritation and tissue inflammation and sensitization of C-polymodal nociceptors occurs, producing hyperalgesia and increased sensitivity to heat within 5 to 10 mm of the injury (Lynn, 1977).

Deep Cervical Pain

Deep pain from the cervical region is dull, aching, and usually poorly localized. It is often associated with primary or secondary muscle spasm and increases with function. Muscular, skeletal, vascular, and neural components are involved in the production of deep somatic cervical pain.

To understand the source of cervical pain and its relationship to referred pain in the face and head, one must know the anatomic distribution of the first three cervical nerves. The first two are primarily sensory and do not exit through vertebral foramina as do other cervical segments. After leaving the spinal canal, C1 and C2 exit between the occiput and atlas and between the atlas and axis, respectively. These nerves traverse between connective tissue and muscle, with the vertebral artery coursing between them, before forming the greater occipital nerve. This nerve innervates the posterior and lateral portion of the scalp. Branches of the third cervical nerve join the first two in forming the greater and lesser occipital nerves. Their sensory innervation extends forward to the frontal and supraorbital region. Any irritation to these cervical nerves in the occipital atlantoaxial region can thus cause pain referred to the frontal area. Irritation may originate from skeletal injury of the myofascial attachments at the base of the skull. The myogenic source of cervical pain can be primary or secondary.

Myogenic Cervical Pain

CERVICAL MYOFASCIAL PAIN-DYSFUNCTION SYNDROME

Myofascial pain and dysfunction of the cervical muscles may exist with or without masticatory muscle or supporting spinal muscle involvement. At some time within the patient's history, however, these structures may have been affected. The pain is usually dull and aching, and the intensity may vary from mild to severe depending on the degree of cervical motion. Localized areas of muscle tenderness may be discerned, especially in the shawl segment of the trapezius muscle. Other deep muscles, such as the splenius capitis, semispinalis capitis, levator scapulae, and sternocleidomastoid, may also be involved. The localized painful areas within the muscle are considered to be caused by asynchronous firing of muscle spindles leading to spasticity or loss of the ability to assume normal muscle resting length. These trigger points within the muscle may elicit predictable patterns of referred pain on pressure or movement (Travell, 1952). The referred pain from the cervical muscles is more prevalent in tense, middle-aged women. Associated physical factors such as sewing, reading, and occupational habits add to the development of the problem. The onset will usually not have a traumatic etiology, although trauma can be the initiator.

FIBROMYALGIA (FIBROSITIS)

This is a painful bilateral muscle disorder involving nonreferring tender points in the masticatory muscles and neck. Muscle ache, fatigue, and stiffness are present. Pain patterns are invariable, and consistently bilateral and symmetrical. Palpation produces local tenderness with no pain radiation or referral. Although

patients do not always have problems with sleeping, they awaken fatigued in the morning.

Those suffering from fibromyalgia may have concurrent MPD syndrome, and patients with MPD syndrome may have fibromyalgia. The profound difference exists in the character of the tender points. Blood tests and radiographs are essentially normal. A secondary form, or concomitant fibromyalgia, may be due to rheumatoid arthritis, ankylosing spondylitis, or systemic lupus erythematosus. Masticatory dysfunction may be a component with this more generalized process and, if present, will necessitate more extensive therapy than would otherwise be needed with MPD syndrome alone (McCain, 1988).

MUSCLE OR TENDON RUPTURE

Rupture of a muscle or tendon, which occurs during sudden acceleration and deceleration as experienced in rear-end car collisions, sports injuries, falls, and blows to the head (Jackson, 1977), may result not only in painful muscle spasm within 24 hours but also in cervical joint dysfunction, internal derangement of the TMJs, traumatic myositis, retropharyngeal hemorrhage, and vertebral fracture (see page 453). Damage to the trachea, spinal cord, and cervical ganglia is also possible.

Injury to the stellate ganglion may lead to diffuse, constant, burning, causalgic pain, which has associated autonomic effects. The pain is usually located within the shoulder and arm, and a unilateral Horner's syndrome (partial ptosis of the upper eyelid, constricted pupil, and absence of sweating on the face and forehead) may develop on the ipsilateral side.

Sports-related injuries, falls, and blows to the head result in trauma similar to rear-end vehicular accidents. Hemorrhage and muscle tears create bruised and tender myositic areas that may become focal trigger points after healing. Such trigger points may be found in the sternocleidomastoid, trapezius, and short neck flexor muscles. Triggering and secondary muscle recruitment may bring about temporalis, masseter, and lateral pterygoid muscle tenderness and dysfunction. Limited neck mobility and mandibular motion may not only occur from muscle hyperactivity but also as a guarding mechanism to reduce pain long after resolution of the injury. Subsequent muscle contracture may make rehabilitation difficult. Internal derangement of the TMJ created by stretching and tearing of the attachments of the disc and capsule further complicate mandibular mobility

(Dolwick, 1983). The history and physical examination, cervical radiographs, CT scan, and MRI will help differentiate this condition from cervical spondylosis, cervical osteoarthritis, and cervical MPD syndrome.

SCALENUS ANTICUS SYNDROME

This syndrome is the result of compression of the neurovascular bundle as it traverses the thoracic outlet to the arm. Compression can be caused by muscle enlargement, spasm, swelling associated with trauma, or anatomic variations such as broad muscle insertions, or an abnormally elevated first rib (Ochsner, 1935). It affects the forearm and hand, producing aching pain, paresthesia, and muscle weakness. Tenderness of the scalenus anticus muscle is found, as well as possible trigger points that refer pain to the shoulder, back, and arm. When the taut and short anterior and middle scalenus muscles entrap the brachial plexus, pain, dysesthesia, and paresthesia are experienced on the ulnar side of the hand. In contrast, pain referred from trigger points in the scalenus muscles is experienced on the radial side of the forearm and hand. Referred pain from this syndrome is relieved by elevation of the arm across the forehead while raising and pulling the shoulder forward. Neurovascular compression can be differentiated by Adson's maneuver (Cailliet, 1977). Pain due to cervical root compression, nerve entrapment in the hand (carpal tunnel syndrome), subclavian artery aneurysm, apical lung involvement, and pathological lymph nodes should be considered in the differential diagnosis.

MUSCLE HEMORRHAGE

Muscle hemorrhage may occur as a result of trauma to the cervical region. Other causes are thrombosis of the intramuscular veins during severe infection, hemorrhagic states resulting from anticoagulant therapy, scurvy, and thrombocytopenic purpura. The extent of these hemorrhages may vary from extravasated streaks between fascicles of muscle to discrete hematomas several centimeters in diameter. The pain may be moderate to severe, throbbing or aching, and worse on palpation. If there are torn muscle fibers associated with the bleeding, the symptoms are more acute, with muscle spasm, stiffness of the neck, and poor localization of the pain.

SECONDARY REFLEX SPASM FROM NOXIOUS STIMULI

Cervical pain related to the neck muscles may originate in other structures. Noxious stimuli from the soft tissue structures of the head can cause a physiologic central spread of excitation, thus producing pain at a distance from the site of the original disturbance. After a long period of noxious stimulation, secondary reflex contraction and spasm of the neck muscles may follow, resulting in a persistent deep ache, with localized stiffness and limitation of motion. Conversely, referred pain of cervical origin also may eventually recruit the muscles of mastication.

Dalessio (1972) has described various sources of secondary muscle contraction pain in the neck. Repeated injections of hypertonic saline in the right temporalis muscle initiated the onset of neck pain on the side of the injection, which became sustained and augmented with subsequent injections. In another experiment, conjunctival irritation of prolonged duration led to cervical and occipital paresthesia and tightness.

Chronic sinus disease, migraine, and prolonged contraction of the intrinsic and extrinsic eye muscles may also cause ophthalmic division pain and a tight or stiff sensation in the trapezius and deltoid muscle region. Chronic sinus disease, migraine, and prolonged anxiety states may also lead to sustained muscle contraction pain in the neck. The pain is usually a deep, persistent ache without throbbing or sharp qualities. There is associated muscle tenderness, with the discomfort being accentuated on neck motion.

A differentiation of soft and hard tissue sources of secondary muscle pain must include tenderness of the cervical vertebral attachments and ligamentous insertions created by a traction periostitis (Cailliet, 1975). Torticollis, scoliosis of the cervical spine due to trauma, and infection of the throat must also be considered. Cervical disc compression leading to encroachment on the foramen magnum may result in a deep, aching pain or a sharper pain superimposed on a dull, aching background. The quality and effects depend on the nerves compressed. Psychogenic habit patterns (a turning away from emotional conflict) must also be considered as a cause of secondary cervical muscle pain (see Chapter 20).

Skeletal Cervical Pain

In determining deep sources of cervical pain, skeletal involvement on an inflammatory, degenerative, metabolic, traumatic, and neoplastic basis must be considered. Much information can initially be obtained from an adequate history. Arthritic diseases, in general, present some difficulty in diagnosis because over 40 per cent of joint complaints are of unknown etiology.

INFLAMMATORY DISEASE (see Chapter 22)

Rheumatoid Arthritis. This disease, which accounts for 10 per cent of all joint disease, has the most severe effects. Cervical spine involvement is common, with the disease affecting primarily the upper cervical discs. The TMJ may also be involved (Fig. 24–7). The atlantoaxial articulations and their associated ligaments are also frequently invaded by the rheumatoid granulation tissues. Pain from atlanto-axial disease radiates along the distribution of the first and second cervical nerves and also to the occiput and vertex. The pain is of varying intensity, from dull to sharp, and is usually constant. Rotation and flexion of the neck are very limited and cause an increase in pain intensity. Radiographic as well as serologic evaluation will aid in the diagnosis.

Ankylosing Spondylitis. Ankylosing spondylitis is another inflammatory disease with cervical involvement. It is associated with the presence of the histocompatability antigen HLA-B27 (present in 90 per cent of Caucasians, 50 per cent of blacks) and is commonly found in young males (Bywaters, 1980). Involvement of the cervical spine may cause a forward protrusion of the head and neck. Spasm of the cervical muscles is pronounced, with subsequent muscle atrophy. The patient may develop recurrent iritis (Bluestone, 1985). Cervical radicular pain is referred to the occipital region. Diminished cervical sensitivity and rigidity may follow. In some instances, either due to the cervical muscle spasm or the inflammatory effects, the TMJ may be painfully involved (Hollander, 1974).

DEGENERATIVE DISEASE

Degenerative diseases of the neck, which may initiate facial pain and masticatory muscle spasm, are osteoarthritis and intervertebral disc syndromes, such as disc herniation and spondylosis. Osteoarthritis is a common disorder found in more than 20 per cent of persons over 35 years of age. Cervical disc degeneration, or spondylosis, may have clinical signs and symptoms similar to osteoarthritis. Disc degeneration is found in over 60 per cent of the population 35 years of age or older.

Osteoarthritis. Osteoarthritis is characterized by cartilage degeneration in the posterior apophyseal joints followed by bony eburnation and osteophyte formation. In contrast, the effects of disc degeneration involve only the fibrocartilage of the intervertebral discs. There may not be a definite relationship between the degree of cervical pain and degree of radiographic change.

The cervical discs most frequently affected by degeneration are C4 through C6. The vertebral bodies also undergo degeneration, with C5 being the most common site of osteophyte formation. Nerve root compression and irritation develop, with pain occurring within the dermatome of the involved nerve as well as the associated muscles and fascia (White, 1955). Head pain is nuchal and occipital (C1 to C2 reference), and may be referred to the ipsilateral frontal and retro-orbital regions. The pain, which occurs most commonly in the morning, is described as a dull ache but may have intermittent stabbing and throbbing qualities. Sudden movements due to flexion and rotation of the neck may bring on excruciating exacerbations, with referred head and jaw pain. Neuralgic pain referred to the occipital area may be intensified by concurrent bombardment of nociceptive stimuli from both degenerative vertebral disease and trigger point muscle pain yielding *occipital myalgia-neuralgia syndrome.* Diagnostic occipital nerve block will help differentiate the neuralgia from the myofascial trigger point (Blume, 1986).

Cervical pain can also be due to a stretching effect upon thickened and contracted periarticular structures. Cold and damp weather increase stiffness and pain. Limitation of motion increases with reflex cervical muscle spasm and may, after a chronic existence, involve the masticatory musculature as a secondary reaction to repeated central excitatory effects and trigger point referral patterns from the trapezius, scalenus, and sternomastoid muscles.

Spondylosis. Spondylosis is a degenerative change that affects the disc and vertebral bodies, usually after 50 years of age. Large anterior spurs in the cervical spine may cause dysphagia, hoarseness, or cough. Compression of the vertebral arteries may produce vertigo, diplopia, scotomata, headache, or ataxia, depending on head position.

Cervical Disc Herniation. Cervical disc herniation, found mainly in young adults, may be due to severe strain or trauma. The onset of severe cervical pain follows nerve root compression and can be accompanied by the development of headache, orbital pain, blurred vision, Horner's syndrome, nystagmus, and paresthesia and motor weakness of the arms. The presence or absence of a normal jaw jerk reflex may help to localize the lesion. As with other cervical pains, chronicity may lead to masticatory muscle involvement due to a central excitatory effect and secondary reflex contraction.

Differential diagnosis of cervical degenerative disease should include MPD syndrome, multiple sclerosis, cervical cord space–occupying lesions, motor neuron disease, cord degeneration and syringomyelia. A good history, radiographic evaluation with vertebral radiographs and a CT scan, neuromuscular evaluation of the neck and extremities, an electromyogram (EMG), and possibly a myelogram will help determine the source of the pain.

TRAUMATIC INJURY: ACUTE CERVICAL STRAIN (WHIPLASH)

Acute cervical strain (whiplash) represents a combination of bony and soft tissue disruption due to trauma to the head and neck. The sudden deceleration or acceleration, depending on the direction of impact, leads to hyperflexion or hyperextension of the neck. The resulting pain is due to irritation of the cervical roots, ligamentous disruption, muscle tears, fascial injuries, and muscle strain. There can also be disc derangement in the TMJ (Ferrar, 1982). Associated autonomic symptoms of tinnitus, postural dizziness, blurred vision, retrobulbar pressure or pain, and dilated pupils may occur. Severe cervical muscle spasm leads to neck rigidity and occipital pain due to occipital nerve entrapment. Irritable myositic foci in the sternocleidomastoid, trapezius, scalenus, deltoid, and rhomboid muscles frequently refer pain to other regions in the head and neck. Compression tenderness exists over C5, C6, and C7. Spinal cord involvement leading to sensory and motor deficit may result, depending on the severity of the trauma.

Recent findings have related the onset of migraine-type headaches to whiplash injury. These headaches responded to treatments considered appropriate for migraine (Winston, 1987). This finding confirms the belief of others that in some way direct trauma or a vasospastic, ischemic reaction of the vertebral arteries that serve this region and the brainstem pain-modulating zone via the basilar artery could lead to the development of migraine-like symptoms (Barlow, 1984).

The biomechanics of disc derangement in the TMJ due to an acceleration-deceleration accident is thought to involve a forward thrust of the body causing hyperextension of the head in which the mandible moves in a posterior direc-

tion less quickly than the cranium (Weinberg, 1987). This creates a downward and forward displacement of the disc-condyle complex relative to the fossa and causes a stretching of the anterior capsule. It is accompanied by a tensing and stretching of the posterior disc attachment and synovial tissues, and loosening or tearing of the medial and lateral condylar attachments of the disc. The stretched posterior attachment becomes suspended between the condyle and fossa, and this may be perpetuated by persistent spasm of the superior head of the lateral pterygoid muscle. This condition, along with concurrent pain referral from cervical and shoulder muscle trigger points, and associated masticatory muscle pain, leads to chronically debilitating, limited mobility of the neck and mandible.

Whiplash injuries can also cause fractures of the vertebrae at the odontoid process, atlantoaxial articular facets, posterior spinous processes, or vertebral body attachments. Degenerative arthritis, spondylitis, and cervical spondylosis may ensue. Displacement of bony articulations and fractures may also cause vertebral artery compression at C1, C2, C3, and C6. It is theorized that transient insufficiency of the vertebral artery, which supplies the lateral spinothalamic tract, may lead to motor and sensory deficits. Transmission of pain impulses to the thalamus from the spinal nucleus of the trigeminal nerve, from the cranial nerves C7, C9, and C10, and from the first three cervical nerves is interrupted when the site of vascular insufficiency is in the upper cervical region (Cailliet, 1975).

A good history and clinical examination, a CT scan, radiographs, and MRI of the TMJ will help differentiate a whiplash injury from primary MPD syndrome, CNS lesions, and primary degenerative spinal disease.

NEOPLASIA

In rare instances, upper cervical vertebral body neoplasia may become a source of neck and face pain and paresthesia. Sensory impairment of the face will occur when lesions compress the descending root of the trigeminal nerve. Benign neoplasms (osteoma, neurofibroma, and angioma), and malignant lesions metastatic from the breast, ovary, prostate, thyroid, or lung, will cause chronic pain referred to the occiput, retro-orbital, and frontal and postauricular regions. Multiple myeloma and infiltrative lesions of Hodgkin's disease or leukemia may also cause pain due to swelling and expansion. Pressure from vertebral collapse leads to encroachment on the intervertebral foramina and nerve root compression. As in other compressive cervical involvements, the type and degree of sensory and motor effects depend on whether higher or lower vertebral bodies are affected, and which of the ventral or dorsal root components are involved. Paget's disease of the upper vertebral bodies and base of the skull has been linked to occipital and frontal head pain.

The history and neuromuscular examination, imaging studies, cerebral spinal fluid evaluation, and myelography will differentiate vertebral neoplasia from demyelinating disease, arthritis, discogenic disorders, and cervical MPD syndrome.

Vascular Source of Cervical Pain

CAROTIDYNIA

Pain originating at the bifurcation of the common carotid artery or in the external carotid area is called carotidynia. Fay (1932) described this pain as involving the carotid artery and its maxillary branches. The syndrome features tenderness, swelling, and occasional conspicuous pulsations of the common carotid artery. Compression of the artery against the transverse cervical process elicits severe pain. With involvement of the maxillary branches, pain may be referred to the eye, malar, and postauricular regions and neck. The cause of carotidynia has been related to transient inflammation, overdistention, relaxation, and increased pulsation of the carotid artery (Lovshin, 1977).

The pain of carotidynia is of high intensity, short duration (11 days on average), intermittent, unilateral or bilateral, and without associated visual disturbance. It occurs more commonly in women and is most prevalent between 40 and 50 years of age (Roseman, 1967). It is usually self-limited and without systemic symptoms. There is sometimes a history of vascular headaches. If systemic symptoms are present, along with visual disturbances and an elevated erythrocyte sedimentation rate, one must rule out cranial arteritis.

CERVICAL MIGRAINE (CERVICOGENIC HEADACHE)

Another cervical pain of vascular origin is cervical migraine. This syndrome may follow trauma, palpation or overmanipulation of the cervical spine, or movement of the neck in various positions, especially flexion. The neck pain is unilateral, with associated paresthesia, and may last for minutes to days. Severe pains

provoke nausea and vomiting. Occipital tenderness and hyperalgesia of the posterior head and neck occur. Occipital neuralgia due to compression of C2, C3, and C4 may be concurrent with bilateral stiffness and pain referred to the neck, occiput, and frontal region. Neck pain is increased with bending and rotation. Tinnitus and vertigo may be present and are also increased with head movement. Transient scotomata, and pain and paresthesia of the upper extremities, also occur. The symptoms result from interference with circulation in the vertebral artery and its branches as they traverse the vertebral canal. Findings reveal abnormalities of the articulation of C2 and C3 (Pfaffenrath, 1984). Complete vertebral artery occlusion in the cervical region will also lead to ischemia of the associated cervical muscles, with concomitant rigidity, tenderness, and pain (Dalessio, 1972).

Neurogenic Source of Cervical Pain

NERVE ROOT COMPRESSION

Compression of the spinal nerves in their foramina and pressure on the cord itself can lead to a combination of motor and sensory deficits. Whether due to trauma, spondylitis, spondylosis, disc compression or protrusion, or neoplasia, interference through pressure and irritation results in deep aching pain of varying intensity. The pain is localized in the proximal regions (neck and shoulder), and paresthesia or numbness is found in the extremities. There may also be intermittent hyperalgesia, muscle wasting in the shoulder and arm, and associated muscle fasciculation.

Cervical and head pain may also be initiated by irritation of the ventral motor roots of the upper five cervical nerves by flexion and rotation of the neck. Frontal, vertex, and occipital paresthesia, with an associated burning scalp sensation, may be present. Severe paroxysms of pain during movement may create muscle contraction headache that, if persistent, will cause reflex muscle spasm through referred pain and excitatory effects and coexisting nerve and muscle pain in the neck and occipital and frontal regions (Cloward, 1963).

NEOPLASIA: EXTRAMEDULLARY AND INTRAMEDULLARY

Lesions that develop within or invade the cervical spinal cord may, by compression or destruction, cause changes in the descending trigeminal root. Alterations in temperature and pain perception then occur (Merritt, 1983). Direct neurogenic involvement by neoplastic invasion may also produce cervical nerve root compression and pain. These neoplasms are either extramedullary or intramedullary. Extramedullary neoplasms are usually metastatic from lung, breast, kidney, prostate, and ovary, or are of leukemic origin. They initially involve the vertebrae and then invade the intervertebral foramina and spinal canal. Extramedullary tumors produce symptoms of pain and paresthesia followed by a sensory loss, weakness, and muscle wasting. Occlusion of the spinal vessels and severe compression necrosis of the cord also may occur.

The most common intramedullary tumors are neurofibromas, meningiomas, and, more rarely, ependymomas. Intramedullary tumors may extend over many segments or be confined to several segments. Because of this variation of involvement, the symptoms can be localized or more general. Meningiomas may involve the foramen magnum and upper cervical segments, and commonly produce pain in the occipital region and stiffness of the neck muscles. Involvement of the upper cervical segments also results in weakness and wasting of the neck muscles. Nystagmus and Horner's syndrome may be found when lesions involve any portion of the cervical cord.

The neck pain and paresthesia and motor involvement associated with cervical neoplasia must be differentiated from acute cervical strain, osteoarthritis and other degenerative diseases, syphilis, multiple sclerosis, syringomyelia, basal brain tumors, and Paget's disease.

PSYCHOGENIC PAIN (see Chapter 20)

Anxiety-Depression

Reaction to pain is a subjective experience influenced by cerebral functions and based on past experience. Pain that arises solely from cerebration may be considered a psychogenic process. Fear and speculation about the cause of one's pain provokes additional worry and preoccupation. Anxiety and depression play a responsible role in individuals who adopt a lifestyle in which suffering is a major factor.

In TMJ patients, Dworkin (1989) has found a greater correlation between continued high levels of pain and anxiety and depression than with physical symptoms. Anxiety as it relates to a psychogenic response may involve a threatened separation from an important person, as in

withdrawal from love, or a reaction to a threatened injury, as occurs with punishment. Therefore, it is the effect of an anticipated happening. Anxiety can lead to acute pain problems such as duodenal ulcer, low back pain, and MPD syndrome. Ignoring unavoidable conflict and elevation of tension levels may also create hyperactive muscle activity leading to MPD syndrome (Olson, 1979). Anxiety will also enhance the perception and response to a painful process. Experimentally induced emotional stress will increase masticatory muscle hyperactivity in MPD syndrome patients two to five times more than in the normal population (Mercuri, 1979).

Depression as it relates to orofacial pain is a more chronic and refractory problem. It occurs frequently in chronic headache patients (Sternbach, 1984). Feelings of inadequacy, anger, and self-punishment are major factors associated with reactive depression. This feeling can be a response to a real, threatened, or fantasized loss of a loved one, job, status, physical strength, attractiveness, or even goals. A lack of motivation, or adequate means to overcome this loss or to regain the missing gratification, exists. Symptoms of weakness, tiredness, loss of appetite, and apathy predominate.

Emotional stress, anger, and unhappiness may create a condition of sustained muscle contraction by somatization of repressed feelings. This can involve the masticatory apparatus. Symptomatically, all the essentials for mandibular dysfunction may be present. Pain, tenderness of the masticatory muscles, limitation of function, and even joint sounds can develop. The patients may relate an endless history of visiting numerous medical and dental specialists who were unable to treat them successfully. In certain instances, examination may reveal a disproportionate response to the symptoms. These emotional factors can theoretically influence the spinal synaptic gate by reducing its inhibitory effects, thus allowing a greater number of incoming small pain fiber impulses to reach the cognitive areas.

Chronic and severe pain sufferers, improperly treated, may develop depression when any hope of success has been abandoned. The real significance of their pain may be lost, and they may become totally absorbed in a world of pain and suffering. A history of past diagnosis and treatment and a thorough evaluation may reveal a reason for the depressive state. A comparison of patients with atypical facial pain, MPD syndrome, and TMJ disc derangement, using the Minnesota Multiphasic Personality Inventory

(MMPI), revealed that MPD syndrome and atypical facial pain patients exhibited considerably more depression, hypochondriasis, and hysteria than did internal disc derangement patients. Additional categorization using this psychometric index may be beneficial (Eversole, 1985). Concern and caution, however, have been expressed about the use of the MMPI as a generally reliable tool for determining personality profile in chronic headache patients. Their tendency to overendorse specific headache questions in the profile significantly elevates the depression, hypochondriasis, and hysteria scores (Dieter, 1988) (see Chapter 20).

Tension Headache (Muscle Contraction or Psychogenic Headache)

Tension headache usually does not have a vascular, inflammatory, or traction component. It constitutes up to 70 per cent of headache patients, with women predominating, and may occur as a complication in 30 per cent of migraine headache patients.

This type of headache is not the typical stress and fatigue-related pressure headache that develops for a short period and is relieved by conventional medication. This headache is a psychophysiological response to anxiety and depression characterized by a steady ache that is described as a tight, band-like, squeezing, or vise-like sensation in the upper back, neck, and around the head. It may be unilateral or bilateral, involving the temporal, occipital, parietal, or frontal region. The masticatory, cervical, and scalp muscles are tender and the patient may complain of soreness and tingling of the scalp, especially when combing the hair. The site and intensity may vary. The symptoms may last for weeks, months, or years without any deterioration of the patient's health. Poor sleep patterns are characteristic, with the patient awakening during the night and early in the morning.

In contrast to migraine, tension headache has no associated aura, photophobia, or visual, nasal, or sleep disturbances. Instead there is a daily, steady, nonthrobbing pain that worsens as the day progresses, leaving the patient's head and neck movement guarded. These headaches occur most frequently between the hours of 4:00 and 8:00 AM and 4:00 and 8:00 PM. Mandibular movement, such as chewing or yawning, may aggravate the headache. The headache also worsens when stress, conflict, or adverse interpersonal relations are experienced. This response fosters some secondary gain, and also helps to obscure a serious emotional disorder, most commonly depression (Martin, 1967). Anxiety and depressive symptoms are converted into physical symptoms that are more apparent and acceptable to the patient. Dullness, apathy, fatigue, and irritability, with possible suicidal undertones, may be elicited during a careful history. Tenderness is present in the trapezius, sternomastoid, temporalis, masseter, occipitalis, frontalis, and other scalp muscles. There also may be referred pain to the orbit, preauricular region, and vertex. Because of the overlap of tenderness and pain referral, muscle contraction headache can be mistaken for primary MPD syndrome.

The mechanism for tension or muscle contraction headache involves cortical influences that alter the gamma efferent system and allow it to continue to fire, thereby permitting an already tightly contracted group of muscles to remain contracted. This continuous reflex contraction also causes ischemia of the scalp muscles that leads to an itching and tingling scalp. EMG activity does not always increase with the onset of pain in tension headache, as it does in migraine headache patients (Phillips, 1982; Sutton, 1982). This finding reinforces the concept that cortical influence and secondary gain may be the provoking factors (Ramirez, 1985). Physical evaluation, blood tests, a CT scan, EEG, and EMG may all be normal. The differential diagnosis includes MPD syndrome, CNS lesions and demyelinating disease, cervical arthritis and spondylosis, cervical MPD syndrome, and primary depression.

Hypochondriasis

Hypochondriasis is a major form of abnormal illness behavior in which an individual inappropriately and unconsciously perceives, evaluates, and acts about his own state of health (Pilowsky, 1978). It involves a fascinated absorption by the experience of a physical or mental impairment (Ladee, 1966). Overconcern with health is disproportionate to any degree of objective disease; minor pains become obsessive concerns, which are unresponsive to any therapy. Neuroticism is characteristic and there may be associated depression. This response may be the result of a real or imagined loss of someone close, the decline of a body function or skill, or disappointment with respect to a job or career (Sternbach, 1974). These exaggerated reactions of concern may be manifested in head and neck pain, which is frequently associated with increased muscle tension. Pain in the temporal, occipital, and frontal regions is associated with muscle tenderness. The degree of dysfunction may not compare with the descriptive history. The spectrum of pain intensity may vary in many patients, but the preoccupation, the fear, and conviction of disease are characteristic.

A prolonged history of illness, with numerous consultations, should alert the practitioner to observe carefully the patient's descriptive response in relation to the clinical findings. Treatment of patients with symptoms of masticatory dysfunction may be difficult, and they usually do not respond to reassurance. With a patient refractory to attempts at treatment, psychological evaluation is recommended.

Conversion Hysteria

Conversion hysteria is another form of abnormal illness behavior in which a psychoneurotic process changes emotional problems into physical symptoms. These symptoms develop as a result of deprivation, frustration, or repressed anger, and constitute a regressive way of relating to others and gratifying an unfulfilled need (MacBryde, 1970). This conversion enables the expression of a forbidden wish, imposes a punishment via the physical symptoms, and provides a new way of relating to others through a sick role. Motor, sensory, and vasomotor disturbances occur as part of the problem.

Pain is a very common conversion symptom related to aggression and punishment. Pain represents an attempt to resolve a personal conflict that cannot be dealt with in a healthy way. Weakness, paralysis, or convulsive movements may occur, as well as changes in cutaneous sensation, dyspnea, dysphagia, anorexia, nausea, and vomiting. Pain and mandibular dysfunction may occur, accompanied by vivid portrayals of severe stabbing, red hot poker-like, or flesh-torn descriptions of pain. Muscle spasm and stiffness preventing mandibular movement may occur in certain instances. This may follow a frightening experience (Thoma, 1969). Indifference to the pain and dysfunction, relation to an emotionally charged situation, pain description that defies neuroanatomic borders, and benefits gained by pain disability should alert the practitioner to this condition. Hypochondriacal patients contrast with conversion hysteria patients by the abnormal intensity of their condition, their fear of an organic cause, and the resolution to solve their problem. Conversion hysteria patients are not overly alarmed, may welcome the existence of an organic cause,

and are resigned to suffering with their problem.

Hysterical trismus may be a response to a recurrence of some previously experienced psychic trauma that has been repressed. The reawakening of this experience precipitates a withdrawal into an intrapsychic conflict with a nonorganic symptomatic response, trismus. The patient is usually unaware of what originally brought on this reaction. When this condition is suspected, a judicious approach to treatment is advised. Abrupt explanation as to the reality of the situation may invoke feelings of hostility and misunderstanding. Differentiation from inflammatory muscle disorders, TMJ disc displacement, ankylosis, contractive muscle disease, and neoplasia must be made by careful history, examination, and radiographs.

Chronic Post-traumatic Pain

Injuries sustained to the head in certain patients result in symptoms that far outlast the healing period. Postconcussion syndrome, which is more common after mild trauma to the head (Merrett, 1977), causes a myriad of symptoms such as headache, dizziness, memory impairment, anxiety, fatigue, irritability, and personality changes. The headache complaint is of the muscle contraction type, causing dull aching extending from the frontal and temporal region posteriorly to the occipital region. The symptoms, in many instances, represent the result of depression due to discouragement, loss, and demoralization (Rimel, 1982). The symbolic effect of the head in securing and maintaining one's control and assertiveness plays a foremost part in magnifying a traumatic experience such as that found in postconcussion syndrome. Post-traumatic anxieties may develop, and humiliation may result from interruption of one's strength and well-being. Inner conflict, fear, and even resentment may occur (Levin, 1982). These ensuing factors lead to a conversion of real symptoms to psychogenic mediators, the result of which is prolonged disability.

Sustained muscle contraction can occur with this entity. Other symptoms will depend on the areas previously injured. Increased EMG activity occurs in patients with chronic post-traumatic headache (Dalessio, 1972). Contraction of head, neck, and skeletal muscles results from noxious stimuli arising inside the head. These contractions may also be due to sustained postural conditions resulting from a pattern of tension, anxiety, and fear. Tenderness of the temporalis and occipital muscles occurs most commonly. Vascular distention pain has also been found in certain post-traumatic conditions. Mandibular dysfunction may or may not be present, depending on the site of injury and the extent of the pain the patient experiences. Differentiation of this conversion reaction from organic disease, such as traumatic neuroma or nerve entrapment syndrome, is difficult and necessitates complete radiographic imaging and a neurological and psychological evaluation.

Chronic Pain

One of the most difficult problems is the diagnosis, treatment, and understanding of the patient with chronic pain. It is defined as persistent or prolonged noxious perception by the body (usually six months or longer) associated with psychologically, emotionally, and physically evoked characteristics of suffering. The patient generally presents a complex history of organic disease that was improperly diagnosed or unsuccessfully treated. With this long-standing pain process, an abnormal illness behavior pattern may surface, leading to obsessive and hypochondriacal behavior. The person's pain and suffering become the daily obsession and motivation to seek treatment despite previously unsuccessful attempts. An entanglement of problems related to family, social acquaintances, and work-related deficiencies may encompass the patient's prolonged suffering.

Chronic pain may produce changes in the central nervous system (Tasker, 1983a). With chronic pain the stimulation of nociceptors seen in acute pain conditions is no longer necessary. It is theorized that injury to the nervous system creates a denervation hypersensitivity (deafferentiation or central pain), or a neuroma formation (Wall, 1979). This produces an alteration in the way the central nervous system processes information and subsequently makes traditional management difficult. The use of medications and therapies that stimulate the release of endorphins, psychotherapy, and strong behavioral modification may reduce the overt suffering. Professional realization should lead one, at best, to expect and accept moderate success. If attempts at appropriate treatment fail, referral for adjunctive psychotherapy may be useful in aiding the patient to cope with the pain.

RELATION OF SYSTEMIC DISEASE TO FACIAL PAIN

Clinicians often approach a specific regional complaint with an isolated view of the specific problem. Although many times this particular approach is adequate for proper diagnosis and treatment, at other times there is failure to make the correct diagnosis because of this limited point of view. Systemic disease can produce a variety of facial pains. Collagen disease, endocrine disturbances, deficiency states, anemias, and infectious diseases may relate to painful syndromes in many parts of the body.

Connective Tissue Disease

Systemic Lupus Erythematosus

Systemic lupus erythematosus (SLE) is a chronic autoimmune connective tissue disease that has familial association. There are several forms of lupus—one generalized with effects upon the kidneys, heart, lungs, joints, muscles, and cutaneous areas; and the other more localized to the face, oral mucosa, chest, back, and extremities. Both are more prevalent in women (9:1) between 20 and 40 years of age.

Erythematous, macular, cutaneous eruptions (50 per cent of patients) may characteristically be found on the face extending across the bridge of the nose to the malar areas, and also on the chest, limbs, palms, and fingertips. Oral ulcerative lesions may occur on the vermilion border of the lips, buccal mucosa, and tongue. Dermal photosensitivity is common, and arthralgia occurs in all cases. Symmetrical polyarthritis, with the appearance of articular osteoporosis and soft tissue swelling, is seen on radiographic examination. The TMJ may be more involved than previously thought, but not as involved as the peripheral joints. Muscle pain and stiffness on mandibular function may be found. Muscle necrosis develops, as in polymyositis, and sometimes there is subsequent weakness. The synovium develops villous synovitis. Joint deformity due to capsular laxity and ligament destruction, as well as degenerative arthritis due to osteonecrosis, may also result.

Evaluation of TMJ symptoms in SLE patients reveals that one-third have current complaints associated with the disease, and two-thirds have a history of severe symptoms. Clinical findings with TMJ involvement are locking or dislocation, muscle and joint tenderness to palpation, and pain with mandibular motion. Radiographic changes in the condyle include flattening, erosion, osteophytes, and sclerosis in 30 per cent of the patients (Jonsson, 1983). The arthralgia of peripheral joints is severe, especially in the proximal and metacarpophalangeal joints of the hand. The wrists, elbows, shoulders, knees, and ankles are also involved. Morning stiffness is a frequent complaint. Neurologic damage may also occur due to small vessel vasculitis, leading to cranial nerve lesions, polyneuritis, and motor signs, including chorea. In one-third of the cases of SLE there is mild to suicidal depression and psychosis.

Hematologic evaluation will aid in the diagnosis; anemia (50 per cent), leukopenia, thrombocytopenia, a constantly elevated erythrocyte sedimentation rate, and abnormal polymorphonuclear white blood cells (lupus erythematosus cells) are found. Serologic examination shows the presence of antinuclear antibodies in over 80 per cent of the cases.

Polyarteritis Nodosa (Systemic Necrotizing Vasculitis)

Polyarteritis nodosa, a connective tissue disease primarily affecting males, is characterized by inflammation and necrosis of small and medium-sized arteries. It is classified with giant cell arteritis, but presents more generalized effects and greater morbidity. The etiology is unknown, although drug hypersensitivity, viral response, allergic phenomena, and hypertension have been suggested as causative factors. Many presenting symptoms are similar to those that occur with SLE as well as other collagen diseases. These include fever, weight loss, arthralgia (50 to 75 per cent), tachycardia, and excruciating headaches due to vascular inflammation and arterial occlusion. Renal necrosis is found in 75 per cent of these patients and, as in SLE, is a major factor in determining prognosis. Subcutaneous nodules coursing along the smaller blood vessels in the skin are found in 25 per cent of the cases.

Sixty-four per cent of the patients develop musculoskeletal effects. Migratory arthralgia is associated with muscle pain and soreness, as well as muscle atrophy and weakness. Degenerative bony changes are not common, but when present suggest concurrent rheumatoid arthritis. Involvement of the TMJ and associated tissues may occur in the later stages. Arteritis in the central nervous system may lead to headache.

Laboratory tests show leukocytosis, anemia, proteinurea, and elevated erythrocyte sedimentation rate. Muscle biopsy underlying a purpuric area may at times confirm the presence of arteritis and muscle inflammation.

Giant Cell Arteritis (Cranial Arteritis, Temporal Arteritis)

Giant cell arteritis is a primary vasculitis syndrome involving major vessels of the head and limbs, as well as the aorta and coronary vessels. A close association exists with polymyalgia rheumatica syndrome, which consists of stiffness, aching, and pain in the muscles of the neck, shoulder, lower back, hips, and thighs (Fauci, 1983). Temporalis and masseter muscle pain and tenderness may be present. With these symptoms, a misdiagnosis of MPD syndrome might be made. Masseter pain becomes intense with function due to claudication (Golding, 1973). The pain may radiate to the angle of the mandible, temporal region, the ear, and TMJ. The temporal artery and scalp become strikingly tender. Headaches with a persistent deep aching or throbbing character and a burning component are common. The pain increases upon lying down and is somewhat reduced with digital pressure over the common carotid artery. Cranial and ophthalmic artery occlusion may lead to stroke and blindness. Between one-third to one-half of patients develop partial or complete loss of vision. Because the symptoms of giant cell arteritis may be confused with those of masticatory dysfunction, and because of the seriousness of the disease, serologic and neurologic evaluation should be done whenever an elderly patient presents with temporal headache, complaints of masticatory dysfunction, orbital pain, and diplopia. Temporal artery biopsy is the best diagnostic procedure because the elevated erythrocyte sedimentation rate is nonspecific.

Polymyositis and Dermatomyositis

Polymyositis and dermatomyositis are relatively uncommon collagen diseases that may occur at any age, and produce chronic inflammatory and degenerative changes of the skin and striated muscle. Their etiology is uncertain. There may be an association with rheumatoid arthritis, SLE, scleroderma, and periarteritis nodosa (Bohan, 1975). The condition is referred to as polymyositis when skin changes are not present. Skin photosensitivity occurs as in SLE, and butterfly-shaped eruptions over the bridge of the nose may be present along with ulcerations of the eyelids and lateral surfaces of the arms. The muscle changes may involve necrosis, fibrosis, and chronic inflammation. Joint and muscle pain and tenderness occur in 15 to

20 per cent of the cases. Muscle weakness and atrophy develop slowly. Masticatory and pharyngeal muscle fibrosis and contracture, with associated masticatory weakness and dysphagia, may make eating difficult. Dysphagia, which occurs in 15 per cent of the patients, may be associated with weakness of the tongue, soft palate, and uvula muscles and concurrent nasal speech. These latter symptoms are associated with severe disease and indicate a poor prognosis (Kagen, 1985).

With the progressive development of the disease, differentiation from localized masticatory muscle involvement becomes easier. Mild anemia, leukocytosis, and elevated serum aldolase, creatine phosphokinase, and transaminase levels are found. The diagnosis is confirmed by biopsy and EMG findings.

Systemic Sclerosis (Scleroderma)

This is a generalized connective tissue disorder characterized by inflammation, fibrosis, and degenerative changes in the skin, synovium, and muscles. Females are more commonly affected, usually between the third and fifth decade, with a familial tendency reported (Medsger, 1983). The etiology is unknown, although endocrine, vascular, and autoimmune factors are possible. The skin becomes indurated and fixed to the underlying connective tissue, with the formation of subcutaneous calcifications. Skin biopsy will show an increase in collagen and atrophy of the epidermis, fibrosis of arterioles, and increased melanin.

Various forms of this disease exist. The diffuse type shows initial signs of pitting edema of the face, hands, and trunk, and with the CREST syndrome type there is Calcinosis, Raynaud's phenomenon, Esophageal dysmotility, Sclerodactyly, and Telangiectasia. Ninety per cent of patients with CREST syndrome initially complain of pallor and cyanosis of the distal two-thirds of the fingers, which become cold and numb (Raynaud's phenomenon). Neuralgia-like and arthritic pains and paresthesia also occur. The tongue, soft palate, and larynx become fibrotic, with complaints of tongue stiffness and difficulty in eating and swallowing. The lips become thin and the mouth small. Muscle contracture leads to limitation in opening of the mouth. The face has a mask-like appearance. Trigeminal sensory neuropathy, as well as other sensory neuropathies, have been reported (Farrell, 1982). Dental radiographs may show extreme widening of the periodontal ligament space. Complaints of TMJ pain and crepitus may occur. Elevated serum glutamic oxalic transaminase, lactic dehydrogenase, and aldolase may be found as a result of the muscle involvement. A latex fixation test is positive in 40 per cent of the patients due to the presence of altered antibodies.

Endocrine Disease
Hypothyroidism

Hypothyroidism is due to a deficiency or lack of thyroid hormone. It may occur in childhood (cretinism and juvenile myxedema) or adult life. The changes in childhood are more pronounced, with malocclusion, retarded tooth eruption, and skeletal deformity. Myopathy occurs, producing slow movements, weakness, muscle cramps, aches, and stiffness. Exposure to cold exacerbates these fibrositis-like symptoms (Wilke, 1981). In the adult type the masticatory muscle reflexes are slower. The patient is lethargic and shows weakness, slow speech, deep voice, hoarseness, dry skin, hypohydrosis, nonpitting edema of the skin, and thinning and brittle hair, especially the lateral one-third of the eyebrows. There is puffiness of the face, especially the nose, lips, tongue, and ears. The enlarged tongue leads to posturing the mandible in an open position and mouthbreathing, which perpetuates gingivitis and dental caries. The patient may complain of headache, cervical myalgia, vertigo, and tinnitus. Facial palsies have occurred, along with difficulty in speaking. Peripheral neuropathy and paresthesia with diminished pain and light touch sensation develop due to abnormal neuronal metabolism (Swanson, 1981). Arthropathy occurs, with synovial effusions, lax joint capsules, chondrocalcinosis, and gout.

Laboratory tests for serum T3 and T4 levels, protein bound iodine, thyroid stimulating hormone, antinuclear antibodies, and rheumatoid factor will differentiate this from other endocrine and connective tissue disorders.

Hypoparathyroidism

A decrease or absence of parathyroid activity can result in a disturbance of calcium and phosphorus metabolism. Two forms of hypoparathyroidism are recognized—idiopathic and postoperative (unintentional removal of the glands during a thyroidectomy). The result is an increase in serum phosphorus and decrease in serum calcium. The chief symptom from this disorder is an increased neuromuscular excitability (Minckler, 1968). Painful muscle spasms occur in the face, larynx, and pharynx, causing a clinical picture that can be mistaken for a seizure disorder. Also present are tingling of the lips and hands, dry skin, brittle nails, and loss of hair. Myopathy is often found, and it is associated with elevated serum creatine phosphokinase levels (Kruse, 1982). Bronchial and laryngeal spasm may cause labored breathing. Tapping of the facial nerve where its main branch exits from the stylomastoid foramen in the preauricular area will cause contraction of the muscles of facial expression (Chvostek's sign). Tetany is present in almost all patients with hypoparathyroidism. Tetanic contraction of the masseter muscles may be pronounced.

Hypoparathyroidism should be differentiated from epilepsy and a brain tumor on the basis of brain calcifications, convulsions, and optic nerve findings. The history and physical evaluation, EEG studies, measurement of parathyroid hormone levels, presence of low serum calcium and high serum phosphorus, and a negative CT scan will aid in diagnosis of this disease.

Hyperparathyroidism

Hyperparathyroidism results from neoplasia (adenomas in 80 per cent of the cases), hyperplasia of the parathyroid gland (15 per cent of the cases), or parathyroid carcinoma (5 per cent of the cases), which cause incompletely regulated secretion of parathormone (Albright, 1948). Due to calcium mobilization (hypercalcemia) and general demineralization, bone cysts with fibrous linings and giant cell or brown tumors result. Pain arising from these lesions is due to secondary infection. The bony lesions in the mandible may precede all other signs by months. Mandibular radiographs revealing lytic bony lesions and loss of dental lamina dura should arouse suspicion. Radiographs of the skull may reveal a ground glass appearance of the calvarium. Malocclusion may occur from increased mobility and drifting of the dentition. Demineralization and possible collapse of the TMJ and surrounding bones may produce an opening of the bite or other malocclusion (Rosenberg, 1962).

Parathormone increases collagenase activity, which may account for the laxity of capsular and ligamentous structures seen so commonly in the vertebral column and other joints. Renal nephrolithiasis is present in 75 per cent of the cases. Fatigue, weakness, and tenderness of the masticatory muscles, as well as peripheral limb muscles, may be present. Cranial nerve neu-ropathy can lead to difficulty in swallowing, fasciculations of the tongue, and sensory loss. Depression and mood alteration cause behavioral changes.

Because of the muscle, bone, and nerve involvement, the differential diagnosis includes TMJ disorders, multiple myeloma, carcinoma, thyroid disease, Paget's disease, osteomalacia, fibrous dysplasia, and Cushing's and Addison's diseases. No tests to date are able to differentiate between neoplasia, hyperplasia, or carcinoma-induced primary hyperparathyroidism (Wallach, 1986). Laboratory tests show elevated serum calcium greater than 12 mg/100 ml, decreased serum phosphorus, anemia, elevated red blood cell sedimentation rate, increased plasma parathormone, increased urinary excretion of cyclic 3':5'-AMP, and a positive radioimmunoassay test against the PTH molecule (Schroeder, 1989).

Diabetes Mellitus

Diabetes mellitus is a multietiological disease that shares the one common cardinal feature of glucose intolerance. It is present in up to 5 per cent of the population. Diabetes mellitus is one of the most common systemic diseases producing pain, paresthesia, motor weakness, and decreased muscle reflex activity.

Diabetes is a disease of carbohydrate metabolism characterized by hyperglycemia and glycosuria (Bunick, 1979). Neuritic changes occur in diabetics and are considered to be due to occlusion of nutrient vessels to the nerves. Headaches and sensory symptoms of severe pain and paresthesia are common. Paralysis of either the third, fourth, or sixth cranial nerves on either one or both sides may occur, leading to weakness of adduction, ptosis of the eyelids, and a dilated pupil with spared light reflex (Vinken, 1968). Mandibular dysfunction is not a common finding, but oral, facial, gingival, dental, and tongue pains may occur. Symptoms of polydipsia, polyuria, polyphagia, fatigue, weight loss, pruritus, and repeated infections, including gingival and periodontal disease, should alert the clinician. Serum (glucose tolerance test) and urine tests should be performed to determine whether there is an elevated blood sugar and glycosuria.

Deficiency States and Anemia

Nerve tissue damage can occur from an inadequate dietary intake. Deficiencies of the B-complex vitamins may cause significant changes in cellular metabolism, leading to loss of dermal and mucosal integrity. Deficiencies of B_1 (thiamine), B_2 (riboflavin), nicotinic acid, folic acid, and B_{12} all produce painful states. The majority of these occur intraorally. B_{12} supplement has been shown to be effective in treating idiopathic glossodynia and some instances of trigeminal neuralgia and burning paresthesias.

Alcoholic–Vitamin Deficiency Polyneuritis

Alcoholism is now considered to be a chronic disease and no longer solely a socially aberrant behavior pattern. Psychological background, personality traits, familial alcohol use patterns, and genetics play an integrated role in its development. It is assumed that 75 per cent of American adults drink alcohol, and that 10 per cent will experience some problem with alcohol abuse.

The nutritional deficiencies that occur in chronic alcoholics are due to inadequate dietary intake, especially of vitamin B_1, toxic effects of large amounts of ethyl alcohol on gastrointestinal absorption, and the development of hepatic cirrhosis. Neurologic symptoms may be an extended effect of long-standing alcohol ingestion. Optic neuritis and ocular, facial, palatal, and pharyngeal paresis may occur. Nerves and muscles may become sensitive to pressure. In Wernicke's encephalopathy there may be paralysis of eye muscles, nystagmus, ataxic gait, and tremor. Korsakoff's psychosis syndrome (confusion, disorientation, and loss of memory) occurs as a chronic sequela to Wernicke's encephalopathy (Victor, 1971).

Although mandibular dysfunction is not a primary condition in the alcoholic, it may develop with progressive involvement of the midbrain. Variants of migrainous pain that occur in the face, such as cluster headache, are frequently brought on or accentuated by alcohol ingestion, possibly due to an increased sensitivity in these patients to vasodilating substances (Schele, 1978). Intoxicated subjects tend to sleep deeply in unusual positions and locations, thereby chronically subjecting the mandible to excursive positions favoring disc displacement and mandibular dysfunction.

The differential diagnosis should include diabetic neuropathy, CNS lesions, nutritional deficiencies, cluster headache, and migraine. An adequate history (keeping in mind the reluctance of alcoholics to admit to their abuse), finding a provokable cause for the headache, and tests for liver enzymes and vitamin B_1 levels

(serum transketolase) may help establish the cause of the problem.

Anemias

In anemia there is a decrease in the oxygen-carrying capacity of the red blood cells due to reduction in hemoglobin concentration. The causes may be numerous and are classified according to extracellular and intracellular factors. Anemias of rapid onset are manifestations of severe blood loss and shock, and are not considered in this discussion. Since anemias may be insidious in development, they usually are tolerated for a long time by most people. Symptoms may not appear until the hemoglobin level or hematocrit values fall below 50 per cent of normal. Signs of weakness, fatigue, pallor, headache, paresthesia, pain, and dyspnea, are characteristic.

The hypoxemia associated with anemias produces cerebral and superficial artery vasodilation, and patients develop unilateral or bilateral pounding headaches. Oxygen deficits, secondary to pulmonary disease, can also produce these symptoms. Visual changes, vertigo, and tinnitus may be present. Aphasia, cranial nerve palsies, stiffness of the neck and jaw muscles, nystagmus, facial paresthesia, glossodynia, glossitis, mucosal atrophy, ulceration, and dysphagia may also develop. Difficulty in wearing artificial dentures results from mucosal intolerance to irritation. Masticatory muscle fatigue may occur in severe anemias due to the relative ischemia, producing persistent tenderness and pain.

Sickle cell anemia is a genetically determined hemolytic anemia predominantly found in blacks (1 in 600). It is due to a rearranged hemoglobin pattern that causes distortion of the red blood cells resulting in reduced blood velocity, increased viscosity, hypoxia, erythrostasis, and sickling. Symptoms of mandibular pain occur due to bone marrow hyperplasia, vascular thrombosis and infarction, infection, osteosclerosis, and hypoxia. There may be secondary osteomyelitis and mental nerve neuropathy. Mandibular pain and paresthesia have been associated with the sickling crisis, and are a result of vaso-occlusive effects on the inferior alveolar nerve (Kirson, 1979). Recovery from this paresthesia may take one to two years. Headaches and cranial nerve palsies develop secondary to cerebral thrombosis. Retrusion of the mandible may occur due to retardation of growth.

A complete blood cell count, evaluation of

red blood cell morphology, and measurement of hemoglobin content and hematocrit will reveal the presence of an underlying anemia. Radiographic lesions (Robinson, 1952) should be differentiated from those associated with an endocrine disturbance, diseases of bone metabolism, or local pathology.

Infectious States

Spirochetal: Syphilis and Lyme Disease

Syphilis affects the head and neck due to invasion of *Treponema pallidum* into the connective tissues, blood vessels, and nerves. Pain is seen in the late stages of the disease; the early stages of syphilis do not cause remarkable pain and dysfunction. In the late nineteenth and early twentieth century, when advanced diagnostic techniques and treatments were not available, the disease progressed to tertiary stages more frequently. Today this is not commonly found. Severe pains may occur in late stages of chronic neurosyphilis. A positive Romberg's sign is also found, the patient being unable to stand erect with the feet together and eyes closed. In the late stage of tabes dorsalis, the pupils may become fixed. The pupils may also fail to react to the light reflex, but will to accommodation.

The effects on the trigeminal nerve can lead to sensory degeneration, but leave the motor root intact. Syphilitic involvement of the masseter and temporalis muscles can cause diffuse interstitial myositis with accompanying pain and tenderness. The onset of the neuropathic component may be gradual, with muscle weakness and loss of tendon reflexes. Loss of taste and paresthesia of the lips, tongue, and cheeks may also be present. In congenital syphilis there is a characteristic appearance of the teeth (Sarnat, 1942). Paresis, tabes, optic atrophy, and deafness may develop.

A history of contact, clinical examination, and serologic tests such as the venereal disease research laboratory (VDRL) test, rapid plasma reagin (RPR) test, *treponema pallidum* immobilization (TPI) test, and more definitively the fluorescent treponemal antibody absorption test (FTA-ABS) aid diagnosis (Sparling, 1971).

Lyme disease, newly recognized, is caused by a spirochete discovered in 1982 called *Borrelia burgdorferi* (Burgdorfer, 1982). This disease was first recognized in 1975 during an outbreak of inflammatory arthropathy in children who lived in the region of Lyme, Connecticut (Benenson, 1989). The clinical onset begins with an expanding red macular or papular rash called erythema chronicum migrans (ECM). The erythema initially occurs at the site of a tick bite, and is followed by smaller multiple secondary lesions, which fade within four weeks. This skin rash is usually accompanied by flu-like symptoms of headache, fatigue, fever, chills, myalgia, and arthralgia (Steere, 1983). The headaches may become intense and are associated with a meningitis-like neck pain and stiffness, not accompanied by a Kernig's or Brudzinski's sign. The head and neck pains are followed by migratory musculoskeletal pains involving the muscles, tendons, bones, and joints. These symptoms last for months and lead to neurologic, cardiac, and arthritic involvement (Steere, 1977). With advancing neurologic symptoms, bilateral facial palsy may occur. Sixty per cent of the patients develop intermittent asymmetrical attacks of joint pain and swelling. About 10 per cent develop chronic joint involvement. Rheumatoid-like inflammation causes pannus formation, erosion of bone and cartilage, synovial hypertrophy, and elevated synovial enzymes.

Laboratory test results are negative for the rheumatoid factor and antinuclear antibodies. The IgM and IgG immunoglobulin antibody titer test against the borrelia burgdorferi spirochete is consistently elevated (Craft, 1984), and helps in differentiating Lyme disease from other rheumatic diseases. Additional test findings show a negative VDRL test, and an elevated erythrocyte sedimentation rate. The differential diagnosis should include systemic lupus erythematosus, rheumatoid arthritis, and multiple sclerosis.

Viral, Fungal, and Parasitic Infections

Viral infections are responsible for numerous constitutional, somatic, and respiratory symptoms. Patients complain of fever, muscular aches, headache, loss of appetite, skin rashes, oral vesiculation and ulceration, gastrointestinal disturbances, upper respiratory symptoms, sinus and ear pain, nasal congestion, and sometimes unilateral or bilateral toothaches. The viral infection of neuromuscular tissues can produce changes that may persist long after the infective period. An example of this process is found in the painful aftermath of a trigeminal herpes zoster infection, causing chronic aching and burning pain and associated dysesthesia for a year or longer. The herpes simplex virus type I (HSV-I) often affects the trigeminal ganglion, the facial nerve, as well as other cranial nerve ganglia (Adour, 1978). Activation of the virus may lead to polyneuritis, demyelination, axon destruction, and even denervation so that the masticatory muscles no longer function normally (myopathy). These effects may result in fasciculation, fibrillation, myotonia, contracture, localized myositis, and atrophy. Bell's palsy may also be caused by the HSV-I, leading to a self-limiting facial paralysis. When involvement of the trigeminal motor fibers occurs, masseter muscle dysfunction may become apparent both clinically and on the EMG recording (McGovern, 1969).

The nerve and muscle response to repeated HSV-I infections and the straining of the TMJ caused by coughing and vomiting may very well be inciting factors for the onset of a chronic temporomandibular disturbance. A careful history of chronicity, prior signs of infection (recurrent oral herpetic lesion), and EMG analysis of the masseter and temporalis muscles may reveal a myopathic dysfunction.

Fungal infection caused by *Actinomyces israelii*, although not common, may also lead to symptoms of masticatory dysfunction. In the cervicofacial type, a periapical infection may spread through the alveolar bone and the periosteum into the adjacent muscles creating severe, painful limitation of movement. Infection also may spread up the ascending ramus and penetrate the middle cranial fossa. Involvement of the gingiva, floor of the mouth, palate, and salivary glands may also occur. Multiple sinus tracts on the skin are characteristic of the disease. The clinical findings, microscopic observation of distinctive sulfur granules, and culture of the fungus will help differentiate this from other infective processes.

Parasitic infections are not a common cause of masticatory dysfunction, although trichinosis due to the *Trichinella spiralis* may involve the masticatory, tongue, laryngeal, extraocular, and neck muscles. The *Trichinella spiralis* is a nematode that infects the hog so that poorly cooked pork, when eaten, will result in infestation of the intestine of man. The larvae develop into worms and after penetrating the intestine eventually migrate to striated muscle, which is a suitable site for their growth and survival. Chills, fever, facial and orbital edema, muscle weakness and tenderness, pain, and fatigue accompany the disease. The facial and orbital edema are due to inflammation of the orbital and facial muscles. Masticatory difficulty occurs in the later stages due to persistent myositis and fatigue of the muscles. Serologic tests, an enzyme-linked immunosorbent assay test, the presence of eosinophilia, and a muscle biopsy

will all help differentiate this condition from rheumatic fever, acute arthritis, polyarteritis nodosa, eosinophilic leukemia, Hodgkin's disease, meningitis, and angioedema.

Epidemic Parotitis (see page 443)

Epidemic parotitis, or mumps, is an acute and painful state caused by an RNA virus that infects only humans. It is characterized by unilateral or bilateral enlargement of the salivary glands. The testicles, ovaries, pancreas, breasts, and brain also may be affected. It is usually found in younger people, although it may occur at any age. The etiologic agent is a myxovirus found in the patient's saliva. Pain on chewing or swallowing may be the earliest symptom. There is tenderness present over the masseter muscle, unilaterally or bilaterally, depending upon the extent of parotid involvement. Occasionally the submandibular and sublingual salivary glands may also be involved, or in rare instances these glands alone may be affected. Elevation of temperature occurs with associated headache, chills, malaise, anorexia, and leukopenia. Both mandibular movement and stimulation of salivary flow increase the pain. The swelling causes the earlobe to be displaced laterally, and the ear is hidden behind the swelling, as opposed to the buccal space abscess in which the ear is not obscured. The papilla of the parotid duct may be swollen and inflamed. The tongue may be elevated when there is involvement of the submandibular gland. The acute pain usually lasts for two to three days, but relapse has occurred after two weeks.

What appears to be a dental infection may cause the patient to seek immediate dental evaluation. Serum tests reveal an elevated serum amylase. Isolation of the virus from the saliva can occur two to four days before and for about one week after the onset of symptoms. Sialography and scintigraphy are not indicated during the acute phase of the disease. The character of the symptoms, the clinical evaluation and, if necessary, laboratory tests will usually differentiate this disease from masticatory muscle pain, masseteric hypertrophy, neoplasia, cat-scratch disease, acute suppurative parotitis, and dental abscess.

SUMMARY

The numerous conditions that may cause craniofacial-cervical pain and masticatory dysfunction have been presented, with intentional duplication because of the regional diagnostic approach. The history, evaluation of the character and quality of the pain, and the use of diagnostic local anesthetic agent blocks usually reduce the number of etiologic possibilities. The most recent advances in CT scanning and MRI techniques also provide information that greatly aids in discovering or ruling out primary or associated pathology. Immunological and biochemical studies further assist in making a diagnosis.

Society's need for expedience and fast pace technology have in some ways added to, or helped propagate, the appearance of certain psychophysiologic pain syndromes. Those who treat chronic pain problems must realize that their obligation is not only to help the patient in successfully overcoming the disease but also to learn to tolerate that which cannot be completely resolved. Successful treatment may indicate a correct diagnosis, but unsuccessful treatment does not necessarily imply an incorrect diagnosis. It may mean only that our therapeutic modalities are limited.

Most importantly, one must be aware of the various conditions that may cause craniofacial and cervical pain so that serious problems are not inadvertently overlooked. If the pain process cannot be successfully managed, or if the problem is beyond one's scope and competence, the patient should be referred to the appropriate specialist for definitive care.

REFERENCES

Adour, K.: Bell's palsy: A complete expression of acute benign polyneuritis. Primary Care 2:717–733, 1975.

Adour, K., Byl, F., Hilsinger, R. L., Jr., et al.: The true nature of Bell's palsy: Analysis of 1000 consecutive patients. Laryngoscope 5:787–801, 1978.

Albright, F., and Reifenstein, B.: The Parathyroid Gland and Metabolic Bone Disease. Baltimore, Williams & Wilkins, 1948.

Alling, C., and Mahan, P. (Eds.): Facial Pain, 2nd ed. Philadelphia, Lea & Febiger, 1977.

Alter, M., and Kurtzke, J. F. (Eds.): The Epidemiology of Multiple Sclerosis. Springfield, IL, Charles C Thomas, 1968.

Archer, W. H.: Oral and Maxillofacial Surgery, vol. 2, 5th ed. Philadelphia, W. B. Saunders, 1975.

Baile, W. Jr., and Meyers, D.: Psychological and behavioral dynamics in chronic atypical facial pain. Anesth. Prog. 33:252–259, 1986.

Barlow, C.: Traumatic Headache Syndromes. Headaches and Migraine in Childhood. Philadelphia, J. B. Lippincott, 1984, pp. 181–197.

Benenson, A.: The continuing saga of Lyme disease. Am. J. Pub. Health 79.9–10, 1989.

Bengtsson, B., and Malmvall, B.: Giant cell arteritis. Acta Med. Scand. 685:1–102, 1982.

Bitoh, S., Hasegawa, H., Ohtsuki, H., et al.: Parasellar metastases: Four autopsied cases. Surg. Neurol. 23:41–48, 1985.

Black, R. G.: A laboratory model for trigeminal neuralgia. In Bonica, J. (Ed.): Advances in Neurology, vol 4. New York, Raven Press, 1974, pp. 651–658.

Block, S. L.: Possible etiology of ear stuffiness (barohypoacusis) in MPD syndrome. Abst. IADR 55:250, 1976.

Bluestone, R.: Ankylosing spondylitis. In McCarty, D. (Ed.): Arthritis and Allied Conditions. Philadelphia, Lea & Febiger, 1985, pp. 819–840.

Blume, H., and Ungar-Sargon, J.: Neurosurgical treatment of persistent occipital myalgia-neuralgia syndrome. J. Craniomandib. Pract. 1:66–73, 1986.

Bohan, A., and Peter, J.: Polymyositis and dermatomyositis. N. Engl. J. Med. 292:344–349, 1975.

Bunick, E., and Lavine, R.: The role of hyperglycemia in the development of complications in the diabetic patient. In Coodley, E. (Ed.): Internal Medicine Update. New York, Grune & Stratton, 1979, pp. 1979–1980.

Burgdorfer, W., Barbour, A., Hayes, S., et al.: Lyme disease—a tick-borne spirochetosis? Science 216:1317–1319, 1982.

Bush, F.: Malocclusion, masticatory muscles and temporomandibular joint tenderness. J. Dent. Res. 64:129, 1985.

Bush, F., and Martelli, J.: Tinnitus and earache: Long term studies in 105 patients with temporomandibular (TM) disorders. J. Dent. Res. 65:65–69, 1986.

Bywaters, E.: Clinico-pathological aspects of ankylosing spondylitis and comparison with the changes in seronegative juvenile polyarthritis and seropositive rheumatoid arthritis. Scand. J. Rheum. 9:61–66, 1980.

Cacioppi, J., Morrisey, J., and Bacon, A.: Condyle destruction concomitant with advanced gout and rheumatoid arthritis. Oral Surg. 25:919–922, 1968.

Cailliet, R.: Neck and Arm Pain. Philadelphia, F. A. Davis, 1975.

Cailliet, R.: Soft Tissue Pain and Disability. Philadelphia, F.A. Davis, 1977, p. 144.

Cameron, C.: The cracked tooth syndrome: Additional findings. J. Am. Dent. Assoc. 93:971–975, 1976.

Chandrasoma, P., and Taylor, G.: Key Facts in Pathology. New York, Churchill Livingstone, 1986, pp. 367–368.

Chun, H.: Temporomandibular joint gout. JAMA 226:353, 1973.

Clarke, T.: Trigeminal neuralgia secondary to brainstem stroke. In Saper, J. (Ed.): Topics in Pain Management, vol. 3. Baltimore, Williams & Wilkins, 10:39–40, 1988.

Cloward, R. B.: Lesions of the intervertebral disc. Clin. Orthop. 27:51–77, 1963.

Cook, A., Woolf, C., Wall, P., and McMahon, S.: Dynamic receptive field plasticity in spinal cord dorsal horn following C-primary afferent input. Nature (London) 325:151–153, 1987.

Craft, J., Grodzicki, R., and Steere, A.: Antibody response in Lyme disease: Evaluation of diagnostic tests. J. Infect. Dis. 149:789–795, 1984.

Cyriax, J.: Textbook of Orthopedic Medicine, vol. 1, ed. 7. Soft Tissue Lesions. London, Baillere Tindall, 1979, pp. 21–88.

Dalessio, D. J.: Wolff's Headache and Other Head Pain, 3rd ed. Oxford, Oxford University Press, 1972.

Dalessio, D. J.: Migraine headache. Hosp. Med. 3:214–247, 1985.

Dalessio, D. J.: Wolff's Headache and Other Head Pain, 5th ed. Oxford, Oxford University Press, 1987.

Desrosiers, J.: Headache related to contraceptive therapy. Headache 13:117–124, 1973.

Desser, E.: Miosis, trismus, and dysphagia: An unusual

presentation of temporal arteritis. Ann. Intern. Med. 71:961–962, 1969.

Diamond, S., and Dalessio, D. J.: The Practicing Physician's Approach to Headache, 4th ed. Baltimore, Williams & Wilkins, 1986.

Dieter, J., and Swerdlow, B.: A replicative investigation of the reliability of the MMPI in the classification of chronic headaches. Headache 28:212–222, 1988.

Dolwick, M.: Surgical Management in Internal Derangements of the Temporomandibular Joint. Helms, C., Katzberg, R., and Dolwick, M. (Eds.): Radiology Research and Education Foundation, 1983.

Dubner, R., Sharav, Y., Graceley, R., and Price, D.: Idiopathic trigeminal neuralgia sensory features and pain mechanisms. Pain 31:23–33, 1987.

Dubois-Delcq, M., Schumacher, J., and Sever, L.: Acute multiple sclerosis: Electronmicroscopic evidence for and against a viral agent in plaques. Lancet 2:1408–1411, 1973.

Dworkin, S.: Dental researchers meet in San Francisco. Jakush, J. (Ed.): Am. Dent. Assoc. News 20:35, 1989.

Eagle, W.: Elongated styloid process: Symptoms and treatment. Arch. Otolaryngol. 67:127–132, 1938.

Eagle, W.: Sphenopalatine ganglion neuralgia. Arch. Otolaryngol. 35:66–84, 1942.

Eversole, L., and Stone, C.: Vasogenic facial pain (cluster headache). Int. J. Oral Maxillofac. Surg. 16:25–35, 1987.

Eversole, L., Stone, C., Matheson, D., and Kaplan, H.: Psychometric profiles and facial pain. J. Oral Surg. 60:269–274, 1985.

Farrell, D., and Medsger, T.: Trigeminal neuropathy in progressive systemic sclerosis. Am. J. Med. 73:57–62, 1982.

Fauchald, P., Rygvold, O., and Oystese, B.: Temporal arteritis and polymyalgia rheumatica: Clinical and biopsy findings. Ann. Intern. Med. 77:845–852, 1977.

Fauci, A.: Systemic vasculitis. In Lichtenstein, I., and Fauci, A. (Eds.): Current Therapy in Allergy and Immunology. Philadelphia, B. C. Decker, 1983, pp. 129–136.

Fay, T.: Atypical facial neuralgia, a syndrome of vascular pain. Ann. Otolaryngol. 41:1030–1062, 1932.

Ferrar, W., and McCarty, W.: A Clinical Outline of TMJ Diagnosis and Treatment. Montgomery, Alabama, Normandie, 1982, p. 84.

Finneson, B. E.: Diagnosis and Management of Pain Syndromes, 2nd ed. Philadelphia, W. B. Saunders, 1969.

Foxen, E. H.: Lectures, Notes on Diseases of the Ear, Nose and Throat. Oxford, Blackwell, 1972.

Friedman, M.: Tenomyositis of the masseter muscle: Report of cases. J. Am. Dent. Assoc. 110:201–202, 1985.

Fulton, J., and Barly, P.: Tumors in the region of the third ventricle. J. Nerv. Ment. Dis. 69:18–24, 1969.

Gerbe, R. W., Fry, T. L., and Fischer, N. D.: Headache of nasal spur origin: An easily diagnosed and surgically correctable cause of facial pain. Headache 24:329–330, 1984.

Goadsby, P., and MacDonald, G.: Extracranial vasodilation mediated by vasoactive intestinal polypeptide (VIP). Brain Res. 329:285–288, 1985.

Gobel, S., and Binck, J.: Degenerative changes in primary trigeminal axons and neurons in the nucleus caudalis following tooth pulp extirpation in the cat. Brain Res. 132:347–354, 1977.

Golding, D.: A Synopsis of Rheumatic Diseases, 2nd ed. Chicago, Year Book Medical, 1973.

Goldstein, N., Gibilisco, J., and Rushton, J.: Trigeminal neuropathy and neuritis: A study of etiology with emphasis on dental causes. JAMA 184:458–462, 1963.

Goose, D.: Cracked tooth syndrome. Br. Dent. J. 2:224–228, 1981.

Gossman, J. R., and Tarsitano, J.: Styloid-stylohyoid syndrome. J. Oral Surg. 35:555–560, 1977.

Graham, J.: Cluster headache. Headache, 11:175–185, 1972.

Hall, E.: Differential diagnosis of glossodynia. J. Oral Med. 42:85–91, 1987.

Hamilton, C., Shelley, W., and Tumulty, P.: Giant cell arteritis and polymyalgia rheumatica. Medicine 50:1–27, 1971.

Hampf, G., Aalberg, V., Tasanen, A., and Nyman, C.: A holistic approach to stylalgia. Int. J. Oral Maxillofac. Surg. 15:549–552, 1986.

Harris, M.: Psychogenic aspects of facial pain. Br. Dent. J. 136:199–202, 1974.

Healy, L., and Wilske, K.: The Systemic Manifestations of Temporal Arteritis. New York, Grune & Stratton, 1979.

Hines, J., and Nankervis, G.: Herpes zoster infection. Hosp. Med. 13:72–84, 1977.

Hollander, J. L., and McCarty, D. J.: Arthritis and Allied Conditions, 8th ed. Philadelphia, Lea & Febiger, 1974.

Hunt, J.: Geniculate neuralgia (neuralgia of the nervus facialis). A further contribution to the sensory system of the facial nerve and its neuralgic conditions. Arch. Neurol. Psychiatry 37:253–258, 1937.

Jackson, R.: The Cervical Syndrome, 4th ed. Springfield, IL, Charles C Thomas, 1977.

Jannetta, P.: Trigeminal accessory fibers rediscovered. World Med. Aug:13–14, 1968.

Jonsson, R.: Temporomandibular joint involvement in systemic lupus erythematosus. Arthritis Rheum. 26:1506–1510, 1983.

Kagen, L.: Laboratory assays useful in assessment of patients with disorders of muscle. In Cohen, A.: Laboratory Diagnostic Procedures in the Rheumatic Diseases. New York, Grune and Stratton, 1985.

Katzberg, R., Bessette, R., Tallents, R., et al.: Normal and abnormal temporomandibular joint: MR imaging with surface coil. Radiology 158:183–189, 1986.

Kazuo, H., Kenjiro, D., Haruhiko, M., and Banri, N.: Factors influencing the duration of treatment of acute herpetic pain with sympathetic nerve block. Pain 32:147–157, 1988.

Kelly, W.: Gout and other disorders of purine metabolism. In Isselbacher, K., Adams, R., and Petersdorf, R. (Eds.): Principles of Internal Medicine, ed. 9. New York, McGraw-Hill, 1980, pp. 479–486.

Kirson, L., and Tomaro, A.: Mental nerve paresthesia due to sickle cell crisis. Oral Surg. 48:509–512, 1979.

Kleinman, H., and Eubank, R.: Gout of the temporomandibular joint. Oral Surg. 27:281–285, 1969.

Kruse, K., Scheunemann, W., Baier, W., and Schawb, J.: Hypocalcemic myopathy in idiopathic hypoparathyroidism. Eur. J. Pediatr. 138:280–282, 1982.

Kudrow, L.: Cluster Headache: Mechanisms and Management. London, University Press, 1980, pp. 10–150.

Ladee, G. A.: Hypochondriacal Syndromes. Amsterdam, Elsevier, 1966.

Lambert, G., Bogduk, P., and Goadsby, P.: Decreased carotid arterial resistance in cats in response to trigeminal stimulation. J. Neurosurg. 61:307–315, 1984.

Laskin, D. M.: Etiology of the pain-dysfunction syndrome. J. Am. Dent. Assoc. 79:147–153, 1969.

Laskin, D., and Block, S.: Diagnosis and treatment of myofascial pain-dysfunction syndrome. J. Prosthet. Dent. 56:75–84, 1986.

Lerner, A.: Infections with herpes simplex virus. In Isselbacher, K., Adams, R., and Petersdorf, R. (Eds.): Principles of Internal Medicine, ed. 9. New York, McGraw-Hill, 1980, pp. 847–851.

Levin, H., Benton, A., and Grossman, R.: Consequence of

Closed Head Injury. New York, Oxford University Press, 1982.

Lovshin, L.: Carotidynia. Headache 17:192–195, 1977.

Lynn, B.: Cutaneous hyperalgesia. Br. Med. Bull. 33:103–108, 1977.

MacBryde, C. M., and Blacklow, R. S.: Signs and Symptoms, 5th ed. Philadelphia, J. B. Lippincott, 1970.

Markoff, M., and Farole, A.: Reflex sympathetic dystrophy syndrome. Oral Surg. 61:23–28, 1986.

Martin, M., Rome, H., and Swenson W.: Muscle contraction headache: A psychiatric review. Res. Clin. Stud. Headache 1:184–192, 1967.

McCain, G., and Scudds, R.: The concept of primary fibromyalgia (fibrositis): Clinical value, relation, and significance to other chronic musculoskeletal pain syndromes. Pain 33:273–287, 1988.

McCarty, D. J.: Arthritis and Allied Conditions. Philadelphia, Lea & Febiger, 1985.

McGovern, F.: Trigeminal sensory neuropathy and Bell's palsy. Arch. Otolaryngol. 94:466–470, 1969.

Medsger, T.: Progressive systemic sclerosis. Clin. Rheum. Dis. 9:655–670, 1983.

Melzack, R.: The Puzzle of Pain. New York, Basic Books, 1973.

Mercuri, L., Olson, R., and Laskin, D.: The specificity of response to experimental stress in patients with myofascial pain-dysfunction syndrome. J. Dent. Res. 58:1866–1871, 1979.

Merrett, J., and McDonald, J.: Sequela of concussion caused by minor head injury. Lancet 1:1–4, 1977.

Merritt, H.: A Textbook of Neurology, 5th ed. Philadelphia, Lea & Febiger, 1983.

Minckler, J.: Pathology of the Nervous System. New York, McGraw-Hill, 1968.

Moskowitz, M.: The neurobiology of vascular head pain. Ann. Neurol. 16:157–168, 1984.

Moss, R., Lombardo, T., Villarosa, M., et al.: Ongoing assessment of oral habits in common migraine and non-headache populations. J. Craniomandib. Pract. 6:352–354, 1988.

Moulin, D., Foley, K., and Ebers, G.: Pain syndromes in multiple sclerosis. Neurology 38:1830–1833, 1988.

Mumford, J.: Teeth and jaws as causes of idiopathic trigeminal neuralgia. Pain (Suppl.) 4:125, 1987.

Ochsner, A., and DeBakey, M.: Scalene anticus (Naffziger) syndrome. Am. J. Surg. 28:669–695, 1935.

Olson, R.: Myofascial pain-dysfunction syndrome: Psychological aspects. In Sarnat, B. G., and Laskin, D. (Eds.): The Temporomandibular Joint: A Biologic Approach to Clinical Practice, 2nd ed. Springfield, IL, Charles C Thomas, 1979, pp. 300–314.

Peter, C., Watson, N., Evans, R., et al.: Post-herpetic neuralgia and topical capsaicin. Pain 3:333–340, 1988.

Pfaffenrath, V., Mayer, E., Pollman, W., et al.: The cervicogenic headache-correlation of the symptomatology with results of a computer aided evaluation of radiographs of the cervical spine, with attention to atlantoaxial articulations. In Proceedings of The Fifth International Migraine Symposium. London, 1984, pp. 19–20.

Phillips, H., and Hunter, M.: A psychological investigation of tension headache. Headache, 22:173–179, 1982.

Pierau, F., Taylor, D., and Fellmer, G.: Convergence of somatic and visceral inputs in the peripheral nerves of the cat and rat. Neurosci. Lett. Suppl. 14:285, 1983.

Pilowsky, I.: A general classification of abnormal illness behaviors. Br. J. Med. Psych. 51:131–137, 1978.

Principato, J., and Barwell, D.: Biofeedback training and relaxation exercises for treatment of temporomandibular joint dysfunction. Otolaryngology 86:766–769, 1978.

Ramirez, J.: A critical analysis of the traditional tension headache model. Headache 25:337–339, 1985.

Reuben, B., and Laskin, D.: Electromyographic analysis of masticatory muscle activity in myofascial pain-dysfunction syndrome (abst). J. Dent. Res. 56:232, 1977.

Riggs, R., Rugh, J., and Barghi, N.: Muscle activity of MPD and TMJ patients and nonpatients. J. Dent. Res. 61:277–283, 1982.

Riley, H. A., German, W. J., Wortis, H., et al.: Glossopharyngeal neuralgia initiating or associated with cardiac arrest. Trans. Am. Neurol. Assoc. 68:28–30, 1942.

Rimel, R., Giordani, B., Barth, J., et al.: Moderate head injury: Completing the clinical spectrum of brain trauma. Neurosurgery 11:344–351, 1982.

Roberts, W.: A hypothesis on the physiological basis for causalgia and related pains. Pain 24:297–311, 1986.

Roberts, W., and Fogelson, M.: Spinal recordings suggest that wide-dynamic range neurons mediate sympathetically maintained pain. Pain 34:289–304, 1988.

Robinson, I. B., and Sarnat, B. G.: Roentgen studies of the maxillae and mandible in sickle-cell anemia. Radiology 58:517–523, 1952.

Roseman, D. M.: Carotidynia, a distinct syndrome. Arch. Otolaryngol. 85:81–84, 1967.

Rosenberg, E., and Guralnick, W.: Hyperparathyroidism: A review of 220 proved cases, with special emphasis on findings in the jaw. Oral Surg. 26:184, 1962.

Rothman, K. J., and Wepsic, J. G.: Side of face pain in trigeminal neuralgia. J. Neurosurg. 40:514–516, 1974.

Round, R., and Keane, J.: The minor symptoms of increased intracranial pressure: 101 patients with benign intracranial hypertension. Neurology 38:1461–1464, 1988.

Rushton, J. G., and Rooke, E. D.: Brain tumor headache. Headache 2:147–152, 1962.

Sarnat, B. G., and Shaw, N. G.: Dental development in congenital syphilis. Am. J. Dis. Child. 64:771–788, 1942.

Schele, R., Ahlborg, B., and Ekbom, K.: Physical characteristics and allergy history in young men with migraine and other headaches. Headache 18:80–86, 1978.

Schellhas, K., Fritts, H., Heithoff, K., et al.: Temporomandibular joint: MR fast scanning. J. Craniomandib. Pract. 6:209–216, 1988.

Schramm, V. Jr., Curtain, H., and Kennerdell, J.: Evaluation of orbital cellulitis and results of treatment. Laryngoscope 92:732–738, 1982.

Schroeder, S., Krupp, M., Tierny, L., et al.: Current Medical Diagnosis and Treatment. Norwalk, CT, Appleton and Lange, 1989, pp. 720–752.

Selby, G., and Lance, J.: Observations on 500 cases of migraine and allied vascular headache. J. Neurol. Neurosurg. Psychiatry 23:23–32, 1960.

Selzer, M., and Spencer, W.: Convergence of visceral and cutaneous afferent pathway in the lumbar spinal cord. Brain Res. 14:331–348, 1969.

Sessle, B. J., Hu, J., Amano, N., et al.: Convergence of cutaneous, tooth pulp, visceral, neck and muscle afferents onto nociceptive and non-nociceptive neurones in trigeminal subnucleus caudalis (medullary dorsal horn) and its implications for referred pain. Pain 27:219–235, 1986.

Sluder, G.: The role of the sphenopalatine ganglion in nasal headaches. NY Med. J. 87:989–990, 1908.

Smith, R., Stern, G.: Muscular weakness in osteomalacia and hyperparathyroidism. J. Neurol. Sci. 8:511–520, 1969.

Solberg, W.: Neuromuscular problems in the orofacial region: Diagnosis-classification, sign and symptoms. Int. Dent. J. 31:206–215, 1981.

Sparling, P.: Diagnosis and treatment of syphilis. N. Engl. J. Med. 284:642–653, 1971.

Spence, J.: Increased prevalence of mitral valve prolapse in patients with migraine. Can. Med. Assoc. J. 131:1457–1460, 1984.

Steere, A., Bartenhagen, N., Craft, J., et al.: The early clinical manifestations of Lyme disease. Ann. Intern. Med. 99:76–82, 1983.

Steere, A., Malawista, S., Hardin, J., et al.: Erythema chronicum migrans and Lyme arthritis: The enlarging clinical spectrum. Ann. Intern. Med. 86:685–698, 1977.

Sternbach, R. A.: Pain Patients. New York, Academic Press, 1974.

Sternbach, R. A.: Acute versus chronic pain. In Wall, P., and Melzack, R. (Eds.): Textbook of Pain. Edinburgh, Churchill Livingstone, 1984, pp. 173–177.

Stookey, B., and Ransohoff, J.: Trigeminal Neuralgia: Its History and Treatment. Springfield, IL, Charles C Thomas, 1969.

Sutton, E., and Belar, C.: Tension headache patients versus controls: A study of EMG parameters. Headache 22:133–136, 1982.

Swanson, J., Kelly, J., and McConahey, W.: Neurologic aspects of thyroid dysfunction. Mayo Clin. Proc. 56:504–512, 1981.

Symonds, C.: Post-traumatic headache: In Brock, S. (Ed.): Injuries to the Brain and Spinal Cord. London, Cassell, 1960.

Tasker, R.: A clinical neurophysiologic investigation of deafferentiation pain. In Bonica, J., Lindblom, U., and Iggo, A. (Eds.): Advances in Pain Research and Therapy. New York, Raven Press. 1983a, pp. 713–738.

Tasker, R., Tsuda, T., and Hawrylyshyn, P.: Clinical neurophysiology investigation of deafferentiation pain. Adv. Pain Res. Ther. 5:713–738, 1983b.

Thoma, K.: Oral Surgery, vol 2, 5th ed. St. Louis, C. V. Mosby, 1969.

Travell, J., and Rinzler, S. H.: The myofascial genesis of pain. Postgrad. Med. 11:425–434, 1952.

Travell, J., and Simmons, D.: Myofascial Pain and Dysfunction. The Trigger Point Manual. Baltimore, Williams & Wilkins, 1983, pp. 4–237.

Vail, H. H.: Vidian neuralgia. Ann. Otolaryngol. 41:837–856, 1932.

Valade, D., and Marquez, C.: A comparison between essential and post-herpetic trigeminal neuralgia. Pain (Suppl.) 4:84, 1987.

Victor, M., Adams, R., and Collins, G.: The Wernicke-Korsakoff Syndrome. Philadelphia, F. A. Davis, 1971.

Vinken, P., and Bruy, G.: Headaches and Cranial Neuralgias, vol. 5, Handbook of Clinical Neurology. Amsterdam, North Holland, 1968.

Waldvogel, F., and Vasey, H.: Osteomyelitis: The past decade. N. Engl. J. Med. 303:360–370, 1980.

Wall, P., Scudding, J., and Tomkiewicz, M.: The production and prevention of experimental anesthesia dolorosa. Pain 6:175–182, 1979.

Wallach, J.: Interpretation of Diagnostic Tests, 4th ed., Boston, Little, Brown & Co., 1986.

Wallach, S.: Paget's Disease of Bone. Phoenix, AZ, Armour Pharmaceutical Co., 1979.

Watson, C., Morshead, C., Van der Kooy, D., et al.: Postherpetic neuralgia: Post-mortem analysis of a case. Pain 34:129–138, 1988.

Wechsler, I.: Multiple peripheral neuropathy versus multiple neuritis. JAMA 110:1910–1913, 1938.

Weinberg, S., and Lapointe, H.: Cervical extension-flexion injury (whiplash) and internal derangement of the temporomandibular joint. J. Oral Maxillofac. Surg. 45:653–656, 1987.

White, J., and Sweet, W.: Pain: Its Mechanism and Neurosurgical Control. Springfield, IL, Charles C Thomas, 1955.

Wilke, W., Sheeler, I., and Makarowski, W.: Hypothyroidism with presenting symptoms of fibrositis. J. Rheumatol. 8:626–631, 1981.

Williams, H., and Elkins, E.: Myalgia of the pharynx. Arch. Otolaryngol. 36:1–11, 1942.

Winston, K.: Whiplash and its relationship to migraine. Headache 27:452–457, 1987.

Youmans, J. R.: Neurological Surgery, vol. 1 and 2. Philadelphia, W. B. Saunders, 1973.

Young, I., Hall, A., Pallis, C., et al.: Nuclear magnetic resonance imaging of the brain in multiple sclerosis. Lancet 1:1063–1066, 1981.

Zohn, D., and Mennell, J.: Musculoskeletal Pain: Diagnosis and Physical Treatment. Boston, Little, Brown & Co., 1976, pp. 126–129.

Zulch, K.: Brain Tumors: Their Biology and Pathology, ed. 2, New York, Springer, 1965.

26

DIFFERENTIAL DIAGNOSIS OF MASTICATORY DYSFUNCTION*

SANFORD L. BLOCK, D.D.S., LL.B.

INTRODUCTION

Masticatory dysfunction involves the inability to achieve mechanical degradation of food, an alteration in mandibular motion, or the presence of those conditions that are the result of masticatory muscle and temporomandibular

joint (TMJ) disharmony (Block, 1980). Any of these disorders may lead to a deficient performance pattern, provoking a patient to seek help from either a dentist or physician.

In this chapter, masticatory dysfunction is separated categorically to aid in understanding etiology and diagnosis. Congenital, neoplastic, traumatic, inflammatory, neuromuscular, metabolic, and psychogenic causes are presented. Some of the conditions are rare or uncommon,

*See Chapters 5, 7–13, 19, 20, 23–25.

469

but each entails symptomatic characteristics that are encompassed in the definition of masticatory dysfunction and may sometimes enter into the differential diagnosis. The most common condition from which these disorders must be distinguished is myofascial pain-dysfunction (MPD) syndrome (Laskin, 1986) (see Chapters 19 and 24).

CONGENITAL AND DEVELOPMENTAL MUSCLE DISORDERS (see Chapter 12)

Muscle Agenesis

The congenital absence of a muscle is rare and results from either nuclear aplasia of muscle cells, a mesodermal defect, or insults to the embryo when differentiation is well advanced. The peripheral and thoracic muscles are most commonly affected. Most deficiencies are unilateral and single, although bilateral involvement has been reported (Adams, 1975). The problem is usually discovered at birth or shortly after.

Agenesis of the facial, masticatory, and neck muscles causes obvious deformities. The diagnosis is made clinically on the basis of defective appearance of the facial profile, asymmetry, and functional difficulty. The definitive diagnosis can be made by biopsy. This aids in distinguishing muscle agenesis from motor nerve involvement in which neural defects prevent adequate muscle development. The absence of the masseter and pterygoid muscles, with a resulting narrow-appearing mandible and open bite, has been reported (Ford, 1960).

Agenesis is frequently associated with other developmental defects and is part of several syndromes. In aglossia-adactylia the tongue is absent and the mandible is small and poorly developed. Congenital facial diplegia (congenital oculofacial paralysis; Möbius' syndrome), in which there is absence of portions of the facial musculature, is characterized by bilateral facial paralysis, inability to abduct the eye, oropharyngeal muscle paralysis, and a mask-like facies (Sprofkin, 1956) (Fig. 26–1). The eyelids and mouth remain open during sleep. The jaw and tongue are underdeveloped, the lips are paralyzed, and the angle of the mouth may droop. Fasciculations of the tongue may be noted, and mastication and deglutition are difficult because of facial, lingual, and masticatory muscle paralysis (Gorlin, 1976). Histologic studies show pontine nuclear atrophy, peripheral nerve lesions, and muscle atrophy (Towfighi, 1979).

Agenesis is also associated with lateral facial dysplasia, a term that encompasses all forms of dysplasia involving the lateral two-thirds of the face (Ross, 1979). The incidence of lateral facial dysplasia is about 1 in 4,000 live births. The most commonly involved regions are the middle and external ear, mandibular condyle and ramus, muscles of mastication, zygomatic arch, and temporal bone. In hemifacial microsomia, a variant of lateral facial dysplasia, the ramus and condyle fail to develop (Kazanjian, 1940). About 70 per cent of these cases are unilateral. The defects occur embryonically at a time when differentiation is well advanced or completed, and the injury (possibly hemorrhage and hematoma from the stapedius artery) is localized (Poswillo, 1973). There may be microtia, dysplasia of the TMJs, less mandibular length with deviation of the midline, macrostomia, and reduced size or absence of the masseter and temporalis muscles. Mandibular dysfunction is usually a result of abnormalities of both the soft and hard tissues.

Benign Masseteric Hypertrophy

Although it does not produce dysfunction, benign masseteric hypertrophy should be considered in the differential diagnosis. Hypertrophy of the masseter muscle may be congenital or functional (Waldhart, 1971). The functional form is relatively common and occurs either unilaterally or bilaterally. There is an associated overgrowth of bone at the angle of the mandible. When this occurs bilaterally, the frontal view of the face appears square. Most patients are seen between 15 and 25 years of age; occurrence is rare in children.

Functional hypertrophy can occur in persons who develop habits of clenching or grinding their teeth (Fig. 26–2). In unilateral hypertrophy, the pathogenesis has been attributed to unilateral chewing due to loss of teeth, painful dental caries, or dysfunction on the opposite side. The history of masseteric hypertrophy is one of slow onset, and the muscle is rarely painful or tender. Associated parotitis has been described by Blatt (1969) and was attributed to partial obstruction of the parotid duct by the hypertrophic muscle. A frontal view radiographic examination shows flaring at the angle of the mandible, with a bony spur at the lower border. Differentiation is necessary from congenital hypertrophy (unilateral enlargement of the tongue, teeth, and mandible) (see Fig. 24–11), hemifacial atrophy (Talacko, 1988) (see Fig. 24–10), and hemimasticatory spasm, in which

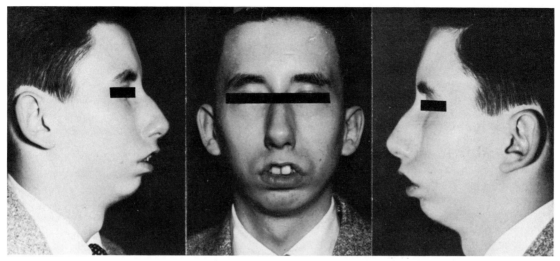

FIGURE 26–1. Prenatal facial diplegia (Möbius syndrome) with underdevelopment of the mandible, bilateral facial muscle weakness, mask-like appearance, and masticatory dysfunction. (From Sarnat, B. G.: Developmental facial abnormalities and the temporomandibular joint. Dent. Clin. North Am. November, 1966, pp. 587–600.)

there is a disturbance of the motor division of the trigeminal nerve (Thompson, 1983). Additional differential diagnoses should include direct muscle involvement from infections (trichinosis or actinomycosis) and tumors (rhabdomyosarcoma, fibrosarcoma, lipoma, and angioma). Parotid tumors and inflammatory diseases must also be considered.

Torticollis

Congenital

Congenital torticollis is frequently noted soon after birth. There is a shortening and rigidity of

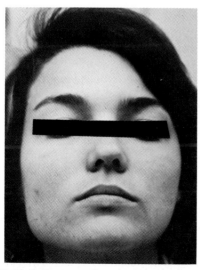

FIGURE 26–2. Benign unilateral masseteric hypertrophy showing squared prominence of the mandibular angles and facial asymmetry.

the sternocleidomastoid muscle and factors such as shortened tendons, fibrotic muscles, and deformed joints cause the head to be rotated and inclined to the involved side (Goldberg, 1978). The condition is generally nonprogressive. The face and skull may be asymmetrical, the face is short, and the eyebrows slope downward (see Fig. 24–9). There may be an exostosis at the clavicular attachment of the sternocleidomastoid muscle, the frontal eminence is flattened, and the ipsilateral occiput bulges. Hereditary factors do not seem to play a role. The usual cause involves birth injury, muscle ischemia, or a fibrous pseudotumor that leads to contracture of the sternocleidomastoid muscle (Middleton, 1930).

A similar condition with a familial relationship, the Klippel-Feil syndrome, involves fusion of some or all of the cervical vertebrae. The neck is short, with a painless limitation of head movement. The facial appearance is relatively symmetrical, with the trapezius muscles appearing flared from the shoulder to the mastoid processes. There may be associated cranial nerve palsy and peripheral nerve paralysis (Gorlin, 1976). Mandibular dysfunction is not pronounced, although patients complain of difficulty in swallowing and esophageal reflux (Lyons, 1968). Neurological evaluation, skull and cervical radiographs, EMG, CT scan, and serum chemistry will help distinguish this condition from cervical degenerative arthritis, cervical disc problems, syringomyelia, spinal cord tumor, torsion dystonia, and drug-induced dystonia (Kiwak, 1983).

Spasmodic

Another form of torticollis, not congenital in origin but clinically related, is spasmodic torticollis. This is a dystonic condition that is associated with intermittent spasms of the neck muscles that typically causes an involuntary deviation of the head from the normal position. Most cases are idiopathic, with psychogenic, traumatic, extrapyramidal disease, and degenerative cervical joint disease also having been implicated as causes (Duane, 1988). Pain of the cervical muscles is common at the onset, with tenderness of the sternocleidomastoid, occipital, trapezius, and nuchal muscles. Nuchal tightness and restricted neck motion are also initial complaints. Symptoms develop over a period of one to two years, with pain becoming more pronounced after the first year. The torticollis is aggravated by stress or fatigue, and corrective gestures are used to straighten the head position. Mandibular dysfunction is usually compensatory, and swallowing is somewhat difficult. However, oromandibular dystonia may sometimes precede the torticollis. Voice disturbances occur due to hyperkinesis of the laryngeal, pharyngeal, tongue, facial, and masticatory muscles. Thyroid disease has been associated with this disorder, but is not an initiator. Degenerative cervical vertebral and intervertebral disc disease may be the cause of the torticollis or it may occur secondarily.

Arthrogryposis Multiplex Complex

Arthrogryposis multiplex complex is a rare congenital deformity characterized by limited joint motion due to muscle atrophy or aplasia, joint dislocation, and ligament contractures. First described in the early nineteenth century, and later reviewed by Hall (1975), only a few cases involving the TMJ articulation have been reported (Heffez, 1985). The term arthrogryposis means curved joint and the general complex is less commonly known as amyoplasia congenita and myodystrophica fetalis deformans. The four extremities are most often affected, although only portions of a limb are involved in some cases. This disease may be present in conjunction with other congenital anomalies such as Möbius syndrome, lower limb and sacral spine agenesis, myelomeningocele, hemivertebrae, rib fusion, and cerebral maldevelopment.

The etiology is unknown, although neurogenic factors causing denervation and in utero muscle atrophy are generally thought to be responsible. Other factors such as metabolic defects, endocrine abnormalities, neurovascular abnormalities, and fetal malposition may contribute to limited joint mobility.

The criteria for the diagnosis of arthrogryposis multiplex complex are joint contractures at birth in at least two different regions; presence of a nonprogressive neurological disorder; diffuse muscle wasting; decreased muscle strength; skin dimpling over the severe joint contractures; webbing of the extremities; and absence of normal skin creases (Fisher, 1970). Histologic findings in primary neurological cases are a decrease in muscle size, absence of muscle spindles, fatty and fibrous muscle infiltration and replacement, and nerve tissue and spinal cord alterations. Primary myopathic cases show no spinal cord neuropathy (Amick, 1967).

The restrictive effects on the TMJ due to ligament and muscle contractures are responsible for failure of the disc, capsule, and articular surfaces to develop normally. The extraarticular contracture is so strong that forceful joint manipulation is ineffective and may lead to discal injury. Retarded mandibular growth leads to antegonial notching and coronoid elongation. Due to the retardation of mandibular growth, midfacial development is also affected, leading to the same type of facial deformity seen in ankylosis, condylar agenesis, and hemifacial microsomia.

NEOPLASTIC DISEASE
(see Chapter 10)

Masticatory dysfunction due to neoplastic disease is most often the result of lesions directly involving the TMJ (Figs. 24–13 and 24–30) or indirectly (Figs. 24–25 and 24–31). Primary tumors involving the muscles of mastication are rare; more common is involvement by extension of lesions from adjacent regions (Cuttino, 1988). This situation should always be considered in cases of limited jaw movement.

Benign Muscle Neoplasms

Rhabdomyoma is a rare benign tumor of striated muscle that can involve the masticatory muscles. It may occur at any age, with a slight predominance in males. The lesion develops as a slow-growing, well-circumscribed, elevated, painless mass that is somewhat firmer than the surrounding tissues. It occurs most commonly in the larynx, pharynx, tongue, floor of the mouth, uvula, and palate (Czernobilsky, 1968).

Masticatory dysfunction is not common unless the lesion interferes with deglutition.

Leiomyoma is a relatively rare tumor developing from smooth muscle. It has been found in the skin, subcutaneous tissue, tongue, lips, buccal mucosa, and uvula. Although it has not been reported in the muscles of mastication, this is a theoretical possibility. The lesion develops as a painless, slow-growing mass that may achieve large size. Dysfunction in swallowing and obstruction of the oropharynx may occur from large lesions at the base of the tongue (McDonald, 1969).

Malignant Muscle Neoplasms

Rhabdomyosarcoma is an extremely malignant tumor of striated muscle with a fairly high incidence in the head and neck (Stout, 1946). It is one of the more common malignant tumors to affect the TMJ. Stout (1946) reported 14 per cent of 245 cases involving the head and neck, and Dito (1962) reported 170 cases in this region, with the face, temple, and mandibular areas involved in 16 per cent of the cases. Tumors of the temporalis muscle, parotid gland, orbit, cheek, palate, and neck have also been reported (Stobbe, 1950).

Clinically, these lesions appear as soft, raised masses. Depending on the location, interference with masticatory function as well as pharyngeal obstruction may occur. Metastases may be either hematogenous or lymphogenous, with lymph node involvement occurring in a high percentage of patients, followed by lung and bone involvement. A common site of metastasis is the ramus of the mandible. Masticatory pain and dysfunction may occur when there is periosteal or neural invasion. Depending on the site of the lesion, abnormal phonation, dysphagia, and aural discharge may also occur. A complete history, clinical evaluation, serum enzyme studies, and radiographs aid in differentiation of this tumor from benign conditions.

MUSCLE TRAUMA

Head and neck injuries can lead to muscle disorders that may persist for many years (Bauerle and Archer, 1951). Trauma can cause tearing of the muscle fibers and their connective tissue sheaths and hemorrhage from associated vessels. The sequelae depend on the extent of hemorrhage, edema, ischemia, and associated skeletal trauma. Extensive muscle trauma may result in replacement with scar tissue, contrac-

ture, and ankylosis. The masseter is the most frequently injured masticatory muscle.

Strenuous exertion of a muscle may also cause rupture, hemorrhage, and edema. Wide yawning, taking large bites of food, or manipulation of the mandible during dental extractions may also cause masticatory muscle trauma. Injury may be at the muscle-tendon junction, tendinous insertion, or in the muscle belly. The most common trauma occurs in the muscle belly, especially following occupational injury (Gilcreest, 1925).

A blow to the mandible or temporal region or sudden mandibular acceleration in rear-end auto accidents are external forces that may lead to chronic masticatory dysfunction. Rear-end vehicular collisions lead to hyperflexion and hyperextension of the head and neck. This sudden backward movement catches the protective muscle reflexes of the neck and mandible unprepared (Cailliet, 1975) and exceeds the limiting influence of the ligaments. Sudden tearing of muscle fibers and fascial attachments may occur, resulting in internal muscle hemorrhage and edema. Masticatory muscle spasm may follow, with pain, tenderness, and functional limitation. The TMJ ligaments and capsule may also be injured, with subsequent periarticular and intra-articular inflammation. This muscle injury may create ischemia, which leads to muscle pain from lack of oxygen and retained metabolites. The presence of both of these conditions initiates inflammation, which may ultimately lead to a fibrous reaction within the muscles (Cailliet, 1975).

Traumatic myositis ossificans may develop in the masticatory muscles at all ages as a result of a single or repeated injury. The masseter and temporalis muscles are involved most frequently. After intramuscular bleeding occurs, organization of the hematoma takes place, with ultimate calcification or ossification that may lead to persistent limitation of mandibular motion. Radiographs show either a diffuse opacity or a solitary area within the muscle. A tender mass may be palpated in the muscle. Serum calcium, phosphorous, and alkaline phosphatase levels are within normal limits.

MUSCULAR AND NEUROMUSCULAR DISEASE

Alteration of masticatory function and deglutition occurs in various muscular and neuromuscular diseases. Disturbance of muscle activity may result from an inflammatory process, general systemic conditions (thyroid and parathyroid disease), primary muscle disorders (muscular dystrophy), neuromuscular junction disorders (myasthenia gravis), central nervous system (CNS) dysfunction (cerebral palsy), and peripheral nerve disorders resulting from lesions or trauma.

Neurological disease causing masticatory dysfunction is characterized by weakness of chewing movements and other functional excursions, continuous spasm of the masticatory muscles, or generalized abnormal mandibular, face, and tongue movements (Earl, 1976).

Various levels of CNS dysfunction produce specific masticatory deficits. Damage to the peripheral motor branches of the trigeminal nerve leads to atrophy, weakness, or total paralysis of the masticatory muscles. If the pyramidal tract and brainstem connections are damaged, the motor nerve and muscles remain intact, but only the basic chewing reflexes exist and the jaw jerk reflex becomes exaggerated. Mandibular dysfunction is manifested by deviation of the mandible to the affected side on opening the mouth and difficulty in mastication.

Inflammatory Disease

Infective Myositis

Infective myositis is an inflammatory disease within muscle due to micro-organisms. Viral, bacterial, mycotic, and parasitic organisms may all be involved. They may spread via the lymphatic or blood vessel systems. Entrance through the oral mucous membrane, lungs, and gastrointestinal and genitourinary tracts has also occurred. The incidence of infective diseases causing mandibular dysfunction is not great.

VIRAL

Viral invasion in influenza, herpetic disease, and coxsackievirus infections may cause fever, headache, and muscle pain and tenderness. The degree of myalgia usually parallels the course of the illness. The influenza A virus (Middleton, 1970) and other viruses may cause muscle necrosis by direct attack upon the cells or secondarily by the formation of virus-antibody complexes on the surface of the cells.

Headache associated with infectious myositis is at times difficult to differentiate from muscle tension headache (Delassio, 1972). Usually there is a history of a recent cold, flu, sore throat, or tonsillitis. Neck pain, exacerbated with movement and stiffness, may precede the head pain. Pain from the cervical muscles is referred to the occipital, temporal, and frontal regions. Tenderness of the sternocleidomastoid, trapezius, and temporalis muscles is present.

Although the masticatory muscles may be directly involved more often, in cases of chronic viral myositis masticatory muscle pain and tenderness occur due to central excitatory effects upon the brainstem and referred pain patterns eliciting secondary muscle contraction. Although the duration of infectious viral myositis is usually brief, the effects may last from six months to a year.

BACTERIAL

Bacterial forms of infectious myositis may be associated with bacteremia, infectious arthritis, dental abscess, and compound jaw fractures. The most common organisms are staphylococci and streptococci. Organisms confined to muscle and fascia may cause local edema and inflammation leading to suppuration. Since striated muscle is not the most suitable tissue for bacterial growth, pure focal bacterial myositis is not common.

Bacterial infections can also be caused iatrogenically by a contaminated needle or surgical instrument carrying organisms to the deep musculature. This is usually associated with swelling that produces facial asymmetry and severe pain and tenderness of the muscle. There may be associated chills and fever, although in more chronic cases this may not occur. With involvement of the muscles of mastication, there is severe limitation of opening of the mouth.

Clostridium tetani produces an often fatal infectious disease, tetanus, in which muscle spasm characteristically appears in the facial and masticatory muscles (Fig. 26–3). The exotoxin produced by this organism exerts its action on the central nervous system rather than directly on the muscle. The tetanus bacilli enter a deep wound where anaerobic conditions afford their best growth. After one to two weeks of incubation, symptoms of restlessness, irritability, and jaw stiffness appear. There are complaints of difficulty in chewing, yawning, and swallowing. The extremities become stiff and functional tasks become difficult. Following this, the masseter muscles become firmly contracted and there is inability to open the mouth. The cervical and abdominal muscles also become spastic and rigid. Convulsions follow and, if not quickly treated with tetanus antitoxin, death ensues.

SYPHILITIC

Infection of masticatory muscles due to invasion by *Treponema pallidum* is rare. Involve-

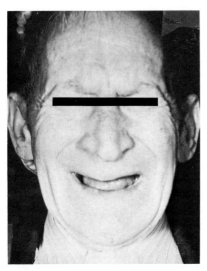

FIGURE 26–3. Characteristic facial expression associated with the advanced stage of tetanus. Note the sardonic smile (risus sardonicus) and elevation of the eyebrows caused by involuntary spasm of the facial muscles. (From Robinson, I. B., and Laskin, D. M.: Tetanus of oral origin. Oral Surg. 10:831–838, 1957.)

ment in the primary and secondary stage has not been reported, but it may occur in the tertiary stage. Gummas have been found as solitary lesions in the tongue and in the masseter, sternocleidomastoid, pharyngeal, laryngeal, and eye muscles (Adams, 1975). Clinically, a gumma initially appears as a firm, circumscribed swelling. Subsequently, there may be necrosis leading to a nodular, ulcerative, nonsuppurating lesion. Pain may be associated with periosteal and nerve involvement. There is also a more diffuse lesion of tertiary syphilis that produces degenerative changes within muscle fibers, along with fatty degeneration and increased fibrous connective tissue formation. Muscle firmness, atrophy, and contracture occur, accompanied by generalized muscle pain. Confirmation of syphilis is by a dark-field examination, and VDRL and treponemal immobilization (TPI) tests.

FUNGAL (MYCOTIC)

Fungal infections involving muscle may occur through direct soft tissue invasion or by hematogenous spread. Actinomycosis clinically manifests itself as a chronic, suppurative, hard swelling of the skin with subsequent draining abscesses and sinus tract formation (Holmes, 1958). Involvement of the underlying masseter muscle and parotid gland may occur, with the muscle being replaced by granulation tissue. This is accompanied by pain and limitation of function. Microscopic examination of the suppurative material and anaerobic culture confirm the diagnosis of a mycotic infection.

PARASITIC

Parasitic myositis is a relatively common disease. Various parasites have an affinity for specific muscles. Since definitive diagnosis of their presence is dependent upon histologic evaluation of biopsy material, and this is not commonly obtained from the face or masticatory muscles, there has been difficulty in establishing the presence of parasites in these regions.

Trichinosis is caused by the *Trichinella spiralis*, a helminth of the Nematoda group. It is estimated that over 20 per cent of the adult population in certain geographic areas may be affected by trichinosis (Most, 1941). Other parasitic diseases such as cysticercosis (pork tapeworm) and protozoal infestations may also produce masticatory muscle symptoms. It is usually contracted either by eating poorly cooked pork or through handling and subsequent ingestion of raw meat. The larvae invade the intestinal wall and deposit embryos. The larvae gain access to the lymphatics and lymph nodes, and then, via the thoracic duct, into the bloodstream. From there, they enter the muscle, liver, pancreas, heart, and brain. The muscles most commonly involved are the tongue, masseter, extraocular, cervical, pectoral, intercostal, and diaphragmatic. Upon invasion, the trichinae cause inflammation and degeneration resulting in muscle damage. Peripheral muscle weakness, with loss of tendon reflexes, may develop. Facial swelling, dysphagia, dyspnea, and hoarseness may also occur. Because clonic spasm and muscle contracture occur with this disease, there may be limitation of mandibular motion associated with pain and tenderness. Although the disease is seldom fatal, myocarditis, with possible cerebral embolism, may cause death.

Blood examination will show eosinophilia, a positive trichinella complement-fixation test two weeks following ingestion, and a decrease in total serum protein and albumin (Wallach, 1986).

Noninfective Myositis—Polymyositis

Polymyositis is a disease of striated muscle of unknown etiology. It may occur in all age groups, with females predominating. Depending on the associated tissues involved, the disease is called polymyositis (muscle only), dermatomyositis (skin and muscle), or neuromyositis (nerve and muscle).

The disease presents primarily as a degeneration of striated muscle fibers accompanied by inflammation. Necrosis of entire groups of muscle fibers may occur, followed by interstitial fibrosis (Hollander, 1974). Initial symptoms consist of lower extremity muscle weakness, followed by pelvic girdle muscle weakness and later inability to raise the arms. Weakness of the laryngeal and pharyngeal muscles causes dysphonia and dysphagia. Weakness of the neck, facial, and extraocular muscles also occurs. Muscle pain may be prominent, but is not consistent. The subcutaneous tissues over the affected muscles may become edematous and diffuse reddening over the face, neck, trunk, and extremities may be seen.

Masticatory muscle weakness and tenderness occur, as well as pain on function. However, these are usually relatively late symptoms. Masticatory and pharyngeal muscle involvement make eating difficult. Pharyngitis and stomatitis are common. Laboratory findings show extremely elevated serum transaminase, creatine phosphokinase, and serum aldolase levels, and reduced urinary creatinine.

Generalized Familial Muscular Dystrophy

Muscular dystrophy is a chronic progressive degenerative disease of striated muscle. The disease is inherited, begins early in life, and occurs predominantly in males. It may be categorized by anatomic involvement, age of onset, and rate of progression. Initial symptoms seen in children are difficulty in climbing stairs, clumsy walking, and weakness of the pelvic and shoulder girdle. Pseudohypertrophic enlargement of the muscles may be seen for years before the disease is recognized. This enlargement of muscle fibers is followed by fibrofatty tissue replacement. The muscle feels firm and rubbery in the hypertrophic stage, but with later atrophy it is difficult to palpate because of overlying fat. In the generalized form, bilateral peripheral weakness is present initially. Later, there is involvement of the facial, masticatory, laryngeal, pharyngeal, and ocular muscles. Facial involvement causes a transverse smile appearance and difficulty in mastication, speaking, and swallowing. The prognosis is poor, with longevity rarely beyond 20 years of age.

Of the various forms of muscular dystrophy that occur, head and neck involvement is found in Duchenne pseudohypertrophic muscular dystrophy and the more restricted facioscapulohumeral dystrophy. The former presents with all the symptoms previously mentioned, as well as additional oral findings of spacing and flaring of teeth as well as tongue enlargement (Table 26–1).

Facioscapulohumeral Muscular Dystrophy

This dystrophy differs from the generalized pseudohypertrophic form in that it may occur at any age, affects either sex equally, is slower in onset, has remissions, does not cause pseudohypertrophy, and shows a predilection for facial muscles and the shoulder girdle; thus, the

TABLE 26–1. Differential Diagnosis of Muscular Dystrophy

	GENERAL FAMILIAL	FACIOSCAPULO-HUMERAL	PROGRESSIVE DYSTROPHIC OPHTHALMOPLEGIA AND OCULOPHARYNGEAL	MYOTONIC
Age of Onset	Childhood	Adolescence	Childhood progressing into 3rd decade	Childhood through 5th decade
Sex	Males	Either	Either	Either
Initial Clinical Signs	Limb, pelvic, and shoulder weakness	Facial, shoulder girdle weakness; winged scapulas	Ptosis of eyelids, dysphagia, and voice changes	Wasting and weakness of distal limbs
Pseudohypertrophy	Yes	Not common	No	No
Facial and Masticatory Muscle Involvement	Weakness of face, pharynx, larynx, and ocular muscles; tongue enlarged	Facial and masticatory muscle weakness; difficult to close eyes or whistle, lips protrude	Weakness of ocular, eyelid, masticatory, pharyngeal, and laryngeal muscles	Facial, masticatory, pharyngeal, laryngeal, and cervical muscle weakness; difficult to swallow, speak, or lift head
Prognosis	Poor	Slow course	Slow course	Slow course

term facioscapulohumeral dystrophy. Due to its slow progression and prolonged remissions, this form is rarely fatal. The onset is usually between six and 20 years of age. Early symptoms are difficulty in raising the arms above the head, facial muscle weakness, and difficulty in closing the eyes. There is an inability to whistle, smile, or purse the lips (Adams, 1975). The lower lip is everted, giving a tapir mouth appearance (Rowland, 1984). Weakness of forehead muscles results in difficulty in wrinkling the brow. During sleep, the eyelids may not be completely closed, and facial expression is absent when laughing or crying. Although involvement of masticatory and pharyngeal muscles may occur, this is not a common finding (Merritt, 1975). Degeneration of the cervical, shoulder, and trunk muscles leads to a winged appearance in which the shoulders are thrown back, with the scapulae and clavicles becoming prominent. Oral findings in facioscapulohumeral dystrophy consist of an anterior open bite, flaring mandibular teeth, and an enlarged tongue (Thayer, 1966). Laboratory tests, as in most muscular dystrophies, show increased serum aldolase, lactic dehydrogenase, serum glutamic oxalic transaminase, and creatine phosphokinase (CPK) levels. Increased urine creatine and decreased creatinine are found. Electromyographic evaluation aids in confirming the diagnosis.

Progressive Dystrophic Ophthalmoplegia: Oculopharyngeal Muscular Dystrophy

Progressive dystrophic ophthalmoplegia is a form of limited degenerative muscle disease primarily involving the extraocular and levator palpebrae muscles. It is a progressive disease, beginning in early childhood and becoming more apparent by the third decade of life. Characteristic symptoms are ptosis, diplopia, weakness of eye movement, and a wrinkled forehead with the head tilted back in an attempt to see beneath the drooping lids. Cases have been reported in which there is paralysis of the masticatory and neck muscles, with wasting that invariably causes masticatory dysfunction (Peterman, 1964).

A related condition is oculopharyngeal muscular dystrophy. It is a familial disease more commonly found in French Canadians and Spanish Americans. Its onset is slow and asymmetrical, and it usually occurs later in life. Dysphagia and voice changes occur, along with flaccid facial paralysis. Atrophy of the masticatory muscles is reflected by sagging of the mandible and hollowing of the temporal areas. The lips droop, and there is ptosis of the eyelids. The latter effect, as in dystrophic ophthalmoplegia, creates a wrinkled brow in an effort to open the eyes (Lewis, 1966). Serum enzymes may be normal, but EMG evaluation characteristically shows myopathy.

Myotonic Muscular Dystrophy

Myotonic muscular dystrophy is an inherited disease occurring in six per 100,000 people, characterized by signs of persistent muscle contraction and hypertrophy followed by atrophy and degeneration of the involved muscles. In myotonia there is a repetitive firing of muscle fibers and a failure of the muscles to relax normally after forceful contraction (Walton, 1981). An acquired form of myotonic muscular dystrophy has also been reported. This form develops following treatment with drugs used to treat hyperlipidemia, such as clofibrate and diazacholesterol, which alter the lipid composition of muscle surface membranes (Furman, 1981). The muscles of the face, jaws, and neck, as well as the extremities are usually involved. There is also associated dystrophy in nonmuscular tissues, such as the testicles and endocrine glands, cardiac dystrophy, and eyes (cataract formation). Early frontal alopecia, ptosis of the eyelids, and conjunctivitis are also present. Mental retardation is frequently found.

Atrophy of the facial muscles gives a lean, expressionless appearance. Wasting of the temporalis, masseters, and sternocleidomastoids is severe, causing a characteristic exaggerated forward curve of the neck (swan-neck appearance) (Adams, 1975). Recurrent subluxation and dislocation of the mandible are common. The muscles of deglutition and phonation become impaired, and the voice may become nasal. Strong or firm movements become sustained, although repetition leads to some relaxation. Gentle movements such as blinking and facial expression may not be hampered. Myotonia of the tongue muscles may be demonstrated by placing a tongue blade below the tongue and gently striking it with a percussion hammer. Malocclusion due to an anterior open bite has been reported (Thayer, 1966). Electromyographic evaluation shows the characteristic after-potentials of myotonia. An ECG reveals that bradycardia and heart block are common. Urine ketosteroids are decreased and urine creatine is increased (Wallach, 1986). The serum may show no abnormalities except for reduction in gamma globulin (Kagen, 1985).

Myasthenia Gravis

Abnormal neuromuscular transmission at the myoneural junction due to an antibody reaction against the acetylcholine receptors (AChR) leads to the disturbance in muscle excitation and contractility seen in myasthenia gravis. The antibodies saturate up to 80 per cent of the AChR sites on the muscle leading to major degradation of the endplates at the neuromuscular junction (Drachman, 1981). Although antibodies are present in 85 to 90 per cent of myasthenia patients, there is no consistent correlation between the titer level and severity of symptoms (Newsom-Davis, 1986).

Myasthenia gravis occurs at any age, but is most common in females between 20 and 30 years of age. The disease is a chronic, but not progressive, process characterized by fluctuating weakness of striated muscles with associated long recovery periods. Recent evidence suggests that although myasthenia gravis rarely recurs within families, patients as well as their relatives often suffer from other autoimmune conditions, which suggests an inherited autoimmune susceptibility (Kerzin-Storrar, 1988).

The initial signs are ptosis and diplopia. This may be followed by weakness of the facial and neck muscles (Fig. 26–4). Inability to lift the head from a pillow without hand support may be an early symptom. Masticatory and glossopharyngeal muscles become involved, resulting in dysphagia and difficulty in speaking. In the early stages of masticatory dysfunction, weakness occurs followed by severe atrophy of the masseter, temporalis, and to a lesser extent, the pterygoid muscles. This atrophy and muscle wasting is due to severe malnutrition that is a

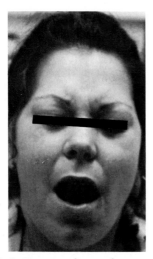

FIGURE 26–4. Patient with myasthenia gravis showing difficulty in opening the mouth.

result of the dysphagia and masticatory weakness. Because of the weakness of the primary elevators, the mandible may droop, with the mouth being partially open.

In advanced myasthenia gravis, the face is expressionless. Diagnostic administration of an anticholinesterase such as neostigmine brings about dramatic improvement within minutes. Routine blood, urine, and cerebrospinal fluid analyses are normal. EMG findings are characteristic, with a rapid decline in the height of the action potential evoked by repetition of a given activity (Grob, 1981). Antibodies to AChR are found in 85 to 90 per cent of patients when muscle is used as the test antigen. Differential diagnosis should include muscular dystrophy, amyotrophic lateral sclerosis, progressive bulbar palsy, hyperthyroidism, and psychoneurosis.

Congenital Myotonia (Thomsen's Disease)

Congenital myotonia is a familial disturbance of muscle conduction characterized by a generalized nonprogressive muscular hypertrophy in which the principal characteristic is delayed relaxation. It usually begins in early childhood, but sometimes it does not produce symptoms until after 20 years of age. The cause may be either a defect in the potassium transfer mechanism or improper formation and utilization of high-energy phosphates (Kent, 1978).

In contrast to myotonic muscular dystrophy, there is extreme muscle hypertrophy and an increase in strength. Stiffness and weakness are relieved by exercise and exaggerated by cold. Because of some slight evidence of muscle dystrophy in the late stages (hollowing of the masseters, absent triceps reflex, cataracts, and testicular atrophy), this disease may be a variant of myotonic dystrophy (Maas, 1950).

Intensified myotonia in adolescence is characterized by persistent painless muscle contraction. Hypertrophy of the shoulder, neck, and masseter muscles gives the patient a Herculean appearance. Strong contractions during sneezing may bring about myotonic contraction of the face, tongue, neck, larynx, and chest (Gellis, 1966). The muscles show myotonia characterized by localized contractions after percussion of the surface. The patient may complain of garbled speech after eating or drinking iced liquids or food. Muscular power, such as in chewing, may be reduced due to inability to relax the antagonists. Open bite deformity has been attributed to hypertrophy of the masseter and suprahyoid muscles caused by abnormal force patterns on the mandible (Kent, 1978). A predilection for the development of malignant hyperthermia following the administration of muscle relaxants has been shown in patients with myotonia congenita, evoking signs of severe masseter spasm and contracture (Heiman-Patterson, 1988). EMG recordings show numerous small, fast, action potentials with delayed relaxation. The CPK is slightly elevated. Urine creatine may be increased, but this is not always specific.

Poliomyelitis

Acute anterior poliomyelitis (infantile paralysis) is a generalized disease of rapid onset, caused by the poliovirus, a picornavirus that is highly cytotoxic and resistant to most forms of inactivation. Destruction of the motor cells in the spinal cord and brain stem occurs with resulting flaccid paralysis and muscle atrophy. In spinal cord disorders, there is destruction of the cells of the anterior horn. A selective affinity of the virus for large motor cells is reflected in the predominant destruction of the motor area of the cerebral cortex and medulla. Before 1956, poliomyelitis was the most common viral infection of the nervous system. Since the development of the Salk and Sabin vaccines the incidence has decreased dramatically from 50,000 to 30 patients per year in the United States.

Acute anterior poliomyelitis may affect either sex and occur at any age, although it is more prevalent in children. The disease spreads from the oropharynx, tonsils, and the gastrointestinal (GI) tract to the cervical and mesenteric lymph nodes and then into the bloodstream. Spread into the nervous system may be either hematogenous, the result of direct neural invasion of sympathetic ganglia, or from invasion of sensory ganglia in the GI tract. The disease begins with fever, malaise, headache, and GI and respiratory symptoms. Muscle soreness appears in the back and neck, and there may be a positive Kernig's sign. Spasm and paralysis of peripheral and spinal muscles follow. In 15 per cent of the cases, the bulbar nuclei are involved. The facial, masticatory, palatal, tongue, and pharyngeal muscles may be paralyzed due to destruction of their respective midbrain nuclei, resulting in dysphagia and dysarthria (Haymaker, 1969). Destruction of these neurons produces a loss of tendon reflexes, atrophy, and flaccid paralysis, which persist for years and result in postpoliomyelitis muscle atrophy (PPMA). Recent evaluation of patients with PPMA using muscle

biopsy specimens revealed mild inflammation in 40 per cent of the specimens, possibly indicating ongoing disease activity (Dalakas, 1988). Recovery of patients with only partial bulbar paralysis results in restoration of normal oropharyngeal function. A diagnosis can be established by a lack of vaccination history and recovery of the virus from the throat, feces, blood, and CSF, as well as a rise in antibody levels in complement fixation tests. The differential diagnosis includes polymyositis, amyotrophic lateral sclerosis, polyneuropathy, and connective tissue disease.

Amyotrophic Lateral Sclerosis

Amyotrophic lateral sclerosis is a motor neuron disease characterized by selective damage to the voluntary motor system in which degeneration of the alpha motor neurons, anterior horn cells, corticospinal tract, and cerebral cortex occurs. The etiology is unknown, although possibilities of a disturbance in the neural enzyme system, slow virus infection (Weiner, 1980), or a carbohydrate metabolism defect have been hypothesized. The disease is relatively common, with an estimated 10,000 cases annually in the United States. It occurs in middle age and has not been proved to be familial.

Degenerative changes in the brainstem affect the fifth, seventh, eighth, eleventh, and twelfth cranial nerves. Muscle weakness, atrophy, loss of tendon reflexes, fibrillations, and fasciculations occur. Pain also occurs in the involved muscles, which are usually affected bilaterally.

With involvement of the hypoglossal nerve and bulbar nuclei, the palatal, pharyngeal, and tongue muscles atrophy (DePaul, 1988; Mulder, 1957). Speech becomes slurred, and there is associated dysphagia, hyperactive jaw reflexes, and dysarthria. Due to substantial tongue weakness, jaw movements compensate for those of the tongue, preserving speech function (Hirose, 1982). Mastication is occasionally involved, and deglutition is impaired because of poor tongue and pharyngeal control (Haymaker, 1969). The muscles of the lower face are weak, giving an expressionless appearance (Fig. 26–5). Laboratory tests show a decreased urinary creatinine. Creatine kinase may be elevated as much as 50 per cent if rapid denervation is occurring. There is also an increase in CSF protein content. The muscle fasciculations characteristically do not stop after motor nerve block with procaine hydrochloride (Adams, 1975). They are intensified by neostigmine and abolished by curare.

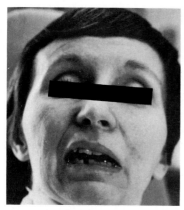

FIGURE 26–5. Patient with amyotrophic lateral sclerosis showing maximum opening of the mouth.

Aspiration pneumonia is the usual cause of death.

When the patient fails to develop spasticity and hyperactive tendon reflexes, the condition is termed *progressive muscular atrophy* rather than amyotrophic lateral sclerosis. In this variant, degeneration is restricted to the ventral horn cells of the spinal cord and the paralysis is completely flaccid (Merritt, 1975). When the muscles of the tongue, mouth, and throat are involved initially and predominantly (bulbar nucleus involvement), the term progressive bulbar palsy is used. Speech is altered, dysphagia occurs, and the jaw reflex is hyperactive. Progressive muscular atrophy and progressive bulbar palsy may both occur in amyotrophic lateral sclerosis.

Pseudobulbar Palsy

Pseudobulbar palsy causes a lesser degree of atrophy than that seen with bulbar palsy of amyotrophic lateral sclerosis. The primary difference between the two conditions is that pseudobulbar palsy causes hypertonia and lack of voluntary control rather than spasticity. The partial paralysis is due to infarction in the corticobulbar system. Arteriosclerosis frequently precedes pseudobulbar palsy. Occlusion of small penetrating arterioles following sustained hypertension leads to cystic cerebral degenerative areas called lacunae. Multiple bilateral frontal lobe lacunae lead to pseudobulbar palsy (Fisher, 1982). Hemorrhage, embolic infarction secondary to mitral valve disease, aneurysms, neoplasms, syphilis, and multiple sclerosis may also cause this condition.

Mandibular dysfunction may occur due to spastic paralysis of the masseter and pterygoid muscles. The mouth may remain in an open position; closure is difficult or impossible (Fig. 26–6). The jaw jerk reflex is pronounced, with an abrupt upward movement. The gag reflex may be absent or diminished. There is an inability to protrude the mandible or perform lateral excursions, and weakness of the masticatory muscles, the tongue, lips, and cheeks make eating difficult. Additional effects on the seventh, ninth, and twelfth cranial nerves lead to speech impairment. Signs of dysphagia, dysphonia, and dysarthria are pathognomonic. If palatal paralysis is complete, nasal speech or aphonia may occur. Loss of control over emotional outbursts leads to spontaneous laughing and crying. Facial muscle spasm may be provoked by the slightest mechanical stimulation. Varying degrees of facial muscle weakness exist, depending on the extent of infarct to the corticobulbar tracts. A CT scan may reveal frontal lobe lacunar hypodensities.

Syringomyelia and Syringobulbia

Syringomyelia, a degenerative disease of the medulla and spinal cord, is characterized by tubular cavitation and excessive formation of neuroglia. This syringomyelic cavity, or syrinx, is found most commonly in the cervical cord, but it may extend over many segments. Communicating and noncommunicating forms are found. The communicating form is designated hydromyelia. Gliosis may lead to the formation of gliomas at various sites. Expansion of the syrinx or cyst occurs slowly, involving both gray and white matter (Olson, 1988). Hydrocephalus is frequent and there is associated cerebellar hypoplasia (Berry, 1981). The onset is usually between 30 and 50 years of age, with both sexes affected equally. Clinically, the disease produces muscle weakness and wasting, with associated sensory deficits and trophic changes in the extremities as well as in the head and neck region.

Cranial nerve involvement leads to loss of pain and temperature sensation within the face, loss of the corneal reflex, atrophy and fibrillation of the tongue muscles, dysphagia, dysarthria, and nystagmus. Due to difficulty in swallowing and manipulating the tongue, mastication becomes dysfunctional.

In syringobulbia, gliosis and cavitation occur only in the medulla, producing symptoms of tongue atrophy and fibrillation, loss of pain and temperature sensation of the face, dysphagia, dysphonia, nystagmus, and laryngeal stridor. The trophic disturbances lead to dermal scars from repeated trauma to the insensitive skin.

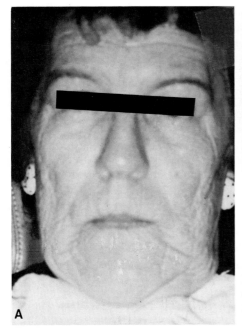

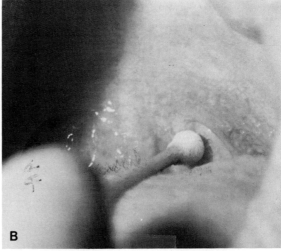

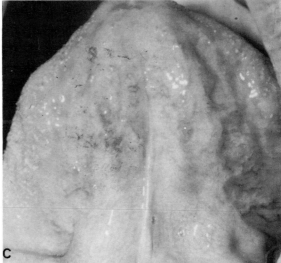

FIGURE 26–6. Pseudobulbar palsy due to infarction of the corticobulbar system may cause extreme mandibular dysfunction with difficulty in closing the mouth. A, Note towel placed under chin to hold mandible in closed-mouth position. B, Absent gag reflex and C, hypertonicity of the tongue muscles with asynchronous movements.

Examination reveals elevation in the CSF pressure due to blockage of the subarachnoid space, with an increase in protein content. Enlargement of the cervical space may be seen in a myelogram. The general muscle wasting, lack of cutaneous alteration, and symmetrical involvement help differentiate amyotrophic lateral sclerosis from this condition.

Parkinson's Disease (Paralysis Agitans)

Parkinson's disease is a dopamine deficiency state resulting from disease, injury, or dysfunction of the dopaminergic neuronal system. It generally affects adults over 40 years of age, although juvenile cases do occur. It may follow damage to the cerebral cortex, basal ganglia, and reticular formation of the brainstem by encephalitis, arteriosclerosis, trauma, and toxic injury from carbon monoxide, manganese, and tranquilizing drugs. Despite its variable causes, a common feature is the loss of pigmented neurons in the substantia nigra and brainstem nuclei.

The primary signs of the syndrome are tremor, rigidity, and bradykinesia or akinesia (Parkinson, 1817). Other signs are mask-like facies, dysarthria, abnormal gait, and cogwheel rigidity of muscle with associated weak movements (Cooper, 1969). These signs are now thought to be due to misregulated impulses from the cerebellum and basal ganglia (globus pallidus, substantia nigra, and other subthalamic nuclei) to the thalamus (Cummings, 1988). Transmission from these nuclei to the thalamus is mediated by dopamine. Patients with Parkinson's disease have been found to have a selective depletion in the dopamine content of these nuclei or an increase in dopamine receptor sites (Goetz, 1987; Papavasiliou, 1972).

Various dysfunctional effects result from involvement of the cranial nerves. There may be prolonged fixation of eye movements and impairment of convergence. Facial expression is fixed and rigid and becomes placid at rest. Facial movements are slow and speech is monotonous and low in intensity. Tapping the bridge of the nose causes repeated orbicularis oculi spasms and increased blinking. Slowness of tongue and masticatory movements prolongs chewing and swallowing. Mandibular tremor occurs because of asynchronous spasticity of opposing muscles. The tongue, face, lips, and head may also show tremors (Steegman, 1970). Masticatory muscle pain and tenderness may accompany the general pain due to muscle rigidity. The tremor and rigidity of the muscles prevent voluntary movements of the mandible. In severe cases, the mandible may remain fixed in either an open or closed position. Retention of artificial dentures is difficult. Excessive salivation may be present.

Current treatment involves L-dopa, a precursor to dopamine, and the use of dopamine agonists that directly stimulate the dopamine receptors without entering their metabolic pathway. High dosages may lead to involuntary tonic contraction of the tongue and masticatory muscles in about 80 per cent of the patients (Mumenthaler, 1977). The differential diagnosis includes amyotrophic lateral sclerosis, drug-induced dyskinesia, hypoparathyroidism, and Wilson's disease.

Huntington's Chorea (Chronic Progressive Chorea)

Chronic progressive chorea is an inherited disease that becomes apparent between 30 and 50 years of age. It is caused by cellular atrophy in the thalamus, basal ganglia (particularly the caudate nucleus), and brainstem. The loss of muscle tone and control results in abrupt and jerky (choreic) movements that are less rapid than in other forms of chorea. Progressive dementia and emotional disturbances are associated with the disease. Chorea minor, a transient form, follows infectious illness, especially rheumatic fever. In a large percentage of the patients with rheumatic joint involvement, the choreic movements are even more rapid than usual.

In the early stages of Huntington's chorea there may be only restlessness and fidgeting. As the disease progresses, there is facial grimacing, smacking lip movements, shoulder shrugging, finger twitching, and minor gait impairment (Huntington, 1872). Abrupt movements of the arms and legs also occur. The gait that develops is due to extension and flexion of the trunk muscles. The intensity of abnormal movement is increased by emotional stimuli and attempting difficult maneuvers. In contrast to Parkinson's disease, which is the result of dopamine deficiency, Huntington's chorea is related to excessive dopamine activity. The degenerative changes in the basal ganglia cause a reduction of gamma-aminobutyric acid (GABA) and acetylcholine (Ach) as well as their synthetic enzymes. It is the reduced GABA and Ach activity that leads to increased dopamine receptor stimulation, yielding the choreiform movements (Bird, 1974).

Spontaneous chewing movements may occur, which interfere with mastication and speech (Earl, 1976). Repetitive buccolingual movements, tongue protrusion, and alternating jaw opening and closing also can occur (Martin, 1986). There is difficulty in speech and swallowing. Sensory innervation is intact. Clenching and bruxing may result in severe attrition of the teeth (Nowak, 1976). Loss of dental proprioception may account for the dyskinetic mandibular movements (Koller, 1983). The EEG is abnormal, and the pneumoencephalogram and CT scan show the characteristic butterfly pattern of enlarged lateral ventricles due to degeneration of the caudate nucleus. The presence of choreiform movements, dementia, and a family history of the disease aid in the diagnosis. Differential diagnosis should include drug-induced tardive dyskinesia, systemic lupus (acute onset with chorea and mental disturbance), hyperthyroidism, and hypoparathyroid disease.

Cerebral Palsy

Cerebral palsy is a broadly descriptive term for the results of injury to the central nervous system that occurs either prenatally, at birth, or in early life. The problem can be related to abnormal implantation of the ovum; structural anomalies during gestation; or brain damage resulting from anoxia, hemorrhage, infection (rubella or bacterial), Rh incompatibility and associated kernicterus, trauma, toxemia of pregnancy, and premature birth (frequently associated with birth weight under 4500 gm). General symptoms of involuntary movements, unilateral or bilateral paralysis, visual loss, mental disturbance, sensory deficits, and aphasia occur. Over half of the children with cerebral palsy have associated mental retardation and epilepsy. The severity of the disease and the extent of disability varies, but the disease is not progressive.

The disease is classified by the type of motor disturbance and its anatomic distribution. Anatomically, the groups are divided according to the area of major damage: the motor cortex, basal ganglia, or cerebellum. The resulting motor disturbances are classified as spastic, dyskinetic, and ataxic, respectively. The spastic form occurs in over 50 per cent of the patients.

Cervicofacial involvement does not predominate unless tetraparesis occurs concurrently with pseudobulbar palsy. Dystonia of the masticatory muscles and dysphagia occur (Low, 1982). Athetosis is the second most frequent problem and results in involuntary and uncoordinated movements of the face, body, and extremities. Grimacing, drooling, and dysarthria are present. When both athetosis and spasticity occur, the facial muscle hypertonicity and abnormal tongue movement produce deformities of the dental arches. Caries and periodontal disease are common. Bruxism and attrition also occur frequently and lead to a closed bite and subsequent TMJ disturbance (Nowak, 1976). Mandibular dysfunction is prominent in all forms of cerebral palsy.

Hepatolenticular Degeneration (Wilson's Disease)

Wilson's disease is familial and results from a defect in copper metabolism. The signs and symptoms usually develop between 11 and 25 years of age. An increase in tissue copper content and urinary copper excretion, and a decrease in serum copper and fecal copper concentration are found. The decrease in serum copper results from a failure to form the copper protein ceruloplasmin. Ceruloplasmin is responsible for transfer of iron from tissue cells to plasma, which explains the low plasma iron-binding levels also found in Wilson's disease. The accumulation of tissue copper affects the brain, kidney, liver, and cornea. Central nervous system damage involves the basal ganglia, cortex, and cerebellum. Degeneration and subsequent cavitation develop in these regions, with loss of neurons, glial cells, and ground substance. The subsequent dystonia that occurs is from faulty regulation by the basal ganglia. Nodular cirrhosis occurs, which causes a decrease in the size of the liver, ascites, and jaundice.

Tremor and muscle rigidity develop early in the course of the disease. Intention tremor, alternating tremor (Parkinson type), and a wing-beating tremor of the upper extremity may occur. The mandible droops, the facial expression becomes rigid, and there is excessive salivation (Rowland, 1984). The persistent mandibular rigidity leads to increased TMJ ligament strain, degenerative joint changes, and subluxation. Laryngeal and pharyngeal spasticity cause dysphagia and hypokinetic dysarthria (Berry, 1974). Torticollis and upper trunk dystonic movements are common. A characteristic greenish-brown pigmentation of the cornea adjacent to the scleral junction is also a frequent finding (Kayser-Fleischer ring).

A familial history of neurologic and hepatic disease, the presence of progressive tremors beginning in the first or second decade, and pigmentation of the scleral margin are diagnostic. Decreased or absent serum ceruloplasmin is found in 96 per cent of the patients, as well as an increased 24-hour urinary copper output (Wallach, 1986). If the diagnosis is inconclusive, a liver biopsy is performed to measure hepatic copper content.

Drug-induced Dyskinesias

Drug-induced dyskinesias can be caused by exposure to various agents used in the treatment of psychotic disorders, nausea, vomiting, and vertigo. Levodopa, anticholinergic medication, high dosages of phenytoin, antihistamines, and antidepressants all can produce some form of oral dyskinesia. By definition, only the dyskinesia produced by antipsychotic medication is called tardive dyskinesia.

Phenothiazines used as tranquilizers, antiemetics, or antipsychotic medications are among the more common drugs capable of causing mandibular motor disturbances (Earl, 1976). Phenothiazines and butyrophenones (Haloperidol) block dopamine neurotransmission and can lead to damage of dopamine receptors and subsequent tardive dyskinesia (Gallager, 1978). This can occur soon after the administration of the neuroleptics so that hypersensitivity of these receptor sites may already be established early in the course of treatment (Goetz, 1984; Klawans, 1981). Haloperidol, used in treating schizophrenia, manic depression, and senile psychosis, has pharmacological properties similar to the phenothiazines and is considered the most frequent cause of general dystonias (Fig. 26-7).

These idiosyncratic reactions are due to the effects upon the brain's extrapyramidal system, the system of nuclei that maintains control over muscular tone and activity. A disruption in any

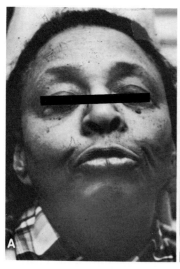 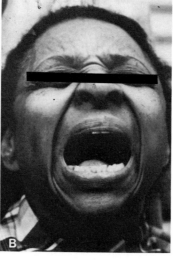

FIGURE 26–7. Drug-induced dyskinesia due to an idiosyncratic effect of prolonged phenothiazine and haloperidol therapy causing extrapyramidal reactions with uncontrolled dystonic movements of the mandible and facial muscles. *A*, Dystonic, involuntary pursing of the lips. *B*, Uncontrolled opening movement due to spasm of the lateral pterygoid muscles.

of these nuclei can lead to transmission of uncontrolled impulses, causing tremor, hypertonic movements, or prolonged contraction (rigidity and akinesia) and akathisia (motor restlessness). The last symptom appears to remain or worsen after withdrawal of the antipsychotic medication.

Toxic dosages of antipsychotic medication may precipitate a Parkinson-type syndrome (Schmidt, 1966). In these patients mandibular tremor and rigidity prevent adequate masticatory movement. The face, tongue, and neck muscles are also involved. Remission of symptoms usually occurs slowly after withdrawal of the medication, but they may persist indefinitely (tardive dyskinesia).

Tardive dyskinesia is characterized by repetitive rapid movements that are most prevalent in the face and manifest as orolingual-buccal movements resembling mastication. The tongue may intermittently protrude from the mouth, and this may be interspersed with puckering and pursing of the lips (see Fig. 26–7). Recent findings suggest that tardive dyskinesia can cause disc derangement and severe degenerative disease in the TMJ (Osborne, 1989). The trunk may develop body-rocking motions, and the fingers and toes incessant flexion-extension maneuvers (Klawans, 1980). Gradual withdrawal of the medication may eliminate the symptoms over a period of weeks or months, although the tendency is for the symptoms to persist. Use of dopamine-depleting medication, such as reserpine, may suppress the symptoms.

The less frequently occurring oromandibular dystonias are the most debilitating. Dystonic spasms (hypertonic spasms) of the orofacial muscles occurring early in the course of drug ther-

apy, and more prominent in younger patients, is called drug-induced or tardive Meige's syndrome (Cramer, 1986). Orbicularis oculi spasms may accompany spasm of the other facial muscles, with the predominant symptoms in the oromandibular region. The simultaneous contraction of the agonist and antagonist muscles becomes interposed with normal movement, causing opening and closing of the mouth and jaw tightening. In addition, there may be irregular, asymmetrical choreiform movements accompanied by facial grimacing, lip smacking, and spontaneous chewing movements, producing dysfunction.

A history of present or prior use of a tranquilizer or other psychotropic medication, without a familial history of neuromuscular disease, may aid in diagnosing this ever-increasing disorder. Differential diagnosis should include Huntington's chorea, Parkinson's disease, hepatolenticular degeneration, and primary Meige's syndrome.

METABOLIC DISORDERS

Thyroid Disease (Hypothyroidism)
(see Chapter 25)

Parathyroid Disease (Hypoparathyroidism and Hyperparathyroidism)
(see Chapter 25)

PSYCHOGENIC DISORDERS

Hysterical Trismus

Hysteria, or conversion reaction, is a dissociative disorder characterized by a variety of somatic and mental symptoms. It is the unconscious process of transforming psychic conflict and anxiety into a somatic condition. The term hysterical trismus refers to a patient developing a sudden inability to mobilize the mandible following a psychologically traumatic or frightening experience, associated with a tonic-clonic contraction of the elevator muscles of mastication. Several cases have been reported (Marbach, 1966; Thoma, 1953; Wilkerson, 1920). Persistence can lead to physical debilitation, muscle weakness, and atrophy.

The myotonia may affect the facial, cervical (spasmodic torticollis) (Merritt, 1975), as well as the masticatory muscles. The contractions, if prolonged, can become painful. In instances in which the trismus is suspected of being psychogenic, the administration of a general anesthetic allows the mandible to move, and maintenance of a bite block between the jaws after recovery allows the patient to recognize the ability to open the mouth. Differentiation from malingering (Munchausen's syndrome), basal ganglia disease, physical limitations of the TMJ, tetanus, and neoplasia is determined by thorough neuropsychiatric evaluation, CT scan, mandibular radiographs, and blood serum chemistry tests.

Tics

Tics are involuntary, inappropriate, and sudden contractions of about 100 to 200 msec involving agonist and antagonist muscles. They are three times more common in males and occur more frequently in children and older persons. Tics may develop in nervous or neurotic individuals and, in these persons, are considered an outward and visible sign of an inner obsession stemming from a particular type of uncontrolled impulsiveness (Mumenthaler, 1977). Organic causes are believed to be prevalent, but are difficult to differentiate from psychogenic causes (Jankovic, 1986).

Dysfunction of the anterior cingulate cortex, which is contiguous with the frontal lobe and interconnects with the limbic system and basal ganglia, is thought to be responsible for many tics. Commonly occurring tic contractions may involve the eyelids (winking, rolling, and lid raising), lower face (chin wrinkling and grimacing), mouth (cheek blowing, biting, and sucking; lip pouting and pursing), tongue (protrusion and flicking), and mandible (chewing and jaw protrusion). Tics are provoked by anger, anxiety, and self-consciousness.

A condition called *Tourette's syndrome* is a chronic, possibly familial disorder involving involuntary tic-like jerks of the face and neck associated with vocalizations, compulsive acts, motor asymmetries, and coprolalia (obscene utterances), echolalia (urge to repeat last syllable, word, or sentence spoken by others), and palilalia (repetition of the patient's last syllable, word, or sentence) (Bruun, 1984). The presence of involuntary vocalizations is a prerequisite for the diagnosis of Tourette's syndrome. It usually occurs during speech rather than silence. In general, these spasmodic contractions interfere with normal mandibular function.

Other forms of facial movement disorders that must be differentiated from tics are hemifacial spasm (unilateral tonic-clonic movement of facial muscles), orofacial dystonia or Meige's syndrome (bilateral writhing tongue, jaw, and neck movements), facial synkinesis (mass movements of many groups of facial muscles occurring when purposeful movement of the face is attempted, usually following Bell's palsy), facial myokymia (rapid unilateral flickering and undulation of the facial muscles from the frontalis to the platysma), focal seizures (complex partial seizure with repetitive movements of the face, with or without limb movement, and associated with abnormal EEG), Parkinson's disease, Huntington's disease, and drug-induced dyskinesias.

SUMMARY

Various abnormalities causing masticatory dysfunction have been described. Although many of these conditions are not common, they must still be considered in any differential diagnosis. In general, masticatory muscle weakness, and weakness of the tongue, pharyngeal and facial muscles can be caused by basilar lesions, peripheral motor nerve lesions, and myasthenia gravis. Spasm of the masticatory muscles is most commonly found in myofascial pain-dysfunction syndrome, but may also be associated with facial trauma, hepatolenticular degeneration, tetanus, and drug-induced dyskinesias. Abnormal mandibular movement may be seen in Huntington's chorea, hemifacial spasm, tics, cerebral palsy, epilepsy, and after phenothiazine and haloperidol therapy. Masticatory dysfunction, which does not respond to standard forms of therapy, and which persists in maintaining muscle and joint disharmony, should encourage the clinician to pursue a thorough neurologic, systemic, and psychologic evaluation of the patient.

REFERENCES

Adams, R. D.: Disease of Muscle: A Study in Pathology, 3rd ed. New York, Harper & Row, 1975.

Amick, L., Johnson, W., and Smith, H.: Electromyographic and histopathologic correlations in arthrogryposis. Arch. Neurol. 16:515–521, 1967.

Bauerle, J. E., and Archer, W. H.: Incidence of subluxation of the temporomandibular joint. J. Am. Dent. Assoc. 43:434–439, 1951.

Berry, R., Chambers, R., and Lublin, F.: Syringoencephalomyelia (Syringocephalus). J. Neuropathol. Exp. Neurol. 40:633–644, 1981.

Berry, W., Darley, F., Aronson, A., and Goldstein, N.: Dysarthria in Wilson's disease. J. Speech Hear Res. 17:169–183, 1974.

Bird, E., and Iversen, L.: Huntington's chorea. Brain 97:457–472, 1974.

Blatt, I. M.: Parotid masseter hypertrophy traumatic occlusion syndrome. Laryngoscope 79:624–637, 1969.

Block, S.: Differential diagnosis of masticatory dysfunction. In Sarnat, B. G., and Laskin, D. (Eds.): The Temporomandibular Joint: A Biological Basis For Clinical Practice, 3rd ed. Springfield, IL, Charles C Thomas, 1980, p. 402.

Bruun, R.: Gilles de la Tourette syndrome. An overview of clinical experience. J. Am. Acad. Child Psychiatry 23:126–133, 1984.

Cailliet, R.: Neck and Arm Pain. Philadelphia, F. A. Davis Co, 1975.

Cooper, I. S.: Involuntary Movement Disorders. New York, Harper & Row, 1969.

Cramer, H., and Otto, K.: Meige's syndrome. Clinical findings and therapeutic results in 50 patients. Neuro-Ophthalmol 6:3–15, 1986.

Cummings, J., Darkins, A., Mendez, M., et al.: Alzheimer's disease and Parkinson's disease: Comparison of speech and language alterations. Neurology 38:680–684, 1988.

Cuttino, C., and Steadman, R.: Myofacial pain syndrome masking metastatic adenocarcinoma: A case report. J. Ala. Dent. Assoc. 72:20, 1988.

Czernobilsky, B., Cornog, J. L., and Enterline, H. T.: Rhabdomyoma: Report of case with ultrastructural and histochemical studies. Am. J. Clin. Pathol. 49:782–789, 1968.

Dalakas, M.: Morphologic changes in the muscles of patients with postpoliomyelitis neuromuscular symptoms. J. Neurol. 38:99–104, 1988.

Delassio, D. J.: Wolff's Headache and Other Head Pain, 3rd ed. New York, Oxford University Press, 1972.

DePaul, M., Abbs, J., Caligiuri, M., et al.: Hypoglossal, trigeminal, and facial motorneuron involvement in amyotrophic lateral sclerosis. Neurology 38:281–283, 1988.

Dito, W. R., and Batsakis, J. G.: Rhabdomyosarcoma of the head and neck: An appraisal of the biologic behavior in 170 cases. Arch. Surg. 84:582–588, 1962.

Drachman, D.: The biology of myasthenia gravis. Ann. Rev. Neurosci. 4:195–225, 1981.

Duane, D.: Spasmodic torticollis. In Jankovic, J., and Tolosa, L. (Eds.): Advances in Neurology, vol. 149: Facial dyskinesias. New York, Raven Press, 1988, pp. 135–150.

Earl, C. J.: Disturbances in mastication associated with neurological disorders. In Anderson, D. J., and Matthews, B. (Eds.): Mastication. Bristol, England, J. Wright, 1976, pp. 221–224.

Fisher, C.: Lacunar strokes and infarcts: A review. Neurology 32:1–6, 1982.

Fisher, R., Johnstone, W., and Fischer, W.: Arthrogryposis multiplex congenita: A clinical investigation. J. Pediatr. 76:255, 1970.

Ford, F. R.: Diseases of the Nervous System in Infancy, Childhood and Adolescence, 4th ed. Springfield, IL, Charles C Thomas, 1960.

Furman, R., and Barchi, R.: Diazacholesterol myotonia: An electrophysiological study. Ann. Neurol. 10:251–260, 1981.

Gallager, D., Pert, A., and Bunney, W. Jr.: Haloperidol induced pre-synaptic dopamine supersensitivity is blocked by chronic lithium. Nature 273:309–312, 1978.

Gellis, S. S., and Feingold, M.: Myotonia congenita (Thomsen's disease). Am. J. Dis. Child. 111:81–82, 1966.

Gilcreest, E. L.: Rupture of muscles and tendons. J. Am. Dent. Assoc. 84:1819–1822, 1925.

Goetz, C., Yanner, C., and Shannon, K.: Progression of Parkinson's disease without levodopa. Neurology 37:695–698, 1987.

Goetz, C., Carvey, P., Tanner, C., and Klawans, H.: Neuroleptic-induced hypersensitivity. Life Sci. 34:1475–1479, 1984.

Goldberg, M.: Torticollis. Curr. Ped. Ther. 8:454–455, 1978.

Gorlin, R. J., Pindborg, J. J., and Cohen, M.: Syndromes of the Head and Neck, 2nd ed. New York, McGraw-Hill, 1976.

Grob, D. (Ed.): Myasthenia gravis: Pathophysiology and management. Ann. NY Acad. Sci. 377:902, 1981.

Hall, J., Trugg, W., and Plowman, D.: A new arthrogryposis syndrome with facial and limb anomalies. Am. J. Dis. Child. 129:120, 1975.

Haymaker, W.: Bing's Local Diagnosis in Neurological Diseases, 15th ed. St. Louis, C. V. Mosby, 1969.

Heffez, L., Doku, H., and O'Donnell, J.: Arthrogryposis multiplex complex involving the temporomandibular joint. J. Oral Maxillofac. Surg. 43:539–542, 1985.

Heiman-Patterson, T., Martino, C., Rosenberg, H., et al.: Malignant hyperthermia in myotonia congenita. Neurology 38:810–812, 1988.

Hirose, H., Kiritani, S., and Sawashima, M.: Patterns of dysarthric movement in patients with amyotrophic lateral sclerosis and pseudobulbar palsy. F. Phoniat. (Basel) 34:106–112, 1982.

Hollander, J. L., and McCarty, D. J.: Arthritis and Allied Conditions, 8th ed. Philadelphia, Lea & Febiger, 1974.

Holmes, P. E.: Cervico-facial actinomycosis in relation to dental treatment: A review with 12 cases. Br. Dent. J. 104:314–317, 1958.

Huntington, G.: On chorea. Med. and Surg. Reporter Phila. 26:317, 1872.

Jankovic, J., and Fahn, S.: The phenomenology of tics. Movement Disorders 1:17–26, 1986.

Kagen, L.: Laboratory assays useful in assessment of patients with disorders of muscle. In Cohen, A. (Ed.): Laboratory Diagnostic Procedures in the Rheumatic Diseases. New York, Grune & Stratton, 1985.

Kazanjian V.: Congenital absence of the ramus of the mandible. Am. J. Orthodont. Oral Surg. 26:175–187, 1940.

Kent, J. N., and Winslow, J. R.: Correction of severe dentofacial deformity associated with myotonia congenita. J. Oral Surg. 36:129–134, 1978.

Kerzin-Storrar, L., Metcalfe, R., Dyer, P., and Kowalska, G.: Genetic factors in myasthenia gravis: A family study. J. Neurol. 38:38–42, 1988.

Kiwak, K., Deray, M., and Shields, W.: Torticollis in three children with syringomyelia and spinal cord tumor. Neurology 33:946–948, 1983.

Klawans, H., Goetz, C., and Perlik, S.: Tardive dyskinesia: Review and update. Am. J. Psychiatry 137:900–908, 1980.

Klawans, H., Nausieda, P., Goetz, C., et al.: Effect of duration of neuroleptic therapy in an animal model of tardive dyskinesia. Neurology 31:103, 1981.

Koller, W.: Edentulous dyskinesia. Ann. Neurol. 13:97–99, 1983.

Laskin, D., and Block, S.: Diagnosis and treatment of myofascial pain-dysfunction (MPD) syndrome. J. Prosthet. Dent. 56:75–84, 1986.

Lewis, I.: Late onset muscle dystrophy: Oculopharyngoesophageal variety. Can. Med. Assoc. J. 95:145–150, 1966.

Low, N., and Downey, J.: Cerebral palsy. In Low, N., and Downey, J. (Eds.): The Child With Disabling Illness, 2nd ed. New York, Raven Press, 1982, pp. 93–104.

Lyons, D. C.: Oral and Facial Signs and Symptoms of Systemic Disease. Springfield, IL, Charles C Thomas, 1968.

Maas, O., and Paterson, A. S.: Myotonia congenita, dystrophia myotonia and paramyotonia: Reaffirmation of their identity. Brain 73:318–336, 1950.

Marbach, J. J.: Hysterical trismus: A study of 6 cases. NY Dent. J. 32:413–416, 1966.

Martin, J., and Gusella, J.: Huntington's disease. Pathogenesis and management. N. Engl. J. Med. 315:1267–1276, 1986.

McDonald, D. G.: Smooth muscle tumors of the mouth. Br. J. Oral Surg. 6:208, 1969.

Merritt, H. H.: A Textbook of Neurology, 5th ed. Philadelphia, Lea & Febiger, 1975.

Middleton, D. S.: The pathology of congenital torticollis. Br. J. Surg. 18:188–204, 1930.

Middleton, P. J., Alexander, R. M., and Szymanski, M. T.: Severe myositis during recovery from influenza. Lancet 2:533–535, 1970.

Most, H., and Helpern, M.: The incidence of trichinosis in New York City. Am. J. Med. Sci. 202:251–257, 1941.

Mulder, D. M.: The clinical syndrome of amyotrophic lateral sclerosis. Proc. Staff Meet. Mayo Clin. 32:427–436, 1957.

Mumenthaler, M.: Neurology. Chicago, Year Book Medical Publishers, 1977.

Newsom-Davis, J.: Myasthenia gravis and myasthenic syndrome. In Appel, S. (Ed.): Current Neurology, vol. 6. Chicago, Year Book Medical Publishers, 1986, pp. 47–52.

Nowak, A. J.: Dentistry for the Handicapped Patient. St. Louis, C. V. Mosby, 1976.

Olson, D., and Milstein, J.: Hydromyelia associated with arrested hydrocephalus. Neurology 28:652–654, 1988.

Osborne, T., Grace, E., and Schwartz, M.: Severe degenerative changes of the temporomandibular joint secondary to the effects of tardive dyskinesia: A review and case report. J. Craniomandib. Pract. 7:58, 1989.

Papavasiliou, P., Cotzias, G., Duby, S., et al.: Levodopa in parkinsonism: Potentiation of central effects with a peripheral inhibitor. N. Engl. J. Med. 286:8–14, 1972.

Parkinson, J.: An Essay on the Shaking Palsy. London, Sherwood Neely and Jones, 1817.

Peterman, A. F.: Progressive muscular dystrophy with ptosis and dysphagia. Arch. Neurol. 10:38–41, 1964.

Poswillo, D.: The pathogenesis of the first and second branchial arch syndrome. Oral Surg. 35:302, 1973.

Ross, R.: Developmental anomalies and dysfunctions of the temporomandibular joint. In Zarb, G., and Carlsson, G. (Eds.): Temporomandibular Joint: Function and Dysfunction. St. Louis, C. V. Mosby, 1979, pp. 119–154.

Rowland, L. (Ed.): Merritt's Textbook of Neurology, 7th ed. Philadelphia, Lea & Febiger, 1984.

Schmidt, W. R., and Jarcho, L. W.: Persistent dyskinesias following phenothiazine therapy. Arch. Neurol. 14:369–377, 1966.

Sprofkin, B., and Hillman, J.: Möbius' syndrome—congenital oculofacial paralysis. Neurology 6:50–54, 1956.

Steegman, A. T.: Examination of the Nervous System, 3rd ed. Chicago, Year Book Medical, 1970.

Stobbe, G. D., and Dargeon, H. W.: Embryonal rhabdomyosarcoma of the head and neck in children and adolescents. Cancer 3:826–836, 1950.

Stout, A. P.: Rhabdomyosarcoma of the skeletal muscles. Ann. Surg. 123:447–472, 1946.

Talacko, A., and Reade, P.: Hemifacial atrophy and temporomandibular joint pain-dysfunction syndrome. Int. J. Oral Maxillofac. Surg. 17:224, 1988.

Thayer, H. H., and Crenshaw, J.: Oral manifestations of myotonic muscular dystrophy: A case report. J. Am. Dent. Assoc. 72:1405–1411, 1966.

Thoma, K.: Trismus hystericus. Oral Surg. 6:449–452, 1953.

Thompson, P., and Carroll, W.: Hemimasticatory spasm—a peripheral paroxysmal cranial neuropathy. J. Neurol. Neurosurg. Psychiatry 46:274–276, 1983.

Towfighi, J., Marks, K., Palmer, E., and Vanucci, R.: Möbius' syndrome: Neuropathologic observations. Acta Neuropathol. 48:11–17, 1979.

Waldhart, E., and Lynch, J. B.: Benign hypertrophy of the masseter muscles and mandibular angles. Arch. Surg. 102:115–118, 1971.

Wallach, J.: Interpretation of Diagnostic Tests, 4th ed. Boston, Little, Brown & Co., 1986.

Walton, J., and Gardner-Medwin, D.: Progressive muscular dystrophy and myotonic disorders. In Walton, J. (Ed.): Disorders of Voluntary Muscle, 4th ed. New York, Churchill Livingstone, 1981.

Weiner, L., Stohlman, S., and Davis, R.: Attempts to demonstrate virus in amyotropic lateral sclerosis. Neurology 30:1319–1322, 1980.

Wilkerson, S. H.: Hysterical trismus and other neuroses of the jaws. Br. Dent. J. 41:318–319, 1920.

Index